Trauma Care Manual

Second edition

Trauma Care Manual

Second Edition

Edited by

Ian Greaves
Visiting Professor of Emergency Medicine
University of Teeside
and
Consultant in Emergency Medicine
British Army

Keith Porter
Chairman of Trauma Care
and
Honorary Professor of Clinical Traumatology
University of Birmingham
and
Consultant Trauma Surgeon
Selly Oak Hospital
Birmingham
and
Immediate Care Practitioner
UK

Jeff Garner
Specialist Registrar in General Surgery
Defence Medical Services
UK

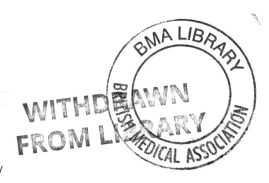
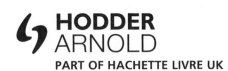
HODDER ARNOLD
PART OF HACHETTE LIVRE UK

Trauma Care

First published in Great Britain in 2001 by
Arnold, a member of the Hodder Headline Group

This second edition published in 2009 by
Hodder Arnold, part of Hachette UK,
338 Euston Road, London NW1 3BH.

http://www.hoddereducation.com

British Library Cataloguing in Publication Data
A catalogue record for this book is available from the British Library

Library of Congress Cataloging-in-Publication Data
A catalog record for this book is available from the Library of Congress

ISBN-13   978 0 340 928 264

1 2 3 4 5 6 7 8 9 10

Commissioning Editor: Gavin Jamieson
Project Editor: Francesca Naish and Eva Senior
Production Controller: Joanna Walker
Cover Designer: Helen Townson
Indexer: Laurence Errington

Typeset in 10/12 pt Minion by Phoenix Photosetting, Chatham, Kent
Printed and bound in the UK by MPG Books, Bodmin, Cornwall
Text printed on FSC accredited material

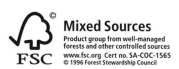

What do you think about this book? Or any other Hodder Arnold
title? Please visit our website: **www.hoddereducation.com**

This edition is dedicated to Professor James M. Ryan.

Contents

Contributors

Professor David A. Alexander MA (Hons) C Psychol PhD FBPS FRSM HonFRCPsych
Professor of Mental Health, Director, Aberdeen Centre for Trauma Research, The Robert Gordon University, Aberdeen, UK

Mr Keith Allison MB ChB MD FRCS(Eng) FRCS(Plast) FIMC.RCSEd
Consultant Plastic Surgeon, Selly Oak Hospital, Birmingham, UK

Mr Ranjeev Singh Bhangoo MB ChB(Hons) FRCS(Eng) FRCS(SN)
Consultant Neurosurgeon, King's College Hospital, London, UK

Dr Stephen Bonner MRCP FRCA
Consultant in Anaesthesia and Intensive Care Medicine, The James Cook University Hospital, Middlesbrough, UK

Dr Stephen J. Brett MD FRCA
Consultant in Intensive Care Medicine, Imperial College Healthcare NHS Trust, Hammersmith Hospital, London, UK

Major M. Leigh Davies MRCS RAMC
Specialist Registrar in General Surgery, Defence Medical Services, UK

Mr Peter Driscoll BSc MD FCEM
Consultant in Emergency Medicine, Hope Hospital, Stott Lane, Salford, UK

Dr J. Michael Elliot MB BS FRCA DipIMC RCSEd
Consultant in Anaesthesia and Intensive Care, Good Hope Hospital, Sutton Coldfield, West Midlands, UK

Major Jeff Garner MB ChB MD MRCS(Glas) FRCSEd(Gen Surg) RAMC
Specialist Registrar in General Surgery, Defence Medical Services, UK; Member of Trauma Care Council

Professor Ian Greaves MB ChB FRCP FCEM FIMC.RCSEd MIHM DipMedEd DMCC DTM&H RAMC
Visiting Professor of Emergency Medicine, University of Teesside; Consultant in Emergency Medicine, The James Cook University Hospital, Middlesbrough; Defence Medical Services, UK; Honorary Secretary of Trauma Care Council

Mr Jonathan Hull MD FRCS(Orth)
Consultant Orthopaedic Surgeon, Frimley Park Hospital NHS Foundation Trust, Camberley, Surrey, UK

Dr Paul Hunt MB BS DipIMC (RCSEd) MCEM MRCSEd DMCC
Specialist Registrar in Emergency Medicine and Critical Care Medicine, Doctoral Research Fellow in Emergency Medicine, The James Cook University Hospital, Middlesbrough, UK

Dr Graham Jay FCEM FACEM
Consultant and Senior Lecturer, Children's Emergency Department, Mater Children's Hospital, Brisbane, Australia

Lt Col S.L.A. Jeffery FRCS (Plast) RAMC
Consultant Plastic Surgeon, Royal Centre for Defence Medicine, Selly Oak, Birmingham, UK

Major Andrew Johnston MRCPI DMCC RAMC
Specialist Registrar in Respiratory and Intensive Care Medicine, University Hospital Birmingham; Defence Medical Services, UK

Dr Tim Jones BA FRCP(UK)
Consultant Rheumatology and Rehabilitation Medicine, Defence Medical Rehabilitation Centre, Headley Court, UK

Dr Susan Klein MA(Hons) Cert [COSCA] PhD
Senior Clinical Research Fellow, Aberdeen Centre for Trauma Research, The Robert Gordon University, Aberdeen, UK

Dr Roderick Mackenzie BSc PhD MRCP FCEM
Emergency Physician, University Hospitals Leicester NHS Trust, Leicester, UK

Dr Paul M. Middleton RGN MB BS FRCS(Eng) DipIMCRCS(Ed) FCEM FACEM
Specialist Emergency Physician, Prince of Wales Hospital; Conjoint Senior Lecturer in Emergency Medicine, Public Health and Community Medicine, University of New South Wales; Visiting Medical Fellow, Biomedical Systems Laboratory, NSW, Australia

Dr Alan Mistlin MRCP(UK) MSc (Sports Medicine) FFSEM
Consultant in Rheumatology and Rehabilitation Medicine, Defence Medical Rehabilitation Centre, Headley Court, UK

Dr Jane S. Mooney BSc (Hons) MB ChB (Hons)
Department of Emergency Medicine, Hope Hospital, Stott Lane, Salford, UK

Dr Peter Oakley MB BChir (Camb) MA MRCGP FFA RCS(Ed)
Consultant Anaesthetist, University Hospital of North Staffordshire, Hartshill, Stoke on Trent, UK

Mr David W. Patton TD FDS FRCS
Consultant/Honorary Senior Lecturer in Oral and Maxillofacial Surgery, Morriston Hospital, Swansea; Honorary Civilian Consultant in Oral and Maxillofacial Surgery to the Army

Dr David Pedley MB ChB MRCP(UK) FRCS(Edin) FCEM
Formerly Consultant in Emergency Medicine, The James Cook University Hospital, Middlesbrough, UK

Professor Keith Porter MB BS FRCS(Eng) FRCSEd FIMC.RCSEd FSEM
Professor of Military Traumatology, University of Birmingham; Consultant in Trauma, University Hospital Birmingham; Chairman of Trauma Care

Lt Col James Ralph FRCA RAMC
Consultant in Anaesthesia and Intensive Care Medicine, Royal
Centre for Defence Medicine and University Hospital,
Birmingham, UK

Lt Col Robert J. Russell MB BS MRCP(UK) FCEM DipIMCRCSEd MIHM RAMC
Senior Lecturer in Military Emergency Medicine, Academic
Department of Military Emergency Medicine, Royal Centre for
Defence Medicine, Birmingham; Consultant in Emergency
Medicine, Peterborough District Hospital; Defence Medical
Services, UK

Dr Karen F. Selby MB ChB MRCOG
Consultant Obstetrician and Gynaecologist, Jessop Wing,
Sheffield Teaching Hospitals NHS Trust, Sheffield, UK

Surg Cdr Jason Smith MRCP(UK) FCEM
Senior Lecturer in Military Emergency Medicine, Academic
Department of Military Emergency Medicine, Royal Centre for
Defence Medicine; Consultant in Emergency Medicine, Derriford
Hospital, Plymouth; Defence Medical Services, UK

Dr Shahana Uddin MB BS FCARCSI
Consultant in Intensive Care Medicine, Barts and The London
NHS Trust, St Bartholomew's Hospital, London, UK

Professor Lee A. Wallis MB ChB FCEM FCEM (SA)
Professor and Head of Emergency Medicine, University of Cape
Town and Stellenbosch University, Republic of South Africa

Mr Jonathan Wasserberg BSc MB BChir Camb FRCS(Eng)
Consultant Neurosurgeon, University Birmingham Foundation
NHS Trust, Birmingham, UK

Dr Rachel Wharton FCEM
Emergency Physician, Queen Alexandra Hospital, Portsmouth
Hospitals NHS Trust, UK

Wing Commander Malcolm Woodcock BSc BM MRCOphth FRCS(Ed) RAF
Consultant Ophthalmologist, Defence Medical Services and
Worcestershire Acute Hospitals NHS Trust, UK

Major Chris Wright MB ChB MCEM DipIMC RAMC
Specialist Registrar in Emergency Medicine and Prehospital Care,
Academic Department of Military Emergency Medicine, Royal
Centre for Defence Medicine, UK

The Editors of this second edition of the *Trauma Care Manual* also gratefully acknowledge those authors who contributed to the first edition:

Mr Gavin Bowyer
Mr Adam Brooks
Dr Danielle Bryden
Dr Gregor Campbell-Hewson
Dr Otto Chan
Mr Charles Cox
Dr Anna Girolami

Dr Carl Gwinutt
Dr Karen Heath
Professor Tim Hodgetts
Mr Andrew Jacks
Mr Alan Kay
Professor Rod Little
Dr Ian Maconochie

Mr Steven Mannion
Dr Bernard Riley
Professor Jim Ryan
Dr Jo Sibert
Mr John Thorne

Preface to the Second Edition

A second edition of the *Trauma Care Manual* has never been more timely than now. The 2007 NCEPOD report *Trauma: Who Cares?* has emphasised once more that there remain significant shortcomings in UK trauma management. The first edition of the *Manual* was intended to begin the process of establishing evidence-based British guidelines for the optimal management of the trauma victim and this aim remains unchanged for the second edition. The editors, authors and Executive Council of *Trauma Care (UK)* have been enormously encouraged by the reception given to the first edition and the enthusiasm of the publishers for a second. We hope that the chapters of this book will continue to provide a system of optimal management of the injured patient that is pragmatic, sensible and, wherever possible, built on a solid evidence base.

We have taken the opportunity of a new edition to completely redesign the manual. The order of the chapters has changed to reflect a more sensible pathway through the trauma victim's journey. Five new chapters have been added and all the remaining chapters have been extensively revised. The use of illustrations has also increased significantly. Most chapters now incorporate case scenarios so that the reader may revisit the information presented in a familiar clinical environment. Although the *Manual* is aimed at UK trauma, we recognise that readers may not be limited solely to the British Isles, and so many chapters also discuss the global perspectives of trauma. We believe that all these additions help maintain the *Trauma Care Manual* as an invaluable reference guide to the multidisciplinary management of trauma.

Perhaps the most dramatic change is not in presentation and format but one of philosophy, with the shift away from the ABCDE paradigm to a new system of <C>ABCDE in which the first component is control of external exsanguinating haemorrhage. We believe this change is simple common sense and strongly commend it and have taken the opportunity of increasing the emphasis on methods of haemorrhage control.

We recognise however that, like all fields of medicine, the management of trauma is an ever-changing area and, while we hope that we have provided a benchmark, we remain committed to reflecting development as their effectiveness is established.

The preparation of a volume of this kind involves an immense amount of hard work. We would like to take this opportunity to thank all our contributors, as well as those who contributed to the first edition. Keith Porter and Ian Greaves would particularly like to express their appreciation of the efforts of our fellow editor, Jeff Garner, in preparing this edition for publication.

Ian Greaves
Keith Porter
Jeff Garner

Teesside, 2009

Preface to the Second Edition

Preface to the First Edition

Trauma Care®, a registered charity, was founded in 1996 by a group of clinicians with an interest in the area, to promote and define best practice in the management of the victims of trauma. This aim has been furthered by a series of successful conferences which have, uniquely, brought together all the professions and specialities involved in trauma care. This programme of conferences continues and is expanding.

The *Trauma Care Manual* has been prepared by Trauma Care in order to begin the process of establishing United Kingdom guidelines for best practice in the management of major trauma. A structured approach is offered which takes into account current British and European clinical practice and is, wherever possible, supported by the available evidence.

We recognize that this is an ambitious project, but believe that the current volume is the first step on a road which will, hopefully, see the regular revision and re-issue of this manual. Future editions will take into account new developments and be based on a reading of the ever-increasing evidence base. As a consequence working groups have been set up, charged with the responsibility of maintaining and developing a current evidence base in their own areas of expertise and working towards the next edition of this manual.

We believe that the establishment of clear practical guidelines reflecting British practice is long overdue and hope that this first edition will grow into – and become recognized as – the definitive statement of best practice.

Dr Ian Greaves
Mr Keith Porter
Prof Jim Ryan

Trauma Care 2000

Trauma Care (UK)

Trauma Care (UK) is a national registered charity founded in 1996. This *Trauma Care Manual* is produced under the authority of the National Council of Trauma Care, which is composed of authorities from across the broad spectrum of the care of the trauma victim. Trauma Care (UK) exists to promote the best integrated trauma care provision by encouraging education and the clinical involvement of all medical specialties and healthcare professions. It is a truly multidisciplinary, multiprofessional organisation.

Trauma Care (UK) organises a national conference each year which is now the biggest trauma conference in the UK and among the biggest in Europe. The annual conference addresses areas of clinical interest in a range of parallel sessions designed to appeal to all professional groups. Every effort is made to reduce costs in order to facilitate the widest possible attendance. One-day seminars on a wide range of topics are also organised around the UK.

As well as the *Trauma Manual*, Trauma Care (UK) also publishes a journal, *Trauma*, which is issued four times each year and contains review articles by international authorities on all aspects of trauma care. Now in its 10th year, *Trauma* is acknowledged to be a leader in its field.

Everybody involved in the management of the trauma victim is strongly encouraged to become a member of Trauma Care (UK). Membership includes subscription to the journal *Trauma* and significantly reduced rates for the conference and study days and regular newsletter. Membership fees allow us to keep the cost of our educational initiatives to a minimum. Membership details and application forms can be obtained from:

Mrs Gillian Robins
Trauma Care (UK) Administrator
Department of Academic Emergency Medicine
Education Centre
James Cook University Hospital
Marton Rd
Middlesbrough TS4 3BW
UK
01642 854186

www.traumacare-uk.com

All proceeds from the sale of the *Trauma Care Manual* are used to support the work of Trauma Care (UK).

The trauma epidemic

OBJECTIVES

After completing this chapter the reader will:
- understand the scale of the global burden of trauma
- understand the differences in impact of this burden of trauma between developed and non-developed countries
- realize the impact of domestic accidents on the UK trauma burden.

INTRODUCTION

Dictionary definitions of *epidemic* include *affecting many persons at the same time* and *extremely prevalent or widespread*. These definitions certainly apply to the worldwide clinical burden of trauma. Although mechanisms change, injuries contribute hugely to the disease burden in all regions of the world, a contribution that is expected to rise in the next 20 years.[1] Injuries kill 5 million people each year, equating to 9% of worldwide deaths and 12% of the worldwide burden of disease in 2000.

Both the cause and effect of traumatic injury differ depending on the population concerned; injuries differ between males and females, between geographical areas, and between low-, middle- and high-income countries. Thus, although injury remains the leading cause of death for those aged between 15 and 44, individual mortality and morbidity may be higher in the elderly.[2] To add to the complexity of understanding the problems caused by trauma, countries with unequal income levels suffer from diverse burdens of disability due to injury; levels of disability due to extremity injury are very high in the developing world, but a greater proportion of disability due to head and spinal cord injuries occurs in high-income countries,[3] suggesting that some types of trauma and their resultant morbidity may be amenable to relatively simple interventions such as improved orthopaedic care and rehabilitation, especially in the developing world.

Deaths due to injury are devastating for families, communities and societies; however, for every death many more are left disabled. The 1990 Global Burden of Disease (GBD) study developed the concept of disability-adjusted life years (DALYs). This concept expresses years of life lost to premature death, but also years lived with a disability of a specified severity and duration. One DALY is one lost year of healthy life. It was calculated in 1990 that injuries caused 10% of worldwide mortality but 15% of DALYs.[4] The effect of changing living patterns, increased mobility and expenditure on motor vehicles, particularly in the developing world, has contributed to a dynamic picture of injury and its effects on populations. A World Bank report projected that the global road death toll will rise by 66% over the next 20 years, but, importantly, this value incorporates a greater divergence between rich and poor nations in the future. An approximate 28% reduction in fatalities is anticipated in high-income countries, but rises of 92% and 147% in fatalities are expected in China and India respectively.[5]

Gender has a great impact on traumatic injury incidence and mechanism. Mortality from road traffic collisions (RTCs) and interpersonal violence is almost three times higher in males than in females. Globally, injury mortality in males is twice that among women, with the highest rates in Africa and Europe; however, in some regions, particularly South-East Asia and the Eastern Mediterranean, females have the highest burn-related deaths at all ages. This distribution is particularly apparent in elderly people in both areas, especially the Eastern Mediterranean, where the risk of burn-related death is seven times higher for females than for males.[1] Age itself has a marked influence on incidence, mechanism and mortality from injury. It is well established that young people between the ages of 15 and 44 account for approximately 50% of global mortality due to trauma.

Injuries have traditionally been viewed as the result of

'accidents' or random events, but in recent years this view has changed, and most injuries may now be viewed as preventable and are widely studied, leading to the implementation of interventions to lessen the related burden of disease in areas as diverse as handgun initiatives to road and water safety education. Other potentially modifiable factors implicated in trauma are the use of drugs and alcohol. Drug intoxication has been associated with interpersonal violence, self-directed violence and vehicular trauma,[6] and alcohol has a significant role to play in many areas of traumatic injury, including interpersonal violence, youth violence, child and sexual abuse, elder abuse and vehicular accidents.[7] The impacts of disasters, however, both natural and man-made, are often profound and far-reaching and are clearly less amenable to prevention. The effects of the 2004 Indian Ocean earthquake and resultant tsunami spread over an immense geographical area from the east coast of Africa to Alaska, and caused approximately 230 000 deaths.[8]

It is pertinent to remember, however, that trauma data are often complete only for high-income, developed nations, with only poor and incomplete data collection in the developing world, where the greatest increase in traumatic injury is occurring. The GBD project found that, although vital registration systems capture about 17 million deaths annually, this is probably only about 75% of the total, as in some regions data are incomplete, for example in Africa data are available for only approximately 19% of countries. The true mortality and morbidity due to injury may be much greater than we imagine.

The World Health Organization (WHO) and the GBD studies base their statistical analyses of health and disease on six geographical regions (Africa, Americas, Eastern Mediterranean, Europe, South East Asia and Western Pacific) and three income levels, high, middle and low. These groups are termed high-income countries (HICs) and low/middle-income countries (LMICs). Injuries are also described as intentional or unintentional (Figure 1.1).

WHO World Health Reports reveal that in 2000 injuries accounted for a mortality rate of 83.7/100 000 population, with more than 90% of the world's deaths occurring in LMICs. European LMICs have the highest injury mortality rates, but the South-East Asia and Western Pacific regions account for the highest number of injury deaths worldwide. Deaths from injury gradually rose in number, from 5 101 000 to 5 168 000 in the years from 1999 to 2002, but remained a constant 9% of overall mortality.[9–12]

In the 2005 updated projections of global mortality and burden of disease, the WHO describes both best and worst predicted figures for mortality and morbidity due to traumatic injury by 2015 and 2030. Overall changes in injury levels range from an optimistic decrease of 4% by 2015 to a pessimistic 4% increase, whereas the figures for 2030 lie between a 5% decrease and a 6% increase in the level of traumatic injury.

INTENTIONAL INJURY

In 2000, intentional injuries accounted for 49% of the annual mortality from injury, one-quarter of all deaths being due to interpersonal violence and suicide.[1] Interpersonal violence caused the deaths of an estimated 520 000 people worldwide in 2000, with 95% of homicides occurring in LMICs. Almost one-third of all deaths took place in the Americas, a region that also accounted for one-third of the total global DALYs lost to interpersonal violence.[1] The highest rates of interpersonal violence are in young males, aged 15–29 years, with the mortality rate in this group in the Americas being twice that of any other region. On a global basis, 60% of mortality occurs in young people aged between 15 and 44 years. Mortality from interpersonal violence is generally lower in women than in men, with the highest female mortality due to interpersonal violence occurring in the African region. The

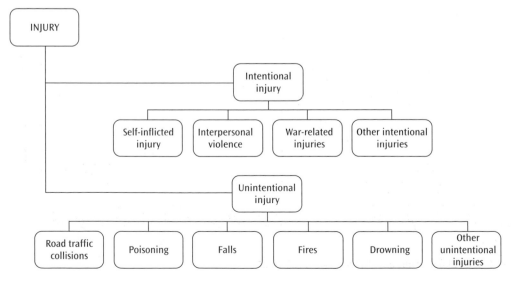

Figure 1.1 World Health Organization/Global Burden of Disease Study classification of injury.

disparity in the incidence of interpersonal violence between HICs and LMICs is striking, even within geographical regions. In the Americas, the rate of interpersonal violence in the HICs was 6.1/100 000 in 2000, compared with 27.3/100 000 in LMICs; in Europe the increase is even more striking, with rates increasing from 1.0 to 15.4 per 100 000.[9–12]

From 1999 to 2002, intentional injury deaths fell from 1689 to 1618 per 100 000, reducing from 3% to 2.8% of total deaths.[9–12] Optimistic WHO predictions suggest that global deaths due to intentional injury will decrease by 3% from baseline by 2015, and by 5% by 2030, whereas in the pessimistic scenario these injuries are predicted to increase by 9% and 13% respectively. Relatively small changes in these rates have a profound effect on the absolute numbers killed or injured in the context of a world population predicted to increase by 2.3 billion people by 2030. Thus, the optimistic prediction of a fall of 5% in deaths by 2030 means that just under 32 million people will die as a result of intentional injury, whereas the pessimistic prediction, a rise of 13%, means total deaths of slightly over 57 million people, equivalent to the entire population of the UK being killed each year.

Homicide and violence

Despite the overall fall in intentional injuries, homicide and violent incidents increased from 527 to 559 per 100 000 but were unequally distributed between men and women, with the rate for women falling from 135 to 114 per 100 000 whilst that for men increased from 392 to 445 per 100 000.[9–12]

In 2000, males accounted for 77% of all homicide deaths.[13] Predictably, the highest rates of homicide occur in young men aged 15–29, with the next highest rates seen in men aged 30–44; gender and age aside, geography, race,

urbanization and poverty all affect the incidence of homicide and violence. Generally, the rates of violent death in LMICs are double those in HICs, with the exception of the USA. The USA is unusual in that it is an established market economy with a relatively high homicide rate. Between 1975 and 1992, the overall annual male homicide rate remained steady at about 16/100 000 population, yet at the same time the rate for 15- to 24-year-old men rose from 21 to 37 per 100 000.[14] The Bureau of Justice statistics, however, reported murder rates using firearms reaching a peak of 6.6/100 000 in 1993, falling to 5.6/100 000 in 1995 – a decrease of 11%. This reached a low of 3.3/100 000 in 2001 but has now risen slightly to stabilize at 3.8/100 000 (Figure 1.2). Although these figures appear to show an encouragingly positive trend towards a reduction in firearm-related homicides, the 2001 *Injury Fact Book*,[15] published by the Centers for Disease Control (CDC), found that homicide was still the second leading cause of death for teenage Americans aged between 15 and 19, and that 85% of these young victims were killed with guns. Overall, the FBI estimates that, although firearms were used in two-thirds of murders in 2004, since 1996 less than 10% of violent crimes have involved guns.[16]

Russia has proved itself able to compete with the USA at many levels, not least in the incidence of interpersonal violence and homicide, which, since the collapse of communism, has increased drastically to 24/100 000 in 1998, three and a half times that of America.[17] The distribution according to age is strikingly different, though, with the homicide rate increasing beyond the 15–24 age group rather than falling as in the USA, to eventually begin falling after the age of 55 years. The rates of homicide in Russia increase the further east one goes, which may result from underlying sociodemographic factors such as poverty or religious belief, but in 1995 homicide rates in 95% of Russian regions were higher than the corresponding US figures[17] (Figure 1.3).

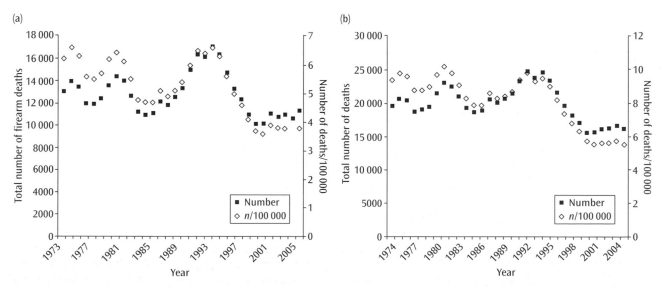

Figure 1.2 Death trends in the USA due to (a) firearms and (b) homicide, 1973–2005.

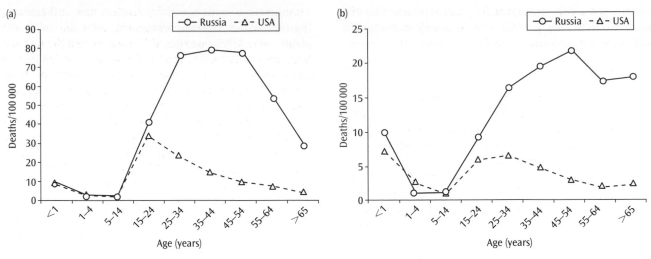

Figure 1.3 Homicide rates per 100 000, Russia vs. USA. (a) Males. (b) Females.

Suicide

A 2002 study by the WHO found that suicide accounts for approximately 1.5% of global mortality and that suicide rates are typically higher than the mortality rates for war and homicide combined. Suicide rates fell between 1999 and 2000/2001, but by 2002 had increased to almost the original level. Once again, however, this general trend obscures gender differences: although both male and female suicide rates showed a similar decrease over 2000/2001, subsequently the rate of suicide among males rose to equal the 1999 figure whilst female mortality from suicide continued to decrease, equating to a decrease in female suicide deaths of 0.5 million but an increase in male suicide deaths over the same period of 1.3 million.[9–12]

As with homicide, age, sex, geography and other factors markedly affect suicide rates. Worldwide, over 50% of suicides occur in people aged between 15 and 44 and over 40% of DALYs attributable to suicide occur in young adults aged 15–29, while the highest suicide rates are found among males in the European region and among both sexes in the Western Pacific region.[1] Although the male suicide rate in European LMICs is twice that found in other regions, women in China have a suicide rate approximately twice that of women in other parts of the world. Eighty-six per cent of all suicides in 2000 occurred in LMICs, with the Western Pacific region not only having the greatest share of deaths relative to other world regions, but also accounting for 38% of the global DALYs lost as a result of suicide.[1]

In 2000, the highest suicide rate in the world was in Lithuania, at 51/100 000, but Russia's rate of 39.7/100 000 was far greater than the Western Europe and North American averages of 5 and 4.1/100 000 respectively[11] and higher even than the suicide rate of 26.4/100 000 in the last year of Soviet government in 1990.[18]

War

Since 1945, 22 million people have been killed and three times as many injured during war or violent conflict.[14] In the 1960s, there were, on average, 11 active conflicts in any one year, in the 1970s there were 14, and in 1996 there were at least 50. Between 1996 and 2006 there were only 15 conflicts that met the definition of war.[19] Modern warfare differs from the 'World Wars'. Between 1989 and 1992, only 3 out of 82 violent conflicts were between nation states; the rest were internal.[14] The aim of modern war is to destabilize the political, social, cultural and psychological foundation of one's opponent, with torture, execution and rape being used routinely as methods of social intimidation. Weapons designed to maim rather than kill are used against civilians as well as combatants, extending the battlefield to the entire society.

Injuries due to war fell markedly in the period between 1999 and 2002 despite the many ongoing conflicts. The overall death rate due to war fell from 269 to 178 per 100 000; as a result, the proportion of global mortality accounted for by war fell from 0.5% to 0.3%. Male mortality decreased from 164 to 161 per 100 000, but the female mortality rate fell by over 5 million per year during this period (from 105 to 18 per 100 000).[9–12]

COMBATANTS IN WARFARE

Fewer troops are now exposed to combat, in contrast to the massed battles of previous wars, but those who are face an increased risk of injury. Penetrating injuries, such as those caused by small arms or exploding munitions, cause 90% of combat trauma, and the advent of effective personal ballistic protection has skewed the distribution of penetrating injuries to involve the limbs rather than trunk. Improved evacuation times and medical care have generally contributed to decreased mortality, with approximately 6% of the wounded dying in the First World War, compared with 3.6% in the Vietnam conflict.[14]

CIVILIANS IN WARFARE

The pattern of warfare continues to change, with large battles fought between standing armies becoming a rarity, being largely replaced by urban combat involving vaguely identified combatants, including sympathetic civilians. This represents the 'asymmetric' battlefield of the future. Approximately 50% of the casualties in the Second World War were civilians; this figure increased to ~80% in the Vietnam War and is ~90% in current wars. Changes in the conduct of war have meant that vulnerable areas such as shelters and hospitals are deliberately targeted, with health workers being interned or executed. According to the United Nations High Commissioner for Refugees (UNHCR), 20.5 million people were refugees by 2005; although data were available on only about a quarter of these people, approximately 44% were estimated to be under 18. United Nations Children's (Emergency) Fund (UNICEF) data suggest that in the 1990s about 2 million children died as a result of war, and 4–5 million were injured or disabled.[14]

The deliberate involvement and targeting of civilian populations may have profound effects, with grave economic and social implications for the victims and their countries. In 1994, 14% of the population of Rwanda was slaughtered within the space of 3 months, leaving nearly 1 million dead. Landmines continue to exact a huge toll, often on the poorest of the world's inhabitants, despite a ban on their use, largely due to the 250 million stockpiled munitions, including 70 million still deployed in over 60 countries. Antipersonnel mines and unexploded ordnance are the best-known weapons that cause superfluous injury or unnecessary suffering, i.e. injury greater than that necessary to put the combatant *hors de combat*,[14] and the SIrUS project of the International Committee of the Red Cross is aiming to clarify this concept (which currently has no legal definition) in order to limit these weapons in accordance with the Geneva Conventions.[20]

Terrorism

Terrorism can be defined as the *systematic use of violence to create a general climate of fear in a population and thereby to bring about a particular political objective.* The apparent randomness of an attack together with the probability of non-combatants being targeted make terrorism an effective weapon, as it engenders fear and dread often out of all proportion to the actual mortality it causes. Global deaths due to terrorism rose to a peak in the late 1980s and then slowly diminished until the attack on the USA on 11 September 2001 (9/11), which killed 2973.[21]

Western Europe benefited from a similar decrease in terrorist attacks from the late 1980s onwards, but also experienced renewed activity in the new millennium, typified by the Madrid bombings in 2004, in which 191 people were killed and over 1700 injured, and the London bombings of 2005, killing 52 and injuring over 700.[21] Asia has witnessed a steady rise in terrorism over the same period, with attacks increasing particularly in South Asia and in the Middle East. The terrorism death toll in South Asia, in countries such as Pakistan, Nepal and India, rose from 297 in 2000 to 1164 in 2005, but the Middle East, particularly Iraq, saw a spectacular rise from 62 deaths in 2000 to almost 6500 in 2005[22] (Figure 1.4). The average annual death rate from RTCs between 1994 and 2003 was 390 times the death rate due to terrorism, and in the USA in 2001 road deaths equalled the total deaths from the 9/11 attacks every 26 days, suggesting a need for terrorist deaths to be considered in a wider context.[23]

Factors contributing to intentional injury

ALCOHOL

Alcohol use is linked to several forms of intentional injury. Self-inflicted injury, particularly suicide, is common in alcohol-dependent individuals, and alcohol dependence is known to increase the risk for suicidal ideation, attempts and completed suicide.[24] People who attempt suicide are often young, single or separated, are likely to have made previous attempts, and have higher levels of substance abuse than non-suicide attempters.[25] Teenagers who drink are five times as likely to be injured in a fight and six times as likely to carry weapons as non drinkers.[26] Young adult males in England and Wales who binge drink are twice as likely, and similar females are four times as likely, to be involved in a fight as are non-binge drinkers.[27] Although males are more likely than females to be both perpetrators and victims of alcohol-related violence, there is evidence of disproportionate increases in violent behaviour among

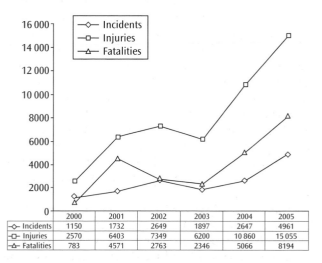

	2000	2001	2002	2003	2004	2005
Incidents	1150	1732	2649	1897	2647	4961
Injuries	2570	6403	7349	6200	10 860	15 055
Fatalities	783	4571	2763	2346	5066	8194

Figure 1.4 Global incidents, injuries and fatalities due to terrorism, 2000–2005.

girls in some countries.[17] In addition, alcohol-related violence may be more likely to result in physical injury to victims, and also in more severe injury.

Illicit drugs have had an enormous effect on the incidence, epidemiology and severity of major trauma. Demetriades et al.[28] found an association between a high rate of alcohol and illicit drug use and patients dying from penetrating trauma, particularly males aged 15–50 and of Hispanic or African American origin. In a UK study of trauma patients, the prevalence of positive toxicology screens, including cannabinoids, cocaine, amphetamine and methadone, was 35%.[29] In a Belgian drug screening study, illicit drugs were detected in the urine of 19% of drivers admitted to hospital after an RTC.[30] In Brazil, the levels of drug-related violence are unprecedented – nearly 4000 children died of gun-related violence in Rio state alone between 1987 and 2001, eight times the number killed in the Israel–Palestine conflict in the same period.[31] Between 1997 and 2003, the Brazilian police force increased in number by 45%, arrests decreased by 31% but deaths due to 'resistance to arrest' increased by 236% – these miscreants each had an average of 4.3 bullet wounds, 61% of which were in the head.[31]

It has been suggested that violence and drugs are related in three ways: first, the pharmacological effects of a drug may result in violent behaviour by the user; second, users may commit violent crime to obtain the money to purchase drugs; and, third, systemic violence is a common feature of the drug distribution system, a finding confirmed by a study showing that violent crime is significantly related to involvement in drug sales, and that most crimes are directly related to the business of drug selling.[32] This violence is compounded by the efforts of the three-quarters of a million street gang members in the USA who routinely use firearms in pursuit of both gang discipline and criminal activity.[33]

UNINTENTIONAL INJURY

The WHO's 2005 projections suggested that in an optimistic scenario global mortality due to unintentional injury would decrease by 1%, and burden of disease by 5%, but that in a pessimistic scenario these rates would increase by 3% and 6% respectively.[5] From 1999 to 2002, however, unintentional injury deaths increased from 3 441 000 to 3 551 000, although this represented an increase in the proportion of total mortality accounted for by unintentional death of only 0.1%, from 6.1% to 6.2%.

Road trauma deaths

In 2005, 63 million cars were produced worldwide, one-sixth of them in the USA,[34] and 77 million babies were born,[35] a ratio of one new car for every 1.2 babies! In 2002, an estimated 1.2 million people died and 50 million were injured in RTCs worldwide, at a global cost of approximately US$518 billion.[5] The economic cost of road crashes and injuries is estimated to equate to 1% of gross national product (GNP) in low-income countries, 1.5% in middle-income countries and 2% in high-income countries. The cost to LMICs amounts to approximately US$65 million, which is more than they receive in development assistance,[36] so the financial burden falls particularly heavily on those countries that can afford it least.

Although deaths due to RTCs decreased from 1 230 000 in 1999 to 1 192 000 in 2002, representing slightly more than 2% of global deaths overall, WHO projections indicate that, despite a 30% decline in RTC deaths in HICs, an 80% increase in RTC deaths in LMICs will generate an overall 65% increase in RTC deaths by 2020 worldwide, making RTCs the sixth most common cause of death. This apparent contradiction is once again explained by a large increase in RTC deaths in LMICs. Experience in HICs has shown that policy initiatives such as seat belt legislation, child car seats, motorcycle helmets, enforcement programmes, alcohol control policies and traffic calming schemes may produce a rapid decline in deaths associated with RTCs, but unfortunately many of these policies are not transferrable to LMICs, often because the patterns of injury are different.[37]

Poisoning

According to WHO data, 350 000 people worldwide died from unintentional poisoning in 2000, making it the ninth most common cause of death among the 15–29 years age group. More than 94% of fatal poisonings occurred in LMICs, making poisoning overall the sixth most common cause of death in India and the ninth most common in China.[38] The contribution of intentional self-poisoning in the context of suicide is difficult to assess globally due to a lack of accurate statistics; however, the WHO suggests that a quarter of the 1 000 000 suicides each year are due to poisoning. In China, as in other developing countries, over 60% of successful suicides each year are due to pesticide poisoning.[38]

The WHO estimates that approximately 2 500 000 people are envenomated in snake attacks each year, posing significant challenges for medical management and resulting in an estimated 125 000 deaths per year.[38] Deaths due to envenomation depend not only on the lethality of the venom, but also on the interaction between the local environment and available medical services. The Inland Taipan has the world's most toxic venom, but it lives in the desert of eastern central Australia and has never caused a recorded fatality. There are approximately 100 adder bites per year in the UK, but only 10 recorded deaths, the last of which was 30 years ago.

Falls and domestic injuries

Falls, excluding those due to assault and self-harm, caused an estimated 283 000 deaths worldwide in 2000, rising to 391 000 in 2002, making falls the second highest cause of unintentional injury death, after RTCs, in that year.[39] Males in the LMICs of Europe have the highest fall-related mortality rates worldwide, with nearly 60% of fall-related deaths occurring in Europe and the Western Pacific region; however, nearly a quarter of fall deaths occur in HICs, and China accounts for twice as many DALYs lost due to falls as any other world region.[1] Falls also have a marked age and sex distribution, with over 40% of fall-related mortality occurring in the over-70s. Conversely, approximately 50% of DALYs lost worldwide are in children under the age of 15.[1]

The home is a major site of unintentional injury and death, with poisoning, falls and fires being the commonest causes. Poor architecture and overcrowding have been suggested to contribute to 11% of injuries among children,[40] and in the UK about 2.6 million accidents occurring in the home are treated in emergency departments each year. In the UK, 4000 people are killed annually as a result of accidents at home, and the total cost has been estimated to be around £30 million a year.[41] Non-fatal home accidents in the UK are projected to increase from 2.5 to 3 million per year by 2010, but accompanied by a fall in deaths from 3400 to 2400.[41] A Department of Trade and Industry (DTI) report[41] in 1999 concluded that *Most home accidents happen when people are doing ordinary, everyday things such as going up or down stairs, cooking, and gardening or when children are playing. Only a small proportion of accidents occur when doing obviously hazardous things such as climbing ladders.* It also suggested that, although accidents usually happen as a result of complex interactions between many factors, such as social and economic circumstances, alcohol, tiredness and safety awareness, human behaviour appears to be the most common cause of home accidents.[42]

Occupational injuries

In 2005 the WHO and the International Labour Office (ILO) estimated that, although the work-related injury toll had reached 2 000 000 cases annually, it continued to rise because of rapid industrialization in developing countries.[43] It was also estimated that the risk of occupational disease had become the most prevalent danger faced by people at their jobs, with disease accounting for 1.7 million work-related deaths annually, or four times the rate for other fatal accidents. In addition, there were approximately 268 million non-fatal work-related accidents each year, on average resulting in at least 3 days of sick time for the victims. The ILO has previously estimated that about 4% of the world's gross domestic product is lost each year as a result of workplace accidents and illnesses.

In many newly industrialized countries, such as Korea, the rate of workplace accidents levels off once the phase of rapid construction changes to a more mature stage of development and the workforce takes up less dangerous service jobs. Where rapid development continues, especially in Asia and Latin America, the death toll is still rising.[43] The estimated number of fatal accidents in China rose from 73 500 in 1998 to 90 500 in 2001, and Latin American countries, particularly Brazil and Mexico, have seen increases in fatal accidents in the construction sector rise from 29 500 to 39 500 over the same period. In 2005, it was estimated that there was a construction industry death somewhere in the world every 10 minutes.[43]

Fires

Fire-related burns were responsible for 238 000 deaths globally in 2000,[1] with more than 95% of these occurring in LMICs. In 2006, in the USA, deaths due to fires and burns were the fifth most common cause of unintentional injury death and the third most common cause of fatal injury at home.[44] Worldwide, mortality due to fire is lowest in European HICs, but four times higher in neighbouring LMICs. Similarly, in the Eastern Mediterranean, death from fires is over three times higher in LMICs than in HICs. However, the highest mortality is in Africa and South-East Asia, with rates in Africa over five times those in European HICs, and Indian and other South-East Asian mortality over eight times as high.[1] Fire-related mortality in the Americas is similar in LMICs and HICs, but in 2005 in the USA someone died in a fire approximately every 2 hours, and someone was injured every half-hour.[43] Smoking is still the leading cause of fire-related deaths in the USA, with cooking the primary cause of residential fires, and the CDC estimates that fire and burn injuries account for 1% of injuries and 2% of the total cost of injuries yearly, to the amount of US$7.5 billion.

As for many other types of unintentional injuries, those most at risk in the USA are children under 4, adults over 65, African Americans, Native Americans, and the poorest Americans, especially those living in rural areas or in substandard housing.[43] These statistics are reflected in the global data, with the groups at highest risk for death from fire being children under 5 and the elderly over 70.[1] Females in South-East Asia have the highest burn-related mortality rates worldwide, followed by males in Africa and females in the Eastern Mediterranean.

Drowning

In 2000, an estimated 409 000 people drowned worldwide, making drowning the second leading cause of unintentional injury death,[45] constituting 8% of the total global mortality from injury. This is an underestimate as the WHO definitions do not include drownings due to cataclysms, transport accidents, assault and suicide. Overall, twice as many males as females are drowned, although this ratio varies from region to region. European and American males are over four times as likely to die from drowning as females, whereas the ratio is 1.5:1 in South-East Asia, 1.8:1 in the Western Pacific and 2.9:1 in Africa. However, the magnitude of the problem is many times greater in these last three regions, which account for, respectively, 22%, 33% and 22% of global drowning deaths; by comparison, Europe and the USA account for only 6.8% and 6% respectively.[45] For example, the death rate due to drowning is eight times higher in Africa than in the USA and Australia, although in these last two countries drowning death rates are higher among indigenous populations than in Caucasians.

Children under 5 have the highest drowning mortality rates worldwide; it is the leading cause of injury death in children in China, the leading cause of unintentional injury death in children under 3 in Australia and the second leading cause of death in US children under 14. Worldwide, children account for over half of deaths from drowning.[1]

Other risks for death from drowning include epilepsy, occupation and alcohol. In Sweden, drowning is the cause of death in 10% of epileptics, 90% of occupational mortality in Alaskan fishermen is caused by drowning, and alcohol is a risk factor for drowning particularly among adolescents and adults. Alcohol or drug use has been implicated in 14% of unintentional drowning deaths in Australia, of which approximately 80% are in males.[43]

Disasters

Natural disaster such as earthquakes, tsunamis, hurricanes and cyclones inflict often incalculable losses on populations, not only in terms of injury and trauma deaths, but also in terms of mortality from subsequent disease and starvation. The risk of disasters is increasing, with data showing a significant increase in the frequency of recorded disasters over the past 50 years, and over 2 billion people affected in the past 10 years.[46] Several factors have been cited to explain this, including global warming, rapid human population changes and urbanization, civil war and conflict, the rise of terrorism, increased technology (with immature safety systems) and improved data collection.[47] Approximately 90% of disasters occur in countries with a per capita income of less than US$760 per annum, and countries in this position tend to have more disasters but less capacity to cope, plan and prepare, with

the frequency of disasters often meaning that there is little time for recovery between events. In the Western Pacific region alone there were 127 major natural disasters between 1990 and 2000, which killed 530 and left over 6 million homeless.[47]

The ability of the population affected by disasters to plan, prepare and respond has a great impact on the scale of death and injury and is demonstrated by the circumstances surrounding the Asian Tsunami of 2004 and Hurricane Katrina in 2005. On 26 December 2004 the second biggest earthquake ever recorded, with a score of 9.3 on the Richter scale, took place with an epicentre close to Sumatra. This earthquake caused devastating tsunamis that spread throughout the Indian Ocean, inundating coastal communities across South and South-East Asia, including parts of Indonesia, Sri Lanka, India and Thailand. Waves up to 30 metres high devastated coastlines in 12 countries, causing serious damage and deaths as far away as the east coast of Africa, and including Somalia, Bangladesh, Tanzania and Kenya. The number of dead and missing approached 250 000, with an estimated half a million injured. The tsunami also destroyed the infrastructure needed to treat the injured and to enable recovery from the disaster, including health facilities. A total of over US$7 billion was provided by nations across the world as aid for damaged regions.[48]

Hurricane Katrina was the sixth strongest Atlantic hurricane ever recorded, and the third strongest on record to landfall in the USA. Hurricane Katrina formed over the Bahamas in late August 2005 and devastated much of the north-central Gulf Coast of the USA, including the city of New Orleans, Louisiana and coastal Mississippi. On 28 August the storm reached its maximum intensity as a category 5 storm with sustained winds of 280 km/h (175 mph). The storm surge caused catastrophic damage by breaching the levees separating Lake Pontchartrain from the city, flooding 80% of New Orleans.[49]

However, owing to the early warning infrastructure in the USA, preparations were made for the arrival of the storm. In Florida, the National Hurricane Center issued hurricane warnings at about 30 and 20 hours before landfall, enabling evacuation orders to be issued. In Mississippi, the state government activated an emergency operations centre and evacuation orders were issued to 41 counties and 61 cities; 88 emergency shelters were established. In Louisiana, three phases of evacuation allowed the removal of approximately 80% of the population of metropolitan New Orleans. Despite these precautions, Hurricane Katrina became the costliest and the deadliest US hurricane on record. The total financial cost from the hurricane, which killed 1836 people (with an additional 705 missing) and injured many more, is estimated at US$81.2 billion.[50]

SUMMARY

- Injuries kill 5 million people each year, equating to 9% of worldwide deaths, and for every death many more are left disabled.
- Injuries are expected to rise in the next 20 years.
- Road traffic collisions caused 1.2 million deaths in 2002 and 50 million injuries at a cost of US$518 billion. This death toll is projected to rise to 1.9 million by 2030. This will be predominantly in low-/middle-income countries, whereas death rates are expected to fall in high-income countries.
- Globally, injury mortality in males is twice that among women, with the highest rates in Africa and Europe. Young people between the ages of 15 and 44 account for approximately 50% of global mortality due to trauma and, although injury remains the leading cause of death for young people, individual mortality and morbidity may be higher in the elderly.
- Intentional injuries account for half of the annual trauma mortality, with one-quarter of all deaths being due to interpersonal violence and suicides.
- Interpersonal violence caused the deaths of an estimated 520 000 people worldwide in 2000, with 95% of homicides occurring in the low middle-income countries.
- Falls were the second highest global injury cause of unintentional death after road traffic collisions. In 2005, there was a construction industry death somewhere in the world every 10 minutes. In 2000, drowning was the second leading cause of unintentional injury death.

REFERENCES

1. Peden M, McGee K, Sharma G. *The Injury Chart Book: a Graphical Overview of the Global Burden of Injuries.* Geneva: World Health Organization, 2002.

2. Aldrian S, Nau T, Koenig F, Vecsei V. Geriatric polytrauma. *Wien Klin Wochenschr* 2005;**117**:145–9.

3. Mock C, Lormand JD, Goosen J, Joshipura M, Peden M. *Guidelines for Essential Trauma Care.* Geneva: World Health Organization, 2004.

4. Murray CJL, Lopez AD. Mortality by cause for eight regions of the world: global burden of disease study. *Lancet* 1997;**349**:1269–76.

5. Ameratunga S, Hijar M, Norton R. Road-traffic injuries: confronting disparities to address a global-health problem. *Lancet* 2006;**367**:1533–40.

6   Carrigan TD, Field H, Illingworth RN, Gaffney P, Hamer DW. Toxicological screening in trauma. *J Accid Emerg Med* 2000;**17**:33–7.

7. WHO Department of Mental Health and Substance Abuse. *Global Status Report on Alcohol 2004.* Geneva: World Health Organization, 2004.

8. http://www.answers.com/topic/2004-indian-ocean-earthquake

9. *World Health Report, Statistical Annex.* Geneva: World Health Organization, 2000.

10. *World Health Report, Statistical Annex.* Geneva: World Health Organization, 2001.

11. *World Health Report, Statistical Annex.* Geneva: World Health Organization, 2002.

12. *World Health Report, Statistical Annex.* Geneva: World Health Organization, 2003.

13. Krug EG, Dahlberg LL, Mercy JA, Zwi AB, Lozano R. *World Report on Violence and Health.* Geneva: World Health Organization, 2002.

14. Greaves I, Porter K, Ryan J, eds. The trauma epidemic. In:*Trauma Care Manual.* London: Oxford University Press, 2000, pp. 1–10.

15. National Center for Injury Prevention and Control. *Injury Fact Book 2001–2002.* Atlanta, GA: Centers for Disease Control and Prevention, 2001.

16. Available at: http://www.ojp.usdoj.gov/bjs/ (accessed 19 October 2006).

17. Pridemore WA. Demographic, temporal and spatial patterns of homicide rates in Russia. *Eur Soc Rev* 2003;**19**:41–59.

18. Webster P. Suicide rates in Russia on the increase. *Lancet* 2003;**362**:220.

19. http://en.wikipedia.org/w/index.php?title=List_of_wars_1990%E2%80%932002&oldid=78601130 (accessed 18 October 2006).

20. McClelland J. The review of weapons in accordance with Article 36 of Additional Protocol I. *Int Rev Red Cross* 2003;**85**:397–415.

21. http://en.wikipedia.org/wiki/Terrorism (accessed 23 October 2006).

22. Memorial Institute for the Prevention of Terrorism; Terrorism Knowledge Base. Available at http://www.tkb.org/Home.jsp (accessed 23 October 2006).

23. Wilson N, Thomson G. Deaths from international terrorism compared with road crash deaths in OECD countries. *Inj Prev* 2005;**11** 332–3.

24. Pirkola SP, Suominen K, Isometsa ET. Suicide in alcohol-dependent individuals: epidemiology and management. *CNS Drugs* 2004;**18**:423–36.

25. Modesto-Lowe V, Brooks D, Ghani M. Alcohol dependence and suicidal behavior: from research to clinical challenges. *Harv Rev Psychiatry* 2006;**14**:241–8.

26. Molcho M, Harel Y, Dina LO. Substance use and youth violence. A study among 6th to 10th grade Israeli school children. *Int J Adolesc Med Health* 2004;**16**:239–51.

27. Matthews S, Richardson A. *Findings from the 2003 Offending, Crime and Justice Survey: Alcohol Related Crime and Disorder.* Findings 261. London: Home Office, 2005.

28. Demetriades D, Gkiokas G, Velmahos GC, Brown C, Murray J, Noguchi T. Alcohol and illicit drugs in traumatic deaths:

prevalence and association with type and severity of injuries. *J Am Coll Surg* 2004;**199** 687–92.

29.   Carrigan TD, Field H, Illingworth RN, Gaffney P, Hamer DW. Toxicological screening in trauma. *J Accid Emerg Med* 2000;**17**:33–7.

30.   Meulemans A, Hooft P, Van Camp L, De Vrieze N, Buylaert W, Verstraete A, Van Snick M. Belgian Toxicology and Trauma Study. 1996. Brussels: Belgian Society of Emergency and Disaster Medicine, Belgian Institute of Traffic Safety, the Toxicological Society of Belgium and Luxembourg. Quoted in: Illegal Drugs and Driving. ICADTS Working Group on Illegal Drugs and Driving. Chaired by: Dr. J. Michael Walsh [USA]. International Council on Alcohol, Drugs and Traffic Safety 2000.

31.   Iulianelli JAS, Guanabara LP, Cesar P, Fraga P, Blickman T. *A Pointless War: Drugs and Violence in Brazil*. Transnational Debate Papers, November 2004; No. 11; TNI Briefing Series.

32.   De La Rosa M, Lambert EY, Gropper B. Drugs and Violence: Causes, Correlates, and Consequences. NIDA Research Monograph 103, 1990; National Institute on Drug Abuse. Available at http://www.drugabuse.gov/pdf/monographs/103.pdf (accessed 24 October 2006).

33.   Drugs and Gangs Fast Facts: Questions and Answers; National Drug Intelligence Center; US Department of Justice. Available at http://www.usdoj.gov/ndic/pubs11/13157/index.htm#relation (accessed 24 October 2006).

34.   http://en.wikipedia.org/w/index.php?title=Automobile&oldid=81870548 (accessed 18 October 2006).

35.   http://www.census.gov/ipc/www/world.html (accessed 15 October 2006).

36.   Peden M, *et al.*, eds. *The World Report on Road Traffic Injury Prevention*. Geneva: World Health Organization, 2004.

37.   Nantulya VM, Sleet DA, Reich MR, Rosenberg M, Peden M, Waxweiler R. Introduction. The global challenge of road traffic injuries: Can we achieve equity in safety? *Inj Contr Saf Promot* 2003;**10**:3–7.

38.   International Program on Chemical Safety; Poisoning Prevention and Management. Geneva: World Health Organization, 2006. Available at http://www.who.int/ipcs/poisons/en/ (accessed 24 October 2006).

39.   http://www.who.int/violence_injury_prevention/other_injury/falls/en/index.html (accessed 28 October 2006).

40.   WHO Regional Office for Europe. Health Evidence Network (HEN). Available from: http://www.euro.who.int/HEN/Syntheses/housinghealth/20050215_1 (accessed 28 October 2006).

41.   *Research on the Pattern and Trends in Home Accidents*. London: Department of Trade and Industry, 1999. Available at: http://www.ecdti.co.uk/cgibin/perlcon.pl (accessed 29 October 2006).

42.   The role of parental supervision and accidents in the home. London: Department of Trade and Industry, 2001. Available at: http://www.ecdti.co.uk/cgibin/perlcon.pl (accessed 29 October 2006).

43.   *Number of Work-related Accidents and Illnesses Continues to Increase*. Geneva: World Health Organization. 2006. Available from: http://www.who.int/mediacentre/news/releases/2005/pr18/en/index.html (accessed 12 November 2006).

44.   National Center for Injury Prevention and Control. *Fire Deaths and Injuries: Fact Sheet 2006*. Atlanta, GA: Centers for Disease Control and Prevention, 2001. Available at http://www.cdc.gov/ncipc/factsheets/fire.htm (accessed 29 October 2006).

45.   Injuries and violence prevention; Drowning Fact Sheet. Geneva: World Health Organization, 2006. Available at: http://www.who.int/violence_injury_prevention/publications/other_injury/en/drowning_factsheet.pdf (accessed 28 October 2006).

46.   Western Australian Department of Health Disaster Preparedness and Management; Health Protection Group. Chamberlain C, ed. Disaster Medical Assistance Teams: A Literature Review. Perth, WA, 2006. Available at http://www.health.wa.gov.au/disaster/DMAT/index/disaster%20medical%20assistance%20teams%20literature%20review%202006.pdf (accessed 29 October 2006).

47.   Answers.Com contributors. Earthquake. Answers.com. Available at http://www.answers.com/topic/earthquake (accessed 29 October 2006).

48.   Russbach R. International assistance operations in disaster situations. *Prehosp Disast Med* 1990;**5**:247–249.

49.   http://en.wikipedia.org/w/index.php?title=Hurricane_Katrina&oldid=84159710 (accessed 29 October 2006).

50.   http://en.wikipedia.org/w/index.php?title=2004_Indian_Ocean_earthquake&oldid=84342510 (accessed 29 October 2006).

Mechanism of injury

After completing this chapter the reader will:
* understand the role of energy transfer in injury pathophysiology
* be able to interpret the mechanism of injury to inform individual patient care.

INTRODUCTION

Mechanism of injury can be defined as the physical circumstances causing an injury event. Assessment of injury mechanism is frequently used to support clinical and resource decision-making in the pre-hospital and emergency department environments. Pre-hospital examples include whether a patient undergoes spinal immobilization or is transported directly to a multidisciplinary trauma centre.[1] In the emergency department, knowledge of the mechanism of injury may be used as a trigger for activation of a trauma team and may alter the thresholds for imaging, intervention or admission. However, there remains some debate regarding whether the mechanism of injury accurately predicts either the severity of injury or the need for specialist resources. The central paradox is that several studies have shown that knowledge of the mechanism of injury does not correlate well with severity of anatomical injury or physiological derangement,[1,2] whereas other studies have demonstrated, conversely, that in certain groups of patients the mechanism of injury does accurately predict mortality and need for specialist care.

> Establish the mechanism of injury with as much accuracy as possible and relate this to the clinical presentation.

The key to this paradox lies in the role of energy transfer in injury pathophysiology and the accuracy of interpretation of the energy transfer in light of individual patient circumstances. Whilst the speed of vehicles involved in a collision is important, it is the resultant energy transfer that injures patients. In this chapter, we explore how an understanding of the physics of energy transfer can inform patient care. It should be emphasized from the outset, however, that, in those with obviously deranged physiology or anatomical evidence of major trauma, time spent analysing the mechanism of injury is unlikely to contribute significantly to the initial clinical assessment and resuscitation (Chapter 4).

PATHOPHYSIOLOGY

Biological tissues, organs and systems can withstand only a limited range of physical, environmental and physiological stresses. Injury is sustained whenever the energy delivered to a tissue exceeds the injury threshold or tolerance of that tissue. The energy can be delivered in any of its different forms:

* kinetic energy
* thermal energy
* electrical energy
* chemical energy
* nuclear energy.

The tolerance of the tissue depends upon factors such as the type of tissue involved and the age and physical health of the patient.[2] It can therefore be understood that the mechanism of injury has two components:

1. the physics of the energy transfer – influenced by the type and magnitude of the energy and the duration of exposure to the energy;

2. the biological response of the human body to receiving such energy – influenced by the tolerance of the tissues, organs and structures involved.

> Consider factors which may reduce the tolerance of human tissues, organs and systems to apparently minimal energy transfer – such as age and pre-existing disease.

Blunt trauma caused by kinetic energy

Kinetic energy (energy related to motion) is the most common type of energy which results in injury. It is responsible for energy transfer in road traffic collisions (RTCs), penetrating trauma, falls and crush injuries. Much of what is understood about kinetic energy stems from Newton's laws of motion. In particular, Newton's first law: a physical body will continue to move at a constant speed and direction (velocity) unless a net force acts upon it.

This law underpins the four collisions recognized during a sudden deceleration (or acceleration) as might be seen in a crash:

- The *first collision* occurs when the vehicle strikes another object and the kinetic energy is absorbed by the crushing metal and other materials.
- The *second collision* occurs when the occupant strikes the interior of the vehicle or another occupant.
- The *third collision* occurs when the occupant's internal organs continue to move and contact hard surfaces, such as the skull and chest wall, creating further potential for injury.
- A *fourth collision* occurs if loose objects in the vehicle continue in motion and collide with the occupant. Even though a car may be stopped from moving by hitting an immovable object, the occupants, their internal organs

and vasculature and other objects within the car will not stop moving until each has encountered its own point of impact.

Another important concept to understand is that the human tolerance to kinetic energy is influenced by both the *magnitude* and the *duration* of exposure. A large energy transfer can be withstood if applied over a prolonged time period, such as when an aircraft lands on a runway, but the same net force may not be tolerated if applied over a very short period, if the aircraft hits the ground in a crash for example. When considering kinetic energy transfer, this exposure can often be described in terms of the rate of change of velocity or the acceleration or deceleration experienced as a result of energy. Most commonly, injury is sustained during excessive deceleration – a falling person decelerates as he or she hits the ground or a motorcyclist decelerates on hitting a tree. Excessive acceleration may also cause injury – the pilot on an ejector seat and the occupant of a stationary vehicle that is hit from behind in a rear end shunt are two examples. The key features that determine the potential effects of energy transferred to the body in these circumstances are the rate of change of velocity, often referred to as ΔV (delta-V), and the magnitude of the energy, often referred to as 'force'.

Historically it was considered essential to 'read the wreckage' in RTCs. Relating the vehicle damage patterns to the different types and directions of energy transfer predicted physical injury patterns in the occupant. Significant frontal impacts may force the engine backwards into the passenger compartment, generating injuries to the lower limbs and pelvis. Side impacts will generate a pattern of trauma on one side, typically including pelvic and rib injury. Mechanism of injury criteria have long formed part of pre-hospital triage criteria and in-hospital trauma team call-out criteria. UK and US criteria are summarized in Table 2.1. It is acknowledged that mechanism of injury criteria overtriage

Table 2.1 Mechanism of injury-related triage criteria from the UK and the USA (anatomical and physiological triage criteria have been omitted)

Royal College of Surgeons of England/British Orthopaedic Association 2000[3]	The Committee on Trauma of The American College of Surgeons 2004[4]
An incident with five or more casualties	Ejection from auto
An incident involving a fatality	Death in the same passenger compartment
High-speed motor crash	Pedestrian thrown or run over
Where the patient has been ejected from the vehicle	High-speed auto crash
Knife wound above the waist	• initial speed >64 mph
Any gunshot wound	• major auto deformity >50 cm
Fall from >8 m	• intrusion into passenger compartment >30 cm
A child pedestrian or cyclist hit by a vehicle	Extrication time >20 min
	Falls >6 m
	Rollover (unrestrained occupant)
	Auto pedestrian injury with >5 mph impact
	Motorcycle crash >20 mph or with separation of rider and bike

a proportion of patients (which has resource implications); however, of more concern is the fact that there is also a significant undertriage rate. It must be remembered that low-energy trauma can still cause serious injury in the vulnerable patient (in particular those at the extremes of age and those with coexistent morbidity).

With the evolution of vehicle construction, materials science and vehicle safety technology, visible damage to the vehicle itself does not necessarily reflect the forces involved in the crash. However, for pre-hospital care providers, reading the wreckage remains important to develop a clear understanding of the sequence of events and recognize hazards to patients and rescue personnel. The presence or absence of energy-dissipating safety features should also be noted (Table 2.2), and it should be understood how these may diminish the risk of serious underlying injuries. Much of the current safety technology is computerized, and many new cars have sophisticated event data recorders (EDRs), which can record, store and even transmit data from the time of a crash. As systems develop it is entirely possible that real-time transmission of the physical circumstances of a crash might be available to the trauma care provider. This could give a precise picture of the magnitude and direction of energy transfer and whether the forces involved are likely to exceed tissue tolerance. Reading the wreckage and establishing the mechanism of injury will, in the near future, become an exact science.

> Successful injury prevention systems reduce energy transfer.

Penetrating trauma caused by kinetic energy

The rules of kinetic energy apply equally to penetrating trauma in that it is the amount of energy transferred to the victim that exerts an injurious effect. This means that descriptions of weapons according to velocity are unhelpful and potentially confusing. When a projectile penetrates the skin, the kinetic energy is transferred to the surrounding cells, which are pushed away from the path of the projectile. In low-energy transfer wounds, typified by stab wounds, this creates a channel of permanent tissue injury. As the degree of energy transfer increases, the process of temporary cavitation becomes increasingly important. Dissipation of kinetic energy pushes the tissues away, creating a large cavity; however, the elasticity of the tissues causes them to recoil into their original position. This temporary cavity is at subatmospheric pressure and will suck in contamination, which is distributed through the tissues previously displaced through cavitation, a fact that should be borne in mind when wound debridement is considered.[5] The degree of kinetic energy transfer is dependent in part on the kinetic energy with which the projectile arrives at the victim, but also upon the retardation offered to that projectile by the tissues. Elastic tissue that will accept the stretch of temporary cavitation and offer little resistance to the passage of the missile may well suffer little permanent damage even from the passage of high-velocity, high-available-energy missiles. Low-available-energy missiles can cause only a low-energy transfer wound, whereas high-available-energy missiles may cause wounds that vary across the spectrum of low to high energy transfer depending on the tissues traversed. If there is no exit wound and the missile is retained within the body, then all the projectile's available kinetic energy must, by definition, have been transferred to the victim's tissues.

The mechanisms of injury in gunshot wounds are discussed fully in Chapter 18, but three common misconceptions warrant correction here.

- Mechanical damage does not necessarily correlate with the degree of clinical injury and the latter is a function of the particular tissues injured. A stab wound from a long, thin blade, such as a screwdriver, will transfer much less energy than a wound caused by a blunt instrument, such as a hatchet, that causes a large gaping

Table 2.2 Safety strategies and how they attempt to minimize injury

Safety strategy	How is injury minimized?
Seat belt	Retaining the occupant in the seat avoids the second collision with the steering wheel or road if ejected
Airbag	Avoids second collision with the steering wheel or dashboard and slows the rate of deceleration
Crumple zone	Energy from the change in velocity is absorbed by deformation of the crumple zone
Collapsible steering column	Energy from the occupant hitting the steering wheel is avoided or absorbed as the column collapses
Head rest	Provides a point of impact for the head as the vehicle accelerates; in its absence the bones of the cervical spine would stop backward motion of the head
Speed limits	Lower speeds reduce the magnitude of change in velocity in the event of a crash
Helmets	The hard exterior absorbs energy by cracking or breaking upon impact and the foam inner absorbs energy by compression
Bark or rubber matting on the ground of play areas	Absorbs the energy of falling by compression

wound, but the clinical consequences of a penetrating wound to the heart are much greater than those of, say, a hatchet wound to the thigh.

- Deciding whether a missile wound is an entrance or exit wound is highly inaccurate and adds little to the management of the patient.
- Penetrating missiles do not always follow a straight path. As they decelerate they are likely to ricochet off internal organs and bones to injure vital structures away from a presumed missile track.

Burns caused by thermal energy

Thermal energy is the kinetic energy of molecular motion, which is measured as temperature and perceived as heat or cold. Thermal energy flows from a hot region to a cold region. In the context of injury this is mostly by conduction – the heat moves directly from molecule to molecule. The severity of the damage to individual cells (the burn) depends upon the duration of exposure, the temperature, the skin conductance and the thermal conductivity of the subcutaneous tissues.[6] The clinical assessment and management of burns is covered in more detail in Chapter 20.

Electric shocks and burns caused by electrical energy

Electrical energy can be defined as a flow of electrical charge. Electrical energy can cause injury in a number of different ways. Heat is the main cause of injury from electricity, as electrical energy is converted to thermal energy. This can cause superficial skin burns or deeper fascial burns either concurrently or independently. Damage can also be caused by the direct passage of electrical energy through tissues. Electricity preferentially travels through tissues offering least resistance – typically skeletal and cardiac muscle and nerves. Wet or sweaty skin is a good conductor whilst dry skin offers a high degree of resistance. As electrical current is conducted from cell to cell the patient may experience muscle contractions, arrhythmias and peripheral or central nerve injury.

Lightning is a unique form of electrical energy that produces different patterns of injury to the more usual injuries sustained from man-made electrical sources. Lightning is extremely high voltage and can cause electrical injury, leading to respiratory or cardiac arrest. In addition, the thermal energy emitted from the lightning rapidly heats the surrounding air, creating a blast wave of moving air molecules that can tear clothing or push a patient to the ground. Moreover, the thermal energy can superheat moisture on the skin or metal objects, causing burns from steam or from melted metal objects in contact with the skin.

Nuclear energy

Nuclear energy refers to the energy released either by splitting atomic nuclei (fission or radioactive decay) or by forcing them together (fusion). This results in the release of different types of energetic particles (neutrons, alpha and beta particles) and electromagnetic rays such as gamma and X-rays. These various forms of radiation have specific physical properties and cause different types of damage to the molecular structure of cells. Rapidly dividing cells are most readily affected – for example those of the gastrointestinal tract, the bone marrow and the skin. If the nucleus is involved, the cell is likely to be irreversibly damaged. The severity of acute radiation poisoning is directly related to the absorbed energy dose, which varies according to the type of radiation and the duration of the exposure. Cutaneous burns are seen only in the context of external exposure. In most cases, and in contrast to other forms of injury, the onset of symptoms occurs from hours to days after exposure and the presentation is predominantly related to underlying cellular damage in the bone marrow, gastrointestinal tract, cardiovascular system or central nervous system.

Contact with nuclear energy as a mechanism of injury may be in the context of occupational or accidental exposure to radiation sources in industry, medicine or research, transport incidents involving carriage of radioactive substances, power station accidents and deliberate release of radioactive substances and nuclear weapons. Despite the association with nuclear weapons, the majority of the energy released by a nuclear explosion is either kinetic or thermal.

Chemical energy

Chemical energy is the energy created or consumed during rearrangement of electric charges in chemical reactions. Acids, alkalis, oxidizing agents, reducing agents, corrosives, desiccants and vesicants can all undergo chemical reactions with tissues and cause direct destruction of cellular proteins and lipids. Chemical reactions which produce thermal energy may also cause more typical thermal burns. The severity of the burn is related to a number of the chemical and physical properties of the agent and the biological nature of the area of contact (Table 2.3). There is more detail on the assessment and management of chemical burns in Chapter 20.

Explosions

An explosion is the phenomenon that results from a sudden release of energy. This can be accidental, for example an exploding petrol tanker, or deliberate, such as

Table 2.3 Features which may influence transfer of chemical energy

Physical and chemical properties of the agent	Biological response of the area of contact
pH	Depth of skin (thin skin is more easily damaged – such as the face or skin creases)
The concentration of the agent	The integrity of the skin (pre-existing areas of skin trauma allow more absorption, or those on steroids may have poor-quality skin)
The length of contact time	
The volume of the agent	Direct application to mucous membranes enhances absorption (for example if ingested)
The physical form of the agent	

a terrorist suicide bomb. Deliberate explosions in the UK are a rare (although extremely high-profile) cause of injury, although experience of explosions in countries affected by civil unrest is growing. The source of the energy is most commonly a chemical reaction, such as occurs with dynamite. Other explosive releases of energy can occur with nuclear reactions, electrical arcs and mechanical overpressure. The same principles of energy transfer apply to explosions, although elucidating the exact mechanism of injury can be complex as multiple types of energy transfer are involved. Injuries from explosions are classically described as being by one of four mechanisms, which are discussed in detail in Chapter 19. More recently, a potential fifth mechanism of injury has been proposed whereby an exaggerated inflammatory response has been noted after exposure to a particular chemical agent, penta-erythritol-tetranitrate, in a series of explosions in Israel.[7] It has not yet been fully accepted.

In addition, explosions can start fires, releasing thermal energy, or disrupt electricity cables, causing electrical injury. Some bombs may contain chemicals or radioactive material, causing additional complications.

SUMMARY

Injury is caused by energy transfer. Understanding the pathophysiology of energy transfer and being able to assess whether human tissue tolerances are likely to have been exceeded by contact with energy is the basis for 'reading the wreckage'. In most cases, very limited information regarding the true forces involved is available to the attending clinician. It may be possible in the near future to access accurate and meaningful data regarding energy transfer and the probability of a patient having sustained serious injuries. In the meantime, a basic knowledge of the mechanism of injury, in terms of the energy type and magnitude and the duration of exposure, may still significantly influence pre-hospital and emergency department decision-making. The mechanism of injury therefore remains a useful adjunct in the care of the trauma patient.

GLOBAL PERSPECTIVES

In the majority of the developed world the safety features described in Table 2.2 are routine in new car production. This is not the case in many parts of the developing world, where there are many older vehicles in use. The Global Burden of Disease study estimated that motor vehicle injuries alone constitute the ninth leading cause of disease burden as measured by the number of associated disability-adjusted life years. In the year 2000 alone, an estimated 5 million people worldwide died from traffic-related injuries – a mortality rate of 83.7 per 100 000 population.[8] Understanding the mechanism of injury on a population basis and introducing relevant and applicable safety strategies (such as enforced speed limits) could have a massive impact on reducing the worldwide morbidity and mortality associated with road traffic collisions.

REFERENCES

1. Hunt RC. Is mechanism of injury dead? *Prehosp Emerg Care* 1999;3:70–3.
2. Shatney CH, Sensaki K. Trauma team activation for mechanism of blunt trauma victims: time for change? *J Trauma* 1994;37:275–82.
3. Royal College of Surgeons of England and the British Orthopaedic Association. *Better Care for the Severely Injured.* London: Royal College of Surgeons of England, July 2000.
4. The Committee on Trauma of the American College of Surgeons. *Advanced Trauma Life Support.* Chicago: American College of Surgeons, 2004.
5. Prehospital Trauma Life Support Committee of The National Association of Emergency Medical Technicians in Cooperation with The Committee on Trauma of The American College of Surgeons. *Prehospital Trauma Life Support.* St Louis: Mosby Elsevier, 2007.
6. Cooper GJ, Dudley HAF, Gann DS, Little RA, Maynard RL. *The Scientific Foundations of Trauma.* Oxford: Butterworth-Heinmann, 1997.

7.   Kluger Y, Nimrod A, Biderman P, Mayo A, Sorkin P. The quinary (Vth) injury pattern of blast. *J Emerg Manage* 2006;4:51–5.

8.   Murray CJ, Lopez AD. Mortality by cause for eight regions of the world: Global Burden of Disease Study. *Lancet* 1997;349:1269–76.

Triage

After completing this chapter the reader will:
- understand that triage is the process in which patients are sorted to ensure optimal care and use of resources
- understand that triage is a dynamic process and must be repeated regularly
- recognize that triage systems must be simple and swift but also reliable and reproducible
- understand that senior staff should be used as triage officers
- acknowledge that triage should never be allowed to delay treatment.

INTRODUCTION

The campaigns of the Napoleonic Wars saw battles that resulted in huge numbers of soldiers being killed or wounded in a single day. At Borodino on 7 September 1812, the worst of these battles resulted in 80 000 French and Russian soldiers being killed; in addition, the Russians inflicted 35 000 wounded on the French.[1] During these campaigns, Baron Dominique Larrey (1766–1842), Chief Surgeon to Napoleon Bonaparte, introduced a system of sorting the casualties arriving at his field dressing stations. Triage comes from the French *trier*, 'to sort or to sieve', and was originally used to describe the selection of coffee beans. It is the process of sorting patients according to priority in order to establish an order for treatment and evacuation. Larrey's primary objective was the swift return of fit men to action and minor wounds were treated early – thereafter his priorities were similar to those in use today. He used senior military surgeons as triage officers, finding that experienced doctors produced more accurate triage.

Triage can take many different forms, and operates at a number of different levels, but at all times its aim is to give the right patient the right care at the right time in the right place. In certain circumstances this may also mean 'doing the most for the most'.

Triage must be a simple procedure that is swift, reliable and reproducible. There are many systems in use worldwide depending on the scenario and the end-point required. A surgeon deciding which of three patients to operate on first will employ a different system from a doctor faced with 80 casualties at a major incident.

The condition of any patient is liable to change because of time or medical intervention, and this is especially true of the seriously injured. An unconscious patient with a moderate isolated head injury may die if his or her airway is not supported but once conscious can be simply observed – this patient's triage priority is initially high, but becomes low. Triage is thus a dynamic process and should be repeated on a regular basis.

WHEN DOES TRIAGE TAKE PLACE?

In pre-hospital medicine, triage is used not only to assign treatment and evacuation priorities to casualties but also to determine which hospital the patient goes to, the means of transport and what sort of team meets him or her on arrival. Triage of the emergency call at ambulance control can also determine the type and speed of the ambulance crew that responds to that call. This is prioritized despatch and is discussed below. Triage to assign treatment and evacuation priorities must take place whenever casualties outnumber the skilled help and other resources available. A two-person ambulance crew attending a two-car motor vehicle crash could have six casualties to deal with. Initially, the crew must assess all those involved, identify those with life-threatening and serious injuries, and develop a plan of action for treatment and transport both before and as other help becomes available. Within an emergency department the same six trauma patients may arrive in a short period of time. Unless the hospital encounters this scenario on a regular basis, it is unlikely that the resuscitation room will have a bay and a full trauma team available for each patient. Using triage principles will help the team leader to determine how to allocate staff and decide which patients are seen in the resuscitation room. Ideally, ambulance control will have triaged some of the patients to other local hospitals, but this may not be possible for geographical reasons. Once the resuscitation has been completed, patients may need further triage for transfer to specialist centres such as neurosurgical or burns units.

WHERE DOES TRIAGE TAKE PLACE?

Before any patient contact, triage at the ambulance control centre may have determined the type of response despatched. Once at the scene, the ambulance crew will triage the patients to determine both the destination hospital and the appropriate mode of transport. In most areas of the UK there is little choice other than a road move to the nearest major emergency department, but, as the use of helicopter ambulances increases, diversion to a specialist centre will become a more frequent option. In the USA triage determines whether the receiving hospital is a trauma centre or a general hospital. During a major incident involving multiple casualties, triage takes place at the scene in order to determine initial priorities for treatment and transport to the casualty clearing station. The patients may be re-triaged for treatment priorities on arrival at the casualty clearing station and again for transport priorities to hospital after treatment. At the hospital another round of triage will take place at the doors of the emergency department to reassign treatment priorities. After initial resuscitation, priorities for surgery will be determined. Many UK emergency departments carry out triage of all patients on arrival. These circumstances are obviously very different from those pre-hospital or at a major incident, but the same principles of triage apply – immediately life-threatening conditions must be treated without delay; serious problems must be identified and given a higher priority than minor ones. A five-category system is used in most departments (Table 3.1).[2] Triage principles have also been used successfully in 'hospital tents' at mass gatherings such as rock festivals and sporting events,[3] to ensure the best use of limited resources.

Table 3.1 Accident and emergency triage categories

Description	Priority	Colour	Target time
Immediate	1	Red	On arrival
Very urgent	2	Orange	Within 10 minutes
Urgent	3	Yellow	Within 1 hour
Standard	4	Green	Within 2 hours
Non-urgent	5	Blue	Within 4 hours

WHO PERFORMS TRIAGE?

The exact nature of the incident and the timing and site of triage will determine the identity of the triage officer or officers. Whenever possible, triage should be performed by experienced senior staff. Although at first sight this might seem to be a waste of a valuable resource better employed in direct resuscitation, accurate triage will help to ensure optimal use of all staff and resources to achieve the best care for all the casualties. Overtriage – awarding a higher priority to a patient than appropriate – will consume staff and resources and dilute or divert them from other high-priority patients. Undertriage will result in the patient receiving the lower priority getting delayed or inadequate care.

> Triage should be performed by experienced senior staff.

PRIORITIES

Different systems of triage are used in the UK, depending on the situation. A working knowledge of the common systems and categories will assist trauma teams to appreciate what may have happened to the patient earlier. The two common pre-hospital systems in use in UK civilian practice are the *Priority 'P' system* and the *Treatment 'T' system*.[4] The significant difference is the inclusion of the expectant priority in the 'T' system (Table 3.2). Each triage priority is conventionally assigned a specific colour. The International Committee of the Red Cross (ICRC) uses its own categories for triage of patients arriving at their hospitals in war zones (Table 3.3).[5]

Expectant priority

This priority is given to casualties with non-survivable injuries, or whose injuries are so severe and their chances of survival so small that their treatment would divert medical resources, thus compromising the survival of other casualties. This priority should be invoked only in a 'mass casualty' situation, when the number of casualties completely overwhelms the medical resources available and rescuers must 'do the most for the most'. The decision to use the expectant priority is taken by the medical and ambulance incident officers acting in concert at the scene. To date, it has not been needed in any major incident in the UK. As a concept, the use of this priority goes against the instincts of all trauma carers, but its appropriate use will save lives. Patients with severe (>80%) burns and comatose patients with compound skull fractures are examples of patients for whom this priority would be appropriate in a declared mass casualty situation. They should still be given analgesia and made comfortable and not just left. If, after all the other casualties have been cared for, they are still alive, treatment should be given.

Table 3.2 UK pre-hospital triage priorities

Description	System P	T	Colour	
Immediate	1	1	Red	Casualties requiring immediate procedures to save life, e.g. airway obstruction, tension pneumothorax
Urgent	2	2	Yellow	Casualties requiring medical treatment within 4–6 hours, e.g. compound fractures
Delayed	3	3	Green	Casualties with injuries that can wait until after 4–6 hours, e.g. small cuts and contusions, minor closed fractures
Expectant		4	Blue	See text
Dead	Dead	Dead	White	Dead casualties must be identified and clearly labelled as such to avoid re-triage

Table 3.3 International Committee of the Red Cross triage categories

Category I	Patients for whom urgent surgery is required who have a good chance of reasonable survival
Category II	Patients who do not require surgery. This includes those for whom reasonable survival is unlikely
Category III	Patients who require surgery, but not urgently

SYSTEMS

Triage systems use anatomical or physiological data as well as information regarding the mechanism of injury, and certain criteria may be used for trauma team activation (Table 3.4). Accurate triage using an anatomical system requires a full secondary survey of an undressed patient so that all injuries are identified and assessed, individually and collectively, before a priority is assigned. Anatomical systems require experienced operators, time and a warm, well-lit environment – all of which are lacking at the scene of an incident. Once the incident has occurred, a patient's injuries will not change. As a result, anatomical systems are static and are of use only in hospital with small numbers of patients to assess. Anatomical information may be used by experience triage officers to modify other triage systems.

Systems using the mechanism of injury promote a high index of suspicion for occult injury. By recognizing and reporting a mechanism of injury associated with a high chance of serious injury, the pre-hospital carers draw the attention of the trauma team to the likely problems. These systems are not of use when dealing with a large number of casualties. In this situation, the mechanism will have been broadly similar for all, and small variations between individuals – such as position within a railway carriage – will not be clear early on. With small numbers of patients, these systems allow the identity of the receiving hospital and activation of a trauma team to be determined.[6] Occasionally, the trauma team will receive a patient without a serious injury when the activation has been based solely on the history;[7] while the disruption is annoying for all concerned, this is a necessary evil if all serious occult injury is to be detected. Some trauma centres use a two-tier graded response to incoming trauma to minimize the nuisance effects and cost of overtriage.[8,9] The pre-hospital information is triaged for either a full or modified trauma call – a senior doctor still leads the modified team, and the response can be upgraded to a full trauma call at any time.

Physiological systems give the best indication of a patient's current condition, although they do not allow for the compensatory mechanisms of children and young adults. When undertriage occurs, it is usually due to the physiological parameters being ignored. Ideally, the triage officer should employ a physiological system and use his or her experience to modify the priority assigned if anatomical or mechanical considerations demand it; hence, the triage officer should be as experienced as possible in dealing with trauma. The most sensitive triage tools combine aspects of all three types of systems but are harder to use in the field.

Table 3.4 Trauma team activation criteria

Anatomical	>1 long-bone fracture – unilateral radius and ulna count as one
	>1 anatomical area injured
	Penetrating injury to head, thorax or abdomen
	Traumatic amputation or crush injury
Mechanism	Fall >6 m
	Pedestrian or cyclist hit by car
	Death of other occupant in same vehicle
	Ejection from vehicle/bicycle
	Major vehicular deformity or significant intrusion into passenger space
	Extrication time >20 min
	Vehicular roll-over
Physiological	Respiratory rate >29/min
	Pulse rate <50 or >130 beats/min
	Systolic blood pressure <90 mmHg
	Glasgow Coma Scale score <13

The triage sieve

The triage sieve[4] (Table 3.5) is a fast, snapshot assessment of the patient that can be used at the scene of a major incident.[10] It is based on mobility, followed by a simple assessment of ABC. The capillary refill time (CRT) is preferred for circulatory assessment as it gives an indication of peripheral perfusion and is simple and rapid to ascertain. Environmental conditions, especially dark and cold, may make the determination of CRT difficult; if this is the case, the pulse should be used. This system will overtriage normally non-mobile patients at the extremes of age and undertriage a mobile but severely injured patient.

The paediatric triage tape, displaying triage sieves adjusted for length, has been developed and validated[11] to address the triage of young children. The severely injured but mobile patient, for example a patient with 40% burns, will eventually cease to be mobile and be re-triaged. In the meantime, this casualty may have been able to move to an area where more help is available, and a more sophisticated triage system can be used which will recognize the significance of the injury. After the rapid and simple first triage, a more sophisticated triage tool can be used. This is often referred to as the 'triage sort'. The Triage Revised Trauma Score (TRTS) is the system currently recommended for this use.

Triage Revised Trauma Score

This modification of the Revised Trauma Score[12] (RTS) allows rapid physiological triage of multiple patients in the field. It uses the unweighted sum of the RTS values to allocate priorities (Table 3.6). This system is used once the patients have been moved from the immediate scene of the incident and a more thorough assessment can be made, for example at the casualty clearing station.

The TRTS was first developed in the USA to help paramedics determine which patients should be taken to a trauma centre and which to a general hospital. Just one point dropped from any of the three parameters signifies increased mortality, and is an indication for the patient to be taken to a trauma centre. Some 97% of all trauma deaths will be identified using this method, the missed deaths being patients with serious injury whose compensatory mechanisms still allow their physiological parameters to remain normal when the first readings are taken by the ambulance crew. This will occur most often when the patient is young and the ambulance arrives quickly. To avoid this problem, the American College of Surgeons' Committee on Trauma devised a Triage Decision Scheme[13] (Table 3.7) that assesses physiological, anatomical, mechanical and pre-morbid factors.

Table 3.5 The triage sieve

Mobility	Can the patient walk?	Yes			→	P3 Delayed
		No			→	Assess A and B
Airway and breathing	Is the patient breathing?	No	→	Open airway, breathing now?		
			No		→	Dead
			Yes		→	P1 Immediate
		Yes	→	Assess rate		
			<10 or >29		→	P1 Immediate
			10–29		→	Assess C
Circulation	CRT	>2s				
		or pulse	>120 beats/min		→	P1 Immediate
	CRT	<2s				
		or pulse	<120 beats/min		→	P2 Urgent

CRT, capillary refill time.

Table 3.6 Triage priorities using the Triage Revised Trauma Score

Respiratory rate (per min)	0	1–5	6–9	30	10–29
Points	0	1	2	3	4
Systolic blood pressure (mmHg)	0	1–49	50–75	76–89	90+
Points	0	1	2	3	4
Glasgow Coma Scale score (total)	3	4–5	6–8	9–12	13–15
Points	0	1	2	3	4
Total score	12	10–11	1–9	0	
Priority	T3/P3 Delayed	T2/P2 Urgent	T1/P1 Immediate	Dead	

Table 3.7 Triage decision scheme

Measure vital signs and level of consciousness

Step 1	RR <10 or >29 SBP <90	Yes	→	Take to trauma centre Alert trauma team
	GCS <13 (i.e. drop one point on TRTS)	No	→	Assess anatomy of injury (Step 2)
Step 2	Flail chest 2+ proximal long-bone fractures Amputation proximal to wrist/ankle All penetrating trauma unless distal to elbow and knee	Yes	→	Take to trauma centre Alert trauma team
	Limb paralysis Pelvic fractures Combination trauma with burns	No	→	Evaluate mechanism of injury (Step 3)
Step 3	Ejection from vehicle/bicycle Death in same vehicle Pedestrian thrown or run over or >5 mph impact speed	Yes	→	Contact medical control Consider taking to trauma centre or consider alerting trauma team
	Motorcycle RTC speed >20 mph (30 km/h) Car RTC speed >40 mph (64 km/h) Major vehicular deformity or intrusion into passenger space Extrication time >20 min Vehicular roll-over Falls >6 m	No	→	Assess pre-morbid state (Step 4)
Step 4	Age <5 or >55 years Pregnancy Immunosuppressed patients Cardiac or respiratory disease	Yes	→	Contact medical control Consider taking to trauma centre Consider alerting trauma team
	IDDM, cirrhosis Coagulopathy, morbid obesity	No	→	Re-evaluate with medical control

When in doubt, take to a trauma centre

IDDM, insulin-dependent diabetes mellitus; GCS, Glasgow Coma Scale; RR, respiration rate (per min); RTC, road traffic collision; SBP, systolic blood pressure (mmHg); TRTS, Triage Revised Trauma Score.

Prioritized despatch

This is a concept that has recently been introduced in the UK. Studies in the USA have shown that prioritized despatch – dividing calls into priorities by using questions about the patient's respiratory and neurological state – improves the efficiency of the ambulance service.[14,15] A motor component of the Glasgow Coma Scale (GCS) <6 and a systolic blood pressure of <90 mmHg have been shown to be significantly associated with the need for a life-saving intervention, but patients with normal blood pressures and motor scores also frequently require these, so further research is needed.[16] Two systems in use are the Advanced Medical Priority Despatch System (AMPDS) and Criteria-Based Despatch (CBD). Both use a fixed sequence of questions to determine the priority. The AMPDS sorts calls into four categories, and CBD into three. As well as ranking emergency calls by urgency, prioritized despatch allows the ambulance control to determine the type and level of response. The target of one paramedic per crew has almost been achieved throughout

the UK, so the choice between the paramedic crew and the all-technician crew is less relevant. Helicopter ambulances are now becoming more widely available for despatch. In France, there is always a doctor in the ambulance control room to monitor calls, and another doctor available to respond to pre-hospital emergencies when despatched. In areas of the UK with a British Association for Immediate Care Scheme (BASICS), a doctor may be asked to attend a scene by ambulance control, or a mobile medical team requested from a nearby emergency department. There are currently few specialized trauma centres in the UK. Nearly all seriously injured patients will therefore be taken to the nearest accident and emergency department. The regionalization of trauma services was recommended in a report on major trauma by the Royal College of Surgeons of England in 1988 but has still to be adopted,[17] although the importance of this development was recently re-emphasized in a National Confidential Enquiry into Patient Outcome and Death (NCEPOD) report, *Trauma: Who Cares.*[18] Such developments would result in a similar system to that in use in the USA.

Labelling triaged patients

Once the casualty is in hospital, a patient number and notes will be assigned; clinical information and decisions must be properly recorded, as must pre-hospital clinical data and triage decisions. The patient report form is a valuable source of information for the trauma team leader during and after a resuscitation; it does not, however, replace listening to the ambulance crew at the handover. In an incident involving a large number of casualties, once a triage priority has been assigned, the triage officer must label the patient appropriately to prevent duplication of effort and confusion among other rescuers as to which patients need treatment and evacuation first.

Unfortunately, there are many different labelling systems available, and there is no accepted national or international standard. This does not matter as long as everyone who is likely to use the local system is familiar with it. Problems are most likely to arise when staff move areas or are operating out of their local region. A labelling system must be dynamic and allow the patient to get better or worse – it should also be simple to use and easily recognized. Part of the label should allow clinical data to be recorded and updated as the patient moves along the chain of care. Labels should be easily visible and robust enough to be of use in dark and wet environments, and must be easily attached to the patient. Ideally, each label should have an identifying number that allows the triage officer to know how many patients have been triaged, and to give the casualty an identifying number by which they can later be traced through the course of the incident.

There is no agreed convention on labelling the expectant priority. Blue is commonly used, but both red and green cards annotated 'expectant' are alternatives. Some cards allow the triage officer to fold the corners of the green card back, showing the red behind. Whatever local alternative is in use, all those who may need to know must be informed as part of major incident planning and preparation.

Many labelling systems use single, coloured cards. Clinical information is recorded on one side of each card. These systems are not ideal as they are not dynamic. If a patient changes priority, a new card needs to be filled out with the clinical data. This wastes time, and there is an attendant risk of transposition errors. As more patients change priority and receive a second card, the triage officer will lose track of the exact number of casualties. If the out-of-date card is thrown away, vital information may be lost, but if it is left with the patient then confusion may occur as to which of the cards is the current one.

The Mettag label is a commonly used system that falls between the single priority and the multiple priority cards. It is a plain white label for clinical information, which has coloured strips at the base of the card that can be ripped off to denote the priority. This system has two major drawbacks. First, it is difficult to tell what category a patient is without getting close up, and, second, the category can only be changed by tearing off further strips in order to indicate a worse category. If the patient improves, a new form is required.

The multiple category card systems are currently the best types available. Data are recorded on the card, which is then folded and replaced in a clear plastic envelope so that only one colour is visible. There is plenty of room for clinical information, and if the category changes then the card is simply refolded. The cards can be tricky to fold and replace in the envelope if the operator is unfamiliar with them. A further disadvantage is that patients might change their own category to ensure earlier evacuation. These cards are relatively expensive, and it is this that has prevented their wider use.

SUMMARY

Triage is the process in which patients are sorted to ensure optimal care and use of resources. It operates at many levels, especially in circumstances with large numbers of casualties and limited resources. Triage systems cannot be applied to single patients. It is a dynamic process and must be repeated regularly; triage systems must be simple and swift, as well as reliable and reproducible. Senior staff should be used as triage officers, and triage decisions must be recorded. It is vital to remember that the overall aim at all times is to give the right patient the right care, at the right time and in the right place.

GLOBAL PERSPECTIVES

The simple triage and rapid treatment system[19] (START) and the triage trauma rule[20] are alternative systems to the triage sieve which are in use in the USA (Tables 3.8 and 3.9).

Table 3.8 The simple triage and rapid treatment system (START)

Is the patient breathing?	No	→	Open airway; breathing now?
	No	→	*Dead*
	Yes	→	*Immediate care*
	Yes	→	Assess rate
	>30	→	*Immediate care*
	<30	→	Check radial pulse
Radial pulse present?	No	→	Control haemorrhage
		→	*Immediate care*
	Yes	→	Assess mental state
Following commands	No	→	*Immediate care*
	Yes	→	*Urgent care*

Table 3.9 The trauma triage rule

Major trauma victim = Systolic blood pressure <85mmHg
Motor component of Glasgow Coma Scale <5
Penetrating trauma to head, neck or torso

REFERENCES

1. Rignault D, Wherry D. Lessons from the past worth remembering: Larrey and Triage. *Trauma* 1999;1:86–9.
2. Manchester Triage Group. *Emergency Triage*. London: BMJ Publishing Group, 1997.
3. Kerr GW, Parke TRJ. Providing 'T in the Park': pre-hospital care at a major crowd event. *Pre-Hospital Immediate Care* 1999;3:11–13.
4. Advanced Life Support Group. *Major Incident Medical Management and Support – The Practical Approach*. London: BMJ Publishing Group, 1995.
5. Coupland RM, Parker PJ, Gray RC. Triage of war wounded: the experience of the International Committee of the Red Cross. *Injury* 1992;23:507–10.
6. Hodgetts TJ, Deane S, Gunning K. *Trauma Rules*. London: BMJ Publishing Group, 1997.
7. Simon BJ, Legere P, Emhoff T, *et al*. Vehicular trauma triage by mechanism: avoidance of the unproductive evaluation. *J Trauma* 1994;37:645–9.
8. Ochsner MG, Schmidt JA, Rozycki GS, Champion HR. The evaluation of a two-tier trauma response system at a major trauma center: is it cost effective and safe? *J Trauma* 1995;39:971–7.
9. Tinkoff GH, O'Connor RE, Fulda GJ. Impact of a two-tiered trauma response in the Emergency Department: promoting efficient resource utilisation. *J Trauma* 1996;41:735–40.
10. Malik ZU, Pervez M, Safdar A, Masood T, Tariq M. Triage and management of mass casualties in a train accident. *J Coll Phys Surg Pakistan* 2004;14:108–11.
11. Wallis LA, Carley S. Validation of the Paediatric Triage Tape. *Emerg Med J* 2006;23:47–50.
12. Champion HR, Sacco WJ, Copes WS, *et al*. A revision of the Trauma Score. *J Trauma* 1989;29:623–9.
13. American College of Surgeons' Committee on Trauma. *Advanced Trauma Life Support for Doctors – Course Manual*. Chicago: American College of Surgeons, 1997.
14. West JG, Gales RH, Cazaniga AB. Impact of regionalisation. The Orange County Experience. *Arch Surg* 1983;18:740.
15. Culley L. Increasing the efficiency of emergency medical services by using criteria based despatch. *Ann Emerg Med* 1994;24:867–72.
16. Holcomb JB, Niles SE, Miller CC, Hinds D, Duke JH, Moore FA. Prehospital physiologic data and lifesaving interventions in trauma patients. *Mil Med* 2005;170:7–13.
17. Royal College of Surgeons of England. *Commission on the Provision of Surgical Services. Report of the Working Party on the Management of Patients with Major Injuries*. London: Royal College of Surgeons of England, 1988.
18. National Confidential Enquiry into Patient Outcome and Death (NCEPOD). *Trauma: Who Cares?* London: NCEPOD, 2007.
19. Super G, Groth S, Hook R. *START: Simple Treatment and Rapid Treatment Plan*. Newport Beach, CA: Hoag Memorial Presbyterian Hospital, 1994.
20. Baxt WG, Jones G, Fortlage D. The trauma triage rule: a new resource-based approach to the pre-hospital identification of major trauma victims. *Ann Emerg Med* 1990;19:1401–6.

Patient assessment

OBJECTIVES

After completing this chapter the reader will:
- be able to explain the tasks of the trauma reception team
- demonstrate the systematic approach to initial trauma care
- demonstrate a method of seamless transition to definitive care.

INTRODUCTION

Trauma care starts at the point of the injury and continues through to the end of rehabilitation. Each link is vitally important, so that both patient and relatives experience the best possible outcome. This chapter concentrates on one of the earliest links in this chain: the initial reception of the trauma patient in the resuscitation room.

Errors are often made in the early management of the trauma patient, for understandable reasons: doctors and nurses are distracted by obvious problems such as a painful deformed leg but miss the subtly developing critical condition such as a bleeding pelvis. Conversely, another common error is to overlook a non-fatal problem such as a carpus dislocation in the desire to save the patient's life. Nevertheless, if these non-fatal injuries are not appropriately managed at the correct time, the patient may develop life-long impairment.[1]

A systematic approach is required in order to identify and treat the immediately and potentially life-threatening conditions before the limb-threatening ones, but without omitting to treat the latter. For the doctor and nurse in the resuscitation room, the first step is usually a call from ambulance control.

PRE-HOSPITAL COMMUNICATION

Warning from ambulance control or, ideally, direct from the crew enables essential information to be transmitted so that the receiving personnel can prepare for the patient's arrival. Without such a system, delays occur and key personnel may not be present when the patient arrives. The essential information is best delivered based around the 'MIST' mnemonic (Table 4.1).

Table 4.1 Essential pre-hospital information

Mechanism of injury
Injuries suspected or known
Signs as recorded
Treatment provided, and its effect
Number, age and sex of the casualties
Estimated time of arrival

The mechanism of the injury provides valuable information about the forces the patient may have been subjected to; similarly, the direction of impact can help the receiving team predict certain injury patterns. Further help can be gained from a description of the damage to the car or the weapon used. In a road traffic collision (RTC), a frontal impact can result in damage to the head, face, airway, neck, mediastinum, liver, spleen, knee, shaft of femur and hips; ejection from a vehicle is another predictor of serious injury, with the victim having a 300% greater chance of sustaining a serious injury than one who remained in the car. Fatalities at the scene following an RTC raise concerns as they imply an increased level of energy transfer and increase the likelihood of serious or life-threatening injuries in those who reach hospital alive. Once this information has been received, the trauma team should be summoned to the resuscitation room – the criteria for trauma team activation are outlined in Chapter 3.

THE TRAUMA TEAM

The exact make-up of this team varies between hospitals, depending upon resources and the time of the day.

Nevertheless, it is recognized that resuscitation is carried out more effectively if the team has certain key features (Table 4.2).

Each member of the team needs to be immunized against hepatitis, and must be wearing protective clothing. Universal precautions should be taken because all blood and body fluids must be assumed to carry human immunodeficiency virus (HIV) and hepatitis viruses.[7] While putting on their protective clothing, team members should be given the pre-hospital information and told their specific tasks during the resuscitation (Table 4.3). These duties are best carried out simultaneously (in parallel) under the direction of a team leader: in this way, any life-threatening conditions can be treated in the shortest possible time.[2,3] It is recognized, however, that the

Table 4.2 Essential features of a trauma team[2-6]

Medical personnel trained in trauma management*
Each person has specific assigned tasks
There is a senior team leader

*For example, Advanced Trauma Life Support® certification.

Table 4.3 Tasks of the trauma team

Role 1: Leader
Coordinates the specific tasks of the individual team members
Questions the ambulance personnel
Assimilates the clinical findings
Determines the investigations in order of priority
Liaises with specialists who have been called
Carries out particular procedures if they cannot be delegated
    to other team members

Role 2: Airway management
Clears and secures the airway while taking appropriate
    cervical spine precautions
Establishes a rapport with the patient giving psychological
    support throughout his/her ordeal in the resuscitation
    room

Role 3: Circulation management
Establishes peripheral intravenous infusions and takes blood
    for investigations
Brings extra equipment as necessary
Carries out other procedures depending on skills level (e.g.
    catheterizations)
Connects the patient to the monitors and records the vital
    signs
Records intravenous and drug infusion

Role 4: Communications
Cares for the patient's relatives when they arrive
Liaises with the trauma team to provide the relatives with
    appropriate information and support
Calls specialists on instructions from team leader

team may (at least initially) consist of only a single doctor and nurse. In such situations the key tasks must be sequentially performed until further help arrives.

RECEIVING THE PATIENT

In most units in the UK the ambulance bay is close to the resuscitation room and the patient can be rapidly transferred by the paramedic personnel. However, when the distance is great, or an airway problem has been identified, a doctor should rapidly assess the patient in the ambulance to see if immediate intervention is required.

If the patient arrives in the resuscitation room on a long spine board, transfer to a hospital trolley will be straightforward, although the board will still need to be removed at the earliest suitable moment, which is usually during the log-roll. When this is not the case, five people will be required to effect a safe transfer; this can usually be achieved by a combination of paramedic and departmental staff. This must be a well-practised procedure to ensure that the spinal cord is protected. During this transfer the patient's head and neck need to be stabilized by one member of the team while three others lift from the side. This allows the fifth member to replace the ambulance trolley cot with a resuscitation trolley. While this is on-going the paramedics should relay their pre-hospital findings using the MIST mnemonic again. The team can now carry out the primary survey and resuscitation of the patient under the direction of the team leader.

In the UK, relatives and friends often arrive at the same time as the patient. It is best that these people are met by a nurse who is not involved in the resuscitation. Then, depending upon their wishes, the relatives can be accompanied to the resuscitation room or to a private room which has all necessary facilities. The decision to admit relatives to the resuscitation room will depend on local policy. If relatives are not admitted to the resuscitation room, information can be passed to them from the resuscitation room on a regular basis, while at the same time information can be sought about the patient's past medical history and current medication.

PRIMARY SURVEY AND RESUSCITATION

The objectives of this phase are to identify and correct any immediately life-threatening conditions. To do this, the activities listed in Table 4.4 need to be carried out. The activities should be performed in parallel if there are enough personnel, but if this is not the case the tasks should be carried out sequentially.

It is essential that problems are anticipated, rather than reacted to once they develop.

Table 4.4 The primary survey and resuscitation

<C>	Control of exsanguinating haemorrhage
A	Airway and cervical spine control
B	Breathing with high-flow oxygen
C	Circulation with haemorrhage control
D	Disability with prevention of secondary injury
E	Exposure with temperature control

Control of exsanguinating haemorrhage

The first component of the primary survey is control of life-threatening external haemorrhage, <C>. This can be achieved by a variety of methods, of which direct pressure and elevation are the simplest. In the majority of cases, direct pressure over a bleeding wound or elevation of a bleeding limb will be all that is required. Occasionally, other interventions will be necessary, including the application of a tourniquet or the use of topical haemostatic agents. The control of exsanguinating haemorrhage is covered in detail in Chapter 5. In the majority of cases, at least temporary control of major external bleeding will have been achieved by the time the patient arrives in the accident and emergency department resuscitation room. If this has not been achieved before arrival in hospital, it should be immediately attended to when the patient arrives in the resuscitation room. It must be remembered, however, that this <C> component of the primary survey is concerned *only with life-threatening external haemorrhage.* The techniques of tourniquet application and use of topical haemostatic agents are as relevant in hospital as out, although they are likely to be used somewhat less frequently in the latter case.

Attempting to clamp vessels in the resuscitation room wastes time and may lead to further tissue damage. This applies particularly in cases of life-threatening haemorrhage – associated hypothermia, acidosis and coagulopathy in these cases will enhance blood loss by preventing haemostatic control other than by direct pressure. It is therefore essential that these patients are identified early so that their appropriate management can be discussed by the surgeons, intensivists and emergency medical personnel. If the decision is taken to use a tourniquet, it is important to note the time that the tourniquet was applied so that neighbouring soft tissue is not jeopardized.

Airway and cervical spine control

A cervical spinal injury should be assumed if the patient has been the victim of significant blunt trauma or if the mechanism of injury indicates that this region may have been damaged, such as the presence of an obvious injury above the clavicles. Consequently, none of the activities described to clear and secure the airway must involve movement of the neck.

One member of the team needs to manually immobilize the cervical spine while talking to the patient. This not only establishes supportive contact, but also assesses the airway. If the patient replies in a normal voice, giving a logical answer, then the airway can be assumed to be patent and the brain adequately perfused. When there is an impaired or absent reply, the airway could be obstructed; in these cases the procedures described in Chapter 6 need to be carried out in order to clear and secure the airway.

The combination of alcohol ingestion and injuries to the chest and abdomen increases the chance of the patient vomiting. Consequently, constant supervision is required since it is impracticable to nurse the trauma victim in any position other than supine. If vomiting does start, no attempt should be made to turn the patient's head to one side unless a cervical spine injury has been ruled out. If a spinal board is in place the whole patient can be turned; however, in the absence of this equipment, the trolley should be tipped head down by 20° and the vomit sucked away as it appears in the mouth.

High-flow oxygen needs to be provided once the airway has been cleared and secured. When the breathing is adequate, the oxygen should be provided at a rate of 15 L/min via a mask with a reservoir bag attached. With a well fitting mask an inspired oxygen concentration of approximately 85% can be achieved. A pulse oximeter should then be attached to the patient. In cases where the SaO_2 cannot be maintained, ventilatory support must be provided mechanically.

The neck should then be inspected for five features which could indicate the presence of an immediately life-threatening thoracic condition (Table 4.5).

When these signs have been excluded, the neck can be immobilized with an appropriately sized semirigid collar and a commercial head block and straps or sandbags and tape. The only exceptions are as follows:

- The restless patient who will not keep still. Since it is possible to damage the neck if the head is immobilized while the body moves, the compromise of using a semirigid collar on its own is accepted.
- The patient with evidence of a significant head injury. The patient should be immobilized with head blocks and tape but *without* a collar. Use of a collar in these circumstances may lead to a significant rise in intracranial pressure.

Table 4.5 Signs in the neck indicating possible life-threatening thoracic conditions

Sign	Condition
Swellings and wounds	Vascular and airway injury
Distended neck veins	Cardiac tamponade, tension pneumothorax
Tracheal deviation	Tension pneumothorax
Subcutaneous emphysema	Pneumomediastinum
Laryngeal crepitus	Laryngeal cartilage fracture

Breathing

When assessing the trauma victim's chest in the primary survey, six immediately life-threatening thoracic conditions must be sought (Table 4.6).

Table 4.6 Immediately life-threatening thoracic conditions

Airway obstruction
Tension pneumothorax
Open chest wound
Massive haemothorax
Flail chest
Cardiac tamponade

Since these conditions require immediate treatment, the examination must be selective but efficient. The examination of the chest begins by inspection to see if there are any marks or wounds. The respiratory rate, effort and symmetry of breathing are then assessed. Percussion and auscultation in the axillae should then be carried out to assess ventilation: listening over the anterior chest mainly detects air movement in the large airways, which can drown out sounds of pulmonary ventilation. Consequently, differences between the two sides of the chest can be missed, especially if the patient is being artificially ventilated.

> The respiratory rate and effort are very sensitive indicators of underlying lung pathology. They should therefore be monitored and recorded at frequent intervals.

If there is no air entry to either side then there is either a complete obstruction of the upper airway or an incomplete seal between the face and mask. The airway and ventilation technique should therefore be checked and treated appropriately. A local thoracic problem is more likely if there is asymmetry in air entry and percussion note. The immediately life-threatening conditions capable of producing this are a tension pneumothorax, an open chest wound and massive haemothorax. The diagnosis and management of each are discussed in detail in the chapter on thoracic injuries.

Examination of the back of the chest requires the patient to be turned on to his or her side. Normally this is carried out at the end of the primary survey (see below), but it can be useful to turn the patient at this stage in order to exclude a posterior chest injury if there are clinical suspicions.

Circulation

The key objectives regarding circulatory care are to stop haemorrhage, assess for hypovolaemia, obtain vascular access and provide appropriate fluid resuscitation.

HAEMORRHAGE CONTROL

Life-threatening external bleeding should have been controlled in the <C> section of the primary survey. Where there is less significant external haemorrhage, direct pressure is the preferred way of managing it.

Long bones should be splinted and circumferential splintage applied where appropriate in cases of pelvic fractures. External pelvic fixation used appropriately can be a life-saving manoeuvre as it can stop exsanguination, but it is a surgical procedure and should normally be performed in an operating theatre. In addition, it is of use only in particular types of pelvic fracture. Consequently, orthopaedic assessment of the patient and his or her radiographs is essential. In the meantime, pelvic splintage can be used to help reduce pelvic bleeding. Simply tying a sheet around the pelvis is effective but this technique should have been largely superseded by the use of a commercially available pelvic splint.

A brief assessment of the abdomen in an attempt to localize bleeding should be carried out as part of C. A precise pathological diagnosis will rarely be possible, but the presence of distension, pain, tenderness and guarding will be suggestive of pathology. Changes in bowel sounds are unlikely to be of assistance in the acute trauma situation.

Assessment for hypovolaemia

Once overt haemorrhage has been controlled, signs of hypovolaemia need to be sought. As with the thoracic examination, this is best done in a systematic fashion. The skin should be observed for colour, clamminess and capillary refill time (CRT). The CRT should be assessed centrally, and is measured by pressing firmly with a finger or thumb for 5 seconds: normal colour should return within 2 seconds. The heart rate, blood pressure and pulse pressure are then measured, and the consciousness level assessed. An automatic blood pressure recorder and ECG monitor should also be connected to the patient at this time so that these vital signs can be recorded frequently.

It is important to be aware that patients have an altered cardiovascular response to haemorrhage after significant skeletal trauma.[8-10] The blood pressure and heart rate tend to be maintained even with significant blood loss, but this is at a cost of increased tissue oxygen debt and higher incidences of multiple organ failure. Isolated vital signs are therefore unreliable in estimating the blood loss or the physiological impairment of the patient, especially at the extremes of age.[10,11] Consequently, when assessing blood loss in the early stages of the resuscitation, the functions of several essential organs need to be taken into account. In this way, reliance is not simply placed on a single vital sign such as blood pressure. Later on, depending upon the clinical situation, these clinical assessments can be augmented by recordings from invasive monitoring devices.

By this time, the presence of significant amounts of blood in the thorax should have been suspected, established or excluded during the airway and breathing phases of the evaluation. Examination of the abdomen and pelvis, including a single attempt at pelvic compression, may give other clues as to the source of haemorrhage. The common sites of occult bleeding are:

- the chest;
- the abdomen and retroperitoneum;
- the pelvis;
- long-bone fractures; and
- externally into splints and dressings.

VASCULAR CANNULATION

Trauma victims require large-bore intravenous access in areas which ideally are not distal to vascular or bony injury. Once cannulation has been obtained, 20 mL of blood should be taken to allow for grouping and cross-match, analysis of the plasma electrolytes and a full blood count. A rapid blood glucose measure (e.g. BM Stix®) should also be taken. If peripheral intravascular access is not possible, then a femoral line should be inserted. Venous cut-down is technically difficult and should be viewed as a last resort. Intraosseous access is an effective alternative in children and increasingly so in adults, using specifically designed intraosseous cannulation devices such as BIG® and EZ IO® (Chapter 8).

> If the patient's name is not known, some system of identification is required, so that drugs and blood can be administered safely.

FLUID RESUSCITATION

The rate of fluid infusion needs to take into account the mechanism of injury. Evidence for this approach comes from both clinical and animal studies[12–15] that have shown an increase in survival by limiting fluid resuscitation until the time of surgery in cases of unrepaired vascular injury following penetrating trauma. In contrast, infusing fluids to achieve a normal blood pressure increases blood loss. The precise reasons for this are not fully established, but it is probably due to a combination of impaired thrombus formation and inhibition of the body's physiological compensatory response to blood loss and physical dislodgment of the clot as the blood pressure increases. It follows that patients who are shocked as a consequence of uncontrollable torso haemorrhage need surgery rather than aggressive fluid resuscitation.

As described previously, the altered cardiovascular response to haemorrhage following tissue injury means that a significant haemorrhage may have occurred by the time the blood pressure falls. Therefore, once any overt bleeding has been stemmed, enough warm crystalloid should be infused to maintain a radial pulse rather than aiming for a target blood pressure. Depending on the patient's response, warmed blood may also be needed. Further clinical assessment and more sophisticated monitoring will then be needed to ensure that there is adequate tissue perfusion (see Chapter 8).

Disability

In the primary survey and resuscitation phase, the AVPU (alert, voice, pain, unresponsive) score, posture, and pupillary response need to be recorded. These tests represent a baseline for the more detailed neurological examination which is carried out in the secondary survey. It is essential that these assessments are monitored frequently to detect any deterioration. There are many possible causes of deterioration, but the most common in the trauma patient are hypoxia, hypovolaemia, hypoglycaemia – especially in the alcoholic and paediatric trauma victim – and raised intracranial pressure.

Exposure

The patient's remaining clothes should now be removed so that a full examination can be carried out. The presence of injuries, and the possibility of spinal instability, mean that garments must be cut along seams so that there is minimal patient movement. It is important to note that the rapid removal of tight trousers can precipitate sudden hypotension due to the loss of the tamponade effect in the hypovolaemic patient. These garments should be removed only when effective intravenous access has been established. At this point a brief head-to-toe assessment designed to identify any significant injuries should be performed.

> Once stripped, trauma victims must be kept warm and covered with blankets when not being examined.

It is important to be aware that trauma victims often have sharp objects such as broken glass and other debris in their clothing and hair and on their skin. Ordinary surgical gloves provide no protection against this, and the personnel undressing the patient must initially wear more robust gloves.

At this stage, a log-roll should be carried out after the substitution of manual for mechanical neck immobilization. This allows assessment of the spine from the base of the skull to the coccyx, the presence of posterior wounds to be noted and a rectal examination to be performed to assess sphincter tone, rectal wall integrity,

Table 4.7 Information from a rectal examination

Is sphincter tone present?
Has the rectal wall been breached?
Can spicules of bone be felt?
Is the prostate in a normal position?
Is there blood on the examiner's finger?

Table 4.8 Mental check at the end of the primary survey and resuscitation phase

Is the airway still secure?
Is the patient receiving high-flow oxygen?
Are all the tubes and lines secure?
Have the blood samples been sent to the laboratories?
Are all the monitors functioning?
Are the vital signs being recorded every 5 minutes?
Is an arterial blood gas sample needed?
Has the radiographer been called?

prostatic position, intraluminal blood and the presence of bony fragments from a pelvic fracture (Table 4.7).

When the primary survey has been completed, the team leader should carry out a quick mental check (Table 4.8) and consider whether the patient is getting better or worse as this can help to determine if urgent surgical intervention is required in those patients not responding to aggressive intravenous resuscitation.

> Only when all the ventilatory and hypovolaemic problems have been corrected can the team continue the more detailed secondary survey.

SECONDARY SURVEY

Once the immediately life-threatening conditions have been either excluded or treated, the whole of the patient should be assessed. This requires a head-to-toe, front-to-back assessment along with a detailed medical history and appropriate investigations. In this way, all injuries can be detected and appropriately prioritized. The common error of being distracted before the whole body has been inspected must be avoided, as potentially serious injuries can be missed – especially in the unconscious patient.

> If the patient deteriorates at any stage, airway, breathing and circulatory state must be immediately reassessed in the manner described in the primary survey.

Examination

THE SCALP

The entire scalp needs to be examined for lacerations, swellings or depressions. This requires the neck support to be removed (when required) and the head to be immobilized manually. The front and sides of the scalp can then be checked. The occipital region should already have been examined during the log-roll. Blind probing of wounds should be avoided, as further damage to underlying structures can result.

It is important to remember that in small children scalp lacerations can bleed sufficiently to cause hypovolaemia; consequently, haemostasis is crucial in these cases, and this is best achieved either by applying direct pressure or by using a self-retaining retractor.

Neurological state

An assessment of the Glasgow Coma Scale, the pupillary responses and the presence of any lateralizing signs should now be recorded. These constitute a 'mini-neurological' examination, which acts as a robust assessment of the patient's neurological state (see Chapter 9). These parameters should be measured frequently so that any deterioration can be detected early.

BASE OF SKULL

The skull base lies along a diagonal line running from the mastoid to the eye. Consequently, the signs of a fracture are also found along this line (Table 4.9).

Because Battle's sign and 'panda eyes' usually take 12–36 hours to appear, they are of limited use in the resuscitation room. A cerebrospinal fluid (CSF) leak may be missed as the CSF is invariably mixed with blood. Fortunately, the presence of CSF in this bloody discharge can be detected by noting the delay in clotting of the blood and the double-ring pattern when it is dropped onto an absorbent sheet. This should preclude auroscopy of the external auditory canal because of the risk of meningitis. As there is a small chance of a nasogastric tube passing into the cranium through a base of skull fracture, these tubes should be passed orally when this type of injury is suspected.

Table 4.9 Signs of a base of skull fracture

Bruising over the mastoid (Battle's sign)
Haemotympanum
Blood and CSF ottorrhoea
Blood and CSF rhinorrhoea
'Panda eyes' (bilateral periorbital bruising)
Scleral haemorrhage with no posterior margin
Subhyloid haemorrhage

CSF, cerebrospinal fluid.

EYES

Inspection of the eyes must be carried out before significant orbital swelling makes examination too difficult. It is important to check for haemorrhages, both inside and outside the globe, for foreign bodies under the lids (including contact lenses), and for the presence of penetrating injuries. If the patient is conscious, the visual acuity can be tested by asking him or her to read a name badge or fluid label. If the patient is unconscious, the pupillary response and corneal reflexes must be determined.

FACE

Most of the significant facial injuries can be detected by gentle, symmetrical palpation and inspection. The presence of lost or loose teeth should be established, as well as the stability of the maxilla, by gently pulling the latter forward to see if the middle third of the face is stable. Middle-third fractures can be associated with both an airway obstruction and base of skull fractures. However, only those injuries coexisting with an airway obstruction need to be treated immediately. Mandibular fractures can also cause airway obstruction because of the loss of stability of the tongue.

THE NECK

If this has not already occurred during the log-roll, the neck should be carefully examined. While in-line manual stabilization is being maintained, the neck should be inspected for any deformity, bruising and lacerations. The cervical spinous processes and neck muscles can then be palpated for tenderness or deformity. The conscious patient can assist in this examination by indicating the site of any pain or tenderness.

Lacerations should never be probed, since torrential haemorrhage can occur if there is an underlying vascular injury. If the wound penetrates the platysma, definitive radiological or surgical management will be needed, the choice depending upon the patient's stability.

THORAX

There are several potentially life-threatening (Table 4.10) and some minor thoracic conditions, such as fractures of the lower ribs, which need to be considered at this stage. The former usually require further investigations to confirm their presence and they should be undertaken only on significant clinical suspicion and after imminently life-threatening injuries have been treated or excluded as the investigations will normally necessitate transfer out of the resuscitation room. Information regarding the mechanism of injury, as well as a detailed examination, is therefore particularly important.

Acceleration and deceleration forces can produce extensive thoracic injuries, including aortic disruption as well as pulmonary and cardiac contusions. However, these often leave marks on the chest wall which should lead the team to consider particular types of injury. For example, the diagonal seat belt bruise may overlap a fractured clavicle, a thoracic aortic tear, pulmonary contusion or pancreatic laceration. The rate, effort and symmetry of breathing should be rechecked. The presence of crepitus, tenderness and subcutaneous emphysema must be noted when the sternum and ribs are palpated. Auscultation and percussion of the whole chest can then be carried out in order to check again if there is asymmetry between the right and left sides of the chest.

ABDOMEN

The key objective of the abdominal examination is to decide if a laparotomy is required and, if so, how urgently. This requires a thorough examination of the whole abdomen, including the pelvis and perineum. All bruising, abnormal movement and wounds must be noted, and any exposed bowel covered with warm saline soaked swabs. As with the scalp, wounds should not be probed blindly as further damage can result. Furthermore, the actual depth of the wound cannot be determined if underlying muscle is penetrated. Consequently, these patients will require further investigations (Chapter 13).

Following inspection, palpation should be carried out in a systematic manner so that areas of tenderness can be detected. Percussion is an ideal way of locating these sites without distressing the patient.

The rate of urine output is the most sensitive indicator of the state of tissue perfusion in the shocked patient, and should be measured in all trauma patients. If this requires catheterization, a transurethral approach should be used if there is no evidence of urethral injury (Table 4.11). Alternatively a suprapubic catheter may be necessary. The initial urine drained should be tested for blood and saved for microscopy and possible subsequent drug analysis.

Marked gastric distension is frequently found in crying children, adults with head or abdominal injuries, and

Table 4.10 Potentially life-threatening thoracic conditions

Pulmonary contusions
Cardiac contusion
Ruptured oesophagus
Disruption of the thoracic aorta
Diaphragmatic rupture
Rupture of the trachea or main bronchi

Table 4.11 Signs of urethral injury in a male patient

Bruising around the scrotum
Blood at the end of the urethral meatus
High-riding prostate

patients who have been ventilated with a bag-and-mask technique. The insertion of a naso- or orogastric tube facilitates the abdominal examination of these patients and reduces the risks of aspiration.

> An intra-abdominal bleed should be suspected if the patient is haemodynamically unstable for no apparent reason, especially if the lower six ribs are fractured or there are marks over the abdominal surface.

Abdominal examination is unreliable if there is a sensory defect due to neurological damage or drugs, or if there are fractures of the lower ribs or pelvis. In these cases further investigation will be required. The choice is dependent upon the resources available and the haemodynamic stability of the patient. Ultrasound and diagnostic peritoneal lavage can be done in the resuscitation room, but may not be diagnostic. Computed tomography (CT) provides greater information, particularly when contrast is used, and is the investigation of choice in the haemodynamically stable patient.

EXTREMITIES

The limbs are examined in the traditional manner of inspection, palpation and active and passive movement. This enables any bruising, wounds and deformities to be detected as well as crepitus, instability, neurovascular abnormalities, compartment syndrome or soft-tissue damage. Wounds associated with open fractures must be swabbed and covered with a non-adherent dressing. Gross limb deformities should also be corrected, and the pulses and sensation re-checked, before any radiographs are taken.

All limb fractures need splintage to reduce fracture movement and hence reduce pain, bleeding, the formation of fat emboli and secondary soft-tissue swelling and damage. In the case of shaft of femur fractures, a traction splint should be used.

Neurological assessment

A detailed neurological examination needs to be carried out at this stage to determine if there are any abnormalities in the peripheral and sympathetic nervous systems. Motor and sensory defects (and, in male patients, the presence of priapism) can help to indicate the level and extent of spinal injury.

SOFT-TISSUE INJURIES

The whole of the patient's skin must be examined to determine the number and extent of the soft-tissue injuries. Each wound needs to be inspected to determine its site, size and depth and the presence of any underlying structural damage. Once the clinical state of the patient stabilizes, superficial wounds can be cleaned, irrigated and dressed. Deeper wounds, and those involving vital structures, will require surgical repair.

THE BACK

Following the initial assessment of the back during the log-roll, this should be supplemented, if clinically indicated, by a more comprehensive assessment. The whole of the back, from occiput to heels, can then be checked and the back of the chest auscultated. The viability of the decubitus skin should be assessed.

Patients who cannot move due to neurological impairment, and also the elderly, have a high risk of developing pressure sores. Preventive steps must therefore be taken from the outset. The spinal board should be removed as soon as possible and the decubitus area moved every 30 minutes, using hip lifts for example.

Analgesia

Pain control is a fundamental aspect of the management of trauma patients. This is not only for humanitarian reasons, but also because pain can reduce the tolerance of the patient to hypovolaemia.[8,16] However, analgesia may mask important clinical signs and symptoms – systemic analgesia can hide a fall in consciousness level from a rise in intracranial pressure for example. Furthermore, in extremity injuries, systemic and regional analgesia can mask the symptoms of rising compartment pressure. Specialist teams involved in the patient's definitive care therefore need to know what analgesia has been given so that subtle early signs are not missed. It is also important to maintain careful monitoring of the patient's status once the analgesia has been administered.

Good communication, explanation and gentle handling are important preliminaries to pain relief. Correct immobilization of injured limbs can also be very effective. In addition, the team should be proficient in providing the other common types of analgesia such as Entonox, morphine and regional analgesia.[17]

Radiography

Around 95% of UK trauma victims will have been subjected to a blunt force. In all these patients, chest and pelvic radiographs should be taken in the resuscitation room. Radiographs of the cervical spine should be taken if clinically indicated. At the end of the secondary survey, further radiographs will be needed to help identify suspected skeletal and spinal abnormalities. The team leader needs to determine which investigations are required, and when. Radiographs of particular sites of

Table 4.12 An AMPLE history

A	Allergies
M	Medicines
P	Past medical history
L	Last meal
E	Events leading to the incident

injury can then be performed on stable patients along with other specialized investigations. The latter may involve transporting the patient to specialized areas where magnetic resonance imaging (MRI), CT or angiography can be carried out. This decision-making process can be helped greatly by discussing the case with the different specialists involved in the patient's care. Consideration should be given to early 'top-to-toe' CT scanning in the haemodynamically stable patient when spiral scans of head, neck, chest, abdomen and pelvis are performed. When this is appropriate, the number of plain films can be significantly reduced.

Medical history

There are five key pieces of information which need to be gathered on all trauma victims. Often, this AMPLE history (Table 4.12) is acquired piecemeal while the patient is resuscitated. Nevertheless, time should be spent as soon as possible to ensure that it is complete.

Details about the patient's past medical history are particularly important in the UK, where there is a high incidence of comorbidity.[18] The most common is cardiovascular disease, followed by psychiatric and respiratory problems. This information can be gained from the patient or his or her relatives, or by inspection of previous hospital records or communication with the patient's general practitioner.

> Pre-existing disease in trauma victims increases their chances of dying.

Assimilation of information

Because the condition of the patient can change quickly, repeated examinations and constant monitoring of vital signs is essential. This enables the following questions to be answered:

1. Is the patient's respiratory function satisfactory? If it is not adequate, then the cause must be sought and corrected as a priority.
2. Is the patient's circulatory status satisfactory? It is essential that the trauma team recognizes shock early in its genesis and intervenes promptly. It is equally important to evaluate the patient's response to the resuscitative measures.

   If less than 20% of the blood volume has been lost, the vital signs usually return to normal after infusion of less than 2 litres of fluid. If the signs then remain stable, the patient is probably not actively bleeding. However, care and constant supervision are needed in these cases because such trauma victims may deteriorate later.

   Transient responders are patients who are actively bleeding or in whom bleeding recommences during the resuscitation. Thus, their vital signs initially improve but then deteriorate. They have usually lost over 30% of their blood volume, and require an infusion of typed blood. Control of the bleeding source invariably requires an operation.

   Little or no response to fluid resuscitation by the shocked patient indicates either that the condition is not due to hypovolaemia or that the patient has lost over 40% of blood volume and is bleeding faster than the infusion rate. The history, mechanism of injury and the physical findings will help to determine which is the most likely. The former requires invasive techniques to monitor the pulmonary and central venous pressures. In the case of major haemorrhage, an operation and a blood transfusion are urgently required. The source of the bleeding is usually in the chest, abdomen or pelvis.
3. What are the extent and priorities of the injuries? The ABC system is used to categorize injuries so that the most dangerous is treated first. For example, problems with the airway must be corrected before those of the circulation.
4. Have any injuries been overlooked? The mechanism and pattern of injury must be considered in order to avoid overlooking sites of damage. Victims of blunt trauma have the injuring force dispersed over a wide area. As a result, trauma rarely 'skips' areas; thus, if an injury has been found in the thorax and femur, but not in the abdomen, then it has probably been missed. The patient must be re-examined.
5. Are tetanus toxoid, human antitetanus immunoglobulin or antibiotics required? These will depend on both local and national policies, which should be known by the team leader.

Documentation and property

Comprehensive medical and nursing notes are required so that the specialist looking after the patient is fully aware of what injuries have been identified and the treatment which has been provided. Many units have a purpose-designed single trauma sheet to help this process. If the patient is unconscious, his or her clothing and belongings should be searched. This may provide clues to the person's identity, as well as essential medical information.

Any possessions brought in with the patient must be logged and kept safe, along with the patient's clothing. This should be with permission if the patient is conscious. Rings and other constrictive jewellery must also be removed as the fingers may swell. If a criminal case is suspected, all clothing, possessions, loose debris, bullets and shrapnel are required for forensic examination. These must be collected in labelled bags and signed for before releasing them to the police.

Relatives

Communication with the relatives usually carries on during the resuscitation, either directly or by the designated 'relatives' nurse'. Nevertheless, once the secondary survey is completed it is useful for the team leader to appraise the relatives of the current findings and management plan. The relatives' nurse should be present at the discussion so that he or she is also aware of what has been said.

TRANSITION TO DEFINITIVE CARE

Once the patient has been adequately assessed and resuscitated, definitive care can start. In many cases this will require either operation(s) or intensive care management or, frequently, both. This requires the patient's injuries to be assigned their correct priority (Table 4.13).

Because around 95% of UK trauma patients are victims of a blunt force, many have sustained multiple injuries.[19] A further consideration therefore is the logistics of carrying out several procedures, and how well the patient can physiologically cope. It may be appropriate in certain cases of significant multiple injuries to use a staged operative procedure, with the patient returning to the intensive care unit between theatre sessions. This will enable the operations to be carried out when the patient's physiological state is optimal.

Finally, the team leader should consider whether there is any advantage in carrying out certain treatments in patients who need to transferred to another hospital for treatment of some of their injuries. For example, it would be essential that a haemodynamically unstable head-injured patient is not transferred to a neurosurgical centre

Table 4.13 Factors affecting the priority of an injury

Are the injuries immediately life-threatening?
Are the injuries potentially life-threatening?
Are the injuries limb-threatening?
What is the physiological state of the patient?
What resources are available in the hospital?
Will the patient require intra-hospital transfer for further specialist care?

until the source of the bleeding has been identified and treated.

> Optimum definitive care requires accurate information on the patient's injuries and physiological state, clinical experience, and a good liaison with all the specialists involved in the patient's care.

SUMMARY

Initial trauma care is best provided by a team of trained staff who are carrying out their tasks simultaneously under the direction of an experienced team leader. In this way, the immediately life-threatening conditions can be identified first and treated appropriately. Subsequently, a full history can be obtained while a detailed head-to-toe examination is carried out. The team leader can then list the patient's injuries, and determine the priorities for both further investigations and definitive treatment.

GLOBAL PERSPECTIVES

Regardless of the expertise or resources available where trauma patients are managed, this simple approach to the patient's assessment will ensure that optimal care can be delivered. In some countries, patterns of trauma differ significantly from those seen in the UK; however, all patients should still be assessed along the lines of the primary survey/secondary survey/transfer to definitive care as outlined in this chapter.

REFERENCES

1. Driscoll P, Monsell F, Duane L, Wardle T, Brown T. Optimal long bone fracture management. Part II. Initial resuscitation and assessment in the accident and emergency department. *Int J Orthop Trauma* 1995;**5**:110–17.
2. Driscoll P, Vincent C. Organising an efficient trauma team. *Injury* 1992; **3**:107–10.
3. Driscoll P, Vincent C. Variation in trauma resuscitation and its effect on patient outcome. *Injury* 1992; **23**:111–15.
4. Burdett-Smith P, Airey G, Franks A. Improvement in trauma survival in Leeds. *Injury* 1995;**26**:455–8.
5. Lecky F, Woodford M, Yates D. Trends in trauma care in England and Wales 1989–97. *Lancet* 2000;**355**:1771–5.

6.   Joint Working Party RCS England and British Orthopaedic Association. *Better Care for the Severely Injured*. London: Royal College of Surgeons (England), 2000.

7.   Walker J, Driscoll P. Trauma team protection from infective contamination. In: Driscoll P, Gwinnutt C, Jimmerson C, Goodall O, eds. *Trauma Resection: The Team Approach*. London: Palgrave Macmillan, 1993.

8.   Rady M, Little R, Edwards D, Kirkman E, Faithful S. The effect of nociceptive stimulation on the changes in haemodynamics and oxygen transport induced by haemorrhage in anaesthetised pigs. *J Trauma* 1991;**31**:617–21.

9.   Driscoll P. Changes in systolic blood pressure, heart rate, shock index, rate pressure product and tympanic temperature following blood loss and tissue damage in humans. Leeds University, MD Thesis, 1994.

10.   Little R, Kirkman E, Driscoll P, Hanson J, Mackway-Jones K. Preventable deaths after injury: why are the traditional 'vital' signs poor indicators of blood loss. *J Accid Emerg Med* 1995;**12**:1–14.

11.   Scalea T, Simon H, Duncan A, *et al*. Geriatric blunt multiple trauma: increased survival with early invasive monitoring. *J Trauma* 1990;**30**:129–34.

12.   Owens T, Watson W, Prough D, Kramer G. Limiting initial resuscitation of uncontrolled hemorrhage reduces internal bleeding and subsequent volume requirements. *J Trauma* 1995;**39**:200–9.

13.   Bickell W, Wail M, Pepe P, *et al*. A comparison of immediate versus delayed fluid resuscitation for hypotensive patients with penetrating torso injury. *N Engl J Med* 1994;**331**:1105–9.

14.   Kaweski S, Sise M, Virgillo R. The effect of prehospital fluids on survival in trauma patients. *J Trauma* 1990;**30**:1215–18.

15.   Krausz M, Bar-Ziv M, Rabinovich R, *et al*. 'Scoop and run' or stabilize hemorrhagic shock with normal saline or small-volume hypertonic saline? *J Trauma* 1992;**23**:6–10.

16.   Kirkman E, Little R. Cardiovascular regulation during hypovolaemic shock: central integration. In: Secher N, Pawelczyk J, Ludbrook L, eds. *The Bradycardic Phase in Hypovolaemic Shock*. London: Edward Arnold, 1994.

17.   Driscoll P, Gwinnutt C, Nancarrow J. Analgesia in the emergency department. *Pain Rev* 1995;**2**:187–202.

18.   Wardle T, Driscoll P, Oxbey C, Woodford M, Campbell F. Pre-existing medical conditions in trauma patients. *40th Annual Proceedings of the Association for the Advancement of Automotive Medicine* 1996:**40**:351–61.

19.   Anderson I, Woodford M, Irving M. Preventability of death from penetrating injury in England and Wales. *Injury* 1989;**20**:69–71.

Control of catastrophic haemorrhage

OBJECTIVES

After completing this chapter the reader will:
- understand the significance of catastrophic haemorrhage in trauma morbidity and mortality
- be aware of the potential methods available for the control of catastrophic haemorrhage
- be able to rapidly and effectively control external haemorrhage.

INTRODUCTION

An estimated 10% of all battlefield deaths are caused by haemorrhage from extremity wounds.[1] Analysis of data from the Vietnam War (from the Wound Data and Munitions Effectiveness Team database) found that bleeding from limb wounds accounted for more than half of *preventable* deaths in combat and that 7% of all combat deaths in Vietnam could have been prevented by using a limb tourniquet.[2] Contemporary experience from the Israeli Defence Force[3] and US and UK experience in Iraq[4] confirms the pivotal role of external haemorrhage control in managing ballistic casualties.

The realization that military casualties were still dying of exsanguinating haemorrhage led to the reassessment of the traditional vertical management priorities of ABC and has resulted in a new casualty treatment paradigm of <C>ABC, where <C> represents immediate control of catastrophic haemorrhage.[5] This has been possible only as a result of a huge increase in the range of equipment and techniques available to manage the trauma casualty. Although exsanguinating haemorrhage is less common in civilian trauma patients, it is undoubtedly important, and many of the techniques used on the battlefield can be applied equally well in such patients, in whom all too often insufficient attention is paid to the control of bleeding. If there is no exsanguinating injury, this phase of the primary survey can be rapidly passed without compromising or delaying care. For this reason the new <C>ABCDE paradigm is as appropriate off the battlefield as on it. The innovations that make effective haemorrhage control more achievable now than ever before include haemostatic dressings, a renaissance in the use of tourniquets and the use of intravascular haemostatic agents.

SITES OF HAEMORRHAGE

Haemorrhage is either external or internal. Internal bleeding is into the chest, abdomen and retroperitoneum, pelvis or thighs from femoral fracture. As a result, when searching for the sources of blood loss it is useful to remember *blood on the floor and four more*. The identification of internal bleeding forms part of the second C and is not a part of <C>.

<C> is concerned only with the identification and management of life-threatening external haemorrhage. If this is not present, <C> can be immediately completed and the next priority – A for 'airway with cervical spine control' – attended to. If catastrophic life-threatening external haemorrhage is present it *must* be controlled before the next stage of treatment can be started.

> Life-threatening external haemorrhage must be controlled before the airway is assessed.

CONTROLLING BLEEDING

A number of methods are available for the control of massive external bleeding. These are:

- direct pressure
- haemostatic dressings

- tourniquets
- positioning
- pressure points.

Which method is used will depend on the location of the bleeding and a combination may be required to achieve control.

Bleeding from limb injuries

It is essential to remember that low-pressure venous bleeding will kill a patient just as fast as an equivalent arterial bleed although it is less dramatic and its significance is more likely to be overlooked; however, no patient should die from limb haemorrhage. Limbs can be elevated to reduce the blood pressure within them. An injured limb should be splinted, and femoral fractures should have traction applied to reduce the internal potential space. Direct pressure and haemostatic dressings can easily be applied to the limbs and, if these measures are likely to be unsuccessful, a tourniquet should be used. A properly applied tourniquet will stop all venous and arterial bleeding. Medullary bleeding from exposed fractures may still continue if the tourniquet level is below the nutrient artery for the bone, but this is usually low pressure and can be stopped with dressings. Bleeding that occurs proximal to the level that a tourniquet can be effectively applied is known as *junctional bleeding* and generally refers to catastrophic bleeding from the groin, the axilla or the neck.

Junctional bleeding

These injuries are challenging to manage. Bleeding from the femoral, axillary and carotid vessels needs to be addressed quickly and aggressively. Direct pressure should be applied immediately to the region of the bleeding vessel while haemostatic dressings are made ready. A haemostatic dressing should be placed inside the wound cavity and pressure reapplied. This pressure may need to be continued until a surgeon can take control of the vessel. Bleeding from the neck requires similar management: where direct pressure fails to control the bleeding then haemostatic dressings must be used. An expanding haematoma in the neck will threaten the patient's airway so consideration of early tracheal intubation must be made during the 'A – airway with cervical spine control' phase of the primary survey.

Bleeding from penetrating wounds of the abdomen or chest

Lacerations to the torso may require direct pressure and the use of haemostatic dressings. True internal bleeding (*non-compressible haemorrhage*) requires urgent surgical assessment and intervention.

HAEMORRHAGE CONTROL TECHNIQUES

Direct pressure

This is the simplest and most immediate way of controlling bleeding. Disposable gloves and personal protective equipment must be worn and pressure applied with the flat of one or both hands, or with a tightly clenched fist, to the area of bleeding. Pressure can be applied through gauze swabs or dressings. The disadvantage of this technique is that it requires at least one practitioner and may need to be continued from the point of wounding all the way to the operating theatre. In addition, the pressure applied tends to reduce as the practitioner tires.

Haemostatic dressings

Traditional cotton gauze dressings simply soak up blood when applied to the point of bleeding although the cellulose fibres in these dressings are known to activate the extrinsic clotting cascade. A number of newer dressings are now available with active haemorrhage control properties.

CHITOSAN

Poly-*N*-acetyl glucosamine (P-NAG) is a naturally occurring, biodegradable, complex polysaccharide found in a variety of marine life and commercially obtained by fermentation or isolated from microalgal cultures. Highly acetylated P-NAG is referred to as chitin whilst the deacetylated form is known as chitosan. Two commercial haemostatic dressings are now available incorporating P-NAG. The HemCon® (HemCon Medical Technologies, Inc., Portland, OR, USA) bandage uses chitosan derived from the exoskeleton of the Arctic shrimp and the dressing is constructed from multiple thin layers of manufactured chitosan mesh. It is distributed as a firm sterile pad up to $10\,cm^2$ in a vacuum-sealed packet that is heat stable and without any particular storage requirements. After application to the bleeding point the chitosan dressing becomes sticky and adherent and is believed to accelerate clotting by ionic attraction of erythrocytes and activation of the clotting cascade, suggesting a mechanism of action potentially unaffected by the consumptive and dilutional coagulopathies encountered in severe trauma.

Animal studies suggest that the HemCon chitosan dressing is effective at reducing haemorrhage and fluid resuscitation requirements, and increases survival.[6] A non-commercial P-NAG preparation was also found to be effective at stopping splenic bleeding in animals with congenital coagulopathies.[7] Field reports of HemCon from both military and civilian pre-hospital environments support its use as an effective haemostat when traditional dressings and pressure fail and tourniquets are impractical.[8,9] The Rapid Deployment Hemostat (RDH™) contains algae-derived chitin and appears to be less effective.[10]

Use of HemCon®

The dressing is removed from the foil packaging. HemCon dressings have two sides: a cream-coloured active side, which goes on the wound, and a darker non-stick side which is helpfully labelled 'THIS SIDE UP'. The bandages will not work with the wrong side down. It is important to apply the dressing directly to the bleeding vessel. The dressing becomes sticky and adherent and slightly malleable. The dressing can be cut up for use with smaller wounds, or multiple dressings can be used for larger wounds. The dressing can be left in place for up to 48 hours and should then be removed with water or saline.

ZEOLITE

The mineral zeolite was originally found as a byproduct of volcanic activity and a range of synthetic zeolite compounds, containing oxides of silicon, aluminium, sodium, and magnesium and small amounts of quartz, are now manufactured for diverse uses in the chemical industry. In its granular form zeolite acts as a molecular sieve and adsorbs water by a hugely exothermic physical process, the extent of which depends upon the ratio of zeolite to water, which may be expressed as the residual moisture (RM) content of the zeolite. The adsorption of water concentrates the platelets and clotting factors around a bleeding wound and promotes rapid clot formation.[11] In an animal model of lethal vascular groin injury specifically designed to recreate a complex junctional injury inaccessible to tourniquet or standard compressive dressings, QuikClot™ (with 1% RM) significantly decreased mortality.[12,13] As the compound in its original formulation is granular, there may be problems with its application as it spills, and the vigorous exothermic reaction in a wound can result in temperatures as high as 50°C above baseline with the possibility of tissue burns.[14] The manufacturers have responded by developing the QuikClot Cool Advanced Clotting Sponge (ACS+™), in which standard zeolite is packaged in porous bags which are easier to apply but which maintain haemostatic efficacy. Experimental mortality is reduced.[15]

Use of QuikClot™

A two-person technique for QuikClot application is recommended. The first operator applies pressure to the wound, whilst the second dries the skin around the wound and opens the QuikClot sachet. The pressure is then removed, the granules poured into the wound by person number two and pressure immediately reapplied to the wound with clean gauze dressings.[16] Any granules that are spilt away from the wound should be cleared up in order to reduce the chances of causing burns to the patient. For this reason QuikClot should not be used on exposed viscera or poured blindly into the abdomen or thorax.

POLYSACCHARIDES

The starch-based haemostatic agent TraumaDEX™ consists of microporous polysaccharide particles made from potato starch which are poured directly into a bleeding wound. The particles are sterile and have a long shelf-life. Like zeolite, the particles exert their haemostatic effect by absorbing water from the blood and plasma, resulting in accumulation and concentration of clotting factors and platelets. In small animal studies, TraumaDEX™ performed well in achieving haemostasis for minor bleeding wounds. However, TraumaDEX™ did not perform well in animal studies involving significant haemorrhage or large arterial bleeding and in some models did not result in any improvement in survival compared with simple compression.[17] Polysaccharide dressings are *not* currently recommended for the control of significant external bleeding.

FIBRIN

Fibrin or fibrin precursors have been recognized as an adjunct to haemostasis for almost a century.[18] Dried fibrin on a gauze dressing has been demonstrated to produce successful haemostasis,[19-21] but widespread use may be deterred by the chances of causing anaphylaxis and the cost of approximately £500 per dressing. It is unlikely that fibrin-based dressings will be in everyday use in the immediate future and their use is not currently recommended.

THE 'IDEAL' DRESSING

The ideal haemostatic dressing has yet to be developed. It should be effective even in large arterial bleeds, easy to use and with minimal side-effects. A long shelf-life and cost-effectiveness are also desirable features. As evidence accrues about these different haemostatics, and experience with the individual products in the field increases, it is clear that there is, in fact, currently no ideal haemostatic dressing and that different products are indicated for different wounds and clinical situations.[22] This demands the development of new guidelines and algorithms.

Tourniquets

The use of a tourniquet to control limb bleeding is not new, having its origins in early eighteenth-century France, but for many years tourniquets have been anathema to trauma surgeons due to the presumed risk of distal limb ischaemia. Other potential complications include compression neuropraxia and reperfusion injury, and a tourniquet applied sufficiently tightly to occlude arterial haemorrhage is often difficult to achieve and painful for the patient. Undoubtedly the inappropriate use of a tourniquet can cause unnecessary harm to the patient, but in a modern trauma system that identifies immediate control of catastrophic haemorrhage as a priority they do have a role to play.[23–25]

Tourniquets improvised from belts, rope or clothing, even when tightened with an improvised windlass, are less effective than commercially produced tourniquets and increase the risk of a limb compartment syndrome by occluding venous return without completely occluding arterial inflow. A wide range of commercial devices are now available with varying degrees of efficacy and ease of self-application.[26] Most can be applied single-handedly and incorporate a windlass to allow complete cessation of distal arterial flow; the British Army has introduced the Combat Application Tourniquet (CAT™).

TOURNIQUET APPLICATION

A tourniquet is used to arrest major limb haemorrhage where direct pressure has been *or is likely to be* ineffective. It is placed as distally as possible, leaving a few centimetres to the wound edge to prevent slippage. Prolonged tourniquet use may necessitate amputation at the level of the tourniquet to prevent life-threatening reperfusion injury, and it is for this reason that the tourniquet is placed as distally as possible. The tourniquet is then tightened *until bleeding stops*, although it is essential to be aware that there may be continued medullary ooze from fracture sites. The tourniquet may need further tightening since the limb volume will decrease as blood drains out of it. As a result, it may be necessary to tighten the tourniquet further after about 15 minutes. Analgesia will be required in the conscious casualty to tolerate the application of a tourniquet, and the time of application must be prominently recorded.

TOURNIQUET TIMES

When a patient is under threat from severe limb haemorrhage, there should be a low threshold for applying a tourniquet. If the patient is then removed from immediate threat (for example extracted from a car wreck) then the requirement for the tourniquet can be re-evaluated as splints and dressings may be enough to control the bleeding. In addition, if transfer to hospital is significantly delayed then the tourniquet can be re-evaluated after 1 hour. The tourniquet should be loosened and the limb observed closely for bleeding. If bleeding recurs, then the tourniquet must be retightened. This is *not* a method for reperfusing the limb as vascular repair and subsequent reperfusion is a job for the trauma surgeon and the anaesthetist. Despite regular use of arterial tourniquets in orthopaedic practice, no clear consensus exists on the upper limit for limb ischaemia times. Applying a tourniquet does not mandate amputation; it does, however, mandate rapid evacuation to a surgeon.

> Always record the time of application of a tourniquet.

Positioning, splinting and traction

Patient and limb positioning is often overlooked. Where possible, the patient should be nursed prone in order to keep the physiological demands on the patient as low as possible. A bleeding limb should be elevated above the level of the heart in order to reduce the systolic pressure within the limb. Elevation may, however, be difficult or contraindicated in long-bone fractures and is certainly contraindicated in leg injuries when there is significant suspicion of an unstable pelvic fracture. There should always be a low threshold for applying splints to injured limbs. Splints will reduce bleeding, allow clot formation and will reduce the analgesic requirements for the patient. If an unstable pelvic fracture is suspected, then it must be splinted (for example, using the SAM Pelvic Sling®), and if a femoral fracture is suspected then some form of traction must be applied to reduce the potential space within the thigh compartment.

Pressure points

If direct pressure, elevation and haemostatic dressings are ineffective, pressure points should be utilized. Pressure points can be found at the brachial artery (midway down the humerus), radial artery (at the thumb side of the posterior wrist), femoral artery (at the groin) and popliteal artery (on the posterior side of the knee joint). Essentially, pressure points are places where an artery runs over a bone and where the artery can be compressed against the bone in order to halt blood flow. The fingertips can be used against the radial or brachial arteries but the fist or even elbow may be needed to apply enough pressure to the femoral artery to stop blood flow.

A SEQUENCE OF HAEMORRHAGE CONTROL TECHNIQUES

The control of exsanguinating external haemorrhage should always follow a logical sequence (Figure 5.1). If each step in this sequence is followed then external haemorrhage *will* be brought under control.

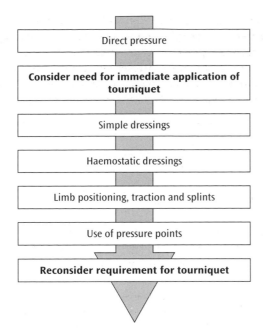

Figure 5.1 Sequence of haemorrhage control techniques.

SUMMARY

As both military and civilian experience with novel haemostatic techniques increases, so new procedures will evolve and new products will appear on the market. Every treatment requires clinical evaluation to determine its efficacy and safety, and it is the immediate care practitioner's responsibility to stay abreast of developments. The products and procedures described above have seen use in the field and when used correctly have made significant improvements in patient outcomes. Practitioners should have the ability to identify a catastrophic haemorrhage and the confidence to treat it first and to treat it aggressively. Inaction in the face of bleeding is inexcusable and, when the equipment is available, then no patient should die from external haemorrhage.

REFERENCES

1.   Champion HR, Bellamy RF, Roberts P, et al. A profile of combat injury. J Trauma 2003;**54**:S13–19.

2.   Bellamy RF. Combat trauma overview. In: Zajtchuk R, Grande CM, eds. Textbook of Military Medicine. Part IV. Surgical Combat Casualty Care: Anaesthesia and Peri-operative Care of the Combat Casualty. Falls Church, VA: Office of the Surgeon General, US Army, 2005.

3.   Lakstein DL, Blumenfeld A, Sokolov T, et al. Tourniquets for hemorrhage control on the battlefield: a 4 year accumulated experience. J Trauma 2003;**54**:S221–5.

4.   Hodgetts TJ, Mahoney PF, eds. Operational Surgical Services Review. Birmingham: Royal Centre for Defence Medicine, 2005.

5.   Hodgetts TJ, Mahoney PF, Russell MQ, Byers M. ABC to <C>ABC: redefining the military trauma paradigm. Emerg Med J 2006;**23**:745–6.

6.   Pusateri AE, McCarthy SJ, Gregory KW, et al. Effect of a chitosan-based hemostatic dressing on blood loss and survival in a model of severe venous hemorrhage and hepatic injury in swine. J Trauma 2003;**54**:177–82.

7.   Schrwaitzberg SD, Chan MW, Cole DJ, et al. Comparison of poly-N-acetyl glucosamine with commercially available topical hemostats for achieving hemostasis in coagulopathic models of splenic hemorrhage. J Trauma 2004;**57**(Suppl. 1):S29–32.

8.   Wedmore I, McManus JG, Pusateri AE, Holcomb JB. A special report on the chitosan-based hemostatic dressing: experience in current combat operations. J Trauma 2006;**60**:655–8.

9.   Brown MA, Daya MR, Worley JA. Experience with chitosan dressings in a civilian EMS system. J Emerg Med 2007 Nov 14; (ePub)18024069.

10.   Pusateri AE, Modrow HE, Harris RA, et al. Advanced hemostatic dressing development program: animal model selection criteria and results of a study of nine hemostatic dressings in a model of severe large venous and hepatic injury in swine. J Trauma 2003;**55**:518–26.

11.   Galownia J, Martin J, Davis M. Aluminophosphate-based, microporous materials for blood clotting. Microporous Mesoporous Mater 2006;**92**:61–3.

12.   Alam HB, Uy GB, Miller D, et al. Comparative analysis of hemostatic agents in a swine model of lethal groin injury. J Trauma 2003;**54**:1077–82.

13.   Alam HB, Chen Z, Jaskille A, et al. Application of a zeolite hemostatic agent achieves 100% survival in a lethal model of complex groin injury in swine. J Trauma 2004;**56**:974–83.

14.   Garner JP, Brown RFR. Recent advances in topical agents for prehospital haemostasis. Trauma 2002;**4**:203–9.

15.   Arnaud F, Tomori T, Saito R, McKeague A, Prusaczyk WK, McCarron RM. Comparative efficacy of granular and bagged formulations of the hemostatic agent QuikClot. J Trauma 2007;**63**:775–82.

16.   Moorhouse I, Thurgood A, Walker N, Cooper B, Mahoney PF, Hodgetts TJ. A realistic model for catastrophic external haemorrhage control. J R Army Med Corps 2007;**153**:99–101.

17.   Bjorses K, Holst J. Various local hemostatic agents with different modes of action; an in vivo comparative randomized vascular surgical experimental study. Eur J Vasc Endovasc Surg 2007;**33**:363–70.

18.   Cushing H. The control of bleeding in operations for brain tumours. Ann Surg 1911;**54**:1.

19.   Holcomb JB, Pusateri AE, Harris RA, et al. Effect of dry fibrin sealant dressings versus gauze packing on blood loss in grade V liver injuries in resuscitated swine. J Trauma 1999;**46**:49–57.

20.   Holcomb JB, Pusateri AE, Harris RA, et al. Dry fibrin sealant dressings reduce blood loss, resuscitation volume, and improve survival in hypothermic coagulopathic swine with grade V liver injuries. J Trauma 1999;**47**:233–42.

21. Morey AF, Anema JG, Harris R, *et al*. Treatment of grade 4 renal stab wounds with absorbable fibrin adhesive bandage in a porcine model. *J Urol* 2001;**165**:995-8.

22. Pusateri AE, Holcomb JB, Kheirabadi BS, Alam HB, Wade CE, Ryan KL. Making sense of the preclinical literature on advanced hemostatic products. *J Trauma* 2006;**60**:674–82.

23. Navein J, Coupland R, Dunn R. The tourniquet controversy. *J Trauma* 2003;**54**(5 Suppl.):S219–20.

24. Lakstein D, Blumenfeld A, Sokolov T, *et al*. Tourniquets for hemorrhage control on the battlefield: a 4-year accumulated experience. *J Trauma* 2003;**54**(5 Suppl.):S221–5.

25. Lee C, Porter KM, Hodgetts TJ. Tourniquet use in the civilian prehospital setting. *Emerg Med J* 2007;**24**:584–7.

26. Calkins D, Snow C, Costello M, Bentley TB. Evaluation of possible battlefield tourniquet systems for the far-forward setting. *Mil Med* 2000;**165**:379–84.

Airway management

After completing this chapter the reader will:
* understand the importance of airway maintenance, ventilation and oxygenation in the trauma patient
* recognize airway obstruction
* understand the principles of basic and advanced airway management techniques
* recognize the importance of simultaneous cervical spine control.

INTRODUCTION

The airway and breathing are the first priorities in trauma resuscitation after control of catastrophic haemorrhage. Airway obstruction is common in trauma victims, and may lead to unnecessary deaths – often preventable by simple, basic measures.[1] Trauma patients die from tissue hypoxia as a result of poor oxygenation, inadequate circulation or both.

> The airway is the first priority in resuscitation in the absence of catastrophic haemorrhage.

In the 'ABC' of resuscitation, 'A' comes before 'B', and 'B' before 'C'! If a problem is found at any stage it must be corrected immediately, before moving on to the next step. An obstructed airway must be cleared immediately, or severe hypoxic brain damage and cardiac arrest will occur within minutes. Likewise, a clear airway does not guarantee adequate ventilation, and any further treatment is futile if hypoxia cannot be corrected. Therefore, the airway, breathing and oxygenation are assessed and managed first, and must not be overlooked even if there are more dramatic injuries. Rarely in civilian practice, but increasingly in military trauma, there is a need to attend to catastrophic exsanguinating haemorrhage first.[2]

Cervical spine injuries may be exacerbated by airway management manoeuvres, and in any trauma patient such interventions must proceed with concurrent cervical spine stabilization unless this significantly impairs the establishment of a protected patent airway.

> Airway and cervical spine control must occur simultaneously.

AIRWAY PROBLEMS IN TRAUMA

Airway problems in the trauma patient may be due to one of a number of causes.

Soft-tissue obstruction

In the unconscious patient, muscle tone in the neck and pharynx is lost, and the tongue 'falls back'. The airway also obstructs at other sites including the soft palate and epiglottis by this mechanism, particularly if the patient is generating negative pressure by respiratory efforts.[3]

Oedema, haematoma or other swelling

These may be due to trauma or burns of the head and neck. Airway burns in particular can cause rapid and severe oedema, which may be fatal without early intubation. Direct trauma to the larynx or trachea may also cause obstruction.[4]

Foreign bodies or foreign material

Teeth, dentures, pieces of tissue, blood clots, semisolid stomach contents or any other foreign matter may block the airway.

Displaced facial bones

A fractured maxilla may displace posteroinferiorly, obstructing the airway by pushing the soft palate against the back of the pharynx. Similarly, a 'flail segment' of jaw from a bilateral mandibular fracture allows the tongue to fall backwards.[5]

Suspected cervical spine injuries

Although cervical spine injuries themselves do not compromise the airway, immobilization makes airway management more difficult. Whilst every effort must be made to ensure that the cervical spine is immobilized, it is important to ensure that the establishment of a patent airway is not compromised by so doing.

Aspiration of gastric contents

Many patients sustain trauma 'on a full stomach', gastric emptying is delayed, and protective laryngeal reflexes may be obtunded in those who are not fully conscious. Regurgitation may lead to potentially fatal aspiration pneumonia.

OXYGEN

Hypoxia

Oxygen is essential for cellular metabolism, and therefore for organ function. In the presence of oxygen, cells metabolize biochemical fuels aerobically to generate energy and carbon dioxide. Under conditions of hypoxia, cells convert to anaerobic metabolism. This cannot be sustained. It is much less efficient in generating energy, and causes progressive metabolic acidosis due to lactic acid production – cells cease to function and eventually are permanently damaged: *lack of oxygen stops the machine and then wrecks the machinery.*[6]

Hypoxia means that there is not enough oxygen getting to the tissues. This can be due to too little oxygen being present in the inhaled air, airway obstruction, too little oxygen getting into the blood due to reduced ventilation, or too little oxygen being carried in the bloodstream (hypoxaemia). It also occurs when cells are unable to use the delivered oxygen, as in carbon monoxide and cyanide poisoning. Hypercarbia is an accumulation of carbon dioxide, has similar causes to hypoxaemia and is not discussed further.

As well as a clear airway, tissue oxygen supply depends on:

- Ventilation – the mechanical process by which air is drawn into the lungs.

- Diffusion – of oxygen across the alveolar–capillary membrane and of carbon dioxide in the reverse direction.
- Perfusion – the circulation carries oxygenated blood to the tissue capillary beds, from which oxygen and carbon dioxide pass into and out of cells.

Normal inspiration results from contraction of the diaphragm and the external intercostal muscles, although in respiratory difficulty the accessory scalene and sternomastoid muscles are also active. However, expiration is normally a passive process, resulting mainly from the elastic recoil of the lungs. During inspiration, muscle tone in the pharynx increases to counteract the negative airway pressure generated, and the vocal cords abduct.[7] This increased tone may be reduced or lost in the unconscious patient, contributing to inspiratory collapse of the pharyngeal walls and consequent airway obstruction.

Airway obstruction and hypoventilation lead to hypoxaemia and hypercarbia. Relief of airway obstruction may be followed by post-obstructive pulmonary oedema.[8]

CAUSES OF HYPOXAEMIA

The causes of hypoxaemia are given in Table 6.1.

A fall in cardiac output will lower mixed venous oxygen saturation, because the body continues to extract oxygen at the same rate from a slower circulation. If impaired alveolar–capillary diffusion is also present, hypoxaemia is

Table 6.1 Causes of hypoxaemia

Low partial pressure of inspired oxygen, e.g. during a fire in an
    enclosed space
Airway obstruction
Apnoea or hypoventilation
    Central nervous system depression (head injury or drugs)
    Spinal cord injury affecting the diaphragm or intercostal
      muscles
    Neuromuscular blocking agents
Mechanical interference with ventilation
    Flail chest
    Tension pneumothorax
    Haemothorax
    Morbid obesity
Impaired diffusion across alveolar–capillary membrane
    Pulmonary oedema
    Lung contusion
    Lung consolidation or collapse
    Aspiration of blood, fluid or vomit
Low cardiac output
    Hypovolaemia
    Myocardial contusion
    Cardiac tamponade
    Tension pneumothorax

exacerbated by systemic 'shunting' of this abnormally desaturated venous blood. This may occur when pulmonary contusions are present.

EFFECTS OF HYPOXAEMIA

Different organs have different sensitivities to hypoxaemia, the heart and brain being the most sensitive. The main effects of hypoxaemia are:

- *Metabolic:* anaerobic metabolism, metabolic acidosis, hyperkalaemia – although in practice hypokalaemia commonly occurs due to the hormonal 'stress response'.
- *Neurological:* cerebral vasodilatation and raised intracranial pressure leading to confusion, agitation, drowsiness, fits and coma.
- *Cardiovascular:* impaired contractility, dysrhythmias. Severe hypoxia leads to serious bradycardia and ultimately asystole.
- *Respiratory:* increased respiratory drive unless hypoxia is due to hypoventilation.
- *Renal:* impaired renal function, acute renal failure.
- *Gastrointestinal:* hypoxic liver dysfunction; increased gut mucosal permeability leading to a systemic inflammatory response.

EFFECTS OF HYPERCARBIA

The main effects of hypercarbia, or too much carbon dioxide in the bloodstream, are:

- *Metabolic:* respiratory acidosis, hyperkalaemia.
- *Neurological:* cerebral vasodilatation and raised intracranial pressure leading eventually to drowsiness and unconsciousness.
- *Cardiovascular:* sympathetic stimulation, causing hypertension, tachycardia and dysrhythmias.
- *Respiratory:* increased respiratory drive unless the hypercarbia is due to hypoventilation.

Oxygen administration

There are very few medical contraindications to high-percentage oxygen, and the risk of CO_2 retention in certain patients with chronic obstructive pulmonary disease (COPD) is often overstated.[9] Correction of hypoxia takes priority: if in any doubt, oxygen must be given and ventilation assisted if necessary.

In the spontaneously breathing patient, oxygen is given by a non-rebreathing reservoir mask (NRRM): this is the best mask for giving high concentrations of oxygen. At flow rates of 10–15 L/min it gives at least 85% oxygen. The standard Hudson-type mask is second best, but can be used if a NRRM is not available. Even high flow rates will give at best 60–70% oxygen. Nasal cannulae give relatively low and unpredictable concentrations of oxygen, and should not be used.

The self-inflating bag–valve–mask (BVM) device (Ambu-type bag) gives at least 85% oxygen, with flow rates of 10–15 L/min and a reservoir bag attached (although hyperventilation reduces the delivered percentage[10]). CO_2 rebreathing is eliminated by the one-way valve.

> In major trauma high-flow oxygen should be given to all patients and the non-rebreathing reservoir mask gives close to 100% oxygen.

ASSESSMENT OF THE AIRWAY AND BREATHING

A thorough and systematic assessment of the airway is essential in order to:

- Identify a compromised airway and breathing.
- Identify the potential for airway compromise. Deterioration may occur as a result of:
  - a decreasing level of consciousness, leading to soft-tissue obstruction
  - increasing oedema especially from burns
  - haematoma
  - accumulation of blood, secretions or regurgitated matter.
- Identify potential risks of airway management such as a cervical spine injury, laryngeal fracture or other airway trauma which may be worsened by intubation.

Airway assessment and management take place simultaneously, but assessment is described separately here for clarity. Continual reassessment is vital because of the risk of deterioration. If the patient deteriorates in any way, it is essential to return to the basic '<C>ABCDE' approach and to reassess the airway (<C> should, by this time, have been adequately controlled). For example, an increased respiratory rate may be due to an obstructing airway, progression of a pneumothorax or deteriorating hypovolaemic shock.

> Continual reassessment is vital.

The 15–second assessment

During this rapid first assessment, it is important to take a 'quick look' for obvious airway problems or respiratory distress. A patient who answers questions sensibly must have a clear airway, reasonable breathing and reasonable cerebral perfusion, as well as being grossly intact neurologically.

Detailed assessment

The detailed assessment of the airway can be divided into three phases: look, listen and feel.

LOOK AT

- The airway for: visible obstruction, oedema, haematoma, foreign body, trauma or burns.
- The neck and chest for: the rate, pattern and depth of breathing, use of accessory muscles, tracheal tug, tracheal deviation, abnormal movement or visible trauma.

LISTEN FOR

- Breath sounds at the mouth, snoring noises suggestive of soft-tissue obstruction, gurgling noises from blood, vomit or saliva in the airway and stridor – an inspiratory 'crowing' sound, signifying partial upper airway obstruction or laryngospasm and hoarseness from possible laryngeal obstruction or injury.

FEEL

- At the mouth for air movement.
- The neck and chest for signs of injury such as tenderness, crepitus and subcutaneous emphysema.

Upper airway obstruction leads to paradoxical see-sawing movement, whereby the chest moves out and the abdomen moves in on inspiration, and the opposite on expiration. The accessory muscles will be active, and tracheal tug may occur. In children, intercostal and subcostal recession are seen. Laryngeal injuries may not be obvious, but signs include swelling, voice change, laryngeal crepitus and subcutaneous emphysema.[4] Most of the above signs demonstrate airway obstruction only if the patient is breathing! If the patient is not breathing the only sign may be difficulty in achieving ventilation.

'Respiratory distress' may be due not only to an airway or breathing problem but also to:

- severe shock activating the respiratory centre;
- head injury causing tachypnoea, bradypnoea or irregular breathing;
- acidosis from hypovolaemia or sepsis.

BASIC AIRWAY MANAGEMENT

> High-flow oxygen should be administered to all trauma patients.

Cervical spine stabilization

If the patient is not already immobilized, the cervical spine should be stabilized immediately if there is any suspicion of spinal injury. It is important to err on the side of caution – immobilization may be removed later if no cervical spine injury is detected.

If the patient is conscious and has a clear airway, after initial manual stabilization, immobilization should be achieved with a semirigid cervical collar, spinal board, head blocks or sandbags, and forehead strapping. If the patient's consciousness level is reduced or the airway is compromised, manual in-line stabilization (MILS) should be performed until the airway is secured.

Basic airway techniques

Once the airway has been cleared of foreign bodies, blood or vomit, simple airway manoeuvres may be used. Both jaw thrust and chin lift relieve soft-tissue obstruction by pulling the tongue, anterior neck tissues and epiglottis forwards. The jaw thrust is preferable, as it can be performed by one person who can simultaneously stabilize the cervical spine. The same person can also modify his or her grip to hold a facemask in position if ventilation is needed. A chin lift requires a second person to stabilize the cervical spine, and prevents application of a tight-fitting facemask.

Oropharyngeal and nasopharyngeal airways are aids to, but not substitutes for, these methods. If using these airways, it is important not to be lulled into a false sense of security and to reassess the patient, and continue the jaw thrust if necessary.

> Without continued jaw thrust, an airway alone may not relieve obstruction.

CHIN LIFT

The chin is gripped between the thumb and forefinger of one or both hands with the thumb(s) anterior to the symphysis menti and pulled forwards (Figure 6.1). Methods of chin lift which involve placing the thumb in the patient's mouth are potentially dangerous, and should be abandoned except in the case of patients with bilateral mandibular fractures, in which case a gloved hand can be used to pull the anterior fragment forwards.

JAW THRUST

Method A

From above the patient's head, both hands are positioned, and the head is stabilized by pressure between the palms of both hands. The mouth is then opened with both thumbs

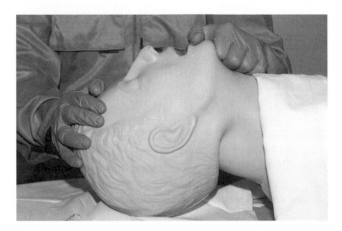

Figure 6.1 The technique for a chin lift.

anterior to the symphysis menti and the jaw pushed anteriorly, with the fingers behind the angles of the jaw on each side (Figure 6.2).

Method B

From above the patient's head or beside the body, the thumbs are placed on the patient's zygomas at each side, while pushing the angles of the jaw forwards with the fingers.

Basic airway equipment

OROPHARYNGEAL (GUEDEL) AIRWAY

This is used in unconscious patients without a gag reflex. The size of oropharyngeal airways used depends on the size of the patient: small adult, size 2; medium adult, size 3; and large adult, size 4.

Alternatively, the airway can be sized using the distance *between the incisors and the angle of the jaw* (Figure 6.3). The mouth is opened and the tip of the airway inserted with the airway inverted (convex downwards). The airway is then passed backwards over the tongue, rotating through 180° as it goes, until the flange lies anterior to the teeth. The patient is then reassessed and jaw thrust maintained if needed.

The complications of an oropharyngeal airway include trauma to teeth and mucosa, worsening of airway obstruction if the tongue is pushed further backwards or if an oversized airway becomes lodged in the vallecula, gagging or coughing, laryngospasm and vomiting and aspiration. If any of these complications occurs, the airway should be removed and a nasopharyngeal airway considered.

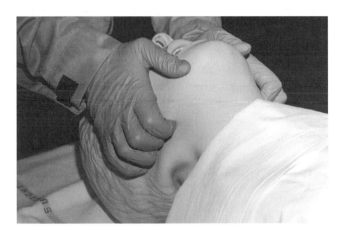

Figure 6.2 The technique for 'jaw thrust'.

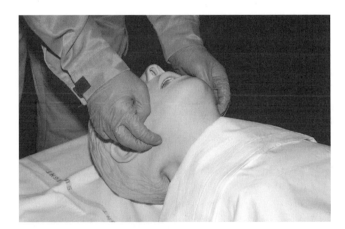

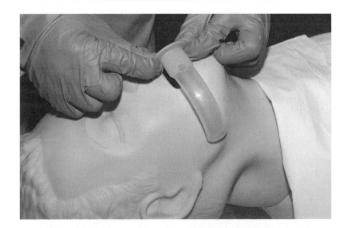

Figure 6.3 The technique for insertion of an oropharyngeal airway.

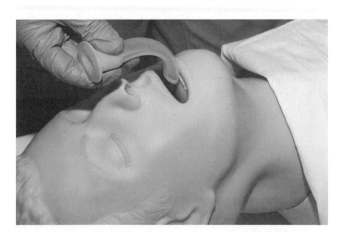

NASOPHARYNGEAL AIRWAY

This may be better tolerated than an oropharyngeal airway in semiconscious patients with a gag reflex, and is useful when trismus or facial swelling prevents the insertion of an oral airway. Suspected base of skull or maxillary fractures are relative contraindications owing to the danger of the airway penetrating the cribriform plate into the cranial vault.[11] However, careful insertion is justified if hypoxia cannot otherwise be relieved – the risk of intracranial insertion is probably overestimated.

Nasopharyngeal airway sizes are as follows:

* adult female: 6.0–7.0 mm (internal diameter);
* adult male: 7.0–8.0 mm (internal diameter).

The nasopharyngeal airway should be lubricated with water-soluble jelly before insertion, and a safety-pin inserted through the flanged end to prevent the airway being inhaled. The airway can be inserted through either nostril, by directing it posteriorly along the floor of the nasopharynx (Figure 6.4). Gentle rotation between the thumb and finger will ease its passage. If resistance is felt on one side, the other nostril or a smaller airway can be tried. The airway is inserted until the flange lies at the nostril. If coughing, laryngospasm or airway obstruction occurs, it should be withdrawn by 1–2 cm. The patient should then be reassessed, and the jaw thrust maintained if necessary.

The complications of a nasopharyngeal airway include trauma to the turbinates and nasal mucosa, bleeding from the nasal mucosa, which may be severe, gagging, vomiting, laryngospasm and airway obstruction if the airway is too long and a risk of intracranial penetration in the presence of basal skull fracture.

FACEMASK VENTILATION

Whichever device is chosen,[12] it is imperative to use an oropharyngeal or nasopharyngeal airway if needed. The mask is held over the mouth and nose, using the thumb and index finger over the hard part of the mask, with one or preferably both hands (Figure 6.5). The remaining fingers are hooked under the jaw, with the little finger if possible behind the angle of the jaw, so that the mask is held by a combined pincer grip and jaw thrust. The patient can then be ventilated with oxygen at 12 breaths/min, enough to cause visible chest expansion. However, achieving a good seal with the facemask with one hand is difficult for an inexperienced operator, therefore a two-person technique should be used in this case (one holds the mask and the other squeezes the bag).

The anaesthetic reservoir bag ('black bag', or 'Waters circuit') delivers close to 100% oxygen at high flow rates. However, the adjustable positive end-expiratory pressure (PEEP) valve makes it difficult to use, and rebreathing of CO_2 can occur. It is therefore best avoided by those not practised in its use.

Complications of facemask ventilation include:

* poor mask seal with inadequate ventilation;
* gastric inflation, leading to diaphragmatic splinting and regurgitation;
* aspiration of regurgitated stomach contents, or matter from the pharynx;
* neck movement, and exacerbation of cervical spine injury;
* pneumocephalus and meningitis in patients with basal skull fracture.[13]

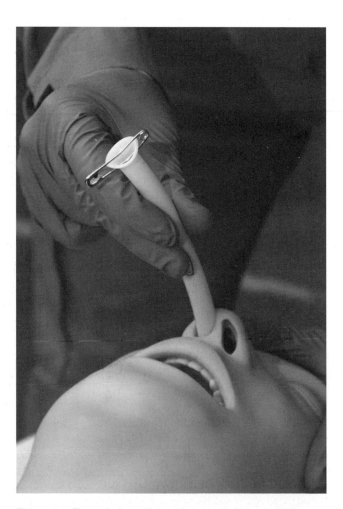

Figure 6.4 The technique of nasopharyngeal airway insertion.

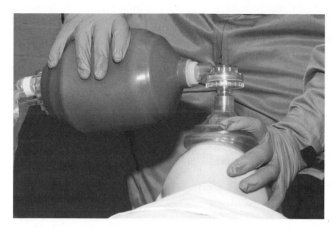 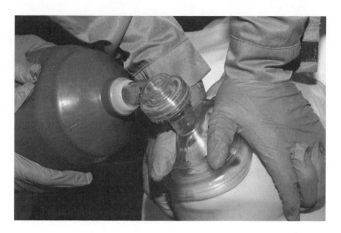

Figure 6.5 The technique for facemask ventilation.

A summary of basic airway management is given in Figure 6.6. Cervical spine immobilization should be carried out if cervical spine injury is suspected. If the patient is breathing adequately, oxygen should be given. In patients in whom breathing is inadequate, as judged by lack of respiratory effort, oxygen saturation by pulse oximetry, hypoxaemia on arterial blood gases or other clinical signs, bag–valve–mask ventilation should be used. This technique requires practice and may be difficult even for experienced operators, particularly in patients with anatomical variations or beards and in edentulous patients. If necessary a two-person technique should be used, with one person holding the mask in place with two hands while another ventilates. If bag–valve–mask ventilation is required, intubation is likely to be necessary. The patient must be reassessed after every intervention. It is important not to assume that an action has had its desired effect.

> Always obtain early expert airway assistance.

ADVANCED AIRWAY MANAGEMENT

Advanced airway management includes the following techniques:

- tracheal intubation;
- laryngeal mask airway;
- oesophageal–tracheal Combitube™;
- needle cricothyrotomy;
- surgical cricothyrotomy.

Advanced airway management is the process of ensuring that the patient is supplied with sufficient oxygen and adequately ventilated. The standard, most familiar and, for most patients, the best method of doing this is to anaesthetize the patient and insert a cuffed endotracheal tube by the oral route.[14] This ensures that the airway is 'secure', i.e. patent and protected from aspiration of stomach contents and secretions. It allows the administration of 100% oxygen and, in the setting of cardiopulmonary resuscitation, the administration of some drugs. However, the technique requires training and experience to perform, and its complications include hypoxia and death from unrecognized oesophageal intubation. Therefore, intubation should never be attempted by those who have not been properly trained. In these circumstances, the airway should be maintained by scrupulous performance of basic techniques until appropriate expertise is available. A cornerstone of airway management is to ensure that once the patient has been intubated the tube does not inadvertently come out. Prompt recognition and management of unplanned extubation or tube displacement is extremely important.

> Unrecognized oesophageal intubation is rapidly fatal. Be alert for tube displacement.

For some patients, awake fibreoptic intubation, gaseous induction of anaesthesia, awake nasotracheal intubation or the formation of a surgical airway under local anaesthesia may be indicated.

Spinal immobilization is assumed in all the airway skills described. However, if cervical spine injury can be excluded, then head extension should be used to facilitate all methods except nasotracheal intubation.

If advanced airway techniques seem to be indicated, expert assistance should be sought sooner rather than later. This may be from an experienced emergency physician, anaesthetist or intensivist. Rates of success and complication rates would appear to be similar between groups.[15]

> Never attempt intubation without proper training.

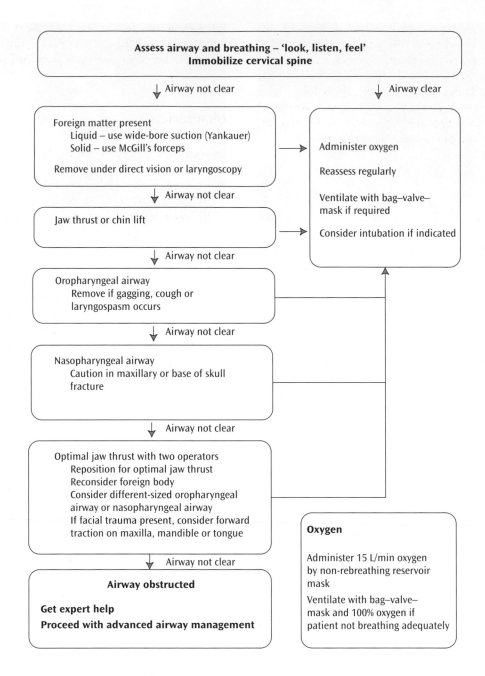

Figure 6.6 An algorithm for basic management of the airway in adult patients. © Difficult Airway Society 2004.

Endotracheal intubation

The indications for intubation are listed in Boxes 6.1 and 6.2 and are all evidence based,[15] whilst the only major contraindication is a lack of training in intubation.

The most dangerous complication of intubation is oesophageal intubation, which, if unrecognized, will cause hypoxia and death in the apnoeic patient. Hypoxia may also be due to:

- tube displacement following successful intubation;
- prolonged intubation attempts;
- intubation of a main bronchus (usually the right) if the tube is inserted too far;
- exacerbation of prior trauma to the airway: following damage to the larynx or trachea, complete airway obstruction may result.[16]

Other immediate complications include trauma to the teeth, tongue, pharynx, larynx or trachea; exacerbation of cervical spine injury; gagging, coughing, laryngospasm, regurgitation or vomiting in the semiconscious patient; exacerbation of raised intracranial pressure in patients with head injury; and cardiac dysrhythmias (tachycardia, bradycardia usually due to hypoxia, or extrasystoles).

Once the airway is controlled by whatever definitive means, ventilation is provided by a self-inflating bag, an anaesthetic reservoir bag or a mechanical ventilator.

Equipment

The equipment required for intubation must be readily available in areas of the hospital that deal with trauma. The exact equipment required will depend on the setting – pre-hospital care will require different equipment from emergency department care and the requirement for adult and paediatric equipment will vary with likely caseload. There must be a robust system in place for daily or more frequent checking of equipment policed by a senior member of the team. An effective mechanism must be established locally for prompt replacement of items that are used, broken or out of date. Anaesthetic drugs should be immediately available in the same areas, along with syringes, labels and ancillary equipment. Some anaesthetic agents are available in pre-filled syringes. A suggested minimum list of equipment is given in Table 6.2.

Monitoring

Oxygenation may be monitored in three ways:

- Clinically, although hypoxaemia is hard to detect.
- By pulse oximetry. This method does not detect hypoventilation if the patient is receiving oxygen, it may not 'pick up' because of poor peripheral perfusion and it may over-read if carboxyhaemoglobin is present. Monitoring the patient's pulse oximetry reading will provide useful information regarding tissue oxygenation; however, it does not provide information about levels of carbon dioxide and can be falsely reassuring in cases of respiratory insufficiency. In addition, it lags behind changes in oxygen delivery or airway problems.
- By arterial blood gas measurement, which should be considered in all major trauma patients.

BOX 6.1 Indications for intubation in trauma

- Airway obstruction
- Hypoventilation
- Severe hypoxaemia despite supplemental oxygen
- Severe cognitive impairment (Glasgow Coma Scale score ≤8)
- Cardiac arrest
- Severe haemorrhagic shock

BOX 6.2 Indications for intubation in burns/smoke inhalation

- Airway obstruction
- Severe cognitive impairment (Glasgow Coma Scale score ≤8)
- Major cutaneous burn ≥40%
- Prolonged transport time
- Impending airway obstruction due to moderate to severe facial, oropharyngeal or endoscopically visualized airway burns
- Severe haemorrhagic shock

Table 6.2 Equipment required for adult orotracheal intubation

Bag–valve–mask with reservoir, connected to high-flow oxygen
Laryngoscope (Macintosh, standard and large adult blades) – preferably two
Suction equipment with wide-bore (Yankauer) catheter
Cuffed tracheal tubes, sizes:
    Males: 8.0–9.0 mm internal diameter; 23–25 cm length
    Females: 7.0–8.0 mm internal diameter; 20–22 cm length
Gum-elastic bougie, or intubating stylet
Water-soluble lubricating jelly
Magill's forceps (to remove foreign bodies, or guide the tube through the cords)
10-mL syringe
Ventilating bag (or mechanical ventilator)
Stethoscope to confirm position
Capnograph
Adhesive tape or tie
Catheter mount (not essential)
Anaesthetic drugs, labels and delivery devices, i.e. syringes and syringe pumps
Difficult intubation equipment, including McCoy laryngoscope, laryngeal mask airways, jet ventilator and emergency cricothyroidotomy kit, should be immediately available.
An assistant trained in applying cricoid pressure and familiar with intubation procedure should be present.
Equipment must be immediately available, checked and functional

Electrocardiographic monitoring is mandatory to detect arrhythmias caused by cardiac complications of trauma, drugs or subclinical cardiac disease unmasked by injury. End-tidal carbon dioxide monitoring is mandatory for intubation and is discussed in more detail below.

Invasive arterial blood pressure monitoring is helpful for more severely injured patients as it allows continuous blood pressure measurement and arterial blood sampling. Radial arterial pressure may be less helpful in the patient who is very cold or hypovolaemic. In this setting, a femoral or brachial arterial line should be considered as long as its insertion does not delay definitive life-saving interventions: insertion once the patient is under anaesthetic should be considered There is evidence that complication rates are low and similar whichever site is used.[17]

Cricoid pressure

Unconscious trauma patients must be assumed to have a full stomach, and to be at risk of aspiration. Cricoid pressure may prevent regurgitation by occluding the oesophagus against the vertebral column. It may also reduce gastric inflation during facemask ventilation and (if applied correctly) improves the view at laryngoscopy.[18] Although usually taught as an advanced airway technique, cricoid pressure should ideally be applied early, as unconscious patients may aspirate at any time.

It should be noted, however, that there is little evidence to prove that cricoid pressure is effective in preventing aspiration.[19] There is also some evidence which suggests that cricoid pressure may displace rather than compress the oesophagus and may reduce the calibre of the airway.[20] However, cricoid pressure does not reduce the success of intubation,[21] and as it may be beneficial it remains standard for rapid-sequence induction (RSI).[11,22] Active vomiting (due to the risk of oesophageal rupture[23]) and laryngeal trauma are contraindications. If the patient vomits, the operator should tell the assistant to release cricoid pressure and should be ready to provide suction to protect the airway.

Firm backwards pressure is applied to the cricoid cartilage with thumb and index finger, and must not be released until the airway is secured and instructed by the operator. Bimanual cricoid pressure may be safer in suspected cervical spine injury, although evidence is lacking.[24] The back of the neck is supported with the other hand, unless support is already given by the posterior half of a rigid cervical collar.

> Never release cricoid pressure until instructed to do so by the person carrying out the intubation.

Anaesthesia for intubation

Patients can be intubated orally without anaesthesia only if they are deeply unconscious. However, the majority of trauma patients needing intubation, for example after head injury, have a preserved gag reflex, muscle tone or clenched teeth. Attempted intubation of such patients without proper anaesthesia may lead to gagging, laryngospasm, regurgitation, hypoxia, bradycardia and raised intracranial pressure in the head-injured.

Oral intubation using RSI is normally used in these circumstances. This involves preoxygenation and cricoid pressure, after which an intravenous anaesthetic induction agent and a neuromuscular blocker ('muscle relaxant') are given. Intubation is performed with cervical spine stabilization as described earlier.

Anaesthetic drugs should be given only by those who are properly trained in their use and who are skilled at intubation. The choice of anaesthetic agent will depend on various factors, including familiarity with the drug, the patient's pattern of injury and comorbidities. The use of unfamiliar drugs in critically injured patients is not advisable unless senior expertise and assistance are available. Their greatest dangers are described below.

LOSS OF MUSCLE TONE

This may lead to complete airway obstruction as well as apnoea. If both intubation and ventilation then prove impossible, catastrophic hypoxia will follow. RSI is therefore contraindicated if a 'difficult airway' is expected, and safer alternatives are awake fibreoptic intubation or cricothyrotomy under local anaesthesia.[25] Guidance on assessment of the likely difficulty of intubation is contained in standard textbooks of anaesthesia and clinical reviews.[22]

HYPOTENSION

Induction agents generally cause vasodilatation and sometimes cardiac depression. Hypotension may be severe in the hypovolaemic patient, who relies on vasoconstriction to maintain his or her blood pressure. Therefore, before RSI is initiated, large-bore venous access should be established and fluid resuscitation according to protocol commenced.

If it is not possible to obtain intravenous access, the intraosseous route may be used to give anaesthetic agents and fluids.[26]

A guide to RSI is given in Table 6.3.

It is vital to prevent hypoxia during intubation, and if pulse oximetry is not available a maximum of 30 seconds should be allowed for the attempt. If unsuccessful, reoxygenation by facemask ventilation is necessary before a further attempt. The time should be marked by asking someone to count time during the intubation attempt.

Intubation difficulties may be due to persistent muscle tone in the semiconscious, swelling, haematoma or foreign material in the airway, the need for cervical spine stabilization and anatomical variations.

Appropriate positioning of the patient's head and neck is extremely important and in some cases will be sufficient to allow intubation. It may be necessary to alter the direction of the pressure on the cricoid cartilage or to release cricoid pressure completely. Laryngeal manipulation by the operator may be helpful. In the case of persistent muscle tone, anaesthetic expertise is needed. Otherwise, an invaluable aid to intubation for those appropriately trained is the gum-elastic bougie,[28] which is a long, flexible guide which can be passed blindly through the cords when laryngoscopy is difficult, and the tube railroaded over it. This should always be available in any resuscitation room, and should be used the moment any difficulty in intubation is encountered. It is probably more effective than the stylet.[29] The McCoy laryngoscope,[30] which has the standard curved blade adapted to lever at the tip, can improve the view of the cords and the laryngeal mask airway (LMA) may also aid difficult airway control.[31] Other techniques, given appropriate experience, include using a fibreoptic laryngoscope, blind nasotracheal intubation and using an alternative technique such as the Combitube™.

Table 6.3 Rapid sequence intubation

Is this likely to be a difficult intubation? Consider both patient anatomy and factors relating to the injuries – if the intubation is predicted to be difficult, call for expert assistance. Guidance on assessing whether intubation is likely to be difficult is available from standard anaesthetic texts and review articles.[22]

1. Check that equipment is available and functioning, including oxygen, suction, bag–valve–mask, laryngoscopes, endotracheal tube (check balloon cuff does not leak), bougie or stylet and syringe. Ensure that the correct drugs are drawn up and labelled. Ensure that resuscitation drugs are available. Ensure that fluid is available for fast-running i.v. infusion to assist drug administration or counter any hypotension secondary to anaesthetic administration.
2. Check that additional equipment is available and functioning, e.g. second laryngoscope, ventilator, reserve oxygen supply, difficult airway equipment.
3. Ensure that monitoring is in place. This should include pulse oximetry, electrocardiogram, capnograph and equipment for non-invasive blood pressure monitoring or, where appropriate, invasive arterial blood pressure monitoring. Monitor alarm limits should be set to appropriate levels and the pulse oximetry signal should be audible to provide an additional cue to alert the operator if oxygenation is impaired.
4. Assistant to apply manual inline stabilization. Remove blocks and front of collar. Position head appropriately.
5. Preoxygenate for 4–8 minutes[27] with a tight-fitting facemask if possible and if circumstances allow.
6. Ask an assistant to apply cricoid pressure firmly – this may be in place already.
7. Give appropriate dose of induction agent into a fast-running i.v. infusion.
8. Give neuromuscular blocking agent into a fast-running i.v. infusion.
9. Wait until the effects of the anaesthetic are evident or for a predetermined time.
10. Position the head as appropriate and with reference to any suspicion of cervical spine injury.
11. Insert the laryngoscope to the right of mouth, sweeping the tongue to the left. Insert the laryngoscope in front of the epiglottis in the vallecula and lift along the direction of the handle. Do not lever the laryngoscope on the teeth! Take care not to cause trauma to the lips, tongue or pharynx.
12. Assess the view of the vocal cords. If the vocal cords are not visible, carry out actions to improve the view. Backward, upward and rightward pressure on the larynx by the assistant may improve the view. Do not attempt intubation if there is no view of the cords!
13. Insert the endotracheal tube from the right side so as not to obscure the view as it passes through the cords. Do not insert the tube too far: just until the cuff is through the cords. Insert the endotracheal tube over the stylet or use a bougie if required.
14. Ventilate manually with 100% oxygen. Inflate the balloon on the endotracheal tube until no leak is present during ventilation. Do not let go of the tube as it may become displaced!
15. Listen in both axillae for breath sounds with ventilation, and over the stomach for the absence of or only faint breath sounds. Asymmetric breath sounds may suggest that the tube is in the right main bronchus. Observe the capnograph tracing for end-tidal CO_2 trace. If there is suspicion of oesophageal placement, remove the tube and carry out failed intubation drills.
16. Secure the endotracheal tube with tape or tie. Insert an oropharyngeal airway to prevent the patient occluding the endotracheal tube by biting when consciousness returns.
17. Ask the assistant to release cricoid pressure only once the tube position is confirmed and the tube is fixed securely.
18. Reassess the patient.
19. Connect to the ventilator if appropriate. Reassess ventilation and oxygenation once connected.
20. Insert an orogastric tube to decompress the stomach and prevent any gas insufflated into the stomach during bag–valve–mask ventilation from causing difficulties with ventilation. Obtain and review arterial blood gases. Obtain and review chest radiograph to confirm tube position. Consider reducing FiO_2 if appropriate. Record the intubation grade and tube position in the patient's notes for future reference.

The above account is no substitute for formal training in anaesthetic techniques.[32] Those who do not perform endotracheal intubation frequently need to recognize that skills fade rapidly, and ensure that they obtain ongoing experience.

In patients with burns to the face, facial swelling may displace the tube tie or cause the tie to cut into the face. An uncut tube may be preferred in this setting to reduce the risk of displacement. Tracheostomy may prove extremely difficult in patients with burns to the neck.

Confirmation of tube position

Confirmation of tracheal tube placement is vital in order to avoid death from oesophageal intubation. The following routine should become second nature. Methods include:

- Seeing the tube pass through the cords at intubation.
- Observing the capnograph tracing.
- Feeling the ventilating bag as you inflate. The lungs normally feel elastic and 'springy': after oesophageal intubation it is usually either impossible to inflate, or the bag deflates with a 'squelch'.
- Watching the chest rise and fall with ventilation (both sides equally), and seeing that the abdomen does not distend.
- Listening to both lungs for breath sounds. Listening in the axillae avoids the auscultation of transmitted tracheal sounds which may be heard and mask intubation of a main bronchus. Auscultate over the stomach for the lack of or very quiet transmitted breath sounds.

Clinical tests for tube placement can mislead, especially in the obese patient.[33] The most reliable clinical sign is to see the tube pass through the cords, although the inexperienced may still mistake the oesophagus for the trachea. Assessing movement and breath sounds over the chest and abdomen is not completely accurate, and condensation inside the tube is not a reliable sign. Oesophageal intubation will eventually cause cyanosis, but this may be delayed for several minutes after preoxygenation, by which time the cause may be overlooked and it is almost certainly too late.

Capnography is mandatory for intubation;[14] however, it is not infallible, and in particular it may show a CO_2 trace from a tube sited in the oesophagus if the patient has recently consumed carbonated drinks.[34] However, in this setting the capnograph should detect CO_2 for only a few breaths before the giving a true reading.[32] If the cardiac output is very low or absent, e.g. in patients with cardiac arrest, the capnograph will not give a trace as CO_2 will not be transported from the tissues to the lungs. This may suggest that the tube is incorrectly positioned when it is in fact in the trachea. Clinical examination and invasive blood pressure tracings should give clues to this.

> If in doubt, take the tube out!

Ventilator management

Ventilation should be managed by a specialist with expertise in the area. There are a large number of things that can go wrong with the ventilator and ventilated patients, including failure of oxygen supply, machine failure, endotracheal tube displacement and dynamic hyperinflation.

Recent trials have suggested that ventilation with traditional tidal volumes of 10–15 mL/kg may contribute to lung injury and increase multiorgan failure and mortality.[35] Alternative ventilatory strategies reduced mortality in all subgroups studied.[36] Patients with pulmonary contusions or severe trauma, and those who have required multiple blood transfusions, are at greater risk of the acute respiratory distress syndrome. Tidal volume settings should therefore be 6 mL/kg where possible. Normal oxygen levels of 8–10 kPa, SpO_2 of ≥93% and normal CO_2 levels should be the goal in most patients, although where lung injury is present hypercarbia may be permitted in patients without brain injury. PEEP or FiO_2 may need to be adjusted to attain these oxygen levels. Caution should be used when increasing PEEP in patients with brain injury as this may adversely affect intracranial pressure; high PEEP may also interfere with venous return and cause a drop in cardiac output.

The ventilated patient must be treated with caution and in a sequential manner:

- Set the ventilator appropriately. Standard initial settings would be a tidal volume of 6 mL/kg, a rate of 12–14 breaths per minute, a peak inspiratory pressure ≤30 cmH_2O and an initial FiO_2 of 1.0, which may be reduced once appropriate.
- Sedate and paralyse the patient if necessary – expertise in administering anaesthesia is essential. Do not use neuromuscular blocking agents if paralysis is not indicated as they increase the risk of critical illness myopathy.[37]
- Ensure that the tracheal tube is not displaced out of the trachea or into a main bronchus, typically the right.
- Ensure that ventilation remains adequate by clinical observation, pulse oximetry, capnography (which may be very effective at guiding ventilation),[38] airway pressure monitoring, frequent arterial blood gas monitoring. An 'arterial line' should be inserted in all ventilated trauma patients and heed should be paid to the ventilator disconnect alarm.

- Use a tracheal suction catheter if airway secretions accumulate.
- Be alert for complications of positive-pressure ventilation (Box 6.3).

Ventilator management during transfer of the patient to imaging areas, the operating theatre or to critical care is covered in another chapter. It should be carried out only by personnel able to identify and manage complications such as unplanned extubation and ventilator failure.

> If a ventilated patient deteriorates in any way, think first of tube displacement.

OTHER ADVANCED AIRWAY METHODS

Laryngeal mask airway

The LMA is a wide-bore tube with a large, spoon-shaped inflatable cuff at the distal end. When inserted blindly into the mouth, the cuff sits above the laryngeal inlet, maintaining the airway and allowing spontaneous or controlled ventilation. Insertion is usually easy, although less so with cervical spine immobilization.[40] Sizes and cuff inflation volumes are listed in Table 6.4.

The LMA may be used as a temporary alternative to tracheal intubation in unconscious patients when intubation is precluded by a 'difficult airway' or lack of expertise, as an alternative to bag-and-mask ventilation as the LMA may allow better ventilation[41] and by the experienced intubationist as an aid to difficult tracheal intubation.[31] Contraindications to the use of the LMA include a lack of training in the technique, patients with active gag reflexes, foreign body airway obstruction, as the

> ### BOX 6.3 The complications of positive-pressure ventilation
>
> - Ventilator disconnection, which is potentially fatal in the apnoeic patient
> - Hypotension due to raised mean intrathoracic pressure and reduced venous return – this may be severe in hypovolaemia or cardiac tamponade
> - Tension pneumothorax which develops easily from a 'simple' pneumothorax during ventilation
> - Inadequate ventilation due to traumatic bronchopleural fistula
> - Dynamic hyperinflation - air trapping due to inadequate exhalation which 'tamponades' the heart in a similar way to tension pneumothorax
> - Air embolism following chest trauma, especially blast injury[39]

Table 6.4 Laryngeal mask airway (LMA) sizes and cuff inflation volumes

Size of LMA	Patient size	Cuff inflation volume (mL)
3	30 kg to small adult	15–20
4	Small to medium adult	25–30
5	Medium to large adult	35–40

LMA may force the object further down into the pharynx, and severe oropharyngeal trauma.

Disadvantages of the LMA include the following:

- It may stimulate gagging, coughing and vomiting in the semiconscious patient.
- It is easily displaced following insertion.
- It does not guarantee a clear airway or adequate ventilation if incorrectly placed.
- It does not protect against aspiration of stomach contents.
- Ventilation with high pressures may lead to gastric distension, regurgitation and aspiration.
- Cricoid pressure may impede insertion.[42]

The LMA may be life-saving, however, when the patient cannot be intubated or ventilated by other means.[43]

> The laryngeal mask does not guarantee ventilation or prevent aspiration.

Nasotracheal intubation

Nasotracheal intubation (NTI) can be performed without laryngoscopy and with minimal neck movement. Unlike oral intubation, it may be possible in semiconscious patients with a gag reflex. Although once thought preferable to oral intubation in patients with suspected cervical spine injury, evidence suggests that it is no safer.[44,45] It also has the following drawbacks:

- The patient must be breathing spontaneously.
- Gagging, vomiting, laryngospasm, hypoxia and raised intracranial pressure may still occur.
- A smaller diameter tube is needed than with oral intubation.
- Oesophageal intubation is a significant risk.
- Basal skull fracture or middle-third facial fractures are relative contraindications, as intracranial passage of the tube through the cribriform plate is possible,[46] and meningitis is also a risk. However, NTI is justifiable if hypoxia cannot be relieved otherwise,[47] provided that care is taken to direct the tube posteriorly.

NTI is an alternative to oral intubation only for those who are skilled in its use and cannot be recommended for more widespread use.

> Blind nasal intubation should be attempted only by those who are specifically trained and skilled in its use.

Surgical airways

A surgical airway is created either by cricothyroidotomy using 'needle' or 'surgical' techniques or by tracheostomy. Tracheostomy is unsuitable in emergency situations as it is technically difficult, time-consuming and may cause serious complications as a result of injury to adjacent neurovascular structures and the pleura. Conversely, the cricothyroid membrane lies superficially in the notch between the thyroid and cricoid cartilages and is relatively clear of major vessels and nerves. Cricothyroidotomy is the only surgical technique discussed here.

NEEDLE CRICOTHYROIDOTOMY

Needle cricothyroidotomy is a temporary life-saving measure, and must be replaced as soon as possible by intubation or tracheostomy. Surgical cricothyroidotomy allows continued adequate ventilation, but is not intended for prolonged use. Cricothyroidotomy by either method is indicated immediately if the airway and ventilation cannot be maintained in any other way, for example in patients with severe facial injury, airway haematoma, oedema or foreign bodies.[48] Surgical cricothyroidotomy may also be considered in patients at risk of impending airway obstruction from burns, oedema or haematoma, in conscious patients in whom general anaesthesia may precipitate irreversible airway obstruction and when awake fibreoptic intubation is not possible, in which case it may be performed under local anaesthesia, or when intubation is otherwise indicated and, although ventilation is possible, a definitive airway cannot be obtained in any other way. It is quicker and safer than tracheostomy.

Laryngeal trauma is a relative contraindication[16] and surgical cricothyroidotomy should be avoided in children as it may cause upper airway collapse.

With either technique, speed is essential to prevent hypoxic brain damage if the airway is completely obstructed. The technique for needle cricothyroidotomy is detailed in Box 6.4. Purpose-designed cricothyroidotomy sets are available, such as the Nu-Trach® or Patil®. Many of these are inserted through a cricothyroid puncture, but allow dilatation to accommodate a larger tube with a 15-mm connector. This allows connection to a self-inflating bag or ventilator.

The complications may be classified as 'early' or 'late' in nature. The early complications include:

- hypoxia and hypercarbia from both failed and prolonged insertion, incorrect placement or subsequent displacement, inadequate ventilation and air trapping;
- haemorrhage, which may be external or internally into the soft tissues of the neck or into the airway, potentially causing hypoxic respiratory arrest;
- air trapping due to inadequate exhalation through the needle cricothyroidotomy, leading to pneumothorax, pneumomediastinum, surgical emphysema, which may also occur from misplacement of the cannula, reduced venous return, reduced cardiac output and hypotension;
- oesophageal perforation.

The late complications are infection, subglottic stenosis, especially in children, and voice dysfunction due to vocal cord or cricothyroid muscle damage.

Although needle cricothyroidotomy appears simple, serious complications arise from CO_2 and air trapping.[48] If the upper airway is not patent, exhalation through the relatively narrow cannula will be inadequate, compromising ventilation even further. Although surgical cricothyroidotomy appears to be more traumatic, it should give adequate ventilation and oxygenation; therefore, needle cricothyroidotomy should be converted to the surgical route urgently if exhalation is inadequate. In addition, needle cricothyroidotomy does not prevent aspiration, or allow spontaneous breathing.

OXYGEN DELIVERY AND VENTILATION SYSTEMS

Needle cricothyroidotomy ventilation systems are difficult to make up 'on the spot', and a suitable jet injector system powered by high-pressure (50–60 psi) oxygen from the wall outlet should always be available in any department

> ### Box 6.4 The steps of needle cricothyroidotomy
>
> - Prepare the equipment: 14G intravenous cannula, syringe, oxygen source, delivery system and connectors (see below), stethoscope.
> - Position the patient, identify the cricothyroid membrane (Figure 6.7) and stabilize the larynx as detailed above.
> - Puncture the skin in the midline over the cricothyroid membrane, using the cannula with syringe attached.
> - Aiming 30–45° caudally, and keeping to the midline, advance the cannula towards the lower cricothyroid membrane while aspirating on the syringe.
> - When air is aspirated, advance the cannula over the needle into the trachea.
> - Withdraw the needle and aspirate again, to confirm tracheal placement.
> - Attach the ventilating system to the cannula hub.
> - Ventilate as appropriate, checking for adequate inflation and oxygenation.
> - Secure the cannula in place – the safest way is to hold it.

that deals with the anaesthesia of trauma patients,[48] along with staff trained in its use.

If a formal jet injector system is not available, a replacement may be improvised. A length of green 'bubble' oxygen tubing is cut so that it fits tightly inside the barrel of a 2-mL syringe, and a hole is cut across the side of the tubing just before the syringe. The syringe is pushed into the cricothyroidotomy cannula hub, and the hole occluded intermittently ('1 second on, 4 seconds off').

These systems are driven by a lower pressure (10–15 L/min oxygen from the wall flowmeter), which means that, although oxygenation may be adequate, CO_2 may accumulate:[49] these methods provide only 20–40 minutes of adequate ventilation before replacement by intubation or tracheostomy is necessary.

However, if none of these is available, ventilation with a self-inflating bag remains possible attached to:

- a 3-mm tracheal tube connector, the smaller end of which is pushed into the cannula hub;
- a 7-mm tracheal tube connector, the smaller end of which is pushed into the barrel of a 2-mL syringe, which is then attached to the cannula hub; or
- an adult-sized cuffed tracheal tube, inserted into the barrel of a large syringe and the cuff then inflated: the syringe is then attached to the cannula hub.

These can be assembled quickly, but give very poor ventilation because of lower pressures and the large compressible volume of gas:[48] CO_2 may accumulate rapidly, and even oxygenation may be inadequate. Anecdotal reports suggest that improvised systems may buy time until a jet ventilator or definitive airway can be inserted orally or surgically.

> Always replace a needle cricothyroidotomy with a definitive airway as soon as possible.

Surgical cricothyroidotomy

As for needle cricothyroidotomy, this is best performed in the stages outlined in Box 6.5 (see also Figure 6.7).

Following surgical tracheostomy the standard 15-mm connector on the tracheostomy or endotracheal tube allows connection of a ventilation system and either spontaneous or controlled ventilation.

The oesophageal–tracheal Combitube™

The Combitube™ is a double-lumen airway which allows airway maintenance, ventilation and protection from aspiration. When inserted blindly into the pharynx, the distal tube usually enters the oesophagus, allowing tracheal ventilation through the proximal lumen.[50] Ventilation should then be possible through the appropriate lumen,

---

Box 6.5 The steps of surgical cricothyroidotomy

- Prepare the equipment: Spencer–Wells forceps, scalpel blade, swab, tube (ideally size 6.0 tracheostomy tube, otherwise tracheal tube), self-inflating bag and oxygen source, 10-mL syringe, stethoscope, tape or bandage.
- Ensure that an assistant stabilizes the head in the midline, and extend the neck if spinal injury is excluded.
- Palpate the cricothyroid membrane between the thyroid and cricoid cartilages, and stabilize the larynx between thumb and fingers of the non-dominant hand.
- Infiltrate local anaesthetic with adrenaline along the borders of the sternomastoids lateral to the cricothyroid membrane if appropriate.
- Make a horizontal midline skin incision over the lower half of the membrane. The small cricothyroid artery runs transversely across the upper third.
- Incise the membrane horizontally, and dilate the opening by inserting the scalpel handle and rotating it through 90° or use forceps if available.
- Insert a suitable lubricated tube as above.
- Inflate the cuff, and ventilate if needed by attaching a self-inflating bag to the tube connector.
- Check for adequate ventilation, as for tracheal intubation.
- Fix the tube securely with a tape or a suture.

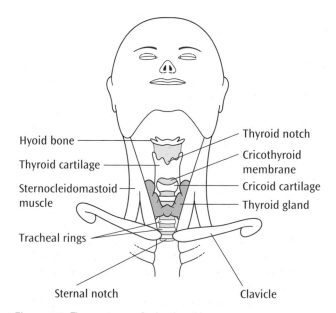

Figure 6.7 The anatomy of cricothyroidotomy.

and the position is confirmed in the same way as for tracheal intubation. Laryngoscopy and intubation are possible past the Combitube™ by deflating the pharyngeal balloon. As with the LMA, it is potentially life-saving in emergency situations.[32,51] The Combitube™ may be used as a temporary alternative to tracheal intubation in unconscious patients when intubation is precluded by a 'difficult airway' or lack of expertise. The contra-indications are similar to those for the LMA.

The disadvantages of the Combitube™ include the fact that it is unsuitable for use in small children and its insertion is more traumatic than that of the LMA. Moreover, gastric inflation may occur if the tube position is not checked carefully, and the pharyngeal balloon may be damaged by sharp teeth on insertion.

Fibreoptic intubation

Fibreoptic intubation may be appropriate for management of some patients by personnel trained in its use. It has a lower success rate and a higher complication rate than other methods of intubation, perhaps because of the type of patients it is used on.[12] It will not be discussed further.

THE DIFFICULT AIRWAY

There are various definitions of a difficult airway, but in essence it refers to the situation that an experienced operator struggles to maintain a patent airway or to intubate the patient.

Personnel involved in airway management should be familiar with guidelines for difficult intubation such as those produced by the Difficult Airway Society[52] and reproduced in Figures 6.8 and 6.9. These guidelines should be read in conjunction with the guidance notes in the article.

For difficult intubation drills to be effective they must be accompanied by practical training by an expert.

The principle of managing the difficult airway or failed intubation is to maintain oxygenation by following a stepwise pathway of various increasingly invasive interventions. In the setting of routine anaesthesia, oxygenation is maintained and the patient is allowed to wake up and breathe spontaneously if possible. This is rarely practical in trauma or burns patients in whom intubation is being carried out to reduce the risk of secondary hypoxic brain injury, prevent airway obstruction or allow life-saving surgery. For this reason, those carrying out airway management must be familiar with the equipment available for difficult airways and have used it previously on simulators or patients.

Finally, if the patient has had a difficult intubation this should be clearly communicated to the receiving hospital unit and documented clearly and in detail in the patient's notes to guide future management.

CERVICAL SPINE STABILIZATION

Cervical spine injury must be assumed in all patients with an appropriate mechanism of injury. Cervical spine injury can be excluded only by a combination of radiological investigation and clinical examination in the conscious patient, therefore:

- Cervical spine radiographs must never be allowed to delay life-saving interventions.
- Cervical spine injury must still be assumed in patients with decreased levels of consciousness unless multislice CT from the occiput to T4 is demonstrably normal.

Adequate methods for cervical immobilization are:

- MILS;
- spinal board, cervical collar, head blocks and strapping;
- cervical collar, sandbags or head blocks, and strapping.

> Intravenous fluid bags are not adequate substitutes for sandbags.

If the patient has not already been immobilized before arrival, MILS must be applied immediately. However, cervical collars make airway management and intubation more difficult, mainly by limiting mouth opening, and also limit access to the neck for cricoid pressure or cricothyroidotomy. Therefore, the following plan is recommended.[8,44]

On arrival in the resuscitation room, the patient must be removed from a long spine board during the primary survey. The risk of developing pressure sores increases with time on the spinal board, particularly in hypotensive patients.[53] The board may also interfere with imaging and cause pain and respiratory compromise.[54]

Sandbags or head blocks and tape should be substituted for MILS only if the patient is conscious and the airway is not at risk; otherwise, MILS should be continued until the airway is secure. If the patient is already in a collar and blocks, these should be removed and carefully replaced by MILS if the airway is at risk. For intubation MILS should be continued and the anterior portion of the cervical collar opened to allow adequate mouth opening. MILS does 'tie down' one person, but the importance of airway control dictates that it should be used when indicated.

> Remove the anterior part of the collar and the sandbags and tape before attempting intubation.

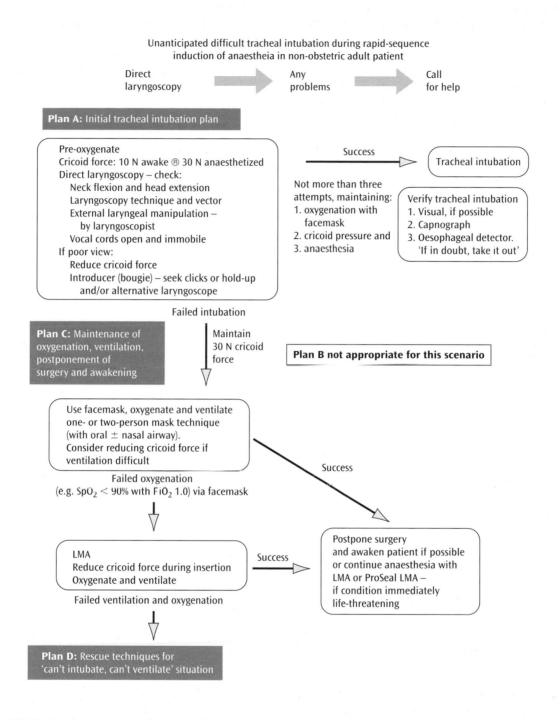

Figure 6.8 Difficult Airway Society guideline for rapid-sequence induction (reproduced with permission). © Difficult Airway Society 2004.

Although cervical spine movement should be avoided if possible, the airway always takes priority. Advanced airway techniques will usually work if basic ones fail, but neck movement must be accepted if the airway cannot be cleared in any other way. Only a small percentage of unconscious trauma victims actually have a cervical spine injury and, even if one is present, small neck movements may not make it worse; conversely, death is certain if the airway remains blocked.

> The airway takes priority over the cervical spine.

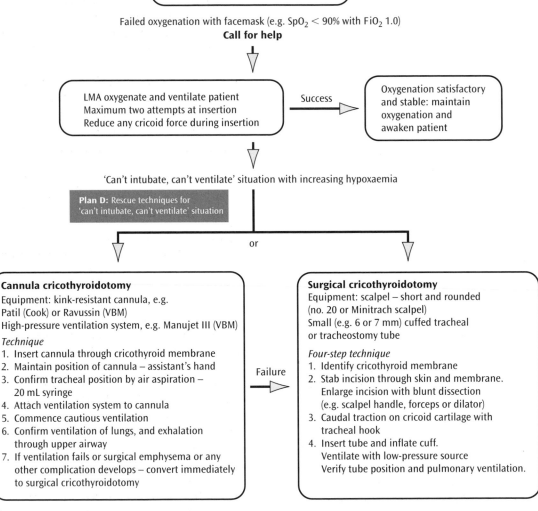

Failed intubation, increasing hypoxaemia and difficult ventilation in the paralysed anaesthetized patient: rescue techniques for the 'can't intubate, can't ventilate' situation

Failed intubation and difficult ventilation (other than laryngospasm)

Facemask
Oxygenate and ventilate patient
Maximum head extension
Maximum jaw thrust
Assistance with mask seal
Oral $\pm$ 6 mm nasal airway
Reduce cricoid force – if necessary

Failed oxygenation with facemask (e.g. $SpO_2 < 90\%$ with FiO_2 1.0)
Call for help

LMA oxygenate and ventilate patient
Maximum two attempts at insertion
Reduce any cricoid force during insertion

Success → Oxygenation satisfactory and stable: maintain oxygenation and awaken patient

'Can't intubate, can't ventilate' situation with increasing hypoxaemia

Plan D: Rescue techniques for 'can't intubate, can't ventilate' situation

or

Cannula cricothyroidotomy
Equipment: kink-resistant cannula, e.g.
Patil (Cook) or Ravussin (VBM)
High-pressure ventilation system, e.g. Manujet III (VBM)

Technique
1. Insert cannula through cricothyroid membrane
2. Maintain position of cannula – assistant's hand
3. Confirm tracheal position by air aspiration – 20 mL syringe
4. Attach ventilation system to cannula
5. Commence cautious ventilation
6. Confirm ventilation of lungs, and exhalation through upper airway
7. If ventilation fails or surgical emphysema or any other complication develops – convert immediately to surgical cricothyroidotomy

Failure →

Surgical cricothyroidotomy
Equipment: scalpel – short and rounded
(no. 20 or Minitrach scalpel)
Small (e.g. 6 or 7 mm) cuffed tracheal or tracheostomy tube

Four-step technique
1. Identify cricothyroid membrane
2. Stab incision through skin and membrane. Enlarge incision with blunt dissection (e.g. scalpel handle, forceps or dilator)
3. Caudal traction on cricoid cartilage with tracheal hook
4. Insert tube and inflate cuff. Ventilate with low-pressure source Verify tube position and pulmonary ventilation.

Notes:
1. These techniques can have serious complications – use only in life-threatening situations
2. Convert to definitive airway as soon as possible
3. Postoperative management – see other difficult airway guidelines and flowcharts
4. A 4-mm cannula with low-pressure ventilation may be successful in patients breathing spontaneously

Figure 6.9 Difficult Airway Society guideline for failed intubation and difficult ventilation (reproduced with permission). © Difficult Airway Society 2004.

SUMMARY

Hypoxia can rapidly kill and in combination with other injuries or hypotension compounds the severity of injury. Airway management is a core skill for those involved in management of the injured patient. Following a systematic, stepwise, escalating strategy for airway management can identify those patients who are at risk from hypoxia and has the potential to prevent disability or death. Ongoing training and experience in airway management is required to prevent skill fade.

GLOBAL PERSPECTIVES

The need to protect the airway of trauma victims and ensure adequate ventilation and oxygenation is universal. What varies around the world are the adjuncts and tools used to accomplish this, the Combitube being more common in North America and the laryngeal mask airway in Europe. Similar differences exist in the use of the stylet and the gum-elastic bougie, with the latter used infrequently in North America. The pre-hospital operator may be an emergency medical technician, an anaesthetic nurse or a physician, again dependent on site. In the military setting, control of catastrophic haemorrhage may take precedence over airway, as extremity haemorrhage may lead to death before hypoxia becomes a factor. In-hospital management in the UK will typically be the responsibility of an emergency physician, anaesthetist or intensivist with advanced airway management training; however, in the USA this may not be the case.[55]

REFERENCES

1. Hussain LM, Redmond AD. Are pre-hospital deaths from accidental injury preventable? *BMJ* 1994;**308**:1077–80.

2. Hodgetts TJ, Mahoney PF, Russell MQ, Byers M. ABC to <C> ABC: redefining the military trauma paradigm. *Emerg Med J* 2006;**23**:745–6.

3. Nandi PR, Charlesworth CH, Taylor SJ, Nunn JF, Dore CJ. Effect of general anaesthesia on the pharynx. *Br J Anaesth* 1991;**66**:157–62.

4. Wilson RF, Arden RL. Laryngotracheal trauma. In: Wilson RF, Walt AJ, eds. *Management of Trauma – Pitfalls and Practice.* Baltimore: Williams & Wilkins, 1996, pp. 288–313.

5. Parkins DRJ. Maxillofacial injuries in immediate care. *J Br Assoc Immed Care* 1996;**19**:34–6.

6. Nunn JF. *Nunn's Applied Respiratory Physiology.* Oxford: Butterworth-Heinemann, 1993, pp. 529–36.

7. Bolton CF, Chen R, Wijdicks EFM, Zifco U. *Neurology of Breathing.* Philadelphia: Butterworth Heinemann, 2004.

8. Willms D, Shure D. Pulmonary oedema due to upper airway obstruction in adults. *Chest* 1988;**94**:1090–2.

9. Bateman NT, Leach RM. Acute oxygen therapy. *BMJ* 1998;**317**:798–801.

10. Davey A, Moyle JTB, Ward CS. *Ward's Anaesthetic Equipment.* London: WB Saunders, 1992, pp. 188–94.

11. Roberts K, Whalley H, Bleetman A. The nasopharyngeal airway: dispelling myths and establishing the facts. *Emerg Med J* 2005; **22**:394–6.

12. Lawrence PJ, Sivaneswaran N. Ventilation during cardiopulmonary resuscitation: which method? *Med J Aust* 1985;**143**:443–6.

13. Klopfenstein CE, Forster A, Suter PM. Pneumocephalus. A complication of continuous positive airway pressure after trauma. *Chest* 1980;**78**:656–7.

14. Dibble C, Maloba M. Best evidence topic report. Rapid sequence induction in the emergency department by emergency medicine personnel. *Emerg Med J* 2006;**23**:62–4.

15. Dunham CM, Barraco RD, Clark DE, Daley BJ, *et al.* for the EAST Practice Management Guidelines Work Group. Guidelines for emergency tracheal intubation immediately after traumatic injury. *J Trauma* 2003;**55**:162–79.

16. Gussak GS, Jurkovich GJ. Treatment dilemmas in laryngotracheal trauma. *J Trauma* 1988;**28**:1439–44.

17. Scheer B, Perel A, Pfeiffer UJ. Clinical review: complications and risk factors of peripheral arterial catheters used for haemodynamic monitoring in anaesthesia and intensive care medicine. *Crit Care* 2002;**6**:199–204.

18. Vanner RG. Cricoid pressure in chaos. *Anaesthesia* 1998;**53**:94–5.

19. Butler J, Sen A. Best evidence topic report. Cricoid pressure in emergency rapid sequence induction. *Emerg Med J* 2005;**22**:815–16,

20. Smith KJ, Dobranowski J, Yip G, Dauphin A, Choi PT. Cricoid pressure displaces the esophagus: an observational study using magnetic resonance imaging. *Anesthesiology* 2003;**99**:60–4.

21. Turgeon AF, Nicole PC, Trepanier CA, Marcoux S, Lessard MR. Cricoid pressure does not increase the rate of failed intubation by direct laryngoscopy in adults. *Anesthesiology* 2005;**102**:315–19.

22. Reynolds SF, Heffner J. Airway management of the critically ill patient: rapid-sequence intubation. *Chest* 2005;**127**:1397–412.

23.   Ralph SJ, Wareham CA. Rupture of the oesophagus during cricoid pressure. *Anaesthesia* 1991;**46**:40–1.

24.   Nolan JP, Parr MJA. Tracheal intubation in trauma. *Br J Anaesth* 1998;**80**:270.

25.   Gwinnutt CL, McCluskey A. Management of the upper airway. In: Driscoll PA, Skinner DV, eds. *Trauma Care. Beyond the Resuscitation Room.* London: BMJ Books, 1998, pp. 19–33.

26.   LaRocco BG, Wang HE. Intraosseous infusion. *Prehosp Emerg Care* 2003;**7**:280–5.

27.   Mort TC. Preoxygenation in critically ill patients requiring emergency tracheal intubation. *Crit Care Med* 2005;**33**:2672–5.

28.   Nolan JP, Wilson ME. Orotracheal intubation in patients with potential cervical spine injuries. An indication for the gum elastic bougie. *Anaesthesia* 1993;**48** 630–3.

29.   Noguchi T, Koga K, Shiga Y, Shigematsu A. The gum elastic bougie eases tracheal intubation while applying cricoid pressure compared to a stylet. *Can J Anaesth* 2003;**50**:712–17.

30.   Gabbott DA. Laryngoscopy using the McCoy laryngoscope after application of a cervical collar. *Anaesthesia* 1996;**51**:812–14.

31.   Baskett PJF, Parr MJ, Nolan JP. The intubating laryngeal mask. Results of a multicentre trial with experience of 500 cases. *Anaesthesia* 1998;**53**;1174–19.

32.   Calder I, Pearce A, eds. *Core Topics in Airway Management.* Cambridge: Cambridge University Press; 2005.

33   Clyburn P, Rosen M. Accidental oesophageal intubation. *Br J Anaesth* 1994;**73**:55–63.

34.   Sum Ping ST, Mehta MP, Symreng T. Reliability of capnography in identifying esophageal intubation with carbonated beverage or antacid in the stomach. *Anesth Analg* 1991;**73**:333–7.

35.   The Acute Respiratory Distress Syndrome Network. Ventilation with lower tidal volumes as compared with traditional tidal volumes for acute lung injury and the acute respiratory distress syndrome. *N Engl J Med* 2000;**342**:1301–8.

36.   Eisner MD, Thompson T, Hudson LD, *et al*; Acute Respiratory Distress Syndrome Network. Efficacy of low tidal volume ventilation in patients with different clinical risk factors for acute lung injury and the acute respiratory distress syndrome. *Am J Respir Crit Care Med* 2001;**164**:231–6.

37.   Gutmann L, Gutmann L. Critical illness neuropathy and myopathy. *Arch Neurol* 1999;**56**:527–8.

38.   Helm M, Schuster R, Hauke J, Lampl L. Tight control of prehospital ventilation by capnography in major trauma victims. *Br J Anaesth* 2003;**90**:327–32.

39.   Gavalas M, Tekkis P. Air embolism. In: Greaves I, Ryan JM, Porter KP, eds. *Trauma.* London: Arnold, 1998, pp. 237–41.

40.   Asai T, Neil J, Stacey M. Ease of placement of the laryngeal mask during manual in-line neck stabilization. *Br J Anaesth* 1998;**80**:617–20.

41.   Alexander R, Hodgson P, Lomax D, Bullen C. A comparison of the laryngeal mask airway and Guedel airway, bag and facemask for manual ventilation following formal training. *Anaesthesia* 1993;**48**:231–4.

42.   Gabbott DA, Sasada MP. Laryngeal mask airway insertion using cricoid pressure and manual in-line neck stabilization. *Anaesthesia* 1995;**50**:674–6.

43.   Calder I, Ordman AJ, Jackowski A, Crockard HA. The Brain laryngeal mask airway. An alternative to emergency tracheal intubation. *Anaesthesia* 1990;**45**:137–9.

44.   Criswell JC, Parr MJA, Nolan JP. Emergency airway management in patients with cervical spine injuries. *Anaesthesia* 1994;**49**:900–3.

45.   Crosby ET. Tracheal intubation in the cervical spine-injured patient. *Can J Anaesth* 1992;**39**:105–9.

46.   Patrick MR. Airway manipulations. In: Taylor TH, Major E, eds. *Hazards and Complications of Anaesthesia.* Edinburgh: Churchill Livingstone, 1987.

47.   Rhee KJ, Muntz CB, Donald PJ, Yamada JM. Does nasotracheal intubation increase complications in patients with skull base fractures? *Ann Emerg Med* 1993;**22**:1145–7.

48.   Benumof JL, Scheller MS. The importance of transtracheal jet ventilation in the management of the difficult airway. *Anesthesiology* 1989;**71**:769–78.

49.   Ryder IG, Paoloni CCE, Harle CC. Emergency transtracheal ventilation: assessment of breathing systems chosen by anaesthetists. *Anaesthesia* 1996;**51**:764–8.

50.   Banyai M, Falger S, Roggla M, *et al*. Emergency intubation with the combitube in a grossly obese patient with bull neck. *Resuscitation* 1993;**26**:271–6.

51.   Eichinger S, Schreiber W, Heinz T, *et al*. Airway management in a case of neck impalement: use of the oesophageal tracheal combitube airway. *Br J Anaesth* 1992;**68**:534–5.

52.   Henderson JJ, Popat MT, Latto IP, Pearce AC; Difficult Airway Society. Difficult Airway Society guidelines for management of the unanticipated difficult intubation. *Anaesthesia* 2004;**59**:675–94.

53.   Mawson AR, Biundo JJ Jr, Neville P, Linares HA, Winchester Y, Lopez A. Risk factors for early occurring pressure ulcers following spinal cord injury. *Am J Phys Med Rehabil* 1988;**67**:123–7.

54.   Vickery D. The use of the spinal board after the pre-hospital phase of trauma management. *Emerg Med J* 2001;**18**:51–4.

55.   Mort TC. When failure to intubate is failure to oxygenate. *Crit Care Med* 2006;**34**:2030–1.

Thoracic injury

OBJECTIVES

After completing this chapter the reader will:
* understand the anatomy and physiology of thoracic trauma
* understand the relationship of thoracic trauma pathophysiology to other organ systems
* be able to recognize and assess thoracic injuries
* be able to initiate the management of the patient with thoracic injuries
* understand which investigations are relevant in thoracic trauma
* be able to outline the practical procedures used in the management of thoracic injuries.

THE EPIDEMIOLOGY OF THORACIC TRAUMA

Thoracic trauma has been recorded for over 5000 years[1] and still accounts for 25–50% of all trauma.[2] It is a contributing cause in 50% of fatal civilian trauma[3] and also a reliable marker of injury severity in multitrauma victims. The aetiology of thoracic injury varies worldwide, with penetrating injury being more common in the USA and South Africa, whilst in the UK blunt trauma is more common. In Europe, the leading cause of civilian thoracic injury is road traffic collisions (RTCs) (Table 7.1).

Many of the deaths from severe thoracic trauma occur immediately at the scene of the injury, although a significant group of patients may be salvaged with early effective management. Improvements in pre-hospital care and the evolution of more efficient transport systems have increased the number of patients arriving at hospital alive following major trauma. Cardiothoracic surgery and resuscitative procedures such as emergency thoracotomy have an important role in the management of thoracic trauma but are indicated in only a small minority of cases. The vast majority of patients can be managed conservatively[5] – careful observation with appropriate fluid replacement and effective analgesia constitutes adequate therapy in up to 90% of such patients. However, compared with patients with severe injuries not involving the chest, patients with thoracic trauma are more likely to be admitted to intensive care, spend longer in hospital and are more likely to die.[6]

The challenge for the management of thoracic trauma in the twenty-first century is the rapid detection and appropriate management of significant intrathoracic injuries and the limitation of secondary organ dysfunction by careful resuscitation and early critical care interventions when necessary. Particularly important are victims of multitrauma and those patients with a combination of blunt and penetrating injury.

ANATOMICAL AND PHYSIOLOGICAL CONSIDERATIONS

The thorax is a musculoskeletal cage comprising the 12 thoracic vertebrae posteriorly, 12 pairs of ribs bilaterally and the sternum anteriorly. The diaphragm makes up the floor of the thorax while the roof of the thorax tapers to the lower neck and thoracic outlet, which is confusingly also referred to as the thoracic *inlet*. The upper thorax is covered mainly by the musculature of the shoulder and upper limb. There are several differences in both thoracic

Table 7.1 Major causes of civilian thoracic injury in Europe[4]

Mechanism	Proportion (%)
Road traffic collision	60
Industrial accidents	15
Domestic injuries	10
Sporting injuries	10
Interpersonal conflict or suicide	5

anatomy and physiology between children and adults. The shape is more or less circular in cross-section in an infant but becomes more flattened anteroposteriorly during growth to adulthood. The flexibility of the musculoskeletal wall is much greater in children as more of the rib cage is cartilaginous and children may sustain severe intrathoracic injuries from blunt trauma with relatively modest signs of chest wall injury.

In infants, the intercostal muscles are underdeveloped and mechanically less efficient than in older children and adults due to the more horizontal alignment of the ribs, relying on the diaphragm for respiration. Thus, infants are more vulnerable to respiratory fatigue.[7] Infants have a higher metabolic rate and oxygen consumption that is up to twice that of adults, resulting in the more rapid development of hypoxia at times of physiological stress. Similarly, a normal infant's respiratory rate is about twice that of an adult (30–40 breaths/min), and infants respond to a higher oxygen demand by further increasing the respiratory rate rather than by increasing tidal volume.

The thorax contains the heart, lungs, great vessels (aorta, inferior and superior vena cava, pulmonary arteries and veins), lower trachea, oesophagus and thoracic duct. The lower ribs overlie the 'intrathoracic abdomen', including the liver, spleen and biliary apparatus. The bulk of the thoracic volume is taken up by the two lungs, with the mediastinum – principally the heart and great vessels – suspended between. Each lung is cloaked in visceral pleura, which is continuous with the parietal pleura that lines the thoracic cage. A tiny amount of fluid between the two layers lubricates the movements of the lungs. The pressure gradient required to generate inspiratory flow is achieved largely by flattening the diaphragm to increase the volume of the thorax, creating a subatmospheric pressure in the lungs. During expiration the intra-alveolar pressure becomes slightly higher than atmospheric pressure and gas flow to the mouth results. The normal adult respiratory rate is 12–16 breaths per minute with a tidal volume (the normal amount of air inhaled and exhaled per breath at rest) of around 500 mL.

The heart is divided into a right and left side, each with an atrium and a ventricle. The atria act as reservoirs for venous blood, with a small pumping action to assist ventricular filling. The ventricles are the major pumping chambers, delivering blood to the low-pressure pulmonary (right ventricle) and high-pressure systemic (left ventricle) circulations. The cardiac output is the product of the amount of blood ejected from the left ventricle with each beat multiplied by the heart rate. It is normally about 5 L/min. The heart is surrounded by a double layer of pericardium analogous to the pleurae of the lungs except the outer fibrous pericardium is unyielding and any collection of pericardial fluid will reduce ventricular filling and decrease cardiac output. This is termed pericardial tamponade.

The anatomical boundaries above and below the thorax include the root of the neck and the upper abdomen and

diaphragm and are referred to as 'junctional zones'. Injuries involving these zones suggest the possibility of multiregional injury, and intrathoracic injury is likely, especially in penetrating trauma. A patient with both intrathoracic and intra-abdominal wounds is much more likely to die and presents a particular challenge for treatment, especially surgical management.[8]

PATHOPHYSIOLOGY

The main pathophysiological consequences of thoracic trauma occur as a result of combined effects on respiratory and haemodynamic function.[9] Death following thoracic injury is often secondary to impairment of oxygen delivery, which is dependent upon pulmonary gas exchange, cardiac output and haemoglobin concentration. Hypoxia may result from a number of different pulmonary and cardiovascular causes, as shown in Table 7.2.

The pathophysiological consequences of thoracic trauma may also be divided into early and delayed effects, as shown in Table 7.3.

For practical purposes it is appropriate to consider the pathophysiology of thoracic trauma by aetiology, the two principal modes being blunt and penetrating trauma.

Blunt thoracic trauma

Blunt trauma occurs largely as the result of rapid deceleration, or crushing, in RTCs, which account for around 70–80% of such injuries. Blast may also result in significant blunt thoracic trauma.[10] Common injuries sustained include haemothorax, great vessel disruption and cardiopulmonary contusions.[11] The severity of injury is directly related to impact velocity and the absence of an

Table 7.2 Causes of hypoxia from thoracic injury

Pulmonary	Cardiovascular
Tension pneumothorax	Tension pneumothorax
Airway obstruction	Massive haemorrhage
Open pneumothorax	Pericardial tamponade
Massive haemothorax	Traumatic disruption of the
Ventilatory failure, e.g.	aorta or great vessels
from a flail chest	Myocardial contusion
Pulmonary contusion	
Tracheobronchial disruption	

Table 7.3 Early and delayed consequences of thoracic trauma

Early	Delayed
Hypoxia	Secondary lung injury
Hypovolaemia	Pulmonary and myocardial contusion
Mechanical	Sepsis

appropriate restraint device such as a seat belt. During profound deceleration, shearing forces may disrupt the great vessels or bronchial tree (the so-called 'bell-clanger' effect), leading to immediate haemorrhage, pneumothorax or a combination of both. Crush injuries may compress the heart between hard bony surfaces such as the sternum and thoracic vertebrae, leading to contusion, or even rupture, of the mycocardium or cardiac valves. Cardiac output may be directly reduced by decreased myocardial contractility, anatomical disruption, reduced venous filling from tamponade or as a result of changes in intrathoracic pressures such as tension pneumothorax.

Pulmonary contusions and chest wall injury lead to impaired ventilation, impairing oxygenation. In the case of chest wall injury it is the loss of mechanical function that contributes to hypoxia. If the chest wall is significantly disrupted it may be impossible to generate a sufficient movement of air to allow adequate gas transfer. Pulmonary contusion is one of the major factors contributing to the increased morbidity and mortality following blunt thoracic trauma. Progressive alveolar haemorrhage and oedema occur, followed by interstitial fluid accumulation and decreased alveolar membrane diffusion. This produces a relative hypoxaemia with increased pulmonary vascular resistance, decreased pulmonary vascular flow and reduced lung compliance. Initial intrapulmonary shunt can reach 30% in the early stages of trauma, although later hypoxia-induced pulmonary vasoconstriction may reduce this. These effects are summarized in Table 7.4 and Figure 7.1.

Penetrating trauma

The principal pathophysiological consequence of penetrating trauma is usually haemorrhage due to damage to major blood vessels. Arterial bleeding from the great vessels is often fatal, although venous bleeding may be arrested by the tamponade effect and the accompanying hypotension. Pericardial tamponade may occur due to direct laceration of the myocardium or coronary vessels and is most commonly seen with a mediastinal entry site.[4] Penetrating trauma may also result in an open pneumothorax, particularly with projectile or fragmentation injuries, when air preferentially enters the pleural cavity through the chest wall during normal respiration. Alveolarvenous injury may also lead to a risk of systemic air embolus, the overall incidence of which in thoracic trauma has been estimated to be 4–14%, with two thirds being the result of penetrating trauma.[13,14] The

Table 7.4 Patterns of injury by mechanism in blunt thoracic trauma

Mechanism of injury	Chest wall injury	Possible intrathoracic injury	Common associated injuries
High velocity (i.e. sudden deceleration)	Sternal and/or scapula and/or bilateral rib fractures with anterior flail segments	Aortic rupture, cardiac contusion, tracheobronchial disruption, rupture of the diaphragm	Head, face, cervical and thoracic spine, lacerations to liver and/or spleen, long-bone fractures
Low velocity (i.e. direct blow)	Lateral impact: rib fractures; anterior impact: sternal fractures	Pulmonary and/or cardiac contusions	Lacerations to liver or spleen if lower ribs are involved
Crush injury	Anteroposteriorly: bilateral rib fractures and/or flail segments; laterally: ipsilateral rib fractures and/or flail segments	Ruptured bronchus, pulmonary and/or cardiac contusions	Fractures to thoracic spine, lacerations to liver and/or spleen

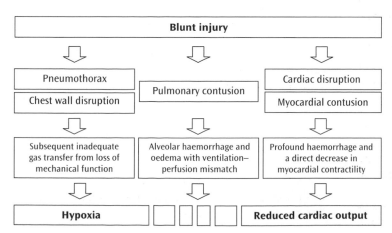

Figure 7.1   Summary of the pathophysiological consequences of blunt thoracic trauma.[12]

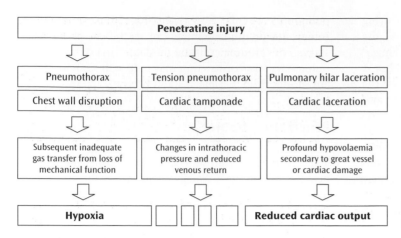

Figure 7.2   Summary of the pathophysiological consequences of penetrating thoracic trauma.

clinical significance of systemic air embolism will depend upon the volume and duration of air entrainment. Figure 7.2 summarizes the consequences of penetrating thoracic injury.

Thoracic trauma and its effects on other organ systems

As already described, thoracic trauma may result in hypoxia, reduced cardiac output or both. The consequence of this is a reduction in the delivery of oxygen to the tissues (DO_2) which, if uncorrected, may result in secondary organ damage and subsequent complications such as acute renal failure. Tissue oxygen delivery may be calculated from the equation:

$$DO_2 = \text{cardiac output (CO)} \times \text{haemoglobin concentration (Hb)} \times \text{oxygen saturation (SaO}_2) \times 1.34$$

Thus, haemoglobin concentration and cardiac output are major determinants of DO_2. Preload optimization by replacement of the circulating blood volume is the most efficient way of increasing cardiac output.[6] Maximal oxygen saturation must be maintained by ensuring effective ventilation and supplementary oxygen therapy.

> Oxygen delivery to the tissues is maximized by restoring blood volume, control of haemorrhage, high-flow oxygen and ventilatory support.

INITIAL ASSESSMENT

The management of thoracic trauma begins, as it does with all trauma victims, outside hospital, and pre-hospital information in the MIST format (see p. 25) should be obtained with particular reference to the need for needle decompression of a tension pneumothorax. Certain wounds or patterns of bruising highlight the likelihood of specific underlying pathology. A seat belt mark on the anterior chest wall should arouse suspicion of fractured ribs, lung contusion or solid organ injury in the abdomen, whereas a penetrating wound medial to the nipple or scapula suggests possible damage to the heart – with the potential for pericardial tamponade – great vessels or hilar structures. However, major intrathoracic injury can occur without obvious external signs. Additionally, fractures of the first and second ribs are associated with major vessel injury. Age greater than 60 years is another predictor of poorer outcome in patients with thoracic trauma.[6]

In the pre-hospital setting, the decision regarding which treatment interventions are appropriate at the scene or during transit to hospital remains a controversial issue. The chances of survival from penetrating thoracic trauma are greater if the time from injury to definitive surgery is minimized[15] and decrease sharply in patients with penetrating cardiac wounds reaching hospital more than 25 minutes after injury.[16]

The primary survey

In every case, management of a trauma patient begins with the systematic examination of the airway, breathing, circulation, disability and exposure/environment (<C>ABCDE) with simultaneous resuscitation interventions as required. Occasionally treatment of catastrophic haemorrhage may take precedence over airway management. This necessity is more common in military trauma.[17] The <C>ABCDE sequence is reviewed with specific reference to thoracic trauma.

<C>

Control of exsanguinating external haemorrhage is unlikely to be a problem in isolated thoracic injury, but significant bleeding from associated injuries must be controlled.

A

The priority is the patency of the airway (Chapter 6). Oxygen therapy should be instituted as soon as possible with high-flow delivery via a suitable mask in order to achieve maximum possible concentration (as near to 100% as possible).

B

Before examining the chest, the neck should also be carefully examined for injuries or physical signs suggestive of intrathoracic pathology. The mnemonic TWELVE may help this assessment:

- **T**racheal deviation
- **W**ounds/bleeding
- surgical **E**mphysema
- **L**aryngeal injury
- **V**enous distension
- **E**xposure – including the removal of a cervical collar with manual in-line stabilization.

The chest must be completely exposed to assess respiratory movement and the quality of ventilation. The respiratory rate should be recorded. Changes to respiratory rate and movement may be due to airway obstruction (a 'see-sawing' chest–abdomen breathing pattern), haemothorax or pneumothorax (reducing the movement on the affected side), pulmonary contusion or pain due to chest wall injury. Impending hypoxia may be indicated by subtle changes such as the appearance of a shallow, rapid breathing pattern.

Visual inspection and palpation of the chest wall may reveal deformity, bruising, abrasions and pathognomonic bruising patterns, penetrating injury, tenderness, instability or crepitus, all of which are markers suggestive of underlying injury. All zones of the lungs, especially the apices, should be percussed and auscultated comparing one side with the other. The back and sides of the thorax should not be forgotten, and in particular there should be a *careful* search for wounds by sweeping for blood on a gloved hand drawn behind the supine patient, from shoulder to buttocks. A more formal assessment of the back of the chest can be completed as part of the log-roll and must be done expeditiously in patients with penetrating trauma so that life-threatening posterior wounds are detected early. Severe burn injuries may result in restriction of respiratory movements due to the formation of a rigid eschar. As a result, surgical intervention may be urgently required to enable normal respiratory movement and adequate ventilation (Chapter 20).

Individual thoracic injuries and life-saving interventions, such as needle decompression and tube thoracostomy, are described later in this chapter. Placement of a radiographic plate on the resuscitation trolley prior to the patient's arrival will facilitate rapid imaging of the chest without interruption of resuscitation. Pneumo/haemothoraces and rib and scapular fractures indicate high-energy transfer to the thorax.

> The respiratory rate and the presence of asymmetrical respiratory movement may be the only evidence of thoracic injury in the pre-hospital setting.

C

The pulse should be assessed for quality, rate and regularity. Blood pressure may be measured by automatic non-invasive devices but the presence of a radial pulse may be considered an indicator of a blood pressure sufficient to perfuse the vital organs. Peripheral circulation may be assessed by skin colour, temperature and capillary return. It should be noted that venous distension in the neck may be absent in a hypovolaemic patient with pericardial tamponade. The heart sounds should be examined for signs of a pericardial tamponade or valvular injury and ECG monitoring is an important adjuvant to circulatory assessment. The patient should be carefully examined for other causes of significant haemorrhage and hypovolaemia such as abdominal and pelvic trauma, burns or long-bone fractures.

> In the pre-hospital setting, the main indicators of a circulatory problem that can be reliably detected without specific monitoring are an elevated pulse rate, loss of radial pulse and increased central capillary refill time of more than 2 seconds.

D

Initially, patients may be confused and combative due to hypoxia or hypercarbia. However, a primary head injury may also cause an altered mental state, which will be compounded by the hypoxia or hypercarbia. The Glasgow Coma Scale (GCS) score should be recorded routinely. In the case of pre-hospital assessment, the AVPU (alert, voice, pain, unresponsive) scale is appropriate (see Chapter 4). Peripheral neurological features may also be present, such as in the case of a high cervical spinal injury. Their recognition is important, as paralysis of the diaphragm will further diminish an already reduced respiratory effort, necessitating respiratory support to prevent hypoxia and hypercarbia.

E

During the primary survey the patient must be fully exposed in order to allow a thorough examination for injuries, although consideration should also be given to temperature control, especially in the case of a lengthy entrapment at the scene or patients with immersion/submersion injuries.

Temperature should be measured and efforts taken to maintain or rewarm the patient as appropriate, such as the use of forced air warmers, prewarmed intravenous fluids or thermally insulating blankets.

> It is vital to prevent hypothermia in trauma patients in order to try and avoid exacerbating post-traumatic coagulopathy.

The secondary survey

Once any immediately life-threatening conditions have been diagnosed and treated, or excluded, the patient can be assessed more thoroughly. This assessment includes taking a detailed history and full examination (Chapter 4).

THORACIC INJURIES

Major thoracic injuries can be divided into those that are immediately life-threatening and those that may be hidden initially but could result in later complications.

Immediately life-threatening injuries

There are six thoracic injuries which can be fatal if they are not recognized and treated immediately. These may be remembered by the well-known mnemonic ATOM FC:

- **A**irway obstruction
- **T**ension pneumothorax
- **O**pen pneumothorax
- **M**assive haemothorax
- **F**lail chest
- **C**ardiac (pericardial) tamponade.

AIRWAY OBSTRUCTION

Obstruction of the pharynx or trachea may occur as a result of anatomical disruption from penetrating or blunt trauma, soft-tissue swelling from airway burns as well as from haemorrhage into the airway or from inhaled material. Complete obstruction of the airway will result in death within minutes if not immediately relieved. The immediate management of airway obstruction is described in Chapter 6. Intrathoracic airway obstruction is fortunately rare. It is difficult to recognize, although the history may be suggestive, and difficult to treat. Vigorous chest compressions may dislodge an obstruction.

TENSION PNEUMOTHORAX

A tension pneumothorax develops when air accumulates in the pleural space. Unlike a simple pneumothorax, the air flow is predominantly unidirectional. Air flows into the pleural space on inspiration, but cannot escape during expiration due to a 'flap valve' effect. This causes a progressive accumulation of air in the pleural space with collapse of the ipsilateral lung, producing hypoxia and eventually shifting of the mediastinum to the opposite side. There is reduced venous return from increased intrathoracic pressure, causing decreased cardiac output. In advanced cases, hypoxia-induced myocardial failure may further reduce cardiac output.

Box 7.1 The procedure for needle decompression of a tension pneumothorax

- High-flow oxygen is administered.
- The second intercostal space in the midclavicular line is identified (Figure 7.3).
- The skin should be cleaned with an appropriate antiseptic solution.
- Using a large-bore cannula (14G/16G), the skin is punctured just above the third rib aiming directly perpendicular to the skin until the pleura is entered. The stylet is removed. The 'rush' of air on puncturing the pleura is often absent or missed, particularly in noisy environments. Signs of clinical improvement are more relevant.
- The cannula should be fixed securely to prevent kinking and left open to the air, and should never be capped off.
- Open or tube thoracostomy should follow as soon as is practical, followed by chest radiography.

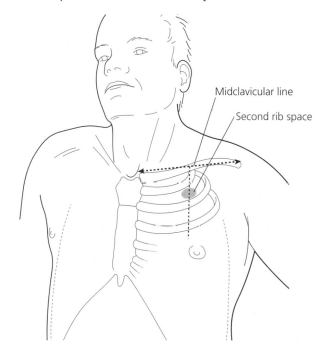

Figure 7.3   Location for needle thoracocentesis (left side).

Box 7.2 The procedure for open and tube thoracostomy

- High-flow oxygen is administered.
- The correct intercostal space on the affected side is identified and the ipsilateral arm may be abducted for improved access and anatomical markings (Figure 7.4).
- The skin is cleaned appropriately (and draped in hospital).
- Consider intravenous analgesia (e.g. morphine) and/or sedation (e.g. ketamine).
- An appropriate local anaesthetic (lidocaine) should be infiltrated under the skin and down to the pleura in the conscious/unsedated patient.
- A 2- to 3-cm skin incision is made in line with the upper edge of the rib – a much larger incision may be required to ensure adequate drainage from an open thoracostomy.
- A track is dissected bluntly through the subcutaneous tissues and muscle layers, staying just above the rib using a blunt artery clip.
- The parietal pleura is punctured with the closed end of a clamp.
- A gloved finger is then inserted through the pleura, and a finger sweep performed to determine the presence of adhesions or bowel. Beware the presence of bony spicules from rib fractures.
- The thoracostomy tube (size 28–32 gauge in adults, or the largest size that will pass easily between the ribs in children) is attached to the drainage bag *with the trocar removed*.
- The tube is inserted in an apical direction through the intercostal tract a sufficient distance to ensure that all the drain holes lie within the pleural space and not so far that the drain may kink inside the thorax – typically 12–15 cm in adults.
- Misting of the tube, or blood-stained fluid drainage, confirms intrathoracic placement.
- The tube should be secured appropriately, usually with sutures, and the incision closed to provide a tight seal on the tube and the area dressed with a number of swabs to prevent kinking outside the body. Leaving untied sutures in place may facilitate wound closure after tube removal.
- Clinical examination is repeated to ensure improvement and the lung fields auscultated to ensure adequate air entry.
- Finally, in-hospital care must include a chest radiograph to confirm positioning.

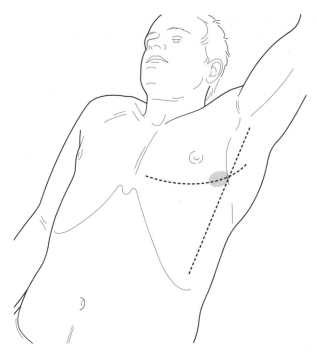

Figure 7.4 Location for open or tube left-sided thoracostomy in the fifth intercostal space just anterior to the midaxillary line. This site is chosen because there is a relative absence of covering muscles, key structures such as the long thoracic nerve are avoided, it is relatively cosmetic and the patient can still lie flat with the drain in. The fifth intercostal space can be identified by placing the patient's hand in the axilla and using the lower border of the hand as a guide, counting from the second space at the sternal angle, or using the nipple level in males.

Tension pneumothorax is purely a clinical diagnosis, recognized by:

- hypotension;
- respiratory distress and increase in respiratory rate;
- over-inflated hemithorax with or without visibly splayed ribs;
- hyper-resonant ipsilateral percussion note;
- reduced or absent ipsilateral breath sounds;
- tracheal deviation;
- distended neck veins.

The last two are late signs. The immediate treatment of a tension pneumothorax is percutaneous needle decompression (Box 7.1). Even if this fails to confirm a tension pneumothorax the needle should still be secured in place to alert emergency personnel that the procedure has been carried out.

The two main complications are failure to puncture the pleura if the needle is too short and the creation of a simple pneumothorax. However, inadvertently creating a simple pneumothorax is far less hazardous than failing to relieve a tension pneumothorax. Both 14G and 16G cannulae are sufficiently long (45 mm) to puncture the pleura in most cases. If signs of a tension pneumothorax remain despite needle thoracocentesis with a 14G/16G needle, a second needle should be placed more laterally to the first. In very muscular individuals the fifth intercostal space anterior to the midaxillary line – the usual location for a 'chest drain' – can also be used.

Following needle decompression a formal thoracostomy and drain should be placed into the affected side as soon as feasible. Thoracostomy is the single most common intervention in patients sustaining thoracic trauma, and may be life-saving. Thoracostomy drainage relieves dyspnoea, improves gas transfer and ventilation–perfusion mismatch as well as identifying continued bleeding and the need for thoracotomy and surgery. It may be either the simple 'open' type or with tube insertion. In the pre-hospital setting, open thoracostomy alone is appropriate in intubated and ventilated patients allowing free drainage of air or fluid to the outside. Formal tube thoracostomy can then be performed once the patient reaches an appropriate setting. The steps taken to carry out an open thoracostomy are the same as for a tube thoracostomy up until the insertion of the drainage tube (Box 7.2).

An underwater seal drainage system is not essential and may be problematic during pre-hospital transfers. A closed drainage bag with a one-way flow system may be used instead. The bag must remain visible to ensure that it is not blocked and has not overfilled. An Asherman® seal can be used to temporarily secure the tube in a pre-hospital setting by placing the tube through the rubber valve of the seal before insertion and using the adherent dressing part to attach this firmly to the skin.

Complications

Possible complications include:

- misplacement which is usually extrapleural due to inadequate dissection;
- damage to thoracic or abdominal organs by instruments (trocars should never be used);
- damage to the intercostal neurovascular bundle under the ribs;
- subcutaneous emphysema due to air leakage around the tube;
- later infection (local, or empyema).

OPEN PNEUMOTHORAX

When a penetrating chest wall injury creates a direct communication between the thoracic cavity and the external environment, an open pneumothorax results. This communication between the thoracic cavity and atmospheric air may lead to preferential influx of air through the chest wall defect as the path of least resistance. Although most penetrating injuries will seal off, larger defects may remain open, with immediate equilibration between atmospheric and intrathoracic pressures. This causes rapid collapse of the lung on the affected side and potentially the

inability to adequately ventilate the uninjured lung. The ipsilateral clinical signs are those of a pneumothorax:

- absent or reduced breath sounds;
- resonant percussion note;
- decreased expansion;
- physical evidence of a penetrating chest wall injury.

Immediate treatment is coverage of the defect with either an Asherman chest seal or a sterile waterproof dressing secured on three sides to act as a flutter valve as a first aid measure. Tube thoracostomies should be placed away from the open wound. Surgical debridement and closure of the wound will be necessary later, and consideration should be given to anti-tetanus protection (for the non-immune) and antibiotic therapy.

MASSIVE HAEMOTHORAX

Massive haemothorax is usually caused by penetrating injury, but it can result from blunt trauma. Life-threatening haemothorax can be due to major lung parenchymal laceration, injury to the pulmonary hilum or direct cardiac laceration. Each hemithorax can accommodate more than half of a patient's blood volume before physical signs become obvious.[18] As well as causing hypotension due to blood loss, a massive haemothorax will also occupy space in the thoracic cavity normally occupied by lung, and the subsequent lung collapse will result in hypoxia. The signs of massive haemothorax are those of hypovolaemic shock together with, on the ipsilateral side:

- dullness to percussion;
- absent or reduced breath sounds;
- decreased expansion.

Immediate treatment begins by achieving large-calibre intravenous access. This must be accomplished before any attempt is made to drain a massive haemothorax. Emergency blood transfusion should be considered early and may necessitate the use of universal donor units until type-specific or fully cross-matched blood is available. Fluid resuscitation should be considered in patients with severe hypotension to ensure adequate organ perfusion. However, until a significant cardiac or vascular injury has been ruled out, the systemic pressure should not be allowed to rise uncontrollably, as this may precipitate further haemorrhage (Chapter 8).

As with pneumothoraces, a haemothorax will require open or tube thoracostomy to allow the lung to reinflate, thereby improving ventilation and oxygenation. A large-bore intercostal drain will be necessary to allow drainage of blood. Initial drainage of greater than 1500 mL of blood, or continuing drainage of 200 mL (3 mL/kg) per hour, indicates the need for an urgent cardiothoracic opinion for consideration of thoracotomy.[19] A temporary chest drain clamp may be appropriate in the interim period before emergency thoracic surgery can be carried out to allow a tamponade effect in the pleural space in order to diminish continued life-threatening haemorrhage. However, this intervention must be balanced against the need to maintain adequate ventilation and oxygenation.

> Always gain intravenous access before draining a suspected massive haemothorax.

FLAIL CHEST

Severe direct chest wall injury may cause extensive disruption, with multiple rib and sternal fractures. When a segment of chest wall loses bony continuity with the thoracic cage, in other words two or more adjacent ribs are broken in two or more places, it becomes flail and will move paradoxically inwards on respiration, reducing tidal volume and compromising ventilation. The principal cause of hypoxia with flail chest, however, is the inevitable accompanying pulmonary contusion. The associated multiple rib fractures may also be accompanied by significant blood loss (estimate approximately 100 mL per rib).

The diagnosis of a flail segment is usually clinical, by observation of abnormal chest wall movement and the palpation of crepitus. Splinting from chest wall muscular spasm may mask the paradoxical movement, and the diagnosis is not uncommonly delayed until these muscles relax from exhaustion. The chest radiograph will not always reveal rib fractures or costochondral separation. An anterior flail chest can be particularly difficult to diagnose, as paradoxical movement (although present) is hard to detect when movement appears symmetrical. A brief and careful inspection from a low level, looking along the chest from the feet, is helpful. The possibility of a central flail should be considered particularly in patients who have sustained steering wheel injuries.

Pain reduces the patient's tidal volume, leading to inadequate ventilation of the basal segments, resulting in atelectasis. Pain also inhibits coughing, allowing secretions to obstruct bronchi and cause acute respiratory failure. Effective pain relief is therefore essential and may include the application of intercostal nerve or paravertebral blockade, although these techniques are most appropriately performed in a hospital setting. Splinting is not an effective management as this will reduce respiratory movement and exacerbate the ventilatory compromise. Operative fixation of rib fractures is very rarely indicated. In severe cases the patient will require intubation and mechanical ventilation. The use of non-invasive ventilation may also be considered.

> The key to management of a flail chest is timely recognition and early respiratory supportive care.

CARDIAC (PERICARDIAL) TAMPONADE

Pericardial tamponade is usually, but not exclusively, caused by penetrating trauma. Myocardial rupture or coronary artery laceration will result in rapid tamponade while more minor injuries, such as contusions, with slower extravasation, will result in a more gradual rise in intrapericardial pressure. Elevated intrapericardial pressure restricts cardiac filling and reduces cardiac output. As the intrapericardial pressure approaches ventricular filling pressure, coronary perfusion will cease, resulting in myocardial ischaemia, infarction and possibly cardiac arrest.

The characteristic features of elevated central venous pressure, hypotension and muffled heart sounds ('Beck's triad') are difficult to illicit in a noisy environment, especially in the pre-hospital setting. More importantly, the combination of a precordial entrance wound with profound hypotension and tachycardia is virtually pathognomonic of pericardial tamponade. The presence of neck vein distension is not a reliable sign as this may be absent in hypovolaemic patients. Low-amplitude complexes may also be seen on the ECG. Aggressive fluid resuscitation may mask the initial signs of a pericardial tamponade, as the temporarily elevated filling pressures achieved may overcome the effect of the raised intrapericardial pressures. However, in the later stages of tamponade, precipitous and profound hypotension will occur as this compensation fails.[14]

The ideal management of pericardial tamponade is surgical decompression and exploration, but pericardiocentesis 'buys time', may be life-saving and can be performed in the pre-hospital setting or the emergency department (Box 7.3). The removal of as little as 20–40 mL of blood can improve cardiac output sufficiently to allow preparations to be made for thoracotomy and surgery. The converse view is that it releases a tamponade without control of the bleeding and may take up valuable time that may be better spent preparing for an urgent thoracotomy. Release of pericardial tamponade is also the main indication for emergency thoracotomy in persistently hypotensive patients following thoracic trauma.[14]

Complications of the procedure include:

- misplacement into the ventricle;
- myocardial injury due to needle puncture;
- dysrhythmias;
- pneumothorax due to pleural puncture;
- puncture of the great vessels.

Potentially life-threatening injuries

Several other thoracic injuries can occur and, although they may not be immediately life-threatening, they may result in severe and possibly fatal complications if not detected and managed quickly. Careful examination may reveal these injuries although the clinical signs may be

Box 7.3 The technique of pericardiocentesis

- Administer high-flow oxygen, obtain large-bore intravenous access and monitor the ECG.
- The site of puncture is marked and cleaned: one finger's breadth inferior to, and just left of, the xiphisternum.
- Local anaesthetic should be infiltrated in the conscious/unsedated patient.
- A large cannula is attached to a 50-mL syringe via a three-way tap and short wide-bore extension.
- The needle is introduced at 45° to perpendicular, aiming towards the tip of the left scapula (Figure 7.5).
- The ECG is continuously monitored while advancing the needle and aspirating. The needle is partially withdrawn if ECG changes appear.
- As much blood as possible is withdrawn from the pericardium. This should be no more than 50 mL; larger volumes suggest intracardiac aspiration.
- Once completed, the capped-off cannula is secured in place.
- Thoracotomy should occur urgently and further aspiration may be needed in the interim.

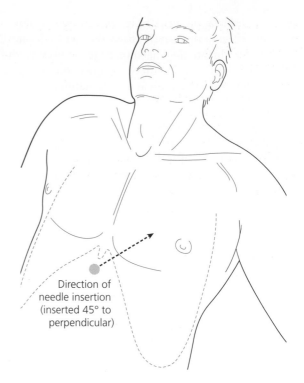

Direction of needle insertion (inserted 45° to perpendicular)

Figure 7.5   Location and direction for pericardiocentesis.

subtle. The mechanism and location of the trauma and observed patterns of wounding can alert the examiner to the presence of one of these conditions:

- cardiac contusion;
- aortic disruption;
- pulmonary contusion;
- simple pneumothorax;
- haemothorax;
- diaphragmatic rupture;
- tracheobronchial disruption and airway injury;
- oesophageal perforation.

CARDIAC CONTUSION

Cardiac contusion is the most commonly missed potentially fatal thoracic injury. It occurs when there is direct compression of the heart, or as a result of rapid deceleration. It is often associated with sternal fracture, and in such cases the right ventricle is more commonly damaged. The diagnosis can be established from the mechanism of injury, serial cardiac enzyme measurements, electrocardiographic changes and echocardiographic evidence of ventricular wall dysfunction and/or pericardial effusion.

Approximately 20% of patients with myocardial contusion suffer from dysrhythmias, including sinus tachycardia, supraventricular tachycardia and ventricular extrasystoles. It is also possible to develop conduction defects ranging from bundle branch block to complete heart block, which may require temporary pacemaker

insertion or external pacing. Myocardial contusion following blunt injury can lead to decreased cardiac contractility and ventricular compliance, resulting in a low-cardiac-output state due to myocardial failure. Cardiogenic shock is rare, but when it occurs conventional protocols should be followed. Associated coronary artery injury or injury to smaller vessels within the contused area can lead to myocardial infarction. Urgent surgical repair with cardiopulmonary bypass may be required in patients with valvular or ventricular septal trauma.

> Cardiac contusions may go unnoticed in the presence of more obvious associated injuries but can be diagnosed using bedside echocardiography in the emergency setting.

AORTIC DISRUPTION

Aortic injuries are immediately fatal in approximately 90% of cases. They occur in high-energy blunt trauma such as deceleration injuries, typically an RTC or fall from height. The aorta may be completely or partially transected, or may have a spiral tear. The commonest site of rupture is just distal to the origin of the left subclavian artery.

The diagnosis should be suspected in survivors of any high-energy chest trauma with a suggestive examination and radiographic findings (Table 7.5), although there is no pattern of skeletal injuries that accurately predicts this condition.[20] The patient may complain of chest and back pain, and examination may reveal absent or reduced pulses

Table 7.5 Radiographic signs consistent with aortic disruption

Widened mediastinum
Apical haematoma
Fractured first or second ribs
Elevation of the right main bronchus
Depression of left main bronchus
Loss of definition of the aortic knuckle
Tracheal deviation to the right
Left-sided haemothorax without any other obvious cause
Deviation of the oesophagus to the right (may be more easily
    seen with a nasogastric tube *in situ*)
Obliteration of the normal aortic window

distally with differential blood pressure between arms and legs. No single radiographic sign absolutely predicts aortic rupture, although a widened mediastinum is the most consistent finding.

Any suspicion of traumatic aortic disruption should prompt further investigation. Patients' survival after reaching hospital depends on early diagnosis followed by urgent surgical repair, unless special circumstances such as a severe operable head injury supervene, when aortic surgery may be delayed under the guidance of cardiothoracic surgeons. Prior to surgery the main objective is to control systolic blood pressure with appropriate medical therapy (for example, beta-blockers or vasodilators) in order to prevent rupture of the remaining flimsy adventitial layer, which would result in fatal haemorrhage. 'Permissive hypotensive' resuscitation may also reduce the risk of disrupting formed clot but may detrimentally compromise organ perfusion pressure elsewhere, particularly in the cerebral circulation.

> Control of the systolic blood pressure is essential in early survivors of traumatic aortic disruption.

PULMONARY CONTUSION

Patients with significant chest wall trauma are likely to have underlying pulmonary contusions. They develop clinically and radiographically over the first 1–3 days, but in severe trauma there may be signs of respiratory failure and radiographic changes such as patchy opacifications on presentation. Computed tomography (CT) is more sensitive than chest radiography for detecting early pulmonary contusions, and a normal early CT has been correlated with absence of later pulmonary contusion.[21] Initial treatment involves high-flow oxygen therapy, appropriate analgesia, judicious fluid replacement and physiotherapy. Serial arterial blood gas analysis should be performed. Mechanical ventilation may be required. Early arterial blood gas analysis may suggest the development of pulmonary contusions as well as providing a baseline for further therapy.

> Pulmonary contusion may present insidiously as respiratory failure several days after the initial injury.

SIMPLE PNEUMOTHORAX

The presence of air in the pleural cavity without penetration from the outside, or evidence of tensioning, constitutes a simple pneumothorax. The ipsilateral chest signs include:

- absent or reduced air entry;
- reduced chest expansion;
- increased resonance to percussion;
- visible air margin on plain chest radiograph.

A small pneumothorax may not be visible on a supine film and an erect, or semierect, chest radiograph should be performed in patients in whom there is clinical suspicion. Treatment of traumatic pneumothorax is by tube thoracostomy, which may be of the smaller 'Seldinger' type to reduce discomfort and scarring. A pneumothorax will increase in size proportionally to increases in altitude during aircraft flight, and tube thoracostomy should be performed before transfer in such patients, unless the aircraft can be pressurized to sea level during flight, but this is unlikely to be of consequence during low level helicopter evacuation.

> An early arterial blood gas analysis is mandatory in all victims of significant trauma.

HAEMOTHORAX

Blood in the thoracic cavity may result from lung laceration or injury to any of the great vessels or the chest wall vasculature. Signs include reduced chest expansion, dull percussion note and decreased air entry on the affected side, although these signs may not be detectable early on in the noisy pre-hospital environment or busy hospital resuscitation room. A supine chest radiograph may fail to identify a small or moderate quantity of blood in the hemithorax, as it will appear as diffuse shadowing instead of a distinct fluid level. An erect or semierect film should reveal blunting of the costophrenic angle and/or a fluid level. A haemothorax may coexist with a pneumothorax, in which case an air margin will also be seen on the affected side. Treatment is the insertion of a large-bore tube thoracostomy in the affected side.

DIAPHRAGMATIC RUPTURE

Penetrating injuries may cause small diaphragmatic perforations that are rarely of immediate significance. By contrast, blunt trauma may produce large radial tears of the diaphragm with subsequent herniation of abdominal viscera. The right hemidiaphragm is relatively protected by the liver, and left-sided ruptures are therefore more common, although if right-sided rupture does occur it has a substantially higher mortality.[22] Left-sided ruptures are more easily diagnosed because of the appearance of gut in the chest on radiography. Bilateral rupture is rare. It can complicate the clinical presentation of polytrauma cases as the combination of abdominal visceral haemorrhage and a diaphragmatic tear may generate excessive drainage from an open or tube thoracostomy, suggesting the need for urgent thoracotomy when, in fact, a laparotomy may actually be more appropriate

The chest radiograph can be misinterpreted as showing a raised hemidiaphragm, acute gastric dilatation or a loculated pneumothorax. Contrast radiography, or identifying an abnormal position of the stomach containing the tip of a nasogastric tube on plain radiography, confirms the diagnosis. In some centres, thoracoscopy is successfully employed, with up to 98% accuracy for diagnosis of diaphragmatic rupture.[23] Laparoscopy is also useful.

Repair of the diaphragm should not be delayed unless more urgent resuscitative or intracranial surgery is required. This is often performed through a laparotomy for associated abdominal injuries, but may equally be performed via thoracotomy or thoracoscopy. Preoperative insertion of a nasogastric tube is mandatory to prevent gastric distension and its sequelae. Pulmonary complications are common in patients undergoing surgery.

> Diaphragmatic rupture is often missed clinically and radiologically. Laparoscopy or thoracosopy are the investigations of choice.

TRACHEOBRONCHIAL DISRUPTION AND AIRWAY INJURY

Evidence of free air in the neck, mediastinum or chest wall, signified by the presence of subcutaneous emphysema, raises the suspicion of major airway damage. Laryngeal fractures, although rare, are indicated by hoarseness, subcutaneous emphysema in the anterior of the neck and local palpable fracture crepitus. Transection of the trachea or a bronchus proximal to the pleural reflection causes extensive deep cervical or mediastinal emphysema, which rapidly spreads to the subcutaneous tissues. Injuries distal to the pleural sheath result in pneumothorax.

Blunt tracheal injuries may not be obvious, particularly if the consciousness level of the patient is depressed. Penetrating injuries are usually apparent, and all require surgical repair. They may be associated with injury of adjacent structures, most commonly the oesophagus, carotid artery or jugular vein. Laboured breathing may be the only indication that there is airway obstruction.

Injury to a major bronchus is usually the result of blunt trauma. There are often severe associated injuries, and most victims die at the site of the accident. For those who reach hospital, there is at least a 30% mortality rate. Signs of bronchial injury include:

- haemoptysis;
- subcutaneous emphysema;
- tension pneumothorax;
- pneumothorax with a large and persisting air leak.

Most bronchial injuries occur within 2.5 cm of the carina and the diagnosis may be confirmed by bronchoscopy.

Severe bronchial disruption accompanied by vascular injury may result in systemic air embolism, which may become apparent only with positive-pressure ventilation or bag–mask ventilation, when the airway pressure overcomes the vascular pressure, allowing air to enter the pulmonary circulation. The consequences are catastrophic if pulmonary venous gas embolizes to the coronary vessels, heart chambers or cerebral arteries.

Endotracheal intubation (or the placement of a surgical airway) is warranted if the airway is completely obstructed or there is severe respiratory distress. The airway may be hazardous to secure and will require urgent senior anaesthetic input for fibreoptic intubation, or immediate tracheostomy, followed by surgical repair. Bronchial tears must be repaired on an urgent basis in the operating theatre, through a formal thoracotomy.

> Sudden circulatory collapse following initiation of positive-pressure ventilation may suggest major bronchial and pulmonary vascular disruption. It is typically unresponsive to conventional resuscitation and requires emergency measures to control air embolism, such as thoracotomy and clamping of the lung hilum.[12]

OESOPHAGEAL PERFORATION

Injury to the oesophagus is usually caused by penetrating trauma. Blunt oesophageal injury is rare, except with sudden compression causing a 'burst' type of defect. This can occur from a severe blow to the upper abdomen, when gastric contents are forced up into the oesophagus, producing a linear tear through which the contents are then able to leak. Mediastinitis, with or without rupture into the pleural space, with empyema formation follows. The clinical picture is identical to that of spontaneous rupture of the oesophagus, but the diagnosis is often delayed.

Treatment is surgical repair with drainage of the pleural space and/or mediastinum. In some severely debilitated patients, a trial of conservative treatment is appropriate. Aggressive, broad-spectrum intravenous antibiotic therapy should be employed immediately in all patients with oesophageal rupture.

> Contrast studies or cautious endoscopy will help diagnose oesophageal rupture.

Fluid resuscitation

Volume replacement is the cornerstone of treating hypovolaemia, although controlled resuscitation in thoracic trauma may often be appropriate. The first priority in treating ongoing significant haemorrhage remains the control of bleeding at source, accepting that in thoracic trauma this may require formal thoracotomy.

Trauma *per se* causes an increased capillary permeability, and pulmonary contusion in particular is characterized by leakage of tissue fluid into the alveoli, leading to pulmonary oedema and respiratory compromise. Excessive intravenous infusion may exacerbate the underlying injury and worsen hypoxaemia. Fluid should not be administered to victims of thoracic trauma if a radial pulse is palpable; if it is impalpable, 250-mL aliquots of fluid should be infused until it returns. In patients with penetrating thoracic trauma, the presence of a carotid or femoral pulse is considered adequate. In polytrauma involving the head, the main therapeutic intervention is the maintenance of satisfactory cerebral perfusion and tissue oxygen delivery.

The choice of resuscitation fluid remains controversial, with the first choice usually being a basic crystalloid such as 0.9% saline. Artificial colloids present a risk of allergic reactions and, while hypertonic saline may have a place in low-volume fluid resuscitation, it has not yet gained universal acceptance.

After initial resuscitation, fluid balance management in severe thoracic trauma is difficult as this represents a balancing act between keeping the patient intentionally dry to prevent pulmonary oedema or ensuring adequate circulatory volume in order to improve cardiac output and accepting that pulmonary oedema is inevitable. The decision of which organ system to prioritize at any one time is always a dynamic one.

> Hypotensive resuscitation to the restoration of a radial pulse is generally appropriate in blunt thoracic trauma: lower pressures are acceptable in penetrating chest injury.

Analgesia

Thoracic trauma causes hypoxaemia directly due to lung injury, but also indirectly through reduced respiratory movement secondary to pain. Adequate analgesia is essential. Opiates are the mainstay of analgesia in trauma and will usually be effective in thoracic trauma, although it is important to remember their negative effects on respiration and blood pressure. An alternative is the dissociative analgesic/anaesthetic agent ketamine, which better maintains cardiovascular stability.

Use of local or regional anaesthesia such as intercostal blocks, paravertebral blocks or epidural infusions can be invaluable for the relief of pain from extensive rib fractures. Epidural administration can provide better analgesia than intravenous morphine patient-controlled analgesia (PCA). However, epidural use may be difficult in the face of coagulopathy, thoracic spinal injuries and patients who are already sedated and mechanically ventilated. Elderly patients with multiple rib fractures may benefit most from epidural analgesia.[6]

The simplest regional method, an intercostal block, is safe and effective. It should be carried out at the level of the injury and at least two levels above and below this in order to adequately cover the region of the injury.[24] The technique is outlined in Box 7.4.

> Adequate analgesia is essential to maximize respiratory effort after thoracic trauma and is possible by many methods.

INVESTIGATIONS

Imaging is essential for accurate diagnosis of most of the conditions mentioned herein.

Plain chest radiography

A plain chest radiograph is the most important investigation in a patient with thoracic trauma and should be carried out as soon as possible during the initial assessment. All victims of penetrating trauma require urgent chest radiographs.[25] An erect film enables the best assessment of lung expansion and free air or blood in the chest cavity. Widening and shift of the mediastinum may be evident. Serious injuries such as pericardial tamponade, traumatic aortic disruption, ruptured diaphragm and major airway injury can usually be diagnosed from the chest radiograph.

Box 7.4 The technique for an intercostal block

- Select the appropriate intercostal level(s) to be blocked.
- Mark each injection point 8 cm lateral to the posterior midline (angle of rib).
- Clean the skin with an appropriate antiseptic preparation.
- 'Walk' the needle to just below the lower edge of the rib.
- Gently draw back to ensure you are not in one of the intercostal vessels.
- Inject 3–5 mL of 0.5% (5 mg/mL) bupivicaine in each space, remembering that the maximum safe dose of bupivicaine is 2–3 mg/kg (lean body mass).

In reality, the radiograph is often performed with a seriously injured patient in a supine, or at best semierect, position. Interpretation of a supine film has many pitfalls: small pneumo- and haemothoraces may be missed due to the air or blood being evenly distributed throughout the hemithorax; the mediastinum usually appears widened, leading to false-positive diagnoses of traumatic aortic disruption; and air under the diaphragm suggestive of a hollow viscus perforation may not be evident. Subcutaneous emphysema may further complicate interpretation. Multiple rib fractures, fractures of the first or second ribs or scapular fractures indicate that severe force has been delivered to the chest, highlighting the need for careful assessment for further unsuspected injuries. Pneumomediastinum, pneumopericardium or air beneath the deep cervical fascia suggests tracheobronchial disruption. Surgical emphysema of the chest wall with haemopneumothorax is generally indicative of pulmonary laceration following rib fractures.

Ultrasound and echocardiography

Portable ultrasound is increasingly being used and, although operator dependent, may be of considerable use in the diagnosis of pericardial and pleural fluid collections. By avoiding ionizing radiation, ultrasound techniques have the advantage of being repeatable as many times as required during the assessment and management of the trauma victim. The greatest benefit is in patients with blunt thoracic trauma, particularly suspected aortic injury, but it can also be used to evaluate intracardiac shunts, valvular injury and pericardial effusions/tamponade.[26]

Transoesophageal echocardiography (TOE) is an ultrasound technique that eliminates the false-positive finding of traumatic disruption of the aorta in patients with a widened mediastinum that commonly occurs on plain chest radiographs. There is evidence to support its use in patients with a high likelihood of aortic disruption based on mechanism of injury and clinical findings, in the presence of a normal chest radiograph,[27] but its usefulness is highly operator dependent. 'Blind spots' such as the aortic arch branches and distal ascending aorta may still be missed, accounting for up to 20% of lesions.[28]

The focused assessment with sonography for trauma (FAST) scan examines the pericardium for fluid and has largely replaced diagnostic pericardiocentesis.

Computed tomography

CT is particularly useful in aiding the diagnosis of aortic injuries. It is recommended as the first-line investigation of stable patients with low or moderate probability of aortic disruption, as it has a high sensitivity and specificity.[29,30] It also allows accurate detection of other thoracic injuries, and it is now common practice for most patients who have sustained significant thoracic trauma to undergo a CT scan of the chest at an early stage of their management, the urgency being dictated by the patient's clinical condition. The newer generation of machines are rapid such that the scan may be completed in a single breath-hold, and can accurately detect pulmonary parenchymal changes, such as haematomas, haemorrhage and changes consistent with acute respiratory distress syndrome (ARDS).

> CT scanning is extremely useful but should not delay or limit resuscitation or surgery.

Angiography

Angiography is the 'gold standard' for the diagnosis of aortic disruption and injury to major thoracic arteries. Almost all imaging is now performed by digital subtraction methods, allowing multiple projections of computer reconstructions of the vessel. However, it is invasive, takes a long time and requires a relatively stable patient. It should be used for investigation of patients in whom the likelihood of traumatic aortic disruption is high, and for those with a CT-confirmed diagnosis that needs to be further localized before surgery at the request of the cardiothoracic surgeon.

Thoracoscopy

Thoracoscopy in trauma is useful to evacuate retained (clotted) haemothoraces, visualize the diaphragm for traumatic ruptures, examine the pericardium, remove foreign bodies and to control intrathoracic bleeding.[14] More recently, its role in the evaluation of mediastinal injuries has been under scrutiny, although only certain patients are suitable and sufficient haemodynamic stability is a necessary precursor. Contraindications include suspected injuries to the heart and great vessels, blunt trauma causing contusion, widened mediastinum on radiography, massive haemothorax or continued bleeding, and inability to tolerate single-lung ventilation.[31]

Digital thoracotomy examination

Digital examination through an open thoracostomy incision into the pleural space may offer diagnostic clues (Table 7.6); it is best performed by an experienced emergency physician or cardiothoracic surgeon. It is part of the technique for tube thoracostomy and should always precede insertion of the drainage tube.

Table 7.6 Possible findings with digital thoracotomy examination

Finding	Clinical relevance
Tense pericardium with reduced cardiac pulsation	Likely pericardial effusion or tamponade
Pleural adhesions	Likely to be secondary to previous trauma or disease
Holes in pericardium or diaphragm	Traumatic injury to thoracic structures, cardiac laceration
Palpable abdominal organs	Diaphragmatic rupture

Laboratory tests

There remains no blood test specific for the assessment of the degree of myocardial injury following trauma. Creatine phosphokinase (CPK) and its myocardial band isoenzyme (CK-MB) are confounded by skeletal trauma and pre-morbid conditions to produce false-positive results. Although sensitive, markers such as troponin I and troponin T have yet to demonstrate specificity as indicators of myocardial contusion.[32,33]

EMERGENCY THORACOTOMY

Thoracotomy is an established procedure in the management of life-threatening thoracic trauma, but it is merely an access technique to allow other procedures to be carried out:

- evacuation of pericardial tamponade;
- direct control of intrathoracic haemorrhage;
- control of massive air embolism secondary to tracheobronchial disruption;
- open cardiac massage;
- cross-clamping of the descending aorta to limit subdiaphragmatic haemorrhage.

There are few indications for its application, and these are specific and evidence based. The procedure is associated with a high mortality and has the best chance of success if performed by an experienced surgeon. Survival rates are directly correlated with the patient's physiological status at presentation. In patients presenting with vital signs after penetrating thoracic trauma, survival from emergency thoracotomy has been quoted to be as high as 38%.[34] However, two large literature reviews have suggested that average survival rates range between 9.1% and 11.2% for penetrating trauma and between 1.1% and 1.6% for blunt trauma.[18,35] It should ideally be performed in an operating theatre, where survival rates are up to six times greater than for emergency department thoracotomy. The potential risk to medical staff includes exposure to blood-borne pathogens such as hepatitis or human immunodeficiency virus (HIV) in this maximally invasive procedure.[36]

Indications for emergency thoracotomy

Since its introduction, indications for emergency thoracotomy have become increasingly selective. The main indications for emergency thoracotomy are:

- cardiorespiratory arrest following isolated penetrating thoracic trauma with definite signs of life at the scene, before arrival in the emergency department;
- post-traumatic persistent hypotension due to intrathoracic haemorrhage, unresponsive to fluid resuscitation;
- persistent severe hypotension, with evidence of tracheobronchial disruption and systemic air embolism or pericardial tamponade;
- requirement for aortic cross-clamping for uncontrollable subdiaphragmatic haemorrhage.

Contraindications to emergency thoracotomy

Perhaps more important than the indications are the contraindications! There is no value in performing emergency thoracotomy in moribund patients with *blunt* trauma. Cardiopulmonary arrest 'in transit', or in the pre-hospital setting, is almost uniformly fatal following trauma,[37] and such patients arriving in the emergency department invariably die, despite all resuscitative attempts.[38]

The contraindications for emergency thoracotomy are:

- the absence of signs of life or a patient in asystole on arrival in the emergency department following blunt thoracic trauma;
- the absence of signs of life at the scene and on arrival, following cardiopulmonary resuscitation for more than 5 minutes;
- 'non-shockable rhythm' arrest for over 10 minutes;
- associated severe head injury or thoracic injury as part of severe multisystem trauma.

Absence of signs of life can be defined as a GCS of 3/15 with absent gag, corneal and pupillary reflexes and no electrical activity on ECG (asystole or ventricular standstill).[39]

Indications for urgent thoracotomy

The best results for thoracotomy are seen in those patients stable enough to undergo thoracotomy in the operating theatre. The indications are listed below:

- ruptured aorta;
- open pneumothorax;
- ruptured diaphragm;
- massive haemothorax;
- oesophageal injury;
- major airway injury;
- penetrating cardiac injury.

Emergency thoracotomy in children

Unfortunately, the hope that emergency thoracotomy may result in a more favourable outcome in children than in adults has not been fulfilled. Comparison of adult and paediatric survival rates shows remarkable similarities. The indications for emergency thoracotomy in children are the same as those currently accepted for adult trauma victims.[14]

Pre-hospital thoracotomy

The chances of survival of patients with thoracic trauma are greater if the time to definitive surgery is kept to a minimum, supporting the concept of 'scoop and run'.[40] On-scene thoracotomies have been abandoned by some,[41] though case series have shown some benefit. Pre-hospital

thoracotomy following loss of pulse should be considered if there is an appropriately experienced, trained and equipped practitioner present and the nearest surgical intervention is over 10 minutes away.[42,43]

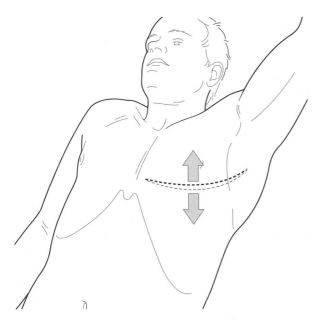

Figure 7.6 Location for emergency thoracotomy incision (left side).

Box 7.5 Technique of clamshell thoracotomy

- The patient is ventilated with 100% oxygen via an endotracheal tube.
- Intravenous (or intraosseous) access should be established, urgent blood transfusion requested and fluid resuscitation started.
- Whilst the thoracostomy tray is being prepared, don apron and sterile gloves.
- Patient is positioned supine with the side to be operated on elevated to 15° by a wedge and the arm abducted.
- Incise through skin and subcutaneous tissue in the fifth intercostal space, starting from the costochondral junction and passing out to the midaxillary line following the upper border of the sixth rib. The inframammary fold may be used as a guide.
- The muscle, periosteum and parietal pleura are then divided in one layer with scissors and blunt dissection. Chest wall bleeding is normally minimal although internal thoracic arteries may need to be ligated later.
- A suitable retractor is then inserted with the handle towards the axilla. Extra distraction may be obtained by dividing the sixth rib posteriorly.
- To extend the incision to the right side, use strong scissors, bone cutters or a Gigli saw to cut through the sternum and into the right fifth intercostal space, mirroring the incision above.
- A bulging pericardium is incised vertically over its anterior surface avoiding the phrenic nerves. The lung may need to be retracted posteriorly to identify the phrenic nerve.
- Place a finger over any cardiac defect, or place a sterile Foley catheter through the cardiac wound and inflate the balloon followed by the application of gentle traction to close the hole. Fluid may be directly infused into the heart if other venous access is unavailable; otherwise keep the catheter clamped.
- The myocardial defects can be closed with buttressed Vicryl sutures avoiding the coronary arteries. Further procedures are undertaken as necessary.
- Hilar clamping may be required in the case of significant lung laceration or air embolism from bronchial–vascular communication.
- Internal cardiac massage is best performed by compressing the heart between two flat hands in a hinged clapping motion. Defibrillate using small internal paddles either side of the heart with energy settings of 15–30 J (or biphasic equivalent).

Procedure for emergency thoracotomy

The best incision for use in emergency thoracotomy should be determined on the basis of the anticipated injury. The left anterolateral thoracotomy (Figure 7.6) is most frequently utilized for resuscitation but in isolation it affords relatively limited access to the thoracic contents and can best be regarded as an initial approach facilitating relief of pericardial tamponade prior to extension into a bilateral anterior thoracotomy (clamshell incision) (Box 7.5). Median sternotomy is the approach of choice for penetrating cardiac injury in the operating theatre; otherwise it is best avoided in the emergency department.

Following emergency thoracotomy the patient needs to be transferred rapidly to the operating theatre for further care. Lower systolic pressures ($\leq$90 mmHg) are acceptable, aiming for critical organ perfusion whilst minimizing risk of additional haemorrhage. Delivery of oxygen can be enhanced by optimization of haemoglobin levels by blood transfusion. Termination of resuscitative measures should be considered on the discovery of irreparable heart, lung or great vessel injuries or lack of self-sustaining rhythm within 15 minutes of starting the thoracotomy.

> Thoracotomies outside of the operating theatre should be limited to those for single penetrating thoracic injuries.

Case scenario

A 26-year-old man was riding a motorbike at 30 mph, swerved to avoid an oncoming vehicle and hit a parked car. The main impact was against the left side of his torso. When the paramedic crew arrived he was slumped against a wall with a bystander giving him first aid. He had removed his own helmet and loosened his jacket. He is pale, sweaty and breathing rapidly with a bleeding open wound and deformity of his left forearm. He is agitated with a respiratory rate of 40. His left chest is bruised, expanding less, has decreased air entry and a high percussion note compared with the right.

What three interventions or procedures would you carry out initially?
The first priority is ensuring airway patency while attempting to maintain in-line stabilization of his cervical and thoracic spine. He is combative but tolerates being laid flat and a mask delivering 100% oxygen. You decide that he may have a tension pneumothorax and carry out a decompression needle thoracocentesis in the left second intercostal space in the midclavicular line with a 14G needle. Within a few moments his breathing rate improves and he becomes more settled. You arrange for careful transfer to the waiting ambulance with a log-roll onto a spinal board with head blocks and cervical collar, establish peripheral intravenous access and tend his arm wound with dressings and bandages. On arrival in the emergency department, the attending doctor organizes three sets of investigations.

What three investigations would you request?
The patient remains stable on arrival to the emergency department and chest radiography is carried out immediately. While the image is being processed the patient is reassessed with a repeat primary survey. A log-roll is performed, demonstrating no tenderness of the cervical or thoracic spine. However, in view of the mechanism of injury and potentially distracting thoracic and limb injuries, the cervical collar is left on. He is given analgesia with 10 mg of i.v. morphine, 1 g of i.v. paracetamol and a 1000-ml Hartmann's solution infusion started. The supine chest radiograph demonstrates a 3-cm rim of air around the left lung, no fluid level and the mediastinal width within normal limits. Patchy opacification of the left middle lobe is noted, consistent with early contusion. Third and fourth rib fractures are seen on the left but there is no flail segment. Arterial blood gases are within normal limits. Baseline blood measurements should also be taken, including full blood count, urea and electrolyte estimation and a random glucose measurement; a blood sample should also be sent to the laboratory for group and save.

What procedure would you carry out next?
With a blunt mechanism of injury, rib fractures and traumatic tension pneumothorax, thoracostomy with a wide-bore tube is the treatment of choice following needle decompression and high-flow oxygen therapy. Placement of the tube thoracostomy results in drainage of 200 mL of bloody fluid initially without further drainage. Chest radiography confirms correct placement of the tube and resolution of the pneumothorax.

Effective analgesia is essential, possibly involving regional anaesthesia such as a thoracic epidural infusion or a morphine PCA. Critical care input may be required with close monitoring due to the evidence of lung contusion. This case requires a low index of clinical suspicion for development of acute lung injury and secondary pneumonia or ARDS. Serial arterial blood gases should be carried out with regular chest physiotherapy. Respiratory support may be required over the next few days.

SUMMARY

Thoracic trauma is common and is usually the most important injury in multitrauma patients, with a high level of associated mortality. The management of thoracic trauma requires good pre-hospital, emergency, surgical, anaesthetic and intensive care decision-making.[6] A logical and systematic approach to examination, assessment and treatment is essential.

Treatment may be prolonged and the initial injury may become of secondary importance to the complications of systemic inflammatory response syndrome, acute lung injury, sepsis and multiorgan dysfunction syndrome. Continued audit of the delivery of care to trauma patients is vital in order to maintain standards and improve morbidity and mortality in the future.[44]

GLOBAL PERSPECTIVES

Much of the experience of severe penetrating thoracic trauma is gained from military medicine and from civilian trauma management centres in the USA and South Africa. During the Vietnam War, the probability of dying from a single assault bullet wound to the chest was 80%. The experience of trauma centres in Europe and the UK mostly involves thoracic injury as a feature of blunt multitrauma from RTCs. However, it has been recognized that there is a growing trend in violent crime in the UK involving stabbing weapons and firearms, which may increase the burden of penetrating thoracic trauma care in the near future.

REFERENCES

1.   Breasted JH. *The Edwin Smith surgical papyrus*. Chicago: University of Chicago Press, 1930.

2.   LoCicero J, Mattox KL. Epidemiology of chest trauma. *Surg Clin North Am* 1989;**69**:15–19.

3.   Odell JA. Thoracotomy. In: Westaby S, Odell JA, eds. *Cardiothoracic Trauma*. London: Arnold, 1999, pp. 138–46.

4.   Westaby S. The pathophysiology of chest trauma. In: Westaby S, Odell JA, eds. *Cardiothoracic Trauma*. London: Arnold, 1999, pp. 3–22.

5.   Leppaniemi AK. Thoracoscopy in chest trauma: an update. *Trauma* 2001;**3**:111–17.

6.   Shirley PJ. Trauma and critical care III: chest trauma. *Trauma* 2005;**7**:133–42.

7.   Phelan PD, Olinsky A, Robertson CF. Lung growth and development. In: *Respiratory Illness in Children*, 4th edn, Vol. 1. Oxford: Blackwell Science, 1994, pp. 1–7.

8.   Asensio JA, Arroyo H, Veloz W *et al*. Penetrating thoracoabdominal injuries: ongoing dilemma – which cavity and when? *World J Surg* 2002;**26**:539–43.

9.   Rooney SJ, Hyde JAJ, Graham TR. Chest injuries. In: Driscoll P, Skinner D, Earlham R, eds. *ABC of Major Trauma*, 3rd edn. London: BMJ Books, 2000, pp. 16–26.

10.   Lavery GG, Lowry KG. Management of blast injuries and shock lung. *Curr Opin Anaesthesiol* 2004;**17**:151–7.

11.   Kemmer WT, Eckert WG, Gathright JB, *et al*. Patterns of thoracic injuries in fatal traffic accidents. *J Trauma* 1961;**1**:595.

12.   Hunt PA, Greaves I, Owens WA. Emergency thoracotomy in thoracic trauma – a review. *Injury* 2006;**37**:1–19.

13.   Yee ES, Verrier ED, Thomas AN. Management of air embolism in blunt and penetrating trauma. *J Thorac Cardiovasc Surg* 1983;**85**:661–8.

14.   Trunkey DD. Initial treatment of patients with extensive trauma. *N Engl J Med* 1991;**324**:1259–63.

15.   Demetriades D, Chan I, Cornwell E *et al*. Paramedic vs private transport of trauma patients. *Arch Surg* 1996;**131**:133–8.

16.   Gervin AS, Fisher RP. The importance of prompt transport in salvage of patients with penetrating heart wounds. *J Trauma* 1982;**22**:443.

17.   Hodgetts TJ, Mahoney PF, Russell MQ, Byers M. ABC to <C>ABC: redefining the military trauma paradigm. *Emerg Med J* 2006;**23**:745–6.

18.   Biffl WL, Moore EE, Harken AH. Emergency department thoracotomy. In: Mattox KL, Feliciano DV, Moore EE, eds. *Trauma*, 4th edn. New York: McGraw-Hill, 2000, p. 245.

19.   Wall Jr MJ, Storey JH, Mattox KL. Indications for thoracotomy. In: Mattox KL, Feliciano DV, Moore EE, eds. *Trauma*, 4th edn. New York: McGraw-Hill, 2000, p. 473.

20.   Lee J, Harris JH, Duke JH, Williams JS. Non correlation between thoracic skeletal injuries and acute traumatic aortic tear. *J Trauma* 1997;**43**:400–4.

21.   Schild HH, Strunk H, Weber W, *et al*. Pulmonary contusion: CT vs plain radiographs. *J Comput Assist Tomogr* 1989;**13**:417–20.

22.   Epstein LL, Lempke RE. Rupture of the right hemidiaphragm due to blunt trauma. *J Trauma* 1968;**8**:19.

23.   Villavicencio RT, Aucar JA, Wall MJ. Analysis of thoracoscopy in trauma. *Surg Endosc* 1999;**13**:3–9.

24.   Fouche Y, Tarantino DP. Anaesthetic considerations in chest trauma. *Chest Surg Clin North Am* 1997;**7**:227–38.

25.   Bokhari F, Brakenridge S, Nagy K, *et al*. Prospective evaluation of the sensitivity of physical examination in chest trauma. *J Trauma* 2002;**53**:1135–8.

26.   Mattox K, Wall M. Newer diagnostic measures and emergency management. *Chest Surg Clin North Am* 1997;**7**:213–26.

27.   Vignon P, Lagrange P, Boncooeur MP, *et al*. Routine transoesophageal echocardiography for the diagnosis of aortic disruption in patients without enlarged mediastinum. *J Trauma* 1997;**42**:969–72.

28.   Ahrar K, Smith DC, Bansal RC, Razzouk A, Catalano RD. Angiography in blunt thoracic aortic injury. *J Trauma* 1997;**42**:665–9.

29.   Gavant ML, Menke PG, Fabian T, *et al*. Blunt traumatic aortic rupture: detection with helical CT of the chest. *Radiology* 1995;**197**:125–33.

30.   Biquet JF, Dondelinger RF, Roland D. Computed tomography of thoracic aortic trauma. *Eur Radiol* 1996;**6**:25–9.

31.   Graeber GM. Thoracoscopy and chest trauma: its role. In: Westaby S, Odell J, eds. *Cardiothoracic Trauma*. London: Arnold, 1999, pp. 110–18.

32.   Hamm CW, Katus HA. New biochemical markers for myocardial cell injury. *Curr Opin Cardiol* 1995;**10**:355–60.

33.   Mair P, Mair J, Koller J, *et al*. Cardiac troponin T release in multiply injured patients. *Injury* 1995;**26**:439–43.

34.   Baxter BT, Moore EE, Moore JB, *et al*. Emergency department thoracotomy following injury: critical determinants for patient salvage. *World J Surg* 1988;**12**:671–5.

35.   American College of Surgeons – Committee on Trauma (Working Group, Ad Hoc Subcommittee on Outcomes). Practice management guidelines for emergency department thoracotomy. *J Am Coll Surg* 2001;**193**:303–9.

36.   Bowley DMG, Robertson SJ, Boffard KD, Bhagwanjee S. Resuscitation and anaesthesia for penetrating trauma. *Curr Opin Anaesthesiol* 2003;**16**:165–71.

37.   Grove CA, Lemmon G, Anderson G, McCarthy M. Emergency thoracotomy: appropriate use in the resuscitation of trauma patients. *Am Surg* 2002;**68**:313–16.

38.   Durham LA, Richardson RJ, Wall MJ, *et al*. Emergency centre thoracotomy: impact of prehospital resuscitation. *J Trauma* 1992;**32**:775–9.

39.   Lorenz HP, Steinmetz B, Lieberman J, *et al*. Emergency thoracotomy: survival correlates with physiological status. *J Trauma* 1992;**32**:780–8.

40.   Smith JP, Bodai BI, Hill AS, Frey CF. Prehospital stabilization of the critically injured patient: a failed concept. *J Trauma* 1985;**25**:65–70.

41.   Purkiss S, Williams N, Cross F, *et al*. Efficacy of urgent thoracotomy for trauma in patients attended by a helicopter emergency medical service. *J R Coll Surg Edin* 1994;**39**:289–91.

42.   Wall MJ Jr, Pepe PE, Mattox KL. Successful roadside resuscitative thoracotomy: case report and literature review. *J Trauma* 1994;**136**:131–4.

43.   Coats TJ, Keogh S, Clark H, *et al*. Prehospital resuscitative thoracotomy for cardiac arrest after penetrating trauma: rationale and case series. *J Trauma* 2001;**50**:670–3.

44.   Brooks AJ, Sperry D, Riley B, Girling KJ. Improving performance in the management of severely injured patients in critical care. *Injury* 2005;**36**:310–16.

Shock

After completing this chapter the reader will:
- be able to define shock
- understand the physiological mechanisms responsible for tissue oxygen delivery
- understand the cellular effects of shock
- understand the body's compensatory responses during shock
- understand the mechanisms of shock following trauma
- be able to recognize, assess and grade the level of shock
- demonstrate a structured approach in the initial management of the shocked trauma patient.

INTRODUCTION

Shock is defined as a clinical state of inadequate organ perfusion and tissue oxygenation. This leads to anaerobic metabolism, the activation of complex cellular and immune-mediated pathways and cellular damage.[1]

Following trauma, shock in the emergency department is often due, in part, to hypovolaemia. However, it is important to be aware that it can arise in delayed presentations from an increase in oxygen demand, for example following sepsis.

CARDIOVASCULAR PHYSIOLOGY

The body normally maintains adequate tissue delivery of oxygen by regulating blood flow and oxygen transportation. The physiological mechanisms preserving these factors need to be appreciated in order to understand the diagnosis and treatment of shock.

Circulatory control

REGIONAL ORGAN PERFUSION

Blood flow through many organs, particularly the kidneys and brain, remains almost constant over a range of blood pressures as a result of organ autoregulation. This is facilitated by changing smooth muscle tone within the arteriolar walls and precapillary sphincters. Arteriolar diameter therefore changes to maintain cellular blood supply as the pressure falls. In addition to the key part played by sympathetic innervation in this regulation, the accumulation of metabolic byproducts, such as H^+ ions, CO_2 and hypoxia, causes a direct relaxant effect on the arterioles.

CARDIAC OUTPUT

The cardiac output (CO) is the volume of blood ejected per ventricle per minute and equates to the product of the stroke volume (SV) and heart rate (HR). In health, typical adult values lie between 4 and 6 litres per minute.

$$CO = SV \times HR$$

The factors that influence cardiac output are directly attributable to its derivation and include those affecting the stroke volume (i.e. preload, myocardial contractility, afterload) and those determining the heart rate.

Factors influencing stroke volume

PRELOAD

This is the volume of blood in the ventricle at the end of diastole. The left ventricular end-diastolic volume (LVEDV) is around 140 mL and the SV 90 mL. Consequently, the end-systolic volume is approximately 50 mL and the left ventricular ejection fraction (SV/EDV) ranges from 50% to 70%.

The greater the preload, the greater the degree of stretch during diastole from the venous return to the heart. This generates an increased force of muscle contraction, elevating the subsequent SV according to Starling's law. However, if the muscle stretch exceeds a critical level, the force of contraction declines and eventually ventricular failure ensues.

The venous network acts as a reservoir for over 50% of the circulating volume. The amount of blood stored is proportional to the size of the vessel lumen, which is controlled by the interplay between local factors and sympathetic tone. A change from minimal to maximal tone, in an adult, can reduce the venous capacitance by approximately 1 litre. Conversely, the dilatation produced by a total loss of tone results in the insufficiency of the normal blood volume to fill it (see Neurogenic shock, p. 88). This, in turn, will lead to a reduction in venous return to the heart.

MYOCARDIAL CONTRACTILITY

Positive inotropes, such as the catecholamines, increase myocardial contractility for a given resting muscle fibre length and, thereby, shift the Starling curve to the left. Antidysrhythmic, anaesthetic and sedative preparations can have a negatively inotropic action. Importantly, in the trauma patient, many of the physiological states resulting from shock, e.g. hypoxia, acidosis and sepsis, also depress myocardial contractility.

AFTERLOAD

This is the resistance opposing the ventricular myocardial ejection of blood. It is significantly different for the two ventricles:

* Left ventricular afterload is mainly due to the resistance offered by the aortic valve and systemic arterial blood vessels and is known as the systemic vascular resistance (SVR).
* Right ventricular afterload is mainly due to the pulmonary blood vessels and is termed the pulmonary vascular resistance (PVR). In the non-diseased state the pulmonary valve has only a small effect.

The walls of the aorta and other large arteries contain a relatively large amount of elastic tissue that stretches during systole and recoils during diastole. The walls of arterioles contain relatively more sympathetically innervated smooth muscle, which is responsible for the α-adrenoceptor-mediated maintenance of vasomotor tone. A combination of local factors and sympathetic innervation continuously influences the arterial system to ensure delivery of blood to where it is most needed. This is exemplified in the shocked patient, in whom differential vasoconstriction maintains supply to the vital organs (brain, heart, kidneys) at the expense of others (skin and gut).

When the afterload is reduced, for example following arterial vasodilatation, and preload maintained, the ventricles contract more quickly and extensively, thereby increasing stroke volume and cardiac output. A good example of this is seen in the patient in the early phase of septic shock. The resulting clinical picture is one of a pink, warm (vasodilated and normovolaemic) patient with a bounding pulse due to the increase in cardiac output.

Factors influencing heart rate

Increases in heart rate, termed positively chronotropic effects, are mediated, both directly and indirectly, by the sympathetic division of the autonomic nervous system. Conversely, stimulation of the parasympathetic division, via the vagus nerve, exerts a negatively chronotropic effect, decreasing the heart rate. Pharmacological inhibition of the sympathetic response, for example with beta-blockers, will also result in a decreased heart rate.

An increase in heart rate usually increases cardiac output at the expense of the duration of diastole, which is the time taken for ventricular filling and myocardial perfusion. If the heart rate continues to increase, diastole is eventually reduced to the point at which filling is compromised and stroke volume and cardiac output decrease. Similarly, as the heart rate falls, the point at which no further filling can occur is reached and cardiac output declines. In the 'normal' healthy individual, stroke volume is relatively unaffected at heart rates between 40 and 150 beats per minute. This range may be considerably reduced by age, pathology and medication, such that a heart rate well within this range may not be tolerated.

PATHOPHYSIOLOGY OF OXYGEN DELIVERY

Interruption of the perfusion of tissues with oxygenated blood is a fundamental process in the pathophysiology of shock. It is therefore important to understand the mechanisms that maintain its integrity in health.

Tissue oxygen delivery (DO_2) is the product of the oxygen content of arterial blood (CaO_2) and the cardiac output. In health, this equates to 500–720 mL/min/m^2.

$$DO_2 = CaO_2 \times CO$$

The DO_2 is, therefore, dependent on the following factors:

* the ability of the lungs to take up oxygen;
* the oxygen-carrying capacity of the blood;
* the cardiac output;
* haemoglobin concentration;
* tissue oxygen consumption;
* blood flow.

The oxygen-carrying capacity of the blood

Blood has a haemoglobin concentration of approximately 15 g/100 mL with, normally, each fully saturated gram (expressed as a proportion with 1 being fully saturated[1]) of haemoglobin carrying 1.34 mL of oxygen. Thus, the oxygen-carrying capacity of fully saturated blood is:

$$Hb\ (15) \times 1.34 \times Hb\ saturation\ (approx.\ 1)$$
$$= 20.1\ mL\ O_2/100\ mL\ of\ blood$$

The relationship between the partial pressure of oxygen available (PaO_2) and haemoglobin oxygen uptake is not linear. This is because the addition of each O_2 molecule to the haem complex facilitates the uptake of the next, producing the sigmoid-shaped oxyhaemoglobin dissociation curve (Figure 8.1).[1] In the normal healthy state, haemoglobin is 97.5% (0.97) saturated at a PaO_2 of 13.4 kPa (100 mmHg). It follows from this curve that further increasing the PaO_2 has little effect on the oxygen-carrying capacity.

An increase in the affinity of haemoglobin for oxygen at a particular PaO_2 means that oxygen is more actively retained, resulting in a leftward shift of the dissociation curve. This is caused by:

- a decrease in H^+ ion concentration (increased pH);
- a decrease in $PaCO_2$;
- a decrease in the concentration of red cell 2,3-diphosphoglycerate (2,3-DPG);
- a decrease in temperature.

At the tissue level, the partial pressure gradient of oxygen is opposite to that found in the alveolar–capillary interface. This drives oxygen from the capillaries into the cells. Normally, intracellular PO_2 averages only 3–3.5 kPa but may be as low as 0.8 kPa. Furthermore, local factors reduce

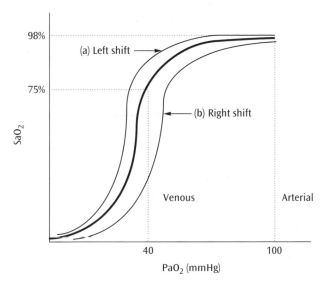

Figure 8.1 The oxyhaemoglobin dissociation curve (thick line). Normal values of haemoglobin oxygen saturation (So_2, %) and partial pressure of oxygen in blood (Po_2, mmHg) are given for arterial and venous blood. The effects of (a) left and (b) right shift in the dissociation curve are shown.

the affinity of haemoglobin for oxygen (shifting the curve to the right), allowing O_2 to be more readily released.

Haemoglobin concentration

The normal haemoglobin concentration (as measured by the haematocrit) is usually just above the point for optimal oxygen transportation (approximately 10 g/dL). Consequently, a slight fall in haemoglobin concentration will actually facilitate oxygen transportation by decreasing blood viscosity.

Approximately 60 times less oxygen is dissolved in the plasma than is combined with haemoglobin. This amount, 0.003 mL/100 mL blood/mmHg, is directly proportional to the PaO_2. Consequently, the total content of oxygen in the blood is equal to the haemoglobin-associated proportion plus the small amount dissolved in the plasma.

Tissue oxygen concentration

In the healthy resting state, the tissues use only 20–25% of the available oxygen. This is known as the oxygen extraction ratio (OER). Thus, body tissues have a tremendous potential to extract more oxygen from the circulating blood. In a healthy subject, the VO_2 remains constant and any increased oxygen demand is met by increasing delivery, usually via a rise in the cardiac output. In the trauma patient with reduced haemoglobin and cardiac output, this may not be possible and the VO_2 is then maintained by increasing the OER. However, this mechanism only operates to a critical level. Below this, VO_2 would then be directly dependent on DO_2 and would, therefore, begin to fall.

THE CELLULAR EFFECTS OF SHOCK

Normally after injury there is a proportional, compensatory, anti-inflammatory response, but this balance can be lost in severe, repeated or prolonged shock. It is also now accepted that certain individuals have a genetic predisposition to manifest these effects. This imbalance can lead to an exaggerated response, known as the systemic inflammatory response syndrome (SIRS).

Shock can give rise to SIRS because ischaemia, and the reperfusion of previously ischaemic tissue, initiates the release of toxic mediators (cytokines, complement, kinins, prostaglandin, leukotrienes and free radicals). Additionally, there may be translocation of gut flora into the circulation due to the breakdown of the normal gastrointestinal mucosal barrier following the compensatory splanchnic vasoconstriction.

In SIRS the inflammatory and anti-inflammatory responses coexist. This leads to further endothelial damage, disseminated intravascular coagulation (DIC), microvascular disturbances and accumulation of tissue leucocytes. These changes result in the sludging of red cells and stagnation of blood flow, further impairing tissue perfusion. In addition, the capillary hydrostatic pressure increases as blood can still perfuse but cannot escape. Consequently, further intravascular fluid is lost to the interstitial space through the leaky capillary wall. Generalized oedema is a good clinical marker of the presence of an inflammatory response and increased capillary permeability. The reduced DO_2 is further compromised by this sequence of events and decreased cellular oxygen consumption can be compounded by mitochondrial dysfunction. The end result of these cascading derangements is an imbalance between oxygen supply and demand, anaerobic metabolism and lactic acidosis.

In an attempt to reduce tissue damage, the body inactivates some of the unnecessary cells via apoptosis (programmed cell death). This mechanism does not augment the inflammatory response, but the presence of cell destruction (necrosis) does. Necrosis, superimposed on a background of ischaemia and reperfusion, is the major cause of cell, tissue and organ parenchyma destruction and the development of SIRS. This condition is one of the commonest causes of late death after trauma. There is also an increased susceptibility to infection.

The key target for the clinician is to avoid delay in correcting shock and, thereby, reduce the likelihood of SIRS.

Compensation

When a sufficient cell mass has been damaged, the shocked state becomes irreversible and the death of the patient inevitable. Fortunately, the body has several compensatory mechanisms that assist in the maintenance of adequate oxygen delivery to the essential organs and help prevent this stage from being reached.

The compensatory response is mediated by three mechanisms that regulate tissue blood and oxygen delivery:

- neurogenic – autonomic nervous system;
- endocrine – vasopressors/vasodilators, hormones (renin, angiotensin, vasopressin, catecholamines);
- inflammatory – cytokines, nitric oxide.

Systemic blood pressure

Blood pressure = cardiac output (CO) × systemic vascular resistance (SVR)

The systolic blood pressure, being the pressure exerted on the walls of the arterial blood vessels, is the maximal pressure generated in the large arteries during each cardiac cycle. Conversely, the diastolic blood pressure is the

minimum. The difference between these two parameters is the pulse pressure.

The mean arterial pressure is the average pressure during the cardiac cycle and approximately equates to the diastolic pressure plus one-third of the pulse pressure. As the blood pressure is the product of the CO and SVR, it is subject to the influence of all the factors that can potentially affect its constituent components.

Preservation of arterial blood pressure

Arterial blood pressure is normally tightly controlled by neural, humoral and metabolic mechanisms to maintain adequate blood flow and perfusion pressure to organs and tissues. Following a fall in arterial blood pressure a number of restorative mechanisms are brought into operation, including the following:

- Baroreceptors in the aortic arch, carotid sinus and heart stimulate the vasomotor centre to dampen down the vagal tone, while promoting sympathetic nerve stimulation to the heart, arteries, veins, adrenal medulla and other tissues. This response helps to maintain the blood pressure despite blood loss of up to 15%.
- The increased sympathetic drive results in vasoconstriction of most blood vessels, increased myocardial contractility and heart rate and the preferential preservation of vital organ perfusion.
- Peripheral vasoconstriction elevates the diastolic blood pressure, causing the pulse pressure to narrow.

Normally, an isolated fall in either cardiac output or SVR results in an increase in the other to maintain the arterial blood pressure. However, if hypovolaemia leads to a marked fall in cardiac output, arterial blood pressure will eventually fall, despite sympathetic activity causing positive inotropic and chronotropic effects on the heart and peripheral vasoconstriction. The clinical picture is of a pale, cold, clammy patient with a weak or absent peripheral pulse.

Following these neural effects, CO and SVR rise in an attempt to normalize the arterial blood pressure. Vasodilatation occurs in skeletal muscle arterioles (via sympathetically stimulated β_2-adrenoceptors) in keeping with the appropriate 'fight or flight' response.

In addition to these neurogenic effects the body also compensates in other ways:

- Selective arteriolar and precapillary sphincter constriction occurs in non-essential organs (e.g. skin, gut). This helps to maintain vital organ perfusion (e.g. brain, heart).
- Specialized cells within the juxtaglomerular apparatus of the kidney respond to a reduction in renal blood flow by releasing renin. This leads to the formation of angiotensin II, a vasopressor and stimulator of aldosterone production.

Aldosterone, secreted by the adrenal cortex, and antidiuretic hormone (vasopressin), released from the pituitary, increase reabsorption of sodium and water by the kidney, reducing urine output to help maintain the circulating volume.

In addition, insulin and glucose are released, promoting the supply and utilization of cellular glucose. The liver also attempts to enhance the circulating volume by releasing osmotically active substances that increase plasma oncotic pressure, thus reducing the osmotic gradient responsible for fluid extravasation from the circulation through leaky capillaries. As a result, CO and SVR rise in an attempt to restore arterial blood pressure back towards its homeostatic set point.

Oxygen delivery

Although sympathetically induced tachypnoea occurs, this does not result in an increased oxygen uptake because the haemoglobin in blood perfusing ventilated alveoli is already fully saturated.

In summary, many of the compensatory mechanisms in shock are catecholamine instigated via the increased sympathetic drive. This is reflected in the clinical features that the shocked patient displays: tachypnoea, tachycardia, reduced pulse pressure and the effects of reduced perfusion on the skin (pallor, sweating and coolness) and gut (leading to ileus).

MECHANISMS OF SHOCK IN TRAUMA

Impairment of each of the following can be responsible for shock:

- venous return;
- cardiac output;
- arterial tone;
- organ autoregulation.

The pathophysiological cardiovascular disorders responsible for the above impairments are categorized below (Figure 8.2):

- hypovolaemic;
- obstructive (impeding venous return, cardiac filling or ejection);
- cardiogenic;
- distributive (inadequate vasodilatation and vasoconstriction – for example in septic, neurogenic and anaphylactic shock);
- dissociative [impairment of haemoglobin oxygen uptake (carbon monoxide, severe anaemia) or impaired uptake of oxygen by cellular poisons (carbon monoxide, cyanide].

These can occur in combination. For example, a patient may be subject to the negatively inotropic effects of a myocardial contusion and be hypovolaemic following a road traffic collision (RTC). However, after trauma, shock usually has a hypovolaemic component, which is easily rectifiable and should be identified and treated before attributing shock to other causes.

When shock is due to major trauma, a reduction in the cardiac output is usually seen, but it may remain normal or increase in the patient with neurogenic or septic shock.

Impaired oxygen utilization is the common denominator resulting from all categories of shock; this progresses to cellular hypoxia, perpetuating cell dysfunction and death. Corrective measures must therefore be identified as being required and applied early

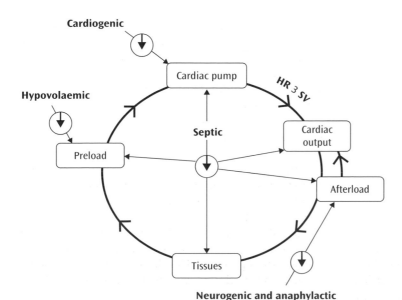

Figure 8.2 Types of shock and their impact on the circulatory system. ↓Decrease/negative effect.

by the clinician in order to minimize the resulting cell damage.

Hypovolaemic and obstructive shock

There are several potential causes of hypovolaemia following trauma. Besides blood loss, intravascular volume can be further depleted via plasma leakage through damaged capillaries into the interstitium. This can account for as much as 25% of the volume loss due to blunt trauma and can be even greater following burns. Irrespective of the cause, the end result in each case is a fall in venous return to the right atrium.

Another reason for impaired return is obstruction due to a tension pneumothorax, cardiac tamponade or massive pulmonary embolus. External thoracic or abdominal compression may also act to obstruct the venous return. In addition, high airway pressures in positive-pressure ventilation cause impedance to venous return, further exacerbating the shocked state.

In the relatively young, fit trauma patient, the compensatory mechanisms described earlier may minimize the effects on cardiac output and arterial pressure after an acute haemorrhage of up to 1–1.5 litres of blood (approximately 20–25% of the total blood volume). Tolerance may be much less in the elderly and those with cardiovascular comorbidity.

It is essential to remember that haemorrhage can be overt, when it is often overestimated, or concealed and commonly underestimated. Concealed haemorrhage occurs into either the body's cavities (thoracic, abdominal and pelvic) or potential spaces (e.g. retroperitoneal, muscles and tissues surrounding long-bone fractures).

Cardiogenic shock

This results from impaired cardiac function and can be caused by:

- cardiac contusion;
- ischaemic heart disease – which may have been the initial cause of the trauma;
- anti-arrhythmic drugs;
- underlying cardiomyopathy.

In cardiogenic shock due to the impact of myocardial trauma and/or ischaemia, the compensatory sympathetic response is often ineffective at restoring cardiac output and arterial blood pressure. The dysfunctional left ventricle is unable to increase its contractility and, despite a tachycardia developing, the cardiac output falls. A compensatory progressive increase in the SVR occurs in an attempt to maintain the arterial blood pressure. Both of these responses, the increased heart rate and SVR, increase myocardial oxygen demand and a vicious cycle

develops, resulting in further myocardial ischaemia and dysfunction.

With each episode of tissue hypoperfusion/hypoxia resulting in cellular destruction, mediators are liberated into the circulation, increasing the risk of SIRS. Cardiac failure is, therefore, frequently accompanied and complicated by autonomic, endocrine and inflammatory responses.

Neurogenic shock

Neurogenic shock results from reduced vascular tone. The sympathetic outflow emanates from the spinal cord between the levels of T1 and L3. A spinal lesion above T4 can impair the nervous system outflow from the cord below this level sufficiently to result in generalized vasodilatation (decreasing the afterload), bradycardia (T1–T4 sympathetically innervates the heart) and loss of temperature control. As this leads to a reduction in the blood supply to the spinal column, it exacerbates nervous tissue damage. In the presence of other injuries both the reflex tachycardia and vasoconstriction responses to hypovolaemia are eliminated.

Hypovolaemia does not occur as a result of intracranial bleeding. In the patient with a cervical cord injury and hypotension, it is essential that the hypotension is not assumed to be due to neurogenic shock. Any injury mechanism of sufficient energy to result in a cervical cord injury is likely to have produced significant injury and haemorrhage elsewhere. Consequently, in the shocked patient with a cervical cord injury, it is essential that any hypovolaemia is excluded before attributing the hypotension to a neurogenic cause.

Anaphylactic shock

In anaphylaxis, antigen-induced IgE-mediated release of vasoactive substances, including histamine, from mast cells causes generalized vasodilatation, reducing the afterload. A coexisting increase in vascular permeability causes fluid to leak into the extravascular space, further compounding this problem.

Septicaemic shock and systemic inflammatory response syndrome

Causes of septicaemic shock in trauma include bacterial translocation across the gut wall, wound infections, aspiration and gastrointestinal perforation.

Trauma is one of the major causes of SIRS, with tissue hypoperfusion, hypoxia and necrosis being the key precipitating factors. This is due to the inflammatory/anti-inflammatory mediators liberated into the circulation that are responsible for the distributive component of shock.

The mediators have a multitude of effects including:

- profound systemic vasodilatation;
- plasma extravasation through leaky capillaries, leading to hypovolaemia and oedema formation;
- depression of myocardial function in some cases;
- impaired tissue autoregulation;
- impairing cellular capacity to metabolize oxygen despite adequate oxygen delivery.

In patients with pre-existing ischaemic heart disease, or poor cardiovascular reserve, and in all patients with advanced sepsis, the situation is further aggravated by the negative inotropic effects exerted by toxins on the myocardium. The relatively high cardiac output, typical of septic shock, becomes compromised and a vicious cycle develops, accelerating the patient's demise.

Estimating volume loss and grading shock

The compensatory mechanisms evoked by shock are related to the decline in function of various organs. It is possible to divide the physiological changes of hypovolaemic shock into four categories depending on the percentage blood loss (Table 8.1).

Limitations in estimating hypovolaemia

Traditional methods of recognizing shock utilize assessment of the physiological response to hypoxia such as heart rate, blood pressure and respiratory rate. These have the advantages of requiring little equipment, permitting rapid, repeated measurement by numerous people with minimal training, and are easily understood. The response to blood loss is, however, not uniform.

Tachypnoea can indicate shock as well as underlying respiratory or metabolic pathology. A tachycardia often occurs early due to the sympathetic response. In grade 2

shock, the diastolic blood pressure rises without any fall in the systolic component, leading to a narrowed pulse pressure. This is due to the compensatory sympathetically mediated vasoconstriction. Consequently, a narrow pulse pressure with a normal systolic blood pressure is an early sign of shock.

A fall in blood pressure will take place only when no further compensation is possible and represents a loss of approximately 30% of the circulating volume.

> In shock, a fall in blood pressure is a late sign as it occurs when no further compensation is possible.

With some patient groups, undue reliance on the clinical signs alone might lead to a gross over- or underestimation of blood loss (Table 8.2). Consequently, it is important that management is based on the overall condition of the patient and not on isolated physiological parameters. Elderly patients are less able to compensate for acute hypovolaemia because of their reduced sympathetic drive, with the loss of smaller volumes resulting in hypotension.

> Use all the parameters to assess and quantify hypovolaemic shock.

A variety of commonly prescribed drugs can alter the physiological response to blood loss. For example, beta-blockers will prevent tachycardia and also inhibit the normal sympathetic positively inotropic response. Thus, a beta-blocked patient is unlikely to become tachycardic after a 15% blood volume loss but will become hypotensive at relatively low levels of haemorrhage.

An increasing number of patients now have pacemakers, and some types allow the heart to beat only at a particular rate irrespective of the volume loss, giving rise to the same errors in estimation of volume loss as occur in patients on beta-blockers. The physiological response to

Table 8.1 Clinical presentation of an adult with hypovolaemic shock[2]

Parameter	Category of hypovolaemic shock			
	I	II	III	IV
Blood loss (litres)	<0.75	0.75–1.5	1.5–2.0	>2.0
Blood volume loss (%)	<15	15–30	30–40	>40
Respiratory rate (per minute)	14–20	20–30	30–40	>35 or low
Heart rate (per minute)	<100	100–120	120–140	>140 or low
Capillary refill time	Normal	Delayed	Delayed	Delayed
Diastolic blood pressure	Normal	Raised	Low	Very low
Systolic blood pressure	Normal	Normal	Low	Very low
Pulse pressure	Normal	Low	Low	Low
Urine output (mL/h)	>30	20–30	5–15	Negligible
Mental state	Normal	Anxious	Anxious/confused	Confused/drowsy

Table 8.2 Pitfalls in assessing blood loss

The extremes of age
Drugs
Pacemakers
The athlete
Pregnancy
Hypothermia
Tissue damage

training will mean that the serious athlete will have a larger blood volume and a resting bradycardia (about 50 beats/min). A pulse of 100 beats/min may represent extreme compensation in these patients.

During pregnancy,[3–7] the heart rate progressively increases so that by the third trimester it is 15–20 beats faster than normal. Blood pressure falls by 5–15 mmHg in the second trimester, and returns to normal during the third trimester when the blood volume will have increased by 40–50%. Supine hypotension due to compression of the inferior vena cava may exacerbate shock and must be prevented by positioning, or insertion of a wedge under the patient, as part of the primary survey (see Chapter 16).

Hypothermia[8] will reduce the blood pressure, pulse and respiratory rate irrespective of any other cause of shock (see Chapter 20). Hypothermic patients are often resistant to cardiovascular drugs, defibrillation or fluid replacement. Estimation of the fluid requirements of these patients can therefore be very difficult and invasive monitoring is often required.

RECOGNITION, ASSESSMENT AND MANAGEMENT OF THE SHOCKED PATIENT

The state of shock is a temporary one – patients either improve or die. Shock can be viewed as *a momentary pause on the way to death*. It is during this pause that the trauma team must take the opportunity to prevent the further deterioration of the patient.

Given the definition of shock, its detection is reliant upon monitoring the consequences of this pathology on certain physical signs.[2] Furthermore, therapeutic intervention for shock must be aimed at restoring adequate oxygen delivery, rather than a normal blood pressure.

The ABC approach to patient assessment, diagnosis and management is paramount, and any information gained from pre-hospital personnel and/or family members is a vital part of this process.

Primary survey and resuscitation

In established shock, the patient will be pale, sweating and distressed, with distended or flat neck veins. However, in the early phases of shock, these clinical abnormalities may be absent and the patient may appear misleadingly well.

CONTROL OF CATASTROPHIC EXTERNAL HAEMORRHAGE

When life-threatening external bleeding is identified, it should be controlled immediately using pressure, elevation, a tourniquet or a topical haemostatic agent as appropriate (see Chapter 5).

AIRWAY AND BREATHING

The next step in the management of any shocked patient is to clear and secure the airway and ensure adequate ventilation with a high inspired concentration of oxygen to optimize oxygen delivery and uptake. Simultaneous immobilization of the spinal column in general, and the cervical spine in particular, should occur if the mechanism of the trauma suggests the potential for injury. The remaining five immediately life-threatening thoracic conditions should then be actively sought and treated when present (see Chapter 7).

CIRCULATION

Hypovolaemia is frequently the sole or principal causative factor of shock found in trauma victims. It is, therefore, essential to examine the trauma patient systematically and establish the location(s) of blood loss. Potential sites for haemorrhage are:

- external ('on the floor');
- chest;
- abdomen and retroperitoneum;
- pelvis
- long-bone fractures.

> Remember 'Blood on the floor and four more'.

Any overt bleeding should be identified and stopped by direct pressure and peripheral venous access gained. Central venous access or a venous cut down may be required if peripheral cannulation is not possible in adult patients.

Basic monitoring should also be commenced and vital signs recorded. The presence of a brady- or tachycardia should be sought. Vasodilatation accompanied by a bounding pulse is suggestive of septic shock. The presence of the radial pulse implies adequate perfusion of essential organs although it is not possible to derive a quantitative estimate of the blood pressure from the presence or absence of peripheral pulses. Additional information should be gained from recording serial pulse oximetry,

ECG, blood pressure and urine output measurements in all trauma patients.

Careful examination of the back is important to identify a posterior injury, and external bleeding into the confines of a splint should be excluded. Major bleeding into the chest should already have been identified during the 'breathing' assessment, but continued observation is necessary to exclude lesser degrees of haemorrhage. Palpation of the abdomen in the conscious patient, or the presence of visible distension, may indicate possible abdominal haemorrhage and the need for further investigation. Owing to the lack of sensitivity of abdominal examination, especially in the presence of other distracting injuries, a high index of clinical suspicion must be maintained based on the mechanism of the injury, physical signs elucidated and specialized investigations.

In the resuscitation room there is no need to spring the pelvis to provide evidence of disruption. An absence of positive findings does not rule out the possibility of pelvic fractures and does not negate the need for a pelvic radiograph.

Significant long-bone fractures, if not already identified, should become apparent during the 'exposure' component of patient assessment. Traction splinting of femoral fractures, in the absence of a pelvic fracture at the proximal point of purchase, decreases the space and volume for potential blood loss. The same rationale applies to the use of pelvic splints.[9] Realignment also facilitates patient analgesia and subsequent patient handling.

Retroperitoneal haemorrhage is invariably occult and may only become apparent once all other sites of bleeding have been excluded or controlled.

> Beware retroperitoneal haemorrhage.

Fluid resuscitation

The team leader's assessment should determine whether the patient's shocked state results from either controlled or uncontrolled haemorrhage. In the former, satisfactory haemostasis and patient resuscitation is achievable prior to any urgent surgery, and where possible blood should be used in these patients

If the bleeding is not controllable, immediate surgical intervention will be necessary and resuscitation should not be allowed to delay this. In these circumstances, no fluids need be given if there is a palpable radial pulse. If the pulse is lost or absent, boluses of 250 mL of crystalloid should be given until it returns. A measurable systolic blood pressure in the region of 80 mmHg is acceptable and avoids the pitfalls of overvigorous resuscitation. However, if there is a significant head injury, a systolic blood pressure of at least 100 mmHg should be maintained in order to promote adequate cerebral perfusion.

> Give fluids in 250-mL aliquots to maintain the presence of a radial pulse.

In cases of uncontrolled haemorrhage bleeding is usually into a major body cavity. Although arterial pressure tends to rise with aggressive, large-volume fluid resuscitation, adverse effects may result. These include dislodgement of haemorrhage-stemming thrombus and dilutional coagulopathy, which can both precipitate further haemorrhage. Hypothermia induced by the administration of cold fluids is also a risk.

All fluids given to trauma patients should be warmed, ideally through storage in a warming cupboard, prior to administration to prevent iatrogenic hypothermia, although this is now thought to instil a protective effect in head-injured trauma patients and cold fluids are being deliberately administered, in some centres, to this patient group. The use of warming coils increases the resistance to flow and prolongs the time required for fluid administration. Another alternative is the use of a level 1 device that rapidly delivers large volumes of warmed fluid although the caveats expressed above regarding the rapid administration of large volumes of fluid should be borne in mind and the device is probably best used simply as a fluid warmer.

It is likely that the administration of recombinant factor VIIa, used to manipulate/facilitate the clotting cascade, may in the future become a standard part of the resuscitation room treatment of severe uncontrollable bleeding, and it has been suggested that this may reduce mortality in trauma patients;[10] however, on the whole, the jury remains out as to how beneficial a treatment this is in this patient group.[11] Further research into this area is undoubtedly required.

What is clear is that shocked patients benefit dramatically from the early administration of blood products and local policies *must* be in place to allow the rapid provision of a 'shock pack' consisting of O-negative red cells and fresh-frozen plasma.

The evidence to support a policy of permissive hypotension is now reasonably strong.[12] For example, mortality among patients with abdominal aortic aneurysm rupture fell from 70% to 23% when preoperative fluids were restricted to maintain a systolic blood pressure of 70 mmHg. The evidence for this approach is far from conclusive in acute hypovolaemic shock. To decide which of these two management options (fluid resuscitation versus emergency surgery) is the most appropriate for each patient treated, an experienced team leader has to evaluate the pros and cons of each approach.

Coagulation abnormalities should be anticipated after massive blood loss due to the dilution of clotting factors by administered fluids. This is exacerbated by the release of tissue factors that inhibit clotting and the low concentration of clotting factors in stored blood.

At the end of the primary survey, the team leader must ensure that the identified tasks required have been/are being carried out. Venous and arterial blood samples should be taken and analysed. Anaerobic metabolism in poorly perfused tissues invariably generates a metabolic (lactic) acidosis. Appropriate management is aimed at:

- increasing cardiac output with fluid administration;
- optimizing PaO_2 and checking the patient is not hypercapnic to ensure adequate tissue oxygen delivery.

The principles of treating sepsis and SIRS are to provide support for failing organ systems and target any infecting organism with appropriate antibiotic or surgical therapy.

TREATMENT

Treatment of shock is subdivisible into the following components:

- control of external haemorrhage;
- intravenous access;
- fluid resuscitation – discussed above;
- investigations and monitoring;
- surgical intervention.

Initial haemostasis and control of external haemorrhage

It is easy to underestimate the extent of blood loss from external sources. A large amount of the evidence may be left at the scene and bleeding – especially from head wounds – can be insidious. Manual pressure applied to bleeding points will normally control venous bleeding, particularly when combined with elevation of the wound above the level of the heart. This is best achieved with the patient lying supine. When dealing with arterial bleeding, however, tourniquets are often necessary. Limb arterial bleeding is best controlled in the resuscitation room by using a sphygmomanometer cuff inflated above systolic pressure. Where this is not possible, a triangular bandage should be applied over the dressing covering the wound such that its knot lies above the bleeding point. If a rigid bar is then incorporated under the knot and twisted, increased pressure can be exerted.[13] Occasionally a topical haemostatic agent may be required (see Chapter 5).

> The time a tourniquet is applied should be clearly marked in the patient's notes so that inappropriately long limb ischaemia is avoided.

Control of external haemorrhage forms an essential part of the primary survey. In cases where the external haemorrhage is associated with compound fractures, appropriate splintage must be applied, although the timing of this must be judged according to clinical priority.

Intravenous access

PERIPHERAL

The largest cannula possible (ideally a 14G or 16G) should be inserted, preferably, in the antecubital fossa; in the shocked patient this can be difficult. The use of an elbow splint will improve flow and decrease the risk of complications, such as loss of the cannula, or clotting of the line. Short, wide cannulae are required as flow is proportional directly to the fourth power of the radius and inversely to cannula length. Ideally, a second cannula should also be placed, although other life-saving interventions should not be delayed while struggling to achieve this. Once intravenous access has been achieved, the cannula must be firmly secured (in the case of femoral or other central lines this means stitching it in place) and 20 mL of blood should be taken for laboratory tests [full blood count, urea and electrolytes, cross-match and, if clinically appropriate, glucose, blood cultures, clotting, pregnancy test (where relevant) and toxicology].

If peripheral intravenous access cannot be effectively achieved, access should be attempted via the femoral vein. Multiple, increasingly fruitless, attempts to cannulate ever smaller veins should be avoided, as should small-bore neck lines. Access to the neck is likely to be difficult due to the need for cervical spine immobilization following blunt trauma, the volumes of fluid which can be infused are small and the procedure is technically difficult. In addition, infraclavicular approaches are associated with a high incidence of complications, such as pneumothorax, which can be potentially catastrophic in the trauma victim. The femoral vein is, therefore, a better site although the external jugular is an alternative in experienced hands.

INSERTION OF FEMORAL VENOUS LINE

The groin is exposed and cleaned. Aseptic technique for ultrasound-guided line insertion is ideal and recommended.[14] The anatomical markings are the anterior superior iliac spine (ASIS) laterally, and the pubic symphysis. Half-way along a line drawn between these landmarks is the surface marking of the femoral artery. The femoral vein lies medial to the artery in a direction pointing towards the umbilicus (Figure 8.3).

In the severely compromised patient there is a degree of urgency in obtaining vascular access, therefore local anaesthetic infiltration over the puncture site may be omitted. The technique described, briefly, below is called the Seldinger method. There are various proprietary kits available for central venous access that differ in lumen number and calibre.

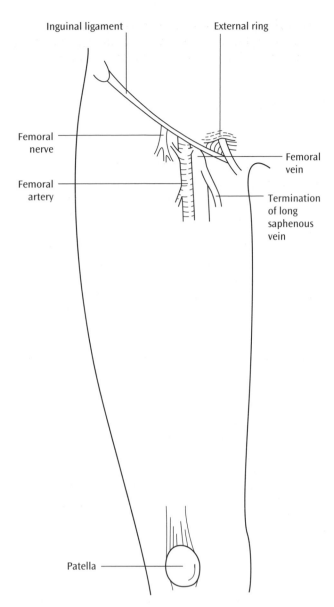

Figure 8.3 Anatomical landmarks for the insertion of a femoral line.

- A wide-bore needle attached to a syringe is inserted over the landmark described and the syringe aspirated until a constant flash-back of venous blood is obtained.
- The syringe is removed from the needle and a guidewire inserted down the needle into the vein. There should be no resistance to the passage of the wire.
- The needle is then removed, leaving the wire in place. The dilator is then passed over the wire and a small nick in the skin is made with a knife to allow easier passage. The dilator is removed, the definitive venous line is inserted over the wire, and the wire is then removed. The line can be used for blood collection and infusion. It is important to keep hold of the wire at all stages so as not to lose it!

In extremis, the insertion of a large-gauge cannula into the femoral vein provides a stopgap until a more definitive line can be placed. The presence of either a pelvic or femoral fracture is not a contraindication to femoral line insertion if this is the only practical option for the rapid infusion of life-saving fluids.

COMPLICATIONS OF PERIPHERAL AND FEMORAL VENOUS ACCESS

These include:

- failed cannulation;
- haematoma;
- extravasation of fluid or drugs;
- damage to adjacent structures;
- air embolism;
- damage to the cannula (usually due to attempts to reinsert the trocar into the cannula).

VENOUS CUT-DOWN

This procedure requires time, surgical skill and anatomical knowledge of the position of suitably placed vessels (antecubital veins, proximal and distal long saphenous vein). It is therefore a technique for experienced personnel in patients who have difficult vascular access when other techniques are used.

- Vascular access for the distal long saphenous vein is sited 2 cm above and anterior to the medial malleolus of the ankle.
- The site should be prepared with aqueous antiseptic solution and towelled to give the operator a sterile area. Local anaesthetic should be infiltrated along the line of the proposed incision in the conscious patient.
- A transverse incision is made over the landmark through the skin.
- The vessel is located and isolated from adjacent adventitia, taking care to avoid the saphenous nerve.
- Using a haemostat, two ligature ties are passed beneath the vessel. The distal one is tied, after which a clip is placed on the tie to allow manipulation of the vessel.
- A transverse venotomy is made and a large-bore intravenous catheter is inserted proximally.
- The proximal tie is then secured around the vessel and catheter, and the overlying cut-down wound is cleaned and dressed with a sterile waterproof dressing.

The complications of intravenous cut-down are similar to those of peripheral venous access.

INTRAOSSEOUS (IO) ACCESS AND INFUSION[15–17]

This procedure was originally used as a means of obtaining vascular access in children. It is now widely used in adults. It is fast, constant, relatively easy and enables fluid and drug administration. There are various anatomical sites, but the most common is the anterior surface of the tibia 2 cm below and medial to the tibial tuberosity or insertion of the patellar tendon. Potential complications of insertion include infection, fracture and growth plate damage.

A conventional intraosseous needle is inserted as follows:

- The site should be prepared with aqueous antiseptic and a small amount of local anaesthetic should be infiltrated into the skin and down to the periosteum of the conscious patient.
- A small incision is made in the skin and, using the intraosseous needle in a twisting and downwards motion, the device is inserted perpendicular to the skin. A loss of resistance is found on entry into the marrow cavity.
- The central trocar is then removed and blood withdrawn for haematology and biochemistry. A three-way tap connected to an extension line is then attached to the needle. This enables fluid and drugs to be administered (via the three-way tap) and so reduces movement of the needle, which is a bulky device and needs to be protected with suitable dressings to avoid displacement.
- A test bolus of 5–10 mL of saline is administered to ensure that the needle is patent and there is no tissuing of fluid. Subsequent infusion cannot rely on gravity flow alone. Instead syringe-administered aliquots are necessary to produce adequate flow rates.

However, in most cases of use in adults, some form of automatic insertion device (examples include the Bone Injection Gun® and EZ IO®) is used. Readers are advised to seek appropriate training on the device they intend to use.

SUBCLAVIAN AND JUGULAR LINES

The insertion of internal jugular and subclavian lines is a difficult technique with a relatively high incidence of complications that occur more frequently in inexperienced hands. In addition, if not performed by someone with considerable experience, unnecessary time can be wasted in the attempt. The narrow-bore lines conventionally used for this approach are not suitable for the rapid administration of fluids and are more appropriately reserved for subsequent patient monitoring. Ideally, these procedures should be performed using an ultrasound-guided approach.[14] For this reason, insertion of these lines blindly is only recommended as a last resort and only then by experienced clinicians (Figure 8.4).

Insertion of a low–approach internal jugular venous line

- The Seldinger technique is used.
- The patient's cervical collar is removed and the patient's head and neck held in neutral alignment. Some head-down tilt of the patient is helpful, but not mandatory.
- The landmark for insertion is the posterior border of the sternocleidomastoid muscle 2–3 cm above the clavicle.
- The needle is advanced just behind the muscle in a direction towards the suprasternal notch. The vein can be reached within the length of a green needle. The needle should be advanced in a straight direction, and if blood is not aspirated then a second pass is made. The advantage of this approach is that arterial puncture can be controlled by direct pressure, unlike the subclavian route.
- Once the definitive line has been inserted and secured, the head blocks and straps may be replaced. Owing to the low placement of the line, this does not interfere with the head blocks.
- A portable chest radiograph should be obtained before the infusion of large quantities of fluid.
- Whichever approach is chosen, it should be performed by experienced staff because of the potential for damaging the vein and neighbouring structures.

Insertion of a subclavian line

- The Seldinger technique is used after removal of the cervical collar and establishment of manual in-line stabilization.
- The area is cleaned and surgical drapes applied.
- The junction of the middle and outer thirds of the clavicle and the suprasternal notch are identified.
- The needle is inserted 1 cm below the clavicle, at the junction of the middle and outer thirds, and advanced towards the suprasternal notch, passing under the clavicle.
- The vein is usually located at a depth of 4–6 cm.

Complications of internal jugular and subclavian lines

These include:

1. arterial puncture;
2. haematoma;
3. haemothorax;
4. pneumothorax;
5. air embolism;
6. loss of the guide-wire;
7. cardiac arrhythmias.

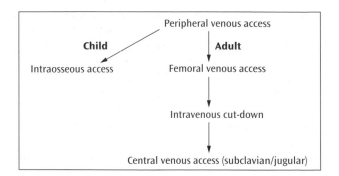

Figure 8.4 A flow diagram for intravenous access.

Table 8.3 Monitored vital signs in hypovolaemic patients

Respiratory rate
Peripheral oxygen saturation
Heart rate
Blood pressure
Pulse pressure
Cardiac monitoring
Temperature
Urinary output
Glasgow Coma Scale

ASSESSMENT AND MONITORING

The shocked patient's vital signs should be continuously monitored (Table 8.3).

Accurate measurement of urinary volume will obviously require the insertion of a urinary catheter. This should be connected to a system permitting accurate volume measurement that can be recorded whenever the other vital signs are measured.

Regular blood gas analysis is an essential component of the management of the shocked patient, allowing the haematocrit as well as the base excess and lactate to be monitored. These last two parameters provide valuable data, being predictive of prognosis, and can be used to evaluate the immediate metabolic status of the patient and the response to resuscitation.

The trend afforded by the repeated monitoring of vital signs also gives essential information regarding the patient's resuscitation status. A 'monitor for shock' providing accurate reproducible, universally applicable data has yet to be developed. Different approaches to attaining this goal have been made and include the use of a transthoracic ultrasound Doppler probe to approximately measure stroke volume; enteral capnography to estimate the reduced mesenteric blood flow due to circulatory diversion to the vital organs; and near-infrared oxygen spectroscopy[18] to determine the tissue oxygen concentration, e.g. in the muscle, gut and brain. Each of these has its advantages and disadvantages and does not, as yet, meet the criteria for a universal 'shock monitor'.

DEFINITIVE HAEMOSTASIS

The only appropriate end-point in the management of ongoing haemorrhage is surgery or embolization by interventional radiology. No procedure should be performed in the resuscitation room that might increase mortality and morbidity by delaying urgent transfer to a place where this can be carried out. Nevertheless, in some cases, procedures such as placement of an external fixator on an open-book pelvic fracture or, rarely, thoracotomy and cross-clamping of the aorta may be life-saving in the moribund patient.

Case scenario 1

A 64-year-old male delivery driver has been taken by paramedic ambulance to the emergency department after having been trapped between a wall and a reversing van. He is conscious, cooperative and maintaining a patent airway. Oxygen is being delivered at a rate of 15 L/min via a non-rebreathe mask. Spinal immobilization has been applied. On examination his respiratory rate is 30, the trachea is central, the chest is non-tender with equal expansion and there is equal bilateral percussion and air entry.

The patient appears pale, clammy and peripherally shut down with a capillary refill time of 4 seconds. Although there are no signs of external bleeding, the patient's lower abdomen and pelvis are markedly tender. Multiple large abrasions overlie this area. His heart rate is 110 beats/min and blood pressure 90/50 mmHg.

How should this man's circulatory disturbance be managed?

This man has been subjected to lower abdominal and pelvic trauma due to the crushing mechanism of his injury. He is maintaining his own airway and is receiving supplementary oxygen. At present there are no signs of intrathoracic pathology but they may coexist. A priority is to reduce any bleeding from his pelvis by the application of a splint. Controlled fluid therapy can then be started following the insertion of two peripheral lines aiming for maintenance of a radial pulse and a urine output of >30 mL/h. Definitive haemostasis will require either interventional radiology or surgery. Prompt pelvic radiography is therefore essential along with a request for specialist advice.

If he had a coexistent head injury, would his fluid therapy be different?

If this man had presented with a head injury in addition to those injuries described above, his fluid management would have differed. Fluid resuscitation in the hypovolaemic, head-injured patient is a balancing act (see Chapter 9). The desire is to temper the volume administered in the patient who is still bleeding prior to haemostasis; however, enough fluid needs to be provided in the head-injured patient to maintain cerebral blood flow and perfuse the brain. As well as the management already mentioned, he would require an urgent CT scan of the head, and possibly neurosurgical input. In general, hypotensive resuscitation is contraindicated in patients in whom the predominant injury is thought to be the head trauma.

Case scenario 2

A 23-year-old male motorcyclist has been involved in a high-speed RTC, finishing up 20 metres from his bike. His spine has been immobilized at scene. On arrival in the emergency department he has a GCS of 10 (eye opening 4, verbal response 5, motor response 1). He is receiving supplemental oxygen (15 L/min, via a non-rebreathe mask), has a respiratory rate of 10 and SpO_2 = 96%. On examination the trachea is central, the neck veins non-distended and there is equal bilateral chest expansion, percussion and auscultation and no sensation below the nipple line.

The patient appears pale and has cool peripheries, making peripheral access more difficult, but essential, to obtain. His heart rate is 50 beats/min, blood pressure 90/50 mmHg and the capillary refill time >4 seconds. No overt bleeding has been detected. Abdominal examination indicates the presence of an unstable pelvis.

What are the likely causes of his hypotension and describe its management?

The forces exerted on this patient, resulting from his high-energy injury mechanism, have been substantial and numerous. He is likely to have an element of hypovolaemic shock attributable to his pelvic fracture; however, the bradycardia and T4 sensory level suggest that he has neurogenic shock. Therapy should be targeted at gaining early invasive monitoring as accurate fluid management will again be a delicate balance aimed at avoiding both hypovolaemia and fluid overload. The consequences of each of these pathologies, if allowed to develop, would compromise the patient's potential recovery. He requires pelvic splint application and definitive haemostasis which, in the case of pelvic haematoma associated with fracture, is best achieved radiologically. Further radiological assessment, in addition to the trauma series of radiographs, will be required to evaluate his spinal column and determine the most appropriate definitive treatment.

SUMMARY

The commonest cause of shock in trauma is haemorrhage. Establishment of the presence and location of haemorrhage is the cornerstone of effective management of shock. Action should be taken to stem any obvious bleeding before administering appropriate intravenous fluids. In many cases the only effective management of bleeding is surgery. If this is necessary, patient management should seek to expedite transfer without increasing morbidity and mortality due to unnecessary procedures being performed. In the patient with ongoing haemorrhage, the presence of a radial pulse or a blood pressure of approximately 80 mmHg – which is sufficient to maintain vital organ perfusion – should be used as an end-point pending definitive control of the haemorrhage. Initial fluid replacement should be with warmed crystalloid, with blood being administered as the second fluid if necessary.

GLOBAL PERSPECTIVES

Shock is a universal condition irrespective of whether the aetiology is trauma, sepsis or any of the other causes; similarly, it matters not whether the cause of the traumatic hypovolaemia is penetrating injury, as is common in the USA and South Africa, or blunt mechanisms (as in Western Europe and the Antipodes). The universal management of the shocked, hypovolaemic patient should be targeted at achieving definitive haemostasis and optimizing tissue oxygenation. The only variation lies in the methods needed to obtain the definitive haemostasis.

REFERENCES

1.   Ganong WF. *Review of Medical Physiology*, 22nd edn. New York: McGraw Hill, 2005.

2.   American College of Surgeons Committee on Trauma. *Advanced Life Support Course for Physicians.* Chicago: American College of Surgeons Committee on Trauma, 2005.

3.   Yeomans ER, Gilstrap LC. Physiologic changes in pregnancy and their impact on critical care. *Crit Care Med* 2005;**33**(Suppl.):S256–8.

4.   Mattox KL, Laura Goetzl L. Trauma in pregnancy. *Crit Care Med* 2005;**3**(Suppl.):S385–9.

5.   Esposito TJ, Gens DR, Smith LG, Scorpio R, Buchman T. Trauma during pregnancy. A review of 79 cases. *Arch Surg* 1991;**126**:1073–8.

6.   Schiff MA, Holt VL. Pregnancy outcomes following hospitalization for motor vehicle crashes in Washington State from 1989 to 2001. *Am J Epidemiol* 2005;**161**:503–50.

7. El Kady D, Gilbert WM, Anderson J, Danielsen B, Towner D, Smith LH. Trauma during pregnancy: an analysis of maternal and fetal outcomes in a large population. *Am J Obstet Gynecol* 2004;**190**:1661–8.

8. Mizushima Y, Wang P, Cioffi WG, Bland KI, Chaudry IH. Should normothermia be restored and maintained during resuscitation after trauma and hemorrhage? *J Trauma* 2000;**48**:58–65.

9. Qureshi A, McGee A, Cooper JP, Porter KM. Reduction of the posterior pelvic ring by non-invasive stabilisation: a report of two cases. *Emerg Med J* 2005;**22**:885–6.

10. Grounds RM, Seebach C, Knothe C, *et al.* Use of recombinant activated factor VII (Novoseven) in trauma and surgery: analysis of outcomes reported to an international registry. *J Intens Care Med* 2006;**21**:27–39.

11. Mittal S, Watson H.G. A critical appraisal of the use of recombinant factor VIIa in acquired bleeding conditions. *Br J Haematol* 2006;**133**:355–63.

12. Kowalenko T, Stern S, Dronen S, Wang X. Improved outcome with hypotensive resuscitation of uncontrolled hemorrhagic shock in a swine model. *J Trauma* 1992;**33**:349–53.

13. Lee C, Porter KM. Prehospital management of lower limb fractures. *Emerg Med J* 2005;**22**;660–3.

14. National Institute for Health and Clinical Excellence (UK). Technology Appraisal Guidance No. 49: *Guidance on the Use of Ultrasound Locating Devices for Placing Central Venous Catheters.* Issued 2002; Reviewed 2005.

15. The International Liaison Committee on Resuscitation. The International Liaison Committee on Resuscitation (ILCOR) Consensus on Science With Treatment Recommendations for Pediatric and Neonatal Patients: Pediatric Basic and Advanced Life Support. *Pediatrics* 2006;**117**:955–77.

16. Smith R, Davis N, Bouamra O, Lecky F. The utilisation of intraosseous infusion in the resuscitation of paediatric major trauma patients. *Injury* 2005;**36**:1034–8.

17. Haas NA. Clinical review: vascular access for fluid infusion in children. *Crit Care* 2004;**8**:478–84.

18. Ward KR, Ivatury RR, Wayne Barbee R, *et al.* Near infrared spectroscopy for evaluation of the trauma patient: a technology review. *Resuscitation* 2006;**68**:27–44.

Head injury

After completing this chapter the reader will:
* understand the difficulties and potential serious consequences of minor head injury
* understand the pathophysiology of head injury
* realize the importance of limitation of secondary insults

* be able to institute appropriate initial treatment to optimize the outcome of head injury
* understand the indications for neurosurgical referral and surgical intervention.

INTRODUCTION

Man has attempted to treat head injuries for thousands of years and, whilst removal of an extradural haematoma in an otherwise uninjured patient remains one of the most satisfying and cost-effective[1] procedures in medicine, neurosurgeons would do well to remember that the greatest single advance in the management of head injury has probably been the introduction of the seat belt. It is vital to realize that there are few conditions whose prevention is so much more desirable than their cure as is the case for head injury. With that proviso, neurosurgeons have still made a considerable contribution to the management of head trauma: the recognition of intracranial pressure (ICP) waveforms,[2] the role of secondary brain injury,[3] the development of the Glasgow Scales[4,5] and the embracing of computed tomography (CT) scanning to reduce time to diagnosis and improve outcome[6] all deserve mention.

Mild and moderate head injury

The most controversial area in the field of mild or minor head injury is the lack of a satisfactory definition. Many definitions of mild and moderate head injury exist but a consensus is now starting to emerge[7] (Table 9.1). Post-traumatic amnesia (PTA), although long accepted as a guide to brain injury severity, is no longer used.[8]

The key issue is identifying those patients who harbour an intracranial lesion that may require neurosurgical input, either observation or active management including surgery. This difficult issue is compounded by the fact that

up to 20% of patients with diffuse head injuries may go on to develop intracranial mass lesions in the 12–24 hours following an early CT scan.[9]

Guidelines are available now to aid this decision-making, the most recent of which in the UK are the National Institute for Health and Clinical Excellence (NICE) guidelines.[10] It is the Scandinavian guidelines, however, that are most easily implemented in the emergency department[7] (Figure 9.1). In addition, consultation with a neurosurgeon is advised when a patient fulfils the criteria for CT scanning but this cannot be done in 2–4 hours, if the patient continues to deteriorate irrespective of the scan findings and if there is a compound or depressed skull fracture, penetrating injury or a cerebrospinal fluid (CSF) leak.[11] If CT is not available, then the 12-hour observation option of the algorithm may be used or a plain skull radiograph obtained and those patients who have a skull fracture moved to a department where CT scanning is available as a patient with a GCS of 14 or 15 and a skull fracture has up to a 10% chance of harbouring an intracranial haematoma.[12]

Table 9.1 Definitions of minimal, mild and moderate head injury

Severity of head injury	GCS	Loss of consciousness	Neurological deficits
Minimal	15	No	No
Mild	14–15	<5 minutes	No
Moderate	9–13	>5 minutes	Yes

For mild and moderate head injury, only one positive criterion is required.

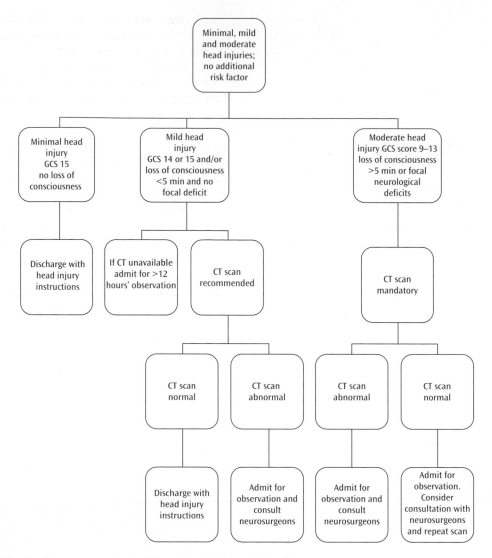

Figure 9.1 Algorithm for the management of mild and moderate head injury.[8]

Mild to moderate head injury has a poorly defined outcome, in part because the majority of patients present to local emergency departments rather than regional neuroscience centres; nevertheless, at least one study has shown a 1.8% mortality rate for such patients,[13] emphasizing the need to implement current relevant guidelines in the emergency department.

> Even mild to moderate head injuries need careful appraisal as they can still result in death.

THE PATHOPHYSIOLOGY OF HEAD INJURY

The uninjured brain

The brain accounts for 2% of body weight but receives 20% of the cardiac output as a result of the enormous amounts of oxygen and glucose required for neurotransmission and maintenance of ionic gradients; 90% of this energy expenditure is neuronal.

To ensure that this critical supply of oxygen and glucose is maintained and responds to changes in demand, cerebral blood flow (CBF) is tightly regulated by at least three forms of autoregulation (pressure, metabolic and viscosity),[14] a mechanism that operates at the level of medium-sized arterioles. Neurosurgical discussions predominantly refer to pressure autoregulation, which maintains a constant CBF for a given metabolic demand at cerebral perfusion pressures (CPPs) in the range 40–150 mmHg (Figure 9.2). Equally important is the response of the brain's medium-sized arterioles to CO_2. Carbon dioxide is freely diffusible across the blood–brain barrier and alters the pH of the brain parenchyma as a result. An increase in CO_2 leading to a decrease in pH produces rapid and profound vasodilatation, thus increasing blood flow. In the face of persistently raised levels of CO_2, however, the 'system' resets its baseline and

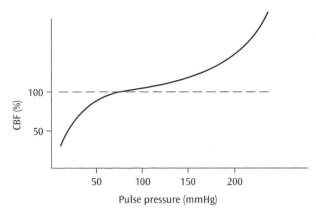

Figure 9.2 The cerebral blood flow curve.

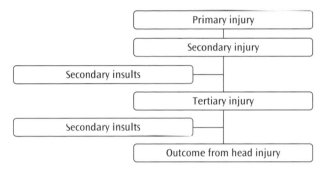

Figure 9.3 The head injury cascade.

vessel diameters return to baseline levels.[15] This critical finding explains why hyperventilation has been found to be mostly detrimental to the patient with a severe head injury.

Following the initial, primary injury, a cascade of events,[16] which remain incompletely understood, is triggered, leading to what are described as secondary and tertiary injuries; these, in turn, can be compounded by secondary insults (Figure 9.3). It is the physician's responsibility to limit this cascade and to minimize the number of secondary insults the patient suffers. Secondary and tertiary injury cascades begin within minutes of the primary injury and continue over several months, and the role of the neurosurgeon who is able to intervene directly in these cascades is to optimize conditions for the patient, to prevent secondary insults and provide the brain with the optimum environment to allow recovery.

> The aim of head injury management is the limitation of secondary injury.

Classification of severe head injury

This may be radiological, anatomical or clinical. The CT classification (Marshall scale) was developed from the data

accumulated from the National Institutes of Health Traumatic Coma Data Bank[17] and was the first to highlight the poor outcome associated with the presence of effacement of the basal cisterns and/or midline shift over 5 mm on the initial CT scan (Figure 9.4). The anatomical classification of head injuries divides them into focal, including contusions and traumatic haematomas, and diffuse injuries, such as concussion and diffuse axonal injury (DAI). These categories are not mutually exclusive as a severe underlying DAI may explain poor recovery following a technically perfect evacuation of an acute subdural haematoma.

Contusions are subpial extravasations of blood and oedema following trauma. They can underlie an area of direct trauma (coup and fracture contusions) or can be placed directly opposite the area of impact and be the result of the brain movement within the skull (contrecoup contusions). Contrecoup contusions classically occur in the orbital gyri, frontal poles, temporal poles and the inferior and lateral surfaces of the temporal lobe, areas of the brain adjacent to particularly uneven internal skull surfaces. The typical CT appearance is of a hyperdense intraparenchymal lesion (Figure 9.5). Classically, bifrontal contusions have the potential to grow 5–10 days after injury and are associated with dramatic patient deterioration – a process referred to as blooming – but blooming can occur unpredictably with almost any contusion and represents the rationale for the neurosurgical advice regarding prolonged inpatient observation. A contusion that is predominantly blood may

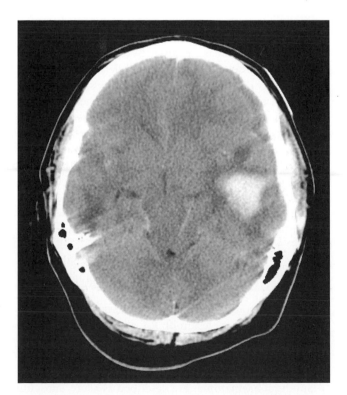

Figure 9.4 A computed tomography scan showing effacement of the basal cisterns.

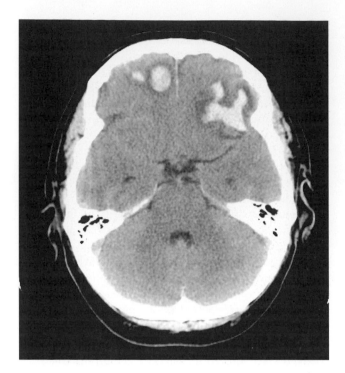

Figure 9.5 A computed tomography scan showing contusions.

be labelled a haematoma and can on occasion be amenable to removal.

Intracranial haematomas occupy a special place in this discussion as they are treatable and prompt efficient surgery, especially in the case of extradural haematomas, can result in remarkable recovery.

A skull fracture is an important risk factor for the presence of a significant haematoma,[12] and up to 85% of extradural haematomas are caused by injury to dural vessels or to a skull vessel as a result of skull deformity, with the vast majority being seen in the under-50s;[18] extradural haematomas are the classic traumatic haematoma of childhood.[19] This is probably due to the increased dural and diploic vascularity of the paediatric skull as well as a more adherent dura. In adult series the incidence is about 2%,[20] with around 50% of cases being due to tearing of the middle meningeal artery as a result of a temporoparietal skull fracture. Delay in diagnosis is common,[21] as the 'classical' presentation of initial loss of consciousness followed by a lucid interval and then increasing drowsiness, contralateral hemiplegia and ipsilateral oculomotor nerve palsy followed by hypertension and bradycardia (Cushing response) with terminal respiratory disturbance and decerebrate rigidity is actually rare.

A typical extradural haematoma presents as a hyperdense biconvex (lentiform) lesion on CT scanning, often in the temporoparietal area (Figure 9.6). Those associated with anticoagulation or active bleeding may have areas of radiolucency, sometimes referred to as the 'swirl effect'.

Subdural haematomas are described as acute, subacute or chronic depending on timeframe and appearances at CT scanning and operation. Nearly all are thought to

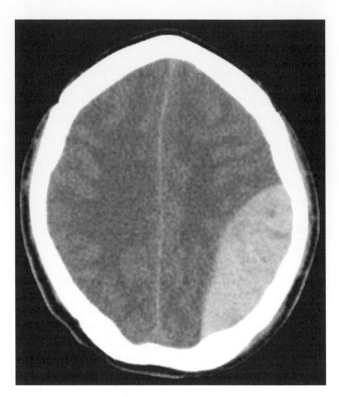

Figure 9.6 A computed tomography scan showing an extradural haematoma.

result from some form of venous injury,[18] the worst involving a cerebral venous sinus. Acute subdural haematomas are composed of clot and blood and occur within 48 hours of injury, classically having a hyperdense concave appearance (Figure 9.7); subacute subdural

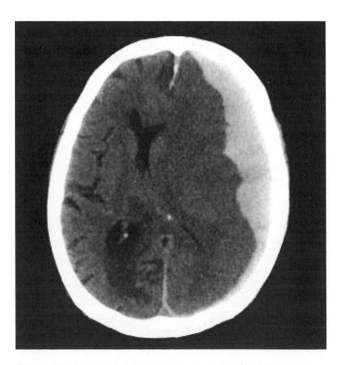

Figure 9.7 A computed tomography scan showing an acute subdural haematoma.

haematomas are a mix of clotted blood and fluid, occur between 2 and 14 days after injury and can be isodense to the brain on CT scanning (Figure 9.8), which can lead to them being missed by the unwary. Chronic subdural haematomas are usually over 2 weeks old and are predominantly fluid; their classical appearance is of a hypodense concave mass lesion (Figure 9.9).

Acute subdural haematomas remain the commonest of the adult post-traumatic haematomas; when seen in conjunction with injury to the temporal lobe, the condition is often termed a 'burst lobe' and is associated with a poor outcome. The rapid venous clot expansion over the surface of the brain produces profound cortical ischaemia, which, in conjunction with the commonly associated DAI, results in very disappointing outcomes.[22] Subacute subdurals are common in the elderly, in alcoholics and in those on anticoagulation and can be missed both clinically and radiologically.

Chronic subdural haematomas are due to minor trauma in the elderly shrunken brain tearing an already stretched bridging vein. However, there is usually no clear history of trauma, rather one of steady cognitive decline over time, attributed to the onset of a dementia, with a CT scan demonstrating the lesion only after a more precipitous drop in consciousness or the development of focal neurology.

The most feared form of diffuse brain injury is DAI, described by Strich,[23] which remains a diagnosis that can be made definitively only by a pathologist. Clinically it is assumed to have occurred when a patient suffers severe neurological injury without gross brain disruption. The only imaging findings of note are the small punctuate

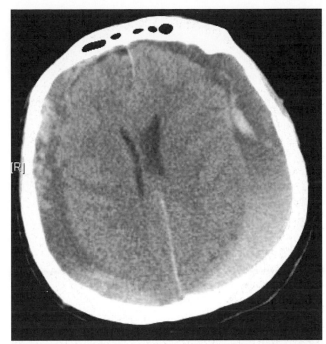

Figure 9.9 A computed tomography scan showing a chronic subdural haematoma.

'Strich' haemorrhages that can sometimes be seen in the corpus callosum, the walls of the third ventricle, basal ganglia and parts of the brain stem.

The only clinical grading system in common use is the Glasgow Coma Scale[4] (GCS) (Table 9.2) and its uniform acceptance has been one of the single greatest advances in neurotrauma; an exacting application of the score in the receiving unit is vital to the patient's care. Two points deserve mention, however: it is the GCS following full resuscitation that is crucial and a score may not be able to be fully assigned due to orbital swelling or pre-hospital interventions such as intubation.[24] Furthermore, abnormal flexion does not equate to decorticate rigidity nor abnormal extension to decerebration – a low GCS score corresponds to injury severity not site.[25]

The injured brain

After severe head injury the brain's consumption of oxygen drops and, paradoxically, the anaerobic glycolytic pathway increases its activity, resulting in acidosis.[26] The reasons for these paradoxical phenomena remain unclear, but there is increasing evidence to suggest that they may be the result of mitochondrial dysfunction, possibly associated with the calcium influx seen in severe head injury.[27]

In addition autoregulation is often significantly non-uniformly deranged throughout the brain, resulting in ischemia despite a reduced cerebral metabolic rate of oxygen ($CMRO_2$). Cerebral blood flow falls resulting in deranged synaptic function initially, but as CBF falls below 40% of normal the sodium/potassium pump fails, the cells

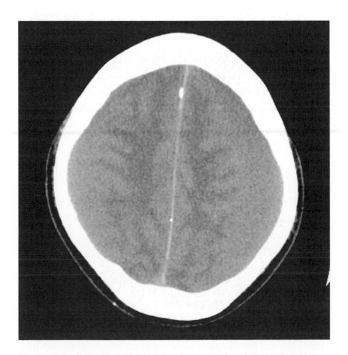

Figure 9.8 A computed tomography scan showing a subacute subdural haematoma.

Table 9.2 The Glasgow Coma Scale and score in adults

Response	Score
Eye-opening	
● Spontaneously	4
● To speech	3
● To pain	2
● None	1
Best verbal response (adult)	
● Orientated	5
● Confused	4
● Inappropriate words	3
● Incomprehensible sounds	2
● None	1
Best motor response	
● Obeys commands	6
● Localizes to a painful stimulus	5
● Withdraws from a painful stimulus	4
● Abnormal (spastic) flexion	3
● Extension	2
● None	1

A modified scale for best verbal response is used in young children less than 4 years of age to allow for their limited comprehension of speech and language development:

● Smiles and follows, interacts	5
● Cries consolably, inappropriate interactions	4
● Cries occasionally consolably, moaning sounds	3
● Irritable, inconsolable	2
● No response	1

swell and ultimately die.[28] Post-mortem studies in patients who died of severe head injury confirm that 80% showed evidence of cerebral ischaemia.[29]

INTRACRANIAL PRESSURE

The brain with all its associated structures, including blood vessels and CSF compartments, is contained within the rigid box of the skull. As a result, the concept of ICP is key to an understanding of brain injury. The Monro–Kellie doctrine states that, as the total volume of the intracranial contents is constant, an increase in the volume of any compartment must be accompanied by a similar reduction in the other compartments or the ICP will rise. Small or very slow increases in the volume of one compartment are well tolerated, but rapid or large increases cannot be accommodated and the pressure–volume curve (Figure 9.10) operates in an exponential way to produce significant rises in ICP.

This has profound effects on CBF. Cerebral blood flow is given by the equation

$$CBF = MAP - ICP$$

where MAP is the mean arterial pressure. Thus, as ICP rises, the CBF must reduce and further affect a brain with already

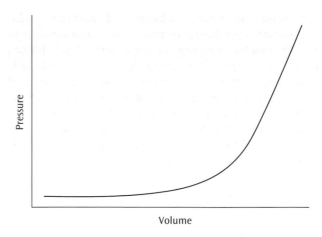

Figure 9.10 The exponential pressure–volume curve.

deranged metabolism and autoregulation. A second effect of a rising ICP is to produce secondary displacement of brain parenchyma, the 'herniation' syndromes which produce specific neurology and are an important cause of secondary insult. Mortality rises as the ICP rises[30] and an ICP of over 40 mmHg is immediately life-threatening.[2] Control of ICP informs much of what is done in the neurosurgical operating suite and in the neurointensive care.

Control of ICP is paramount.

Herniation syndromes

As ICP rises, the brain parenchyma can be forced through the rigid internal openings defined by the skull and the internal folds of the dura. These patterns of herniation are associated with specific radiological and clinical findings, which typically progress from one herniation syndrome to the next more severe one if they are not treated. Atypical presentations and rapid unpredictable deteriorations may be more common in the emergency department and vigilance is required.

SUBFALCINE HERNIATION

Subfalcine herniation results from a mass lesion pushing the cingulate gyrus under the free edge of the falx cerebri. Although usually only a radiological diagnosis associated with dilatation of the contralateral lateral ventricle secondary to occlusion of the foramen of Monro, it can injure the pericallosal arteries with resultant leg weakness.

UNCAL HERNIATION

Uncal herniation is the syndrome seen when an expanding mass lesion compresses the temporal lobe, pushing the uncus over the free edge of the tentorium cerebelli. This compresses the cerebral peduncle and ipsilateral oculomotor nerve, producing contralateral hemiparesis/plegia and an ipsilateral oculomotor nerve palsy. The latter can present as just pupillary dilatation or progress to include ptosis and a 'down and out' pupil secondary to paralysis of the ocular muscles innervated by the third nerve. Kernohan's notch refers to uncal herniation presenting with weakness ipsilateral to the mass lesion and results from compression of the contralateral cerebral peduncle against the contralateral tentorial edge.

CENTRAL HERNIATION

Central herniation follows on from uncal herniation and refers to the downward movement of the brain stem, associated radiologically with the presence of small brain stem haemorrhages on the CT scan from damage to the stretched perforating vessels that supply the brain stem. This impairment of the blood supply to the brain stem produces the depressed levels of consciousness, hypertension, bradycardia and respiratory abnormalities seen with this syndrome. Again it is emphasized that the absence of Cushing's response does not mean that such a herniation is not proceeding 'on the quiet'.

CEREBELLAR TONSILLAR HERNIATION

Cerebellar tonsillar herniation through the foramen magnum is the end stage of this whole process. Death ensues from apnoea as the obliterated cisterna magna compresses the medulla oblongata and the respiratory centre. Occasionally, in the context of trauma, tonsillar herniation may present following a seizure with little in the way of preceding neurology.

Secondary insults

This is a critical concept in the management of the head-injured patient. It refers to conditions such as hypoxia, hypotension and hyperglycaemia which are common in the head-injured patient and lead to further injury to an already damaged brain. They are potentially preventable, and the major role of the physician looking after a head-injured patient is to prevent secondary insults. Up to 90% of patients suffer some kind of secondary insult, half of which are severe; more worryingly, 50% of head-injured patients suffered a secondary insult whilst being transported around the hospital, for example during transfer from intensive care unit (ICU) to the CT scanner.[31]

The relationship of secondary insults to outcome was clearly demonstrated by the Traumatic Coma Databank, which showed that a single systolic blood pressure measurement below 90 mmHg and hypoxia (PaO_2 <60 mmHg) were major predictors of poor outcome;[32] a systolic blood pressure of less than 90 mmHg was associated with a 150% increase in mortality;[33] and patients who suffered similar insults in the ICU also went on to have poorer outcomes.[34] Five insults are consistently associated with poor outcomes:

- arterial hypotension
- reduced CPP
- raised ICP
- hypoxaemia
- pyrexia.[35]

A reduced CPP reduces delivery of oxygen to an already injured brain, but also produces compensatory cerebral vasodilatation, increasing ICP in a vicious cycle of secondary injury. Pyrexia produces its poor outcome by increasing the brain's metabolic demands with a 10% rise for every 1°C rise in temperature in a brain with deranged autoregulation, unable to meet this demand. Furthermore, hyperglycaemia is also clearly associated with a poorer outcome,[36] probably because the increased glucose is metabolized anaerobically by the ischaemic cells, resulting in the production of lactate. It is important to add that, in practice, prevention of secondary insults means preventing the conditions that can lead to these insults, such as limiting seizures or eliminating sepsis.

Managing the head-injured patient

The key is to get the patient to the emergency department quickly without exacerbating or producing any secondary insult. An efficient primary and secondary survey in the emergency department and institution of definitive specialist treatment as soon as possible are essential.

ON THE SCENE

Rigid neck immobilization is used as a routine in all trauma patients but where possible should be achieved using head block or sandbags and tape rather than a cervical collar as the latter may increase intracranial pressure as a result of reduced venous return. The Brain Trauma Foundation[37] directs that the airway should be secured in all patients with a severe head injury. Ideally, this should follow the administration of sedation and muscle relaxants, but it may be possible without drugs, although at least one study found that mortality among patients intubated at the scene without anaesthesia reached 100%.[38] The underlying aim is to avoid hypoxia and maintain SaO_2 >90%. An occluded airway produces both hypoxia and raised ICP as the patient struggles to breathe. Neck movement must be avoided in order to prevent exacerbation of a potential cervical spine injury. Intubation should be performed using a second assistant to provide manual in-line stabilization during the procedure. Further assistants will also be needed to apply cricoid pressure and administer anaesthetic drugs.

Intubation is necessary in patients with severe head injury.

IN THE EMERGENCY DEPARTMENT

The GCS score that counts is the score after adequate resuscitation, as many of the early pupil changes seen in severe head injury relate to brain stem hypoperfusion rather than brain stem compression.[39] Hypotonic fluids such as Ringer's or dextrose/saline should be avoided.[40]

During the secondary survey it is important to make a thorough examination of the whole head by removing the head blocks and collars whilst an assistant maintains manual in-line stabilization. Lacerations at the back of the head, skull step-offs indicating a fracture, foreign bodies, CSF or blood leaking from the nose or ear including behind the tympanic membrane should be identified. Bruising over the mastoid (Battle's sign), periorbital ecchymosis (racoon eyes) and unilateral facial nerve palsy are indicative of a possible base of skull fracture but tend to occur relatively late and after the patient has left the emergency department.

A nasogastric tube should not be placed in any patient with a suspected base of skull fracture, in which case an orogastric tube should be inserted instead. If the patient has been intubated prior to arrival of the neurosurgeon, a prior GCS with breakdown of the individual scores is helpful; once intubated the verbal component is scored as 'T', e.g. E2, M5, VT.

Aside from the GCS, assessment of pupillary size and reactivity is vital. A difference of up to 1 mm (one size) between pupils is seen in up to 20% of the healthy population, but pupillary inequality after resuscitation mandates a CT scan of the head. Unequal pupils may be due to local trauma resulting in a traumatic mydriasis, exposure to pharmacological agents, or a Horner's syndrome caused by trauma to the sympathetic chain at any level from the hypothalamus to the cervicothoracic cord, making the unaffected pupil appear dilated. Bilateral absence of the pupillary light reflex is a very poor prognostic sign,[37] and mortality rates of 56% for patients with bilateral fixed pupils and an extradural haematoma and 88% for such patients with an acute subdural haematoma are quoted.[41] Examination must specifically exclude the lateralizing signs of the herniation syndromes.

The use of mannitol to maintain CBF remains important though controversial.[42] Its acute effects are likely to be rheological rather than osmotic. North American practice is to administer a 100-mL bolus of 20% mannitol to any severely head-injured patient with unequal pupils. Plasma osmolality must remain <320 mOsm/L to avoid the risk of acute tubular necrosis,[43] although recent work suggests higher doses may be needed.[44] Hypertonic saline is a potential alternative to mannitol[45] – if either is used a urinary catheter is required.

Hyperventilation is no longer recommended as it worsens outcome[46] – the aim is normocapnia.

Acute subdural, penetrating injuries, cortical contusions, a history of significant alcohol abuse and epilepsy in the first 24 hours after admission are all indications for prophylactic anticonvulsants[47] – if no further seizures have occurred then anticonvulsants should be tapered off. There is no role for routine anticonvulsants otherwise. Seizures in the emergency department must be controlled as they increase cerebral oxygen consumption and raise ICP. Lorazepam (4 mg i.v. over 2 minutes, repeated after 5 minutes if necessary) is the drug of choice. Airway support including intubation may be required. The maintenance anticonvulsant of choice in trauma is phenytoin, administered as an i.v. loading dose of 18 mg/kg over half an hour in adults. Since phenytoin is cardioactive, cardiac monitoring must be instituted. More recently, fosphenytoin has been advocated as an easier and safer phenytoin prodrug. In a patient with an unexpectedly prolonged post-ictal state the possibility of non-convulsive status epilepticus should be considered and an electroencephalogram (EEG) may be required.

Agitation can lead to hypoxia and raised ICP and is often the result of pain – adequate analgesia including opiates should be administered. If there is no obvious source of pain or the patient does not respond to analgesia, raised ICP should be considered as a cause and intubation and sedation may be required prior to CT scanning. In these circumstances the team should be prepared to wake the patient in the presence of a normal CT scan.

Any scalp wounds should be cleaned and covered with antiseptic swabs until investigations are completed and wounds definitively treated. Heavy bleeding from scalp wounds is common and can be controlled with rapid through-and-through sutures until a definitive closure can be performed. The routine use of antibiotics is not recommended, including in patients with base of skull fractures, unless there is an obviously contaminated wound with an underlying skull fracture or a penetrating injury.[48] In these cases a broad-spectrum cephalosporin is recommended; metronidazole should be added if a sinus injury is suspected.

All patients with a moderate or severe head injury require a head CT scan interpreted by an experienced radiologist, who, in conjunction with the neurosurgeon, can ask for any additional investigations that might be required. A non-enhanced study with 1.5-mm cuts through the posterior fossa and 5-mm cuts through the supratentorial compartment with bony and brain windows is adequate. The head CT scan can be combined with CT imaging of the cervical spine if the C1/C2 and C7/T1 junctions have not been adequately visualized on plain films.

If CT facilities are not available even after interhospital transfer then a plain skull radiograph may still be useful. The presence of a linear skull fracture in an adult correlates with a risk of developing an intracranial haematoma that is 3–175 times greater than in the absence of the skull fracture[12] – but a haematoma may still develop in the absence of a fracture.

CT scanning is the investigation of choice in all patients with moderate or severe head injury.

WHEN TO CALL THE NEUROSURGEON

It is prudent to ask for an urgent neurosurgical consultation during the primary survey in the presence of a compound depressed skull fracture, an injury with visible brain tissue or where there is obvious lateralizing neurology. Otherwise it is unusual to need neurosurgical advice prior to completion of the primary and secondary surveys and all immediate investigations and interventions have taken place. Neurosurgical advice should be sought when:[49]

- There is a positive head CT.
- A patient fulfils criteria for CT scanning but this cannot be done for 24 hours.
- The patient continues to deteriorate irrespective of CT scan findings or if there is a compound depressed skull fracture, penetrating injury or CSF leak.

The order of treatment priorities in polytrauma has traditionally placed neurosurgical actions after thoracoabdominal intervention, but it is worth noting that the commonest cause of trauma death within the first 72 hours is neurological injury.[50]

The CRASH trial[51] has clearly shown that steroids have no place in the current management of the head-injured patient.

SURGICAL INTERVENTIONS

The Traumatic Coma Data Bank series found that only 37% of patients in coma as a result of head injury underwent surgery,[52] but these are the patients that the neurosurgeon can help the most, and there is anecdotal evidence that those units with improved outcomes in severe head injury are those that treat well-chosen cases of head injury aggressively with early surgery.

Exploratory burr holes by the non-neurosurgeon are a temporizing measure of last resort.

Exploratory burr holes

These are now rarely required, and evacuation of a clot through a burr hole is a temporizing measure which should only be performed to allow transfer to a neurosurgical centre for definitive treatment. The placement of exploratory burr holes is shown in Box 9.1.

Box 9.1 The technique of exploratory burr holes

- Shave and prepare the head.
- Explore the side ipsilateral to a 'blown' pupil or contralateral to a hemiparesis/plegia. In the absence of lateralizing signs, place the first burr hole on the side of the scalp trauma.
- Place the burr hole just above the zygomatic arch 1 cm anterior to the tragus.
- If this is negative and a small cruciate durotomy reveals no underlying clot, place a further burr hole above the apex of the pinna.
- If this too is negative, a burr hole should be placed in the midpupillary line just behind the hairline avoiding the midline. This placement will allow a neurosurgeon to subsequently fashion a trauma flap if needed using these burr holes.
- If this is also negative, then similar burr holes should be placed on the opposite side of the skull.
- If these also prove negative, posterior fossa burr holes can be considered, but this is a high-risk procedure for the non-neurosurgeon and is not recommended.

Indications for neurosurgical intervention

Extradural haematomas always require removal except for trivial 'fracture haematomas' associated with linear skull fractures, which are only 1–2 mm in thickness and exert no mass effect. Occasionally, such haematomas can expand, sometimes silently, especially if the first scan was performed soon after injury.[9] This explains why neurosurgeons may request a further scan 'the morning after the night before' in such cases.

Acute subdural haematomas need to be removed, although it should be remembered that the outcome from large acute subdural haematomas in the elderly or those with fixed pupils is nearly always death, or at best severe lifelong disability.[53]

Brain contusions are usually managed conservatively unless they are associated with significant mass effect and midline shift of more than 5 mm. If a contusion expands in association with a decline in consciousness or a rise in ICP, then surgery is often performed. Multiple contusions in association with an extra-axial haematoma may need to be removed, as will even small contusions in the temporal lobe owing to their propensity to cause uncal herniation.

Skull fractures are usually managed conservatively. Depressed skull fractures will need to be repaired if compound, depressed more than the thickness of the surrounding skull table or cosmetically unacceptable. Focal neurological deficits in association with depressed skull fractures are considered by some to be an indication for elevation, but there is no evidence that surgery helps the deficit. Cerebrospinal fluid leaks that do not resolve with conservative management will require repair of the dural defect associated with the base of skull fracture.

Penetrating injuries and craniofacial trauma are discussed separately below.

Chronic subdural haematomas which produce significant headache, depressed levels of consciousness, confusion, and focal neurology are amenable to surgery, even in the very elderly.

Conservative management of extra-axial lesions is possible.[41] In a fully conscious patient with no other significant lesion, no mass effect or midline shift (<5 mm), no effacement of the basal cisterns and a clot thickness of less than 10 mm, conservative management may be attempted. This entails a long period of inpatient stay followed by an even longer period of surveillance as an outpatient with multiple scans. Furthermore, it is the experience of most neurosurgeons that patients with conservatively managed extradural haematomas nearly always come to surgery as a result of profound incapacitating headache associated with the haematoma. Many small acute subdural haematomas, particularly those over the tentorium cerebelli and the interhemispheric fissure, are best managed conservatively.

Preoperative protocols

Even in the case of urgent neurosurgery some investigations and procedures are mandatory though they can usually be performed as the patient is being wheeled into theatre, prepared and anaesthetized. Included in this list are:

- four units of cross-matched or O-negative blood;
- clotting studies including platelets;
- full blood count;
- blood gas analysis (which will also allow analysis of the urea and electrolytes);
- effective venous access usually including a central line;
- arterial access;
- a Foley catheter;
- informed consent (if the patient is capable);
- access to the patient's scans;
- plain radiographs including a chest radiograph may also be required.

Craniotomy

Most neurosurgical procedures in trauma can be performed through the classical question mark flap. The patient is positioned supine on the operating table with the shaved head fixed in a head clamp or ring and 15–20° of head elevation to reduce venous bleeding. The incision commences at the zygoma 1 cm anterior to the tragus and curves backward over the auricle to the midline, finishing anteriorly just behind the hairline. Haemostasis is achieved by the application of Raney clips or curved artery forceps applied to the wound edges to evert them. A myocutaneous

flap is then raised using the cutting diathermy. Burr holes are now placed as for exploratory burr holes, and any clot is rapidly evacuated using suction. The burr holes are joined together with a craniotome to raise a free bone flap that extends to 2–2.5 cm short of the midline. Bone rongeurs are used to nibble bone, removing the lateral part of the sphenoid wing and some temporal bone to gain adequate access to the middle fossa. The details of the neurosurgical procedures achievable through this exposure are beyond the scope of this manual, but suffice it to say that clots, whether extradural or subdural, should be evacuated. The bone flap should be secured if at all possible after the procedure.

Chronic subdural haematomas

There is no consensus on the treatment of chronic subdural haematomas. Treatment options include a short course of steroids, standard burr holes, twist drill drainage, which can be done at the bedside, shunting and craniotomy. This variety of procedures reflects the fact that the recurrence rate can be up to 20% following any form of chronic subdural drainage barring craniotomy. The most commonly used procedure is burr hole drainage.

Injuries to the frontal sinus

Non-depressed linear fractures through the anterior wall of the frontal sinus can be treated conservatively. Fractures involving the posterior wall of the sinus are nearly always associated with dural tears even if not evident on CT. They are notorious as a cause of delayed infection even years after an injury, and thus formal exploration and repair should be undertaken within a few days of injury.[54] It is usually approached thorough a bicoronal flap in conjunction with the craniofacial team.

Base of skull fractures

Base of skull fractures, even in conjunction with CSF leaks, are managed conservatively as the majority of leaks will stop spontaneously.[55] The patient is nursed 20–30° head up, reducing ICP whilst not overly encouraging the entry of air into the cranial vault. Antibiotics are withheld. The patient is observed closely and any deterioration mandates CT scanning and lumbar puncture to exclude hydrocephalus, pneumocepahlus and meningitis. Should the leak persist beyond 7–10 days, then the patient can undergo a trial of therapeutic lumbar punctures (following CT to exclude obstructive hydrocephalus) in an attempt to reduce ICP and allow the leak to heal or be considered for surgical repair. Delayed presentation of CSF leak following trauma or meningitis associated with a CSF leak is an absolute indication for repair, although, paradoxically, the inflammation associated with a bout of meningitis usually stops the leak. Surgery for persistent leak may be performed through a bicoronal skull base approach or more commonly by utilizing an endoscopic approach as most non-healing leaks are through the floor of the frontal cranial fossa. Preoperative thin-slice CT contrast and radioisotope studies may be needed to localize the leak.

Penetrating injuries

Penetrating head injuries, predominantly gunshot wounds, are becoming increasingly common, especially in the USA. Bullet wounds to the head – as elsewhere – are either low energy transfer wounds, in which the damage is confined to the bullet track, or high-energy transfer, in which cavitation and contamination distant to the wound track become considerations. The American Association of Neurological Surgeons has produced recommendations regarding the role of surgery in penetrating head injury.[56] Patients with fixed pupils or decerebrate/decorticate posturing (if not shocked or hypoxic) should not be operated on as the hopes of a meaningful recovery are close to zero. If surgery is embarked upon it should be confined to entry and exit wound toilet; the track should not be explored to recover bone or missile fragments unless there is a mass lesion that needs to be removed. If the patient recovers, then vigilance is required to detect the late development of abscesses or pseudoaneurysms, both of which are well-recognized complications of gunshot wounds to the head. Removal of a foreign body such as a screwdriver or arrow that remains embedded in the brain should be done in theatre and, if the trajectory passes close to named vessels or a large clot is shown on the CT scan, then angiography is prudent prior to surgery.

Intensive care management of the head-injured patient

The keys to successful ICU management of the head-injured patient are ventilation, sedation, attention to the features outlined above that may contribute to secondary brain injury and close monitoring. In addition to standard ICU monitoring, two other modalities are commonly employed in head injury cases.

TISSUE OXYGENATION MONITORING

Mixed venous jugular bulb oxygen saturation (SjO_2) is measured by the retrograde placement of an oximetry catheter within the internal jugular vein so that the tip lies at the jugular bulb and samples the average saturations of all the cerebral venous blood flow (normally between 50% and 70%). From this, cerebral oxygen consumption can be estimated as:

$$SjO_2 = SaO_2 - (\text{oxygen consumption/cardiac output} \times Hb \times 1.39)$$

Thus, SjO_2 will change if there is an imbalance between oxygen consumption and delivery. If SjO_2 <50% and the SaO_2 is normal, then there is either a decreased CBF or increased $CMRO_2$. If CPP is maintained then a fall in CBF is due to an increase in cerebral vascular resistance. Global desaturation <50% is associated with neuronal damage and must be actively managed.

ICP MONITORING

An ICP of 20–25 mmHg is associated with poor outcomes,[57] although there is no convincing evidence that actively treating raised ICP produces an improved outcome.[41] Nevertheless it is accepted that *comatose head injury patients with abnormal CT scans should undergo ICP monitoring*, with a value of 20–25 mmHg being the threshold for initiating new interventions to lower ICP. Intracranial pressure monitoring may also be beneficial in patients with a GCS of 8 or less following resuscitation but in whom a CT is normal and in patients aged over 40 or those with systolic blood pressure below 90 mmHg or motor posturing.[58]

The two devices most commonly used to monitor ICP are the external ventricular drain (EVD) and the intraparenchymal monitor, usually referred to as an ICP bolt. The EVD remains the gold standard, is relatively cheap and allows therapeutic CSF drainage; its major disadvantage is the need for considerable skill in placing it in the frontal horn of the right lateral ventricle. Intracranial pressure bolts require less skill in placement, but do not allow CSF drainage and are prone to drift in their ICP readings. They are placed with a twist drill and the site of placement is the same as for the EVD.

In the absence of selective treatments for the different causes of raised ICP, a staircase of non-specific therapies are used as ICP becomes increasingly difficult to control, aiming to maintain a CPP of 60–70 mmHg.[41] This staircase includes the non-specific measures already outlined, such as nursing head up, ensuring freedom from seizures, normocapnia and treatment of sepsis. Boluses of mannitol, mannitol with frusemide or hypertonic saline can be given to raise plasma osmolality and reduce ICP. Failure to control ICP with these measures requires consideration of repeated CT scanning to exclude new or recurrent intracranial collections, which must be drained if present. If no new collections are identified and ICP is still uncontrolled, then neuromuscular paralysis must be considered, accepting that repeated assessment becomes difficult and complications such as myoneuropathies and respiratory problems increase. Finally, novel treatments such as barbiturate coma, hyperventilation to 'buy time', decompressive craniectomy in the absence of a mass lesion or deliberate hypothermia (core temperature of 32–33°C) can be considered. There are, in addition, certain novel more targeted protocols, but these are not commonly used in the UK.[59,60] In addition to managing the patient's head injury, all the other principles of intensive care apply, including the early use of enteral feeding.

OUTCOME FROM HEAD INJURY

The mortality after severe head injuries still runs at 30–35%[52] and, of those who recover, a significant number will be left dependent on lifelong care. The long-term consequences in those who appear to recover well from mild or moderate injury are less well recognized, often leaving those who suffer from what is increasingly called the 'post-concussive' syndrome feeling as though they are malingerers. These symptoms can be myriad, ranging from headache and poor memory to personality change (often manifest as aggression), tinnitus and disruption of the sleep–wake cycle.

In recognition of this 'neglect' and the resultant distress caused, Alves and Jane[61] have developed a screening methodology for those patients with symptoms of what they refer to as 'post-traumatic' syndrome. For most people working in less resource-rich environments, acknowledging these symptoms as being real and troubling – and indeed explaining what the patient and his or her family may expect over the coming months (symptoms can persist for over 1 year) when they are discharged from acute care – is often as effective.

SUMMARY

Although the incidence of serious head injury has markedly decreased in the UK since the introduction of seat belt legislation, it remains a significant problem in terms of both mortality and morbidity. Minor or mild head injuries should be managed according to a recognized treatment algorithm to minimize post-injury sequelae. The priorities in managing severe head injury are the limitation of secondary brain injury, identification of surgically remediable lesions and control of intracranial pressure. Surgical intervention of any kind is virtually never required outside of a specialist neurosurgical unit. Despite marked improvements in neurosurgical technique and head injury management in general, the mortality rate after serious head injury remains a disappointing 30–35%.

Case scenario

A 24-year-old car driver has been involved in a roll-over RTC at approximately 70 mph. He was not wearing a seat belt, was trapped in the vehicle and it took nearly 2 hours to extricate him. His head struck the windscreen. He was conscious at the scene and complained of headache and right-sided abdominal pain. By the time he has been transported to the emergency department he is making incomprehensible sounds, does not open his eyes to any stimuli and withdraws from a painful stimulus. He is cold with a pulse rate of 100 beats/min, blood pressure of 70/30 and a respiratory rate of 24 per minute. He has bruises and abrasions over the right side of his abdomen

What is his immediate emergency department management and what is his GCS?

He is managed according to <C>ABCDE principles. In the absence of catastrophic haemorrhage, attention turns to his airway and he requires intubation. His GCS is 7 (E1, V2, M4) and he cannot protect his own airway. This must be done while maintaining manual in-line stabilization. His breathing has settled to 18 per minute with analgesia. He has intravenous fluids running through two large-bore cannulae with a target pressure of 100 mmHg. A focused assessment with sonography for trauma (FAST) scan reveals a large amount of free fluid in the right upper quadrant. His trauma series radiographs do not adequately cover his cervical spine, his chest is normal and his pelvis is intact. His haemoglobin is 9.2 g/dL.

What emergency department treatment can help this man's head injury?

Following intubation he needs high-flow supplemental oxygen and intravenous fluids to maintain a systolic blood pressure of over 100 mmHg to maintain cerebral perfusion. Tight glycaemic control, avoidance of fitting and analgesia will help.

He stabilizes sufficiently to undergo CT scanning. This shows a large extradural haematoma and a normal cervical spine and chest. There is a grade III liver injury with approximately 1500 mL of blood in the abdominal cavity – the other viscera are intact. His blood pressure has fallen again since his CT scan and his haemoglobin is now 7.1 g/dL.

Describe the approach to his liver and head injuries

A grade III liver injury is potentially manageable conservatively, but he appears to be becoming more unstable with a falling haemoglobin, which would suggest that conservative management is inadvisable. His extradural haematoma requires craniotomy and removal – this would preclude frequent reassessment of his abdomen and therefore he requires laparotomy for his liver injury. Ideally the two procedures could be performed concurrently.

GLOBAL PERSPECTIVES

On-scene interventions do make a difference. A study comparing head injury mortality in two geographical locations (Charlottesville, USA, and New Delhi, India) found a mortality of 11% in India compared with 7.2% in USA – the difference being predominantly in those with a Glasgow Coma Scale score >5 (12.5% vs. 4.8%). Of the Indian patients, only 2.7% received first aid at the scene and 6.9% were in hospital within the hour, whereas in Charlottesville 84.3% received on-scene interventions and 50.2% were in hospital in 1 hour.[62]

REFERENCES

1.   Pickard JD, Bailey S, Sanderson H, et al. Steps towards cost-benefit analysis of regional neurosurgical care. BMJ 1990;301:629–35.

2.   Lundberg N. Continuous recording and control of ventricular fluid pressure in neurosurgical practice. Acta Psychiatr Neurol Scand 1960;149(Suppl.):1–193.

3.   Andrews PJ, Piper IR, Dearden NM, Miller JD. Secondary insults during intrahospital transport of head-injured patients. Lancet 1990;335:327–30.

4.   Teasdale G, Jennett B. Assessment of coma and impaired consciousness: a practical scale. Lancet 1974;2:81–4.

5.   Jennett B, Bond M. Assessment of outcome after severe brain damage: a practical scale. Lancet 1975;1:480–4.

6.   Seelig JM, Becker DP, Miller JD, et al. Traumatic acute subdural haematoma: major mortality reduction in comatose patients treated within four hours. N Engl J Med 1981;304:1511–18.

7.   Ingebrigsten T, Romner B, Kock-Jensen C. Scandinavian guidelines for initial management of minimal, mild and moderate head injuries. J Trauma 2000;48:760–6.

8.   Dikmen SS, Levin HS. Methodological issues in the study of mild head injury. J Head Trauma Rehabil 1993;8:30–7.

9.   Smith HK, Miller JD. The danger of an ultra early computed tomographic scan in a patient with an evolving intracranial haematoma. Neurosurgery 1991;29:258–60.

10.   National Institute of Health and Clinical Excellence. Head Injury: Triage, Assessment, Investigation and Early Management of Head Injury in Infants, Children and Adults. Manchester: NICE, 2003.

11.   Royal College of Surgeons of England Working Party. Report of the Working Party on the Management of Patients with Head Injuries. London: Royal College of Surgeons of England, 1999.

12.   Servadei F, Merry GS. Mild head injury in adults. In: Winn, HR, ed. Youman's Neurological Surgery, 5th edn, Philadelphia: WB Saunders, 2003, pp. 5065–81.

13.   Seravedi F, Ciucci G, Loroni L, et al. Diagnosis and management of minor head injury: a regional multicentre approach in Italy. J Trauma 1995;39:696–701.

14.   Lassen N. Cerebral blood flow and oxygen consumption in man. Physiol Rev 1959;39:183–238.

15.   Muizelaar JP, van der Poel HG, Li ZC, et al. Pial arteriolar vessel diameter and CO_2 reactivity during prolonged hyperventilation in the rabbit. J Neurosurg 1988;69:923–7.

16.   Graham DI, Gennarelli TA. Pathology of brain damage after head injury. In: Reilly P, Bullock R, eds. Head Injury, 4th edn. New York: Arnold Publishing, 1997, pp. 133–53.

17.   Marshall LF, Marshall SB, Klauber MR, et al. The diagnosis of head injury requires a classification based on computed axial tomography. J Neurotrauma 1992;9(Suppl. 1):S287–92.

18.   Marshall L, Gautille T, Klauber M. The outcome of severe closed head injury. J Neurosurg 1991;75:S28–36.

19.   Gallagher JP, Browder EJ. Extradural haematoma: experience with 167 patients. J Neurosurg 1968;29:1–12.

20.   Lindenberg R. Trauma of meninges and brain. Pathol Nerv Syst 1971;2:1705–65.

21.   Heiskanen O. Epidural hematoma. Surg Neurol 1975;4:23–6.

22.   Jamieson K, Yelland J. Surgically treated traumatic subdural hematomas. J Neurosurg 1972;37:137–49.

23.   Strich S. Diffuse degeneration of the cerebral white matter in severe dementia following head injury. J Neurol Neurosurg Psychiatry 1956;19:163–85.

24.   Gale J, Dikmen S, Wyler A. Head injury in the Pacific North-west. Neurosurgery 1983;12:487–9.

25.   Greenberg RP, Stablein DM, Becker DP. Noninvasive localization of brain-stem lesions in the cat with multimodality evoked potentials: correlation with human head injury data. J Neurosurg 1981;54:740–50.

26.   Anderson BJ, Marmarou A. Post-traumatic selective stimulation of glycolysis. Brain Res 1992;585:184–9.

27.   Xiong Y, Gu Q, Peterson PL, et al. Mitochondrial dysfunction and calcium perturbation induced by traumatic brain injury. J Neurotrauma 1997;14:23–34.

28.   Schroder ML, Muizelaar JP, Kuta AJ, et al. Thresholds for cerebral ischemia after severe head injury: 28. Relationship with late CT findings and outcome. J Neurotrauma 1996;13:17–23.

29.   Adams J, Graham D. The pathology of blunt head injury. In: Critchley M, O'Leary J, Jennet B, eds. Scientific Foundation of Neurology. London: William Heinemann, 1972, pp. 488–91.

30.   Miller JD. Physiology of trauma. Clin Neurosurg 1982;29:103–30.

31.   Andrews PJ, Piper IR, Dearden NM, Miller JD. Secondary insults during intrahospital transport of head injured patients. Lancet 1990;335:327–30.

32.   Chesnut RM, Marshall SB, Piek J, et al. Early and late systemic hypotension as a frequent and fundamental source of cerebral ischemia following severe brain injury in the Traumatic Coma Data Bank. Acta Neurochir 1993;59(Suppl.):121–5.

33.   Chesnut RM, Marshall LF, Klauber MR, et al. The role of secondary brain injury in determining outcome from severe head injury. J Trauma 1993;34:216–22.

34.   Piek J, Chesnut RM, Marshall LF, et al. Extracranial complications of severe head injury. J Neurosurg 1992;77:901–7.

35.   Miller J, Piper I, Jones P. Pathophysiology of head injury. In: Narayan RK, Wilberger JE, Povlishock JT, eds. *Neurotrauma.* New York: McGraw-Hill, 1996, pp. 61–9.

36.   Lam AM, Winn HR, Cullen BF, Sundling N. Hyperglycaemia and neurological outcomes in patients with head injury. *J Neurosurg* 1991;**75**:545–51.

37.   Brain Trauma Foundation. Guidelines for prehospital management of traumatic brain injury. *J Neurotrauma* 2002;**19**:111–74.

38.   Lockey D, Davies G, Coats T. Survival of trauma patients who have prehospital tracheal intubation without anaesthesia or muscle relaxants: observational study. *BMJ* 2001;**323**:141.

39.   Ritter A, Muizelaar JP, Barnes T, *et al.* Brain stem blood flow, papillary response, and outcome in patients with severe head injuries. *Neurosurgery* 1999;**44**:941–8.

40.   Shackford SR, Zhuang J, Schmocker J. Intravenous fluid tonicity: effect on intracranial pressure, cerebral blood flow and cerebral oxygen delivery. *J Neurosurg* 1992; 76: 91–98.

41.   Brain Trauma Foundation, The American Association of Neurological Surgeons, The Joint Section on Neurotrauma and Critical Care. Guidelines for the management of severe head injury. *J Neurotrauma* 2000;**17**:457–595.

42.   Schot RJ, Muizelaar JP. Mannitol in acute traumatic brain injury. *Lancet* 2002;**359**:1633–4.

43.   Feig PU, McCurdy DK. The hypertonic state. *N Engl J Med* 1977;**297**:1444–54.

44.   Cruz J, Minoja G, Okuchi K. Major clinical and physiological benefits of early high doses of mannitol for intraparenchymal temporal lobe hemorrhages with abnormal pupillary widening: a randomized trial. *Neurosurgery* 2002;**51**:628–38.

45.   Bayir H, Clark RS, Kochanek PM. Promising strategies to minimize secondary brain injury after head trauma. *Crit Care Med* 2003;**31**(Suppl.):S112–17.

46.   Muizelaar J, Marmarou A, Ward J, *et al.* Adverse effects of prolonged hyperventilation in patients with severe head injury: a randomized clinical trial. *J Neurosurg* 1991;**75**:731–9.

47.   Temkin NR, Dikmen SS, Wilensky AJ, *et al.* A randomized, double-blind study of phenytoin for the prevention of post-traumatic seizures. *N Engl J Med* 1990;**323**:497–502.

48.   The 'Infection In Neurosurgery' Working Party of the British Society for Antimicrobial Chemotherapy. Use of antibiotics in penetrating craniocerebral injuries. *Lancet* 2000;**355**:1813–17.

49.   Tolias C, Wasserberg J. Critical decision making in severe head injury management. *Trauma* 2002;**4**:211–21.

50.   Acosta JA, Yang JC, Winchell RJ, *et al.* Lethal injuries time to death in a level I trauma centre. *J Am Coll Surg* 1998;**186**: 528–33.

51.   The Crash Trial Collaborative Group. Final results of MRC CRASH trial, a randomised placebo-controlled trial of intravenous corticosteroid in adults with head injury – outcomes at 6 months. *Lancet* 2005;**365**:1957–9.

52.   Foulkes MA, Eisenberg HM, Jane JA, *et al.* The Traumatic Coma Data Bank: design, methods, and baseline characteristics. *J Neurosurg* 1991;**75**:S8–13.

53.   Narayan RK, Greenberg RP, Miller JD, *et al.* Improved confidence of outcome prediction in severe head injury. A comparative analysis of the clinical examination, multimodality evoked potentials, CT scanning, and intracranial pressure. *J Neurosurg* 1981;**54**:751–62.

54.   Sataloff RT, Sariego J, Myers DL, *et al.* Surgical management of the frontal sinus. *Neurosurgery* 1984;**15**:593–96.

55   Mincy JE. Posttraumatic cerebrospinal fluid fistula of the frontal fossa. *J Trauma* 1966;**6**:618–22.

56.   American Association of Neurological Surgeons and the Brain Trauma Foundation. Surgical management of penetrating brain injury. *J Trauma* 2001;**51**:S16–25.

57.   Marmarou A, Anderson RL, Ward JD, *et al.* Impact of ICP instability and hypotension on outcome in patients with severe head injury. *J Neurosurg* 1991;**75**:S59–64.

58.   O'Sullivan MG, Statham PF, Jones PA, *et al.* Role of intracranial pressure monitoring in severely head–injured patients without signs of intracranial hypertension on initial computerized tomography. *J Neurosurg* 1994;**80**:46–50.

59.   Rosner MJ, Rosner SD, Johnson AH. Cerebral perfusion pressure: management protocol and clinical results. *J Neurosurg* 1995;**83**:949–62.

60.   Eker C, Asgeirsson B, Grade PO, *et al.* Improved outcome after severe head injury with a new therapy based on principles for brain volume regulation and preserved microcirculation. *Crit Care Med* 1998;**26**:1881–6.

61.   Alves WM, Jane JA. Post-traumatic syndrome. In: Youmans JR, ed. *Neurological Surgery*, Vol. 3, 3rd edn. Philadelphia: WB Saunders, 1990, pp. 2230–42.

62.   Colohan AR, Alves WM, Gross CR, *et al.* Head injury mortality in two centres with different emergency medical services and intensive care. *J Neurosurg* 1989;**71**:202–7.

Maxillofacial injuries

OBJECTIVES

After completing this chapter the reader will:
- understand the significance of facial injuries in airway obstruction and haemorrhage
- be able to provide a systematic approach to the assessment of facial injuries
- be able to describe simple and effective methods of treating maxillofacial emergencies in the resuscitation room.

INTRODUCTION

Since the Second World War, interpersonal violence has overtaken road traffic collisions (RTCs) to become the most common cause of maxillofacial injuries. A study of facial injuries in the UK found that half were caused by assaults, 19% by playing sports, 16% by RTCs, 11% by falls and 2% by industrial accidents.[1] Home Office statistics record that violent crime against the person more than doubled between 1974 and 1990, and it continues to rise.

The most common facial injury following assault is a laceration, seen in almost 40% of all assaults.[2] Those most commonly assaulted are young men between the ages of 18 and 25 years, of whom about half test positive for blood alcohol. Alcohol and, increasingly, recreational drugs are the most important contributory factors in assault cases, and may also complicate the initial management of the injuries. Thirty per cent of all assault victims have fractures, 83% of which are of the facial skeleton.[2] Midface fractures are more common in RTCs, whereas nasal bone fractures and fractures of the mandible and zygoma are more common in assaults.

> Interpersonal violence is now the most common cause of a facial injury in the UK and half of all assault victims with facial injuries will test positive for alcohol in the blood.

ANATOMICAL CONSIDERATIONS

The airway

The commonest preventable cause of death in facial injuries is airway obstruction, which is often due to the tongue falling backwards in the unconscious patient and usually occurs at the scene of the injury before qualified help is available. This is more likely in patients with bilateral fractures of the mandible, when the tongue may lose its anterior support. Facial injuries are also commonly associated with fractures of the teeth or dentures, resulting in bleeding into the mouth. This also compromises the airway when the patient is lying on his or her back. Conscious patients with orofacial injuries are generally more comfortable sitting up, with the head forward, to allow blood and saliva to drain out of the mouth.

The middle third of the facial skeleton

The middle third of the facial skeleton is a complex three-dimensional structure consisting mainly of the two maxillae and nasal bones centrally and the zygomatic bones laterally (Figures 10.1 and 10.2). It is attached to the base of the skull and may usefully be regarded as a 'crumple zone' like that incorporated into the design of a car. In a frontal impact, the middle third of the face will crumple and absorb some of the force that would otherwise be transmitted to the skull and brain. As it is pushed backwards, the middle third slides down the

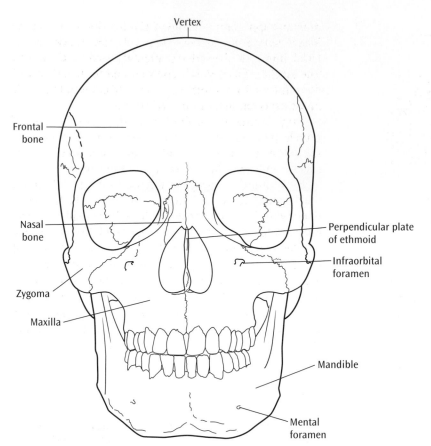

Figure 10.1 Anterior view of the skull and facial bones.

sloping base of the skull, obstructing the airway and causing an anterior open bite in which the front teeth are gagged open. Pulling the upper jaw forwards in this situation may therefore relieve the airway. The maxilla tends to separate from the skull base at one of three levels originally described by Le Fort[3] (Figure 10.3). On clinical examination only the tooth-bearing segment of the upper jaw moves in a Le Fort I fracture, whereas in a Le Fort III fracture the whole mid-third of the face moves, including the cheekbones (zygomas). In a Le Fort II fracture the nose moves with the tooth-bearing segment of the maxilla.

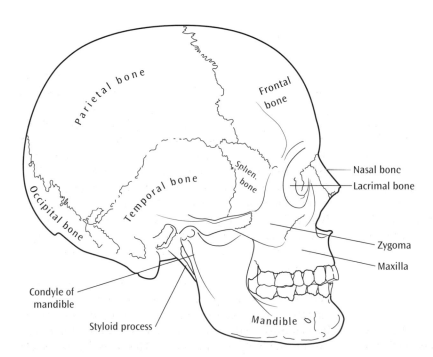

Figure 10.2 Lateral view of the skull and facial bones.

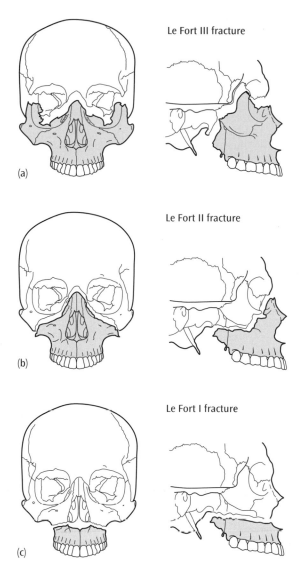

Le Fort III fracture

(a)

Le Fort II fracture

(b)

Le Fort I fracture

(c)

Figure 10.3 Le Fort fracture lines of the maxilla.

The mandible

The mandible, together with its attached structures, forms the lower third of the facial skeleton, and is slung beneath the skull base, articulating with the temporal bones at the temporomandibular joints. The necks of the condyles just inferior to the temporomandibular joints are a point of weakness, and fractures commonly occur here from force transmitted through the mandible from a blow on the chin. The combination of a laceration on the chin and bilateral condylar fractures is sometimes called the 'guardsman fracture', as it might occur when fainting on parade and falling forwards onto the chin.

Soft tissues

The soft tissues which cover the facial skeleton have an excellent blood supply which, when associated with the

dramatic appearance of some facial injuries, may lead the inexperienced to attribute hypovolaemic shock to the facial injury, and overlook internal bleeding elsewhere. The excellent facial blood supply also means that tissues of doubtful vitality may often be preserved at the initial repair in the expectation that they will survive.

Large lacerations of the face tend to gape because of muscle pull, and may give the erroneous impression of tissue loss. Soft-tissue wounds of the lower neck, such as stab wounds, may involve the apex of the lung

Facial injuries, particularly those to the middle third, may cause rapid soft-tissue swelling which masks underlying fractures. Gross swelling of the eyelids may also hide significant damage to the globe of the eye, which frequently remains undetected.[4] The zygoma forms part of the orbit and affords protection to the globe, and the greatest proportion of missed eye injuries are associated with fractures of the orbitozygomatic complex. The branches of the facial nerve (seventh cranial nerve) spread across the face like the fingers of a hand and branches are frequently damaged in facial lacerations.

The cervical spine

The head is supported on the cervical spine, which is easily damaged in deceleration injuries or falls and there is a relationship between facial injuries, head injuries and injuries to the cervical spine.

> An unconscious patient who has a fracture of the middle third of the facial skeleton has a 10–15% chance of having an injury to the cervical spine.

The teeth

Teeth are frequently knocked out or fractured in facial injuries and may be inhaled, especially in the unconscious patient, causing pulmonary complications if not removed bronchoscopically at an early stage. The anatomy of the airways is such that a tooth is more likely to be impacted in the right main bronchus and demonstrated on chest radiographs near the right border of the heart shadow. Smaller fragments of teeth may slip down into the more peripheral airways, making their recovery more difficult. Ingested teeth will generally pass through the alimentary tract uneventfully. Unsuccessful endoscopic recovery of a tooth or part of a tooth may necessitate thoracotomy for its recovery.

Avulsed teeth may also be displaced into the soft tissues, particularly of the lip. Lip lacerations should be carefully explored before closure in the presence of missing or broken front teeth. A fracture of the crown of a tooth may expose the pulp of the tooth. This may be extremely painful and is frequently the main complaint of a patient with a facial injury.

MANAGEMENT

The initial management of a facial injury follows the principles described earlier in this manual. Particular care should be taken to stabilize the cervical spine. The primary survey is intended to detect and remedy immediately life-threatening injuries and the exact diagnosis of the type of facial injury is unnecessary during the primary survey. Those aspects of the primary and secondary survey particularly relevant to maxillofacial injuries are detailed below.

THE PRIMARY SURVEY

Catastrophic haemorrhage control

Exsanguinating external haemorrhage from the maxillofacial region is uncommon, but may not be amenable to compression or tourniquet control. Hypotensive resuscitation and the use of novel topical haemostatic agents such as Quikclot™ or HemCon™ may be useful to control difficult bleeding in head and neck trauma although evidence is currently not available.

Airway with cervical spine control

The patency of the airway is vital, as airway obstruction is the commonest cause of death in patients with facial injury. While the airway is being assessed and re-established, cervical spine immobilization is necessary if not already performed. Ask the patient his or her name as the response affords immediate information on the level of consciousness, patency of the airway and ability to breathe.

> Many patients with facial injuries will be under the influence of alcohol or drugs. Never assume that confusion, abusiveness or lack of cooperation is due to alcohol unless all other causes have been excluded.

It is essential to look for agitation due to hypoxia, cyanosis and the use of the accessory muscles of respiration and to listen for the stridor, snoring or gurgling characteristic of airway obstruction or hoarseness suggestive of laryngeal injury.

ESTABLISH THE AIRWAY

Although severe facial injuries look intimidating, it is usually possible to establish an airway with relatively simple manipulations. It is unusual to have to resort to an immediate surgical airway unless a foreign body is impacted in the vocal cords or there is direct damage to the larynx.

The important stages in airway establishment are to sequentially:

- Clear debris such as broken teeth or dentures from the mouth with a careful finger sweep and suction.
- Perform a chin lift and jaw thrust – which may be difficult when the face is covered with blood.
- Pull the tongue forward – this is often easier with a towel clip or suture passed through the posterior dorsum of the tongue.
- Disimpact a displaced maxilla in a Le Fort injury suggested by the front teeth not meeting vertically. The upper jaw is held and pulled firmly forward.
- Pull a displaced mandible forwards if a bilateral mandibular fracture has allowed the central portion, to which the tongue is attached, to fall back.

If the airway cannot be established by these simple methods, a laryngoscope should be used to check that there is no foreign body impacted in the vocal cords, and, if there is, to remove it. If it cannot be removed quickly and easily, it should be left and a surgical airway performed. If no foreign body is seen and it is possible to pass an endotracheal tube, this should be done. If there is oedema around the glottis, or the degree of bleeding is too great to enable the operator to see the vocal cords, a surgical airway should be performed.

Cricothyroidotomy

A cricothyroidotomy is the preferred surgical airway in an emergency.[5] It is inadvisable in children under the age of 12 years, because of the risk of damaging the cricoid cartilage, which is the only circumferential support for the upper trachea in this age group – an alternative is needle cricothyroidotomy and jet insufflation.

Tracheostomy

In laryngeal fractures, tracheostomy is preferred to needle cricothyroidotomy because of anatomical disruption. This should always be performed by an experienced surgeon.

> Cricothyroidotomy is the surgical airway of choice unless in a child or patient with laryngeal trauma.

MAINTAIN THE AIRWAY

Once an airway has been established, it must be maintained and frequently reassessed. The airway may be maintained by:

- posture
- oropharyngeal airway
- nasopharyngeal airway
- intubation
- surgical airway
- tongue suture.

An oropharyngeal airway is easily dislodged, and poorly tolerated in a responsive patient, while a nasopharyngeal airway is better tolerated and less likely to be dislodged. Neither will prevent the aspiration of blood or debris and either may become blocked with blood clot.

Care is required when passing a nasopharyngeal airway in a patient with fractures of the middle third of the facial skeleton, as these may be associated with skull base fractures. The tube should be passed horizontally through the nostril, and not upwards towards the skull base. Once in position, a nasogastric tube can be passed through it to aspirate the stomach contents.

In patients with severe facial injuries, the main threat to the airway is bleeding into the mouth and oropharynx. Endotracheal intubation with a cuffed tube is preferable, as this protects the lower airways and facilitates ventilation. Depending on the level of consciousness, this may require the use of sedation and muscle relaxants. However, intubation can be difficult when there is uncontrolled bleeding into the mouth. A surgical airway should not be delayed by repeated attempts to intubate.

> Great care is required when passing a nasopharyngeal airway in the presence of a skull base fracture; oropharyngeal tubes, although easily dislodged, may be preferred.

IMMOBILIZE THE CERVICAL SPINE

The cervical spine should have been immobilized prior to arrival in the emergency department; despite this the neck should be examined for the following, temporarily removing the collar and maintaining manual in-line stabilization:

- swelling
- wounds
- surgical emphysema
- tracheal deviation
- laryngeal crepitus
- raised jugular venous pressure.

Breathing

The assessment, control and treatment of breathing difficulty are described elsewhere in this manual (Chapter 6), and are not modified in the presence of facial and neck

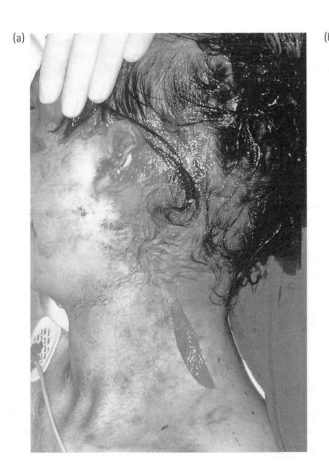

(a)

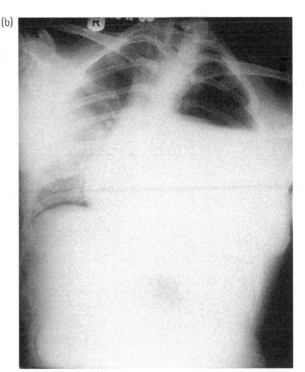

(b)

Figure 10.4 (a) Stab wound to the left supraclavicular neck. (b) The resultant left-sided haemopneumothorax on a chest radiograph.

injuries. It must be remembered that facial injuries sustained in RTCs are frequently associated with chest and abdominal injuries, including diaphragmatic rupture. In addition penetrating injuries to the lower part of the neck may involve the apex of the lung, causing a haemopneumothorax (Figure 10.4). Damage to the phrenic nerve in the neck will also paralyse the diaphragm.

Circulation

The tissues of the head and neck have a good blood supply. However, in the absence of damage to the major vessels in the neck, or severe middle third facial fractures, the degree of bleeding is usually insufficient to cause hypovolaemic shock and hypotension. It is easy for attention to be diverted by a severe facial injury, and to miss covert bleeding elsewhere; similarly, scalp injuries may also bleed profusely, but again are rarely the cause of hypovolaemia. The exception is in children, in whom scalp bleeding may be life-threatening.

> Never assume that hypovolaemic shock is due solely to facial or scalp bleeding.

Post-nasal bleeding into the oropharynx in severe middle third facial fractures may be torrential, difficult to control and often signifies a base of skull fracture. The assessment and control of bleeding follows the principles outlined elsewhere in the manual (Chapters 5 and 8). The following apply specifically to maxillofacial injuries.

Major bleeding from the soft tissues of the head and neck can usually be controlled by direct pressure to the bleeding site. Once the bleeding has stopped, the wound should not be probed, particularly if it is in the neck, until the casualty is in an operating environment where bleeding can be controlled surgically.

> Probing penetrating wounds in the neck may precipitate severe recurrent bleeds.

In the emergency department bleeding vessels in the neck should not be clamped unless they can be clearly seen and cannot be controlled with pressure. Inappropriate attempts at clamping vessels may tear them and inadvertently damage other structures such as the vagus or accessory nerves.

Bleeding inside the mouth is often inaccessible to direct pressure, other than biting on a swab. If the general condition of the casualty permits, he or she should be sat up to reduce venous bleeding and to allow blood to escape through the mouth rather than falling to the back of the throat and compromising the airway. Bleeding from the inferior alveolar artery within the mandible is usually controlled by reduction of the mandibular

fracture and immobilization. It may be helpful to pass a wire around the teeth on either side of a bleeding mandibular fracture, tightening it to pull the ends of the fracture together; in this case, maxillofacial assistance will be required. Torrential bleeding from the region of the nasopharynx following trauma to the middle third of the facial skeleton is difficult to manage, and often signifies a fracture of the skull base. Massive resuscitation may be required.

> In catastrophic bleeding, intubation or a surgical airway may be necessary to secure the airway. A cuffed 6- or 7-mm trachesotomy tube will usually fit into a cricothyroidotomy to stop ingress of blood.

The following interventions may help to control severe bleeding into the nasopharynx:

* Even with good suction, blood accumulates in the back of the throat and obstructs the airway; the head of the bed should be raised to reduce the venous pressure at the skull base if possible.
* Anterior and posterior nasal packs. Alternatively, pass a Foley catheter through each nostril until visualized behind the soft palate, after which the catheter balloon can be inflated and pulled forward to impact in the nasopharynx. A variation is the Epistat™ device with anterior and posterior balloons, which can be inflated to apply pressure to the anterior nasal cavity as well (Figure 10.5). If the maxilla is very mobile, the nasopharyngeal balloons or packs may simply press the posterior maxilla downwards, rather than apply pressure to the skull base. If this happens, it will be necessary to push firmly upwards with a finger at the back of the palate.

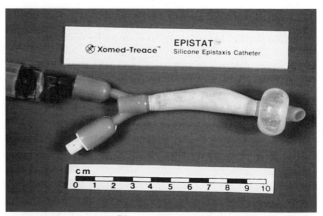

Figure 10.5 An Epistat™ used to control haemorrhage from the nose and nasopharynx.

Disability: brief neurological examination

The assessment of the level of consciousness in the primary survey by the AVPU (alert, voice, pain, unresponsive) method is unchanged in the presence of maxillofacial injuries, remembering that:

- Pupillary signs may be misleading in the presence of cranio-orbital trauma as a traumatic mydriasis may be present.
- The presence of blindness in one or both eyes should be established at an early stage as prompt surgical decompression of the orbit or optic nerve may be effective. Even if the eyes are closed by swelling, it is possible, in the conscious patient, to put a pen torch against the swollen eyelid, and ask whether the casualty can see the light.
- Approximately half of all maxillofacial injuries are caused by assault, and half of those assaults are alcohol related. The level of consciousness, agitation and confusion may be caused by alcohol or drugs, but a hypoxic aetiology must be excluded. Facial fractures, a swollen tongue and dental malocclusion will also contribute to poor speech.

Whilst accepting the additional difficulties of AVPU assessment in the presence of maxillofacial injuries, a baseline level of deficit should be recorded which can be regularly reassessed to detect deterioration at an early stage.

Exposure and environmental control

This remains unchanged following maxillofacial trauma.

SECONDARY SURVEY

Only the maxillofacial secondary survey is described here. In the absence of airway obstruction, or uncontrolled bleeding, the definitive treatment of maxillofacial injuries may usually be delayed until the patient is completely resuscitated and life-threatening injuries have been dealt with.

The head, face and scalp

The head, face and scalp should be inspected for swelling, bruising and lacerations. Swelling may mask the deformity associated with underlying fractures of the facial bones. The bruising and swelling of a 'black eye' may mask fractures of the orbitozygomatic complex, or damage to the globe of the eye. Scalp lacerations should be gently probed with a gloved finger to detect underlying depressed skull fractures, but it is dangerous to probe penetrating neck injuries which have pierced the platysma muscle as this may precipitate severe bleeding, particularly below the angle of the mandible.

Ensure that the branches of the facial nerve are undamaged (Figure 10.6). The branches of the nerve should be tested by asking the casualty to raise his or her

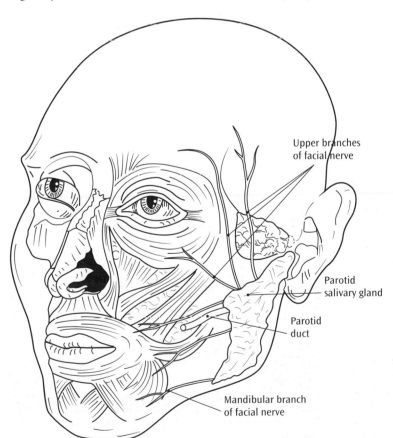

Upper branches
of facial nerve

Parotid
salivary gland

Parotid
duct

Mandibular branch
of facial nerve

Figure 10.6 The main branches of the facial nerve and the position of the parotid duct.

eyebrows, screw up the eyes and show the teeth. Microneural repair of the damaged branches is much easier if carried out at initial wound exploration in the operating theatre.

> When examining facial lacerations, always test the branches of the facial (seventh cranial) nerve.

Parotid duct injuries in cheek lacerations require repair. If facial lacerations are sutured in the emergency department, the wounds should be explored to exclude the presence of foreign bodies and appropriate radiographs taken. All wounds should be thoroughly cleaned to prevent tattooing with debris[5] (Figure 10.7).

> If there is any possibility of a foreign body in a wound such as teeth or glass always perform an appropriate radiograph.

The skull base

Evidence of a skull base fracture should be sought. 'Panda eyes', bruising over the mastoid (Battle's sign) and subconjunctival haemorrhage associated with skull base fractures may take some hours to develop. Le Fort II and III fractures of the maxilla, and nasoethmoid fractures, are often associated with fractures of the cribriform plate of the ethmoid, leading to a leak of cerebrospinal fluid (CSF) down the nose. This may be difficult to detect in the early stages as the CSF is mixed with blood. A clue may be given by the 'tramlines' left by mixed blood and CSF running down the cheek. Blood tends to separate from the CSF to leave two lines of blood separated by CSF. Subsequently,

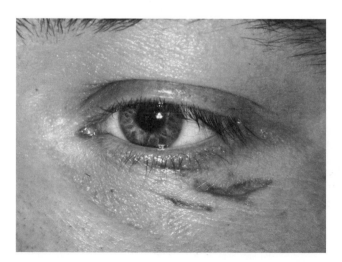

Figure 10.7 Tattooing of a scar as a result of inadequate debridement of a facial laceration.

further investigations may be required to confirm the presence of CSF leak.

The ears

The ears should be examined for haematoma, lacerations of the external canal and evidence of skull base injury. Blood in the external auditory canal is often due to a tear in the anterior wall following a blow to the mandible that has forced the head of the condyle back into the canal. If the tympanic membrane is intact in the presence of a skull base fracture, CSF will not be seen, but the tympanic membrane will bulge outwards and have a blue appearance due to blood in the middle ear.

The eyes

The eyes should always be examined to detect globe damage or fractures of the orbital walls. The reactivity of the pupils, originally noted as part of AVPU in the primary survey, should be rechecked, looking for deterioration. When the eyelids are swollen, it is painful to force them open to allow examination of the fundus; by shining a pen torch held against the lids, the casualty will be able to say whether he or she sees light, indicating whether the visual pathway is intact or not. It may be necessary to delay a full ophthalmological assessment until the swelling has reduced. The incidence of missed injuries to the globe associated with fractures of the orbitozygomatic complex is high, and in these circumstances a full eye assessment should be performed by an ophthalmologist.

> Remove the patient's contact lenses prior to eye examination.

Subconjunctival haemorrhage is noted and, if the posterior limit of the bleeding cannot be seen, indicates that it is blood tracking forwards from a fracture. This sign may take some hours to develop. Subconjunctival bleeding with a visible posterior limit is due to direct trauma to the conjunctiva. Double vision should be recorded, as this may indicate oedema of the orbit or a blow-out fracture of the

Table 10.1 The signs and symptoms of an orbital blow-out fracture

Swelling and bruising around the eye

Diplopia, usually on upwards gaze, which may be painful

Tethering or backwards retraction of the globe when looking up

A sunken eye (enophthalmos), although this may take time to develop and may not be initially apparent

Numbness over the cheek and upper lip on that side in the distribution of the infraorbital nerve

orbital walls (usually the floor) (Table 10.1). Blow-out fractures are commonly missed as they are not readily seen on standard radiographs. In general, a blow-out fracture of the orbit should be suspected when double vision is associated with numbness of the skin in the distribution of the infraorbital nerve, even if no fracture is seen on the 15° occipitomental radiograph. There will usually be blood in the maxillary sinus, however, causing opacity on the radiograph. If the sinus is not too opaque, the 'hanging-drop sign' may be present. This is a small bulging opacity below the shadow of the infraorbital margin on the occipitomental radiograph, representing herniation of the periorbital fat down through the fractured orbital floor. In practice, this injury is usually confirmed on a coronal CT scan.

Facial bones

The facial bones should be palpated to detect fractures. Painful bruising and swelling may mask any underlying step deformity. Fractures of the zygoma and orbit are particularly easy to miss when there is a swollen black eye.

> Beware of the black eye! It is easy to overlook an underlying fracture of the orbitozygomatic complex, or damage to the globe of the eye.

Table 10.2 summarizes the common clinical features of the common facial bone fractures and identifies which is the

Table 10.2 The clinical features of common facial bone fractures

	Facial bone				
	Mandible	Maxilla	Zygoma	Nasal bones	Larynx/trachea
Clinical features	Pain on movement; Swelling and bruising; The teeth do not meet properly – a change in dental occlusion; A step in the occlusal plane of the teeth; Numbness of the chin and lower lip on that side; Bleeding from the mouth	Gross swelling (ballooning) of the face; Disruption of the dental occlusion; Nosebleed; The upper jaw can be moved: Le Fort I – the tooth-bearing portion of the maxilla moves; Le Fort II – the bridge of the nose moves with the maxilla; Le Fort III – both cheekbones move with the maxilla; In maxillary fractures, the middle of the face may look flat, and CSF may leak from the nose if the cribriform plate is fractured. If the maxilla has been displaced backwards there may be an anterior open bite	Black eye; Subconjunctival haemorrhage; Flat cheek unless masked by swelling; Possible double vision; Numbness of the skin of the cheek in the distribution of the infraorbital nerve; Unilateral nosebleed	Swollen and tender bridge of the nose; Nose deformity; Bleeding from the nose; Deviation of the nasal septum with a reduced nasal airway; If the nasoethmoid complex is fractured, the angle between the forehead and nose is deepened, and fractures may be felt on the infraorbital margin on each side. There may also be a CSF leak	Evidence of direct trauma to the neck; Noisy breathing – snoring, gurgling or croaking; Hoarseness of the voice; Crepitus
Appropriate radiograph	Orthopantomogram and posteroanterior view of the mandible	15° occipitomental view CT scan for Le Fort II and III fractures	15° occipitomental view CT scan if orbital blow-out fracture suspected	Nil for broken nose. CT scan for nasoethmoid fractures to determine frontal sinus and orbital wall involvement	CT scan

CSF, cerebrospinal fluid; CT, computed tomography.

most appropriate imaging to request. Computed tomography scanning of Le Fort fractures should be done only after discussion with the maxillofacial surgeon.

Teeth and mouth

If the upper and lower teeth do not seem to meet properly, this may indicate a fracture of the maxilla or mandible. Some dental malocclusions are pre-existing and are developmental in origin. A haematoma in the floor of the mouth strongly suggests a mandibular fracture. Fractured teeth exposing the pulp may be very painful and require early dental management. Broken or avulsed teeth should be accounted for. They may be:

- lost at the scene of the accident;
- intruded into the gum;
- inhaled;
- ingested
- lying in the soft tissues, particularly the lip, as a foreign body.

Case scenario

A 22-year-old man was brought in to the emergency department having been thrown over the handlebars of his bicycle and striking his face on the road. He lost consciousness for less than 1 minute.

Detail the emergency department management of this patient
He should be assessed according to a <C>ABCDE protocol. The primary survey reveals no airway, breathing or circulatory problem. The secondary survey below the clavicles is normal. Assessment of the head and face reveals the appearance in Figure 10.8.

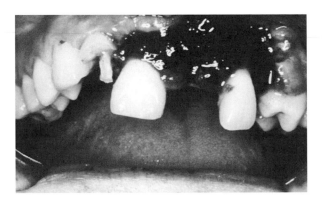

Figure 10.8 Several broken or missing teeth were evident on orofacial examination. Some of these fragments could not be accounted for.

What radiographs are appropriate at this stage?
He should undergo chest radiography to exclude inhaled teeth fragments and, if there is any suspicion of an associated mandibular fracture, an orthopantogram should be taken.

A plain chest radiograph is taken (Figure 10.9). What does it show and what further treatment should he have?

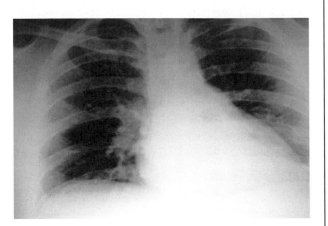

Figure 10.9 Chest radiograph showing tooth in right main bronchus.

His chest radiograph shows a tooth fragment in the lower lobe of the right lung. This was successfully recovered with a bronchoscope (Figure 10.10).

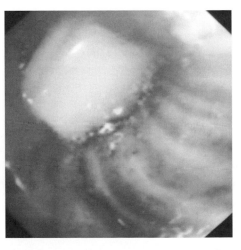

Figure 10.10 Endoscopic view of the tooth in the bronchus.

If a tooth cannot be accounted for, a chest radiograph should be taken to exclude its presence in a bronchus, or smaller fragments further down the bronchial tree. Tooth fragments in the lung should be referred for a specialist opinion and attempted bronchoscopic removal. Retained teeth fragments may lead to chronic thoracic infection.

SUMMARY

Facial injuries, whether in isolation or in combination with other injuries, should be managed in accordance with the principles emphasized throughout this manual. Significant facial injuries often appear more serious than they are, but, if the primary and secondary surveys are carried out carefully, more serious life-threatening conditions will not be overlooked. When death occurs from a facial injury, it is nearly always from airway obstruction.

REFERENCES

1.   Crosher RF, Llewelyn J, MacFarlane A. Should patients with facial fractures be regarded as high risks for HIV? *Br J Oral Maxillofac Surg* 1997;**35**:59–63.

2.   Shepherd JP, Shapland M, Scully C, Leslie IJ. Pattern, severity and aetiology of injury in assault. *J R Soc Med* 1990;**83**:75–8.

3.   LeFort R. Étude experimentale sur les fractures de la machoire supérieure. *Rev Chirurg Paris* 1901;**23**:208–27, 360–79, 479–507.

4.   Al-Qurainy A, Stassen LFA, Dutton GN, Moos KF, El-Attar A. The characteristics of midface fractures and the association with ocular injury: a prospective study. *Br J Oral Maxillofac Surg* 1991;**29**:291–301.

5.   Brantigan CO, Grow JB. Cricothyroidotomy: elective use in respiratory problems requiring tracheostomy. *J Thorac Cardiovasc Surg* 1976;**71**:72–81.

Ophthalmic injuries

After completing this chapter the reader will:
* understand the importance of ophthalmic injury
* be able to take an ophthalmic history and interpret ophthalmic signs

* be able to identify ophthalmic injuries which indicate neurological damage
* understand management decisions
* be able to triage ophthalmic injuries.

INTRODUCTION

Ocular trauma is a significant cause of ocular morbidity that, because of the generally unilateral nature of the condition, does not figure highly on blindness registers. Although ocular trauma accounts for only a small proportion of cases of bilateral blindness, it is the leading cause of monocular blindness.[1] There are 2.4 million ocular and orbital injuries annually in the USA alone.[2] Approximately one-quarter of all eye injuries are work related, and they account for up to 12% of all workplace injuries.[3,4]

THE MULTIPLY INJURED PATIENT

The first priority is a thorough correctly performed primary survey with appropriate attention to haemorrhage control, airway, breathing, circulation and disability. Obvious eye injuries will be noted under E of the primary survey, or during the performance of airway and other interventions.

> The first priority is always <C>ABC with cervical spine stabilization.

An essential part of trauma management is the secondary survey, which must be thorough and include an assessment of the eyes. If this is difficult, then ophthalmic assistance should be sought, since the signs can be subtle and may be missed. If the face is injured, the eye may also be injured, and if the eye is injured the brain may also be injured, particularly with penetrating injury.

HISTORY

An appropriate history should be taken from the patient if possible, or a reliable adult in the case of a young child or an unconscious patient. The AMPLE history:

* **A**llergies
* **M**edication
* **P**ast medical history
* **L**ast meal
* **E**vent leading to injury and the environment

is a useful system to help ensure that all the important factors are covered.

Such information may not be readily available in the early stages of the management of multisystem trauma. In every case, however, the key ophthalmic questions remain the same:

* Does the patient have any visual symptoms or pain?
* Was there a chemical injury or burn?
* Was the trauma blunt or potentially penetrating/ perforating?
* Was there a high-energy transfer injury?
* Is there a possibility of penetrating injury – either ocular or cranial?
* Is there a history of spectacle or contact lens wear?
* Is there a past history of ophthalmic disease?
* Is the patient taking any eye medication?

EXAMINATION

A formal and detailed examination of the eyes and surrounding structures forms part of the secondary survey; however, signs of significant ophthalmic and facial trauma should be noted as part of the primary survey and investigations should be directed accordingly. The examination should follow a predefined format:

- Record the visual acuity.
- Check the pupil light reflexes for a relative afferent pupillary defect (RAPD) by the swinging torch test.
- Check facial, lid and ocular symmetry and appearance.
- Examine the eye movements and check for diplopia.
- Examine the anterior and posterior segments of the globe.

In patients with severe periorbital swelling or haematoma, direct examination of the eye may not be possible, making it difficult to exclude serious pathology. In this situation, the patient's case should be discussed with an ophthalmologist and a computed tomography (CT) scan with at least 2-mm slices of the orbit should be considered.

Visual acuity

The most basic assessment of visual function is the visual acuity,[5] and this is measured by asking the patient to read a standard Snellen reading chart. Visual acuity is recorded as a fraction, with the distance from the chart recorded as the numerator and the best line achieved on the chart as the denominator. The patient should wear his or her spectacles, but if they are not available then a pinhole should be used to overcome any spectacle error. The eyes are tested one at a time, with one eye carefully occluded. Very poor vision is recorded as the ability to count fingers, see hand movements or perceive light. Reduced vision that does not improve with a pinhole is indicative of pathology, whereas reduced vision that is overcome by using the pinhole simply indicates a refractive (glasses) error.

In the patient with polytrauma, early formal assessment of visual acuity using a Snellen chart is rarely possible, and a less formal estimation will be required pending a later reassessment.

The swinging torch test

This tests for a relative afferent pupillary defect (Gunn's pupillary phenomenon),[6] which assesses optic nerve function and gross retinal function.

- In reasonable general illumination, the direct and consensual reflexes of each pupil are checked with a bright light. The pupils should be of equal size, and both should react to light. It is important not to forget the effects on pupillary activity of any drugs that might have been given previously (Table 11.1).
- The light is shone onto the first pupil for 2 seconds, and then swung to the other pupil, taking 1 second to swing across. The light is then swung back to the first pupil after 2 seconds. This movement is repeated for several cycles and the reaction of the pupils is observed. The pupils should react equally, but if either pupil dilates when the torch is shone on it then that eye has poor retinal or optic nerve function (a relative afferent pupillary defect).

In order to carry out this test accurately a number of principles apply:[7]

- To avoid pupillary constriction associated with accommodation (the near response), the subject should fixate on a distant target.
- Each eye must be stimulated identically in an alternating fashion, with the brightness, incident angle and duration of the light stimulus the same for both eyes.
- The alternating swing interval from one eye to the other should be equally rapid in both directions.

Assessment of facial appearance

The majority of patients will have a generally symmetrical face. Trauma can cause fractures of the facial skeleton in and around the orbit as well as significant soft-tissue swelling. This may distort the bony and soft-tissue structure, resulting in facial asymmetry. In craniofacial trauma, the incidence of ocular damage is high, ranging from 15% to 60% in published series.[8]

The face should be inspected and palpated for possible facial and nasal fractures. For example, malocclusion or difficulty opening the jaw may indicate the presence of a zygomatic fracture or cerebrospinal fluid rhinorrhoea may result from a fracture of the anterior cranial fossa. Further orbital evaluation (after assessment of visual acuity and pupils) includes an assessment of eyelid and canthal position, globe position, orbital rim palpation, facial sensation and ocular motility.

Almost invariably there will be eyelid oedema and ecchymosis, in some cases sufficient to shut the eye completely. A mechanical ptosis may occur simply as a result of the oedema or from damage to the levator muscle/aponeurosis. The horizontal alignment of the pupils and lateral canthi is checked by careful inspection. A more formal method, which is not usually appropriate in the resuscitation room, can be performed by holding a transparent ruler in front of the face. The eyes and lateral canthi should be level. Lateral canthal displacement can occur in soft-tissue injuries such as lacerations. They may also result from fractures involving the lateral orbital rim, for example following a zygomatico-orbital fracture causing an inferior displacement of the lateral canthus. Lacerations

Table 11.1 Drugs affecting the pupil

Pupillary action	Substance	Pharmacological action
Mydriasis (dilation)	Alcohol (ethanol)	Sedative and hypnotic
	Amitriptyline	
	Imipramine	
	Nortriptyline	
	Protriptyline	Antidepressant
	Amphetamine	
	Dextroamphetamine	
	Methamphetamine	
	Phenmetrazine	Anorexiant
	Amyl nitrate	Antianginal agent
	Atropine	
	Belladonna	
	Homatropine	Antispasmodic (systemic)
		Mydriatic (topical)
	Cannabis	
	Hashish	
	Marihuana	
	Tetrahydrocannabinol	Psychedelic agent
	Carbamazepine	Antidepressant
	Cimetidine	Gastrointestinal agent
	Clomiphene	Ovulatory agent
	Dipivefrin	
	Adrenaline	Adrenergic agent (topical)
		Vasopressor (systemic)
	Droperidol	
	Haloperidol	
	Trifluperidol	Antipsychotic agents
	Ephedrine	Vasopressor
	Hexamethonium	Antihypertensive agent
	Isoniazid	Antitubercular agent
	Phenylephedrine	Vasopressor (systemic)
		Adrenergic agonist (topical ophthalmic)
	Phenytoin	Anticonvulsant
	Scopolamine	Adjunct to anaesthesia
Miosis (constriction)	Bupivacaine	
	Chloroprocaine	
	Lidocaine	
	Mepivacaine	
	Prilocaine	
	Procaine	
	Propoxycaine	Local anaesthetics
	Ergonovine	
	Ergotamine	
	Methylergonovine	
	Methysergide	Agents used to treat migraine
	Morphine (opiates)	Analgesics
	Neostigmine	
	Physostigmine	
	Pilocarpine	Miotic

and fractures of the medial nasoethmoidorbital region can cause displacement of the medial canthus. Fractures in this region may result in telecanthus (widening of the distance between the medial canthi). Hypertelorism (increased intraorbital distance) may be seen in patients with severe facial injury in whom lateral dislocation of the entire bony orbit has occurred. With injuries in the area of the medial canthus and lateral aspect of the nose, damage to the nasolacrimal system (canaliculi, lacrimal sac and nasolacrimal duct) should be suspected and investigated further by specialist diagnostic canalicular probing and irrigation.

Hypo-ophthalmos (a downward displace of the globe) is the most common non-axial type of globe displacement and is associated with a fracture of the orbital floor. Subluxation of the entire globe into the maxillary sinus has been described in extreme orbital floor disruption.[9] The anteroposterior position of the globe should be assessed.[10] Outward expansion of the orbital walls (blow-out fractures) can produce enophthalmos (a sunken eye). In the early stages following blunt orbital trauma, oedema and haemorrhage can increase the orbital volume, causing a transient exophthalmos (protruding eye) or masking of a potential for enophthalmos. The degree of proptosis or enophthalmos should initially be assessed by careful observation, although subsequent formal assessment with an exophthalmometer will be required following specialist referral. Viewing the axial projection of the globes from above and/or below can help to establish their gross position in relation to each other.

The orbital rim should be palpated for areas of local tenderness, deformity (step defect), loss of continuity (for example, separation of frontozygomatic suture) and crepitus owing to surgical emphysema. Orbital and subcutaneous eyelid emphysema occurs as a result of open communication with the perinasal sinuses (typically ethmoidal) allowing air to dissect into the soft tissue. Usually this does not produce any significant complications although patients should be instructed to avoid straining or blowing their nose (including sneezing if possible) for about 4 weeks after the injury or any subsequent surgery. They should be given prophylactic antibiotics. Rarely sufficient air may accumulate in the orbit to cause a mass effect that can potentially result in a compressive optic neuropathy and severe visual loss.[11]

Anaesthesia or paraesthesia of the facial skin can follow the fracture of bones through which branches of the trigeminal nerve pass to the skin. A blow-out fracture of the maxilla may affect the infraorbital nerve as it runs along the inferior orbital wall, resulting in anaesthesia of the cheek and upper lip.

Lid injuries

Blunt injury can cause a ptosis from avulsion of the levator palpebrae superioris tendon. These patients are treated conservatively. However, it is important to be aware that a third nerve palsy can also cause a ptosis, and therefore the ocular movements and pupils should be examined in order to exclude this.

LID LACERATIONS

The possibility of foreign bodies in the wound or trapped subtarsally should be considered. The lids should be everted if possible and the wound must be searched for foreign bodies and radiographs taken if necessary, being aware that small wounds can hide large foreign bodies. The threshold for performing radiographs should be low.

The contour of the lid margins, which should be smooth and continuous, should be inspected. An assessment of the depth of the wound should be made. The presence of orbital fat in the wound is an indicator of orbital involvement and the possibility of occult injury to the globe, optic nerve and extraocular muscles should be considered.[12] It is also important to consider that the paranasal sinuses and brain may be penetrated if the eyelids have received a penetrating injury, especially if caused by glass or a knife; such cases will require systemic antibiotics in order to prevent infection.[13–15] The lids should be gently retracted in order to examine the eye. This should be done very carefully and may require ophthalmic referral and surgical lid retractors. It is vital not to press on the eye as it may also be penetrated.

> Always consider damage to underlying structures.
> Examine the eye very gently.
> If suturing is required, ask the ophthalmologist to do this.

Eye movements

Ocular motility should be examined, looking especially for restriction of eye movement in any direction. The presence of diplopia (double vision), either in the primary position or gaze evoked, is a useful symptom, but it should be remembered that not all people have binocular vision (for example, those with a history of squint or a lazy eye). The presence of double vision on upwards or downwards gaze and loss of sensation in the area of the infraorbital nerve are suggestive of an orbital floor fracture with involvement of the inferior rectus muscle and infraorbital nerve.[16] In some cases, a degree of neurological trauma may also accompany orbital injuries, and the possibility of higher level disruption of ocular motility, for example from cranial neuropathies or brain stem damage, should be considered. Any ocular motility findings should be taken in the context of the broader picture and correlated with other clinical findings.

Fractures of the facial skeleton will require semiurgent specialist referral unless they involve the airway, or are associated with neurological problems or an orbital haematoma – all of which require urgent intervention. Orbital haematoma is associated with blunt trauma and often with a fracture of the facial skeleton. Most occur in the potential subperiosteal space. On CT examination the lack of adjacent sinus opacification and the absence of systemic toxicity differentiate this entity from a subperiosteal abscess, which can have a similar appearance.[17] Although often only a mild problem, the haematoma can cause a pressure rise in the posterior part of the orbit sufficient to cause an orbital compartment syndrome, compressing the optic nerve; this is a sight-threatening problem and requires urgent ophthalmic referral.[18] The orbital apex is particularly crowded with nerves, thus bony disruption here, along with the associated oedema, can produce a superior orbital fissure syndrome, manifested by ipsilateral ptosis of the upper eyelid, proptosis, ophthalmoplegia, reduced sensation in the ophthalmic branch of the trigeminal nerve and dilation/fixation of the pupil, or an orbital apex syndrome (add reduced visual acuity and RAPD to the above). Again, this situation requires urgent specialist referral for prompt reduction of inwardly displaced orbital fractures. Adjunctive high-dose corticosteroids can also be considered.[19] The signs of orbital haematoma, superior orbital fissure syndrome and orbital apex syndrome are listed in Table 11.2.

Orbital tension is assessed by gently palpating over the swelling through the upper lid. It is important never to press on a penetrated eye as the pressure rise may cause the intraocular contents to extrude.

Table 11.2 The signs of orbital haematoma, superior orbital fissure syndrome and orbital apex syndrome

Sign	Orbital haematoma	Superior orbital fissure syndrome	Orbital apex syndrome
Proptosis with tense orbit	✓	✓	✓
Reduced or absent ocular movements	✓	✓	✓
Reduced visual acuity with RAPD	±	–	✓
Dilatation/fixation of pupil	✗	✓	✓
Ipsilateral ptosis of upper eyelid	✗	✓	✓
Hypaesthesia of ophthalmic branch of trigeminal nerve	✗	✓	✓

RAPD, relative afferent pupillary defect.

> Never press on a perforated eye.

Investigations of facial fractures, which include plain radiography and CT scanning, are unlikely to be a high priority in the patient with multisystem trauma. Nevertheless, appropriate plans should be made for the correct initial and definitive investigations. Definitive investigations will be arranged following referral to the appropriate specialist surgical team.

Facial radiographs can be difficult to read, and if there is any doubt then expert advice should be sought and followed. As well as showing soft-tissue swelling and fractures, the presence of fluid (blood) in the sinuses and the so-called teardrop sign, due to prolapse of the orbital fat pad through an orbital floor fracture, are useful indicators of orbital trauma. A CT scan is particularly good at demonstrating fractures of the floor of the orbit and the optic canal, which can compress the optic nerve – the patient will have reduced vision and a RAPD. If there is a history of high-energy transfer injury, for example following hammering, drilling or blast injuries, the possibility of an intraocular foreign body (IOFB) or bodies should be considered. There should be a very low threshold for ordering at the very least orbital radiographs, although orbital CT with at least 2-mm slices is the best form of investigation in such circumstances.[20]

Anterior and posterior segments: the globe

Examination of the globe of the eye requires practice and, ideally, the use of a slit lamp. If the use of a slit lamp is not possible, as in the case of major multisystem trauma, a bright penlight and close inspection of the eye, or a magnifier such as the plus 10 lens in the ophthalmoscope, should be used. The fundus should always be examined using an ophthalmoscope. An informal assessment of whether the intraocular pressure is raised can be made by the application of gentle pressure to the closed eye. However, this should never be attempted in the penetrated eye.

> Never apply an eye pad to a ruptured globe, since this may inadvertently apply pressure and cause extrusion of the contents of the eye.

The anterior segment

The conjunctiva should be smooth and transparent, but blood may have collected underneath it. Following blunt trauma, if the posterior aspect of the haemorrhage cannot be seen, this indicates that blood may have tracked forward from a base of skull fracture. A CT scan should be considered to exclude this, as base of skull fractures are associated with long-term morbidity, and there may be intracranial injury.[21] Subconjunctival blood may also hide a penetration or a rupture of the globe.[22] If there is any suspicion that this may be the case, expert assistance should be sought.

The cornea should be transparent and perfectly smooth, and should give off a bright, even reflection of light. The cornea should be examined carefully for abrasions, lacerations or foreign bodies. Fluorescein drops should be used with a blue light (cobalt blue filter on the slit lamp biomicroscope) to aid the diagnosis of a corneal abrasion. Iris pigment may be seen where it has prolapsed forward to plug a hole in the cornea.[23]

The upper lid should be everted in order to check for foreign bodies. This should not be attempted if the eye is perforated. Eversion of the upper lid should be carried out in stepwise fashion:

1. Ask the patient to look down.
2. Grasp the lashes between the thumb and forefinger.
3. Place a cotton bud at the top of the tarsal plate (10mm from the lid margin).
4. Push the cotton bud down and pull the lashes up; the upper lid should then evert.

> Do not evert the eyelids if the globe is perforated.

The iris should be flat and have a round pupil at its centre. A distorted iris indicates significant damage to the anterior segment of the eye. Blunt trauma can result in a dilated pupil due to rupture of the sphincter pupillae muscle. Occasionally blunt trauma will cause miosis (pupil constriction).[24]

The presence of blood in the anterior segment indicates damage to the iris, lens, ciliary body or drainage angle. This is called a hyphaema and requires urgent ophthalmic assessment as an uncontrolled rise in intraocular pressure can develop.[25]

Assessment of hyphaema

Hyphaema is most commonly seen in children, and 75% of cases occur in males.[26,27] The timing and exact cause of the injury should be recorded accurately to give additional insight into the likely degree of associated ocular damage. Resist the temptation to focus entirely on the globe. There should be a thorough assessment of the tissues around the eye, including an examination of sensation looking for areas of hypaesthesia and anaesthesia, as blow-out fractures frequently accompany hyphaemas.[28] An accurate drawing should be made of the size and shape of the clot/hyphaema. A note should be made of whether the iris and lens details are visible beyond the hyphaema. If they are, a careful search should be made for signs of iris damage such as an irregular pupil, iris sphincter tears or dialysis (iris root torn away from anterior chamber angle or seemingly the peripheral cornea as you look at it). The lens should be clear; this is best assessed by looking at the red reflex with an ophthalmoscope. Any opacity will appear as a dark area in the reflex. More formal assessment can be carried out with a magnifier or a slit lamp. Afro-Caribbean and Mediterranean patients should be screened for sickle cell disease/trait. Non-steroidal anti-inflammatory drugs (NSAIDs) should be avoided.

THE POSTERIOR SEGMENT

The fundus should be examined with an ophthalmoscope. Blunt trauma can cause:

* vitreous haemorrhage and a cloudy view;[29]
* commotio retinae, seen as greyish oedema and haemorrhages;[30]
* retinal tears and detachment (this usually occurs 2 weeks post trauma).[31]

If it is impossible to examine the eye as a result of severe periorbital swelling, specialist advice should be sought from an ophthalmologist.

* Always suspect a ruptured globe.
* Always consider cranial penetration.[32]
* Always record the Glasgow Coma Scale score.
* Always perform an appropriate neurological examination.

SPECIFIC CONDITIONS

Chemical injuries

Chemical injuries from acid, alkali, solvents, detergents and irritants are an absolute emergency[33–35] and require immediate and copious irrigation with sterile normal saline, even before testing vision.

* The lids should be held apart and the eye irrigated immediately with the nearest water source for 15 minutes. Ideally, saline solution should be used, but non-sterile water can be used if it is the only liquid available.
* A topical anaesthetic should be instilled and eyelid retractors used if available.
* Particles (such as lime or cement) should be sought and removed with a cotton bud or blunt forceps.
* Irrigation must continue until the pH is normal (tested with litmus paper). If the pH is persistently elevated, the fornices should be rechecked for particles.
* Visual acuity must be assessed and recorded.
* A topical antibiotic should be instilled. Ointment is preferable to drops because of its lubricant properties.

* A mydriatic/cycloplegic should be used to prevent pupil spasm. Phenylephrine must be avoided because of its vasoconstrictive properties.
* A sterile pad is applied.
* The patient should be referred to an ophthalmologist.

Superglue

Rapidly setting superglues harden quickly on contact with moisture. These adhesives are generally non-toxic, but, nonetheless, treatment for acidic or basic pH should be carried out as above. No more than gentle pressure should be applied to try and separate the eyelids. Glued lashes may need to be cut to facilitate this. Any easily accessible bits of loose glue can be removed with fine forceps. Treatment from this point should be essentially supportive. Misdirected lashes and hardened glue may abrade the cornea, causing an epithelial defect. Topical antibiotic ointment should be applied to prevent infection and lubricate the eye. Residual glue that cannot easily be removed should be left; it will eventually come away after a few days as the epithelium in contact with it sloughs off.

> Do not attempt to forcibly pull or cut superglue away from bonded tissues.

Foreign bodies

All ocular foreign bodies should be treated as being potentially intraocular, and there should be a low threshold for performing radiography or CT of the eye and orbit in such cases. If a view of the fundus is not possible, an ultrasound scan can provide details of retinal detachment, intraocular foreign body or posterior scleral rupture.

Corneal or subtarsal foreign body

Corneal or subtarsal foreign bodies should be removed carefully with a needle, using the slit-lamp biomicroscope. Corneal foreign bodies may be buried in the corneal stroma and require quite vigorous debridement, which is a specialist procedure. If there is any doubt about the situation, ophthalmic assistance should be sought.

Intraocular foreign bodies

If there is a history of high-energy transfer injury, for example following hammering, drilling or blast injuries, the possibility of an intraocular foreign body or bodies should be considered. Hammering metal on metal (for example, nails and chisels, etc.) is the most common cause of IOFB injury.[36,37] Most IOFBs will be identified radiographically, but investigation (ideally CT) should still be performed even in cases where the IOFB is clearly visible on clinical examination. It is possible that there may be further hidden IOFBs that will only be discovered on radiological examination. All patients with IOFBs should be treated with prophylactic antibiotics (oral ciprofloxacin 750 mg twice daily for 7 days). If the IOFB is small, the entry site may be self-sealing, although larger IOFBs are likely to leave the globe open. Thus, topical medications should not be applied once the diagnosis of an IOFB has been established until an ophthalmologist has assessed the patient. However, it is important not to worry if topical dilating drops have been instilled as part of the examination before an IOFB was identified as the Minims™ eye drops in most general use are preservative free and are unlikely to cause any significant toxicity.

Corneal abrasions

These are very painful but heal quickly. The pupil should be dilated in order to ease ciliary muscle spasm, antibiotic ointment instilled, and a firm double eye-pad applied. The eye must be shut before the pad is applied. The patient can remove the pad the next day and instil antibiotic drops four times a day. Topical anaesthetic drops should not be given for use at home since they inhibit corneal epithelial cell division and healing.[38]

Penetrating and perforating injuries[39]

A penetrating injury refers to a partial thickness wound whereas a perforating injury is one in which there is a full-thickness wound through the tissue concerned (which should be specified).

A penetrating eye injury with perforation of the sclera or cornea is a surgical emergency. The patient should not have topical medication applied to the eye. The eye should be covered with an eye shield rather than a pad as a pad will press on the eye and cause the contents to extrude.

The patient should be nursed sitting up, and adequate pain relief should be given. A tetanus booster must be given if it is appropriate[40] and the patient should also be given systemic antibiotics as with IOFBs. Ciprofloxacin penetrates the eye well and has a broad spectrum of activity. The patient must remain nil-by-mouth, and arrangements should be made for the ophthalmologist to take the patient to the operating theatre as soon as possible.

Orbital haematoma

This is usually a mild problem that requires only conservative management. If the orbit is very tense,

especially if associated with limitation of eye movements or reduced vision, urgent ophthalmic advice should be obtained. A tense orbital haematoma does not need urgent CT scanning, as this will delay the appropriate management – which is urgent decompression of the orbit and/or high-dose systemic steroids. These patients can be difficult to assess, and ophthalmological assistance is essential.

Orbital fractures

Patients with orbital fractures should be told not to blow their nose, and treatment with systemic antibiotics with a broad-spectrum antibiotic (including anti-anaerobic cover) should be started. Further management can be delayed if there is no airway compromise.

Hyphaema

The presence of a hyphaema indicates significant intraocular trauma and is often associated with a blow-out fracture. As such, all patients with hyphaema should be assessed by an ophthalmologist. The management includes bed rest sitting up, pupil dilatation with atropine drops and, if the intraocular pressure is raised, appropriate medical management. If necessary, anterior chamber washout can be considered, although this is potentially hazardous.

Lid lacerations[41]

These all require appropriate plastic surgical techniques for effective closure; therefore, they should be referred after the administration of a tetanus booster and systemic antibiotics as indicated. The position and depth of lid lacerations is important and consideration should be given to more serious concurrent injury (see Assessment of hyphaema, p. 129).

Non-accidental injury

Although fortunately relatively rare, non-accidental injury to children does take place, with direct ocular trauma occurring in 20–25% of such cases.[41,42] There are a number of specific ophthalmological manifestations that should not be missed. Infants generally do not get black eyes accidentally, and corneal cigarette burns may be deliberately inflicted despite apparently plausible explanations.[43] Bruises that appear of different ages may help to reveal inconsistencies in the history.

Retinal haemorrhages occur in shaken babies. It is important to be aware that children do not 'malinger', and reduced vision with a normal examination may indicate psychological problems. If there is any doubt, the child should be admitted and the ophthalmologist and the paediatrician involved.

Associated intracranial injury

If there is intracranial injury, then the intracranial pressure can rise. This may be identified by the presence of swollen optic discs, which should always be sought.[44] The pupils can enlarge because of uncal herniation through the tentorium cerebelli pressing on the third nerve,[45] and so the pupil reactions must always be recorded. The pupils should not be dilated, but if this is done the neurosurgeons should be told as it may mislead them!

The cranial nerves can be damaged, and the ocular movements should be assessed to identify intracranial injury. The patient may not be conscious or cooperative, so these tests may have to be performed later. The cranial nerves and general nervous system should always be examined for associated signs.

The polytrauma patient

Although the immediately life-threatening problems should be addressed first, ophthalmic injury can lead to severe lifetime disability, and the presence of an ophthalmic injury should be sought in all polytrauma patients.

It is important to note that the eyes may be damaged by remote injury. For example, crush injuries to a limb or the chest can result in retinal damage from emboli or Purtscher's retinopathy. Episodes of hypotension can result in infarction of the occipital cortex or the optic nerves.[46]

USEFUL OPHTHALMIC PREPARATIONS

For the prescription of ophthalmic preparations, prefixes are used to denote whether the formulation is an ointment (Oc) or should be used as drops (Gutt or G). Topical preparations contain preservatives, which are toxic to the inside of the eye and thus should not be applied to eyes that may have been penetrated. The most common ophthalmic drugs used in the casualty department (and their uses) are listed in Table 11.3.

SUMMARY

The eye should always be assessed in a careful and systematic fashion. This can be difficult and may require specialist skills. A low threshold for seeking ophthalmological assistance is appropriate. The priorities in the management of the multiply injured patient remain those of the primary survey, but it is important to remember that ophthalmic injury can lead to lifetime visual disability that may be prevented by appropriate timely intervention. Thus, it is vital to judge the management priorities appropriately.

Table 11.3 Ophthalmic preparations

Drug	Use
Amethocaine, benoxinate	Topical anaesthetic. For examination of the patient with corneal foreign body or corneal abrasion. Stings on application
Fluorescein	Orange dye which adheres to areas of cornea with no epithelium. This fluoresces as yellow/green under a blue light when dilute, and is adherent to de-epithelialized cornea. Will stain soft contact lenses yellow
Cyclopentolate, tropicamide	Dilate the pupil. Pale irises dilate quickly and dark irises dilate slowly. Always record in the notes which drug was used to dilate pupils and when it was given
Chloramphenicol,* fucithalmic	Broad-spectrum topical antibiotics. Used as prophylaxis in cases of corneal abrasion and foreign bodies
Ofloxacin	Broad-spectrum, strongly bactericidal antibiotic used in cases of severe corneal infection
Betagan, acetazolamide, pilocarpine	Used to reduce intraocular pressure. Betagan can cause asthma; acetazolamide is a systemic preparation and should not be used in patients with renal failure. Pilocarpine will cause the pupil to constrict
Dexamethasone	Steroid used to reduce anterior segment inflammation. Beware side-effect of raised intraocular pressure
Ciprofloxacin	Broad-spectrum bactericidal systemic antibiotic which penetrates the eye through the blood–retinal barrier. Used in penetrating ocular injury
Cefuroxime, metronidazole	Systemic antibiotics used in orbital fractures and lid lacerations. Note that metronidazole is useful in sinus injury. Cefuroxime may not cover streptococci

Note: atropine and homatropine last for a long time (up to several days) and should not be used in the accident and emergency department.
* See Global perspectives.

GLOBAL PERSPECTIVES

The aetiology, diagnosis and management of eye trauma are the same throughout the world. The only significant difference is the availability and usage of chloramphenicol in eye trauma, specifically in the USA. Whilst topical chloramphenicol can be prescribed in the USA, there is a general Food and Drug Administration warning that it should be used only if there is no alternative treatment available. This is because of the clear association of systemic chloramphenicol with blood dyscrasias, such as anaplastic anaemia, although there are only 23 reported cases of blood dyscrasias potentially attributable to *topical* chloramphenicol. There is no consensus about the safety risk of the ocular use of topical chloramphenicol although there have been some papers warning against this.[47,48] Outside the USA it remains in widespread use as a first-line treatment.

REFERENCES

1. Wong TW, Tielsch JM. Epidemiology of ocular trauma. In: Tasman W, ed. *Duane's Ophthalmology 2002*, Vol. 5. CD-ROM edition. Philadelphia: Lippincott, Williams & Wilkins, 2002.
2. Parver LM, Dannenburg AL, Blacklow B, *et al.* Characteristics and causes of penetrating eye injuries reported to the National Eye Trauma System Registry, 1985–1991. *Public Health Rep* 1993;**108**:625–30.
3. Morris RE, Witherspoon CD, Helms HA Jr, Feist RM, Byrne JB. Eye injury registry of Alabama (preliminary report): demographics and prognosis of severe eye injury. *South Med J* 1987;**80**:810–16.
4. Saari KM, Parvi V. Occupational eye injuries in Finland. *Acta Ophthalmol* 1984;**161**(Suppl.):17–28.
5. Westheimer G. Visual acuity. In: Moses RA, Hart WM, eds. *Adler's Physiology of the Eye: Clinical Application*. St Louis: Mosby, 1987, pp. 415–28.
6. Levatin P. Pupillary escape in disease of the retina or optic nerve. *Arch Ophthalmol* 1959;**62**:768–79.
7. Skarf B, Glaser JS, Trick GL, Mutlukan E. Neuro-ophthalmologic examination: the visual sensory system. In: Tasman W, ed. *Duane's Ophthalmology 2002*, Vol. 2. CD-ROM edition. Philadelphia: Lippincott, Williams & Wilkins, 2002.
8. Gossman MD, Roberts DM, Barr CC. Ophthalmic aspects of orbital injury, a comprehensive diagnostic and management approach. *Clin Plast Surg* 1992;**19**:71–85.
9. Berkowitz RA, Putterman AM, Patel DB. Prolapse of the globe into the maxillary sinus after orbital floor fracture. *Am J Ophthalmol* 1981;**91**:253–7.
10. American Academy of Ophthalmology. *American Academy of Ophthalmology Basic and Clinical Science Course*. Section 7: Orbit, eyelids, and lacrimal system. San Francisco: AAO, p. 113.
11. Hunts JH, Patrinely JR, Holds BJ, Anderson RL. Orbital emphysema. *Ophthalmology* 1994;**101**:960–6.
12. Spoor TC. Penetrating orbital injuries. *Adv Ophthalmic Plast Reconstr Surg* 1987;**7**:193–216.
13. Mono J, Hollenberg RD, Harvey JT. Occult transorbital intracranial penetrating injuries. *Ann Emerg Med* 1986;**15**:589–91.
14. Mutlukan E, Fleck BW, Cullen JF, Whittle IR. Case of penetrating orbitocranial injury caused by wood. *Br J Ophthalmol* 1991;**75**:374–6.
15. Fanning WL, Willett LR, Phillips CF, Wallman LJ. Puncture wound of the eyelid causing brain abscess. *J Trauma* 1976;**16**:919–20.
16. Dutton JJ. Management of blow-out fractures of the orbit. *Surv Ophthalmol* 1991;**35**:279–80.
17. Harris GJ. Subperiosteal abscess of the orbit. *Arch Ophthalmol* 1983;**101**:751–7.
18. Liu D. A simplified technique of orbital decompression for severe retrobulbar haemorrhage. *Am J Ophthalmol* 1993;**116**:34–7.
19. Rohrich RJ, Hackney FL, Parikh RS. Superior orbital fissure syndrome: current management concepts. *J Craniomaxillofac Trauma* 1995;**1**:44–8.
20. Woodcock MGL, Scott RAH, Huntbach J, Kirkby GR. Mass and shape factors in intraocular foreign body injury. *Ophthalmology* 2006;**113**:2262–9.
21. Kylstra J. Preparation of the eye trauma patient for surgery. In: Shingleton BJ, Hersh PS, Kenyon KR, eds. *Eye Trauma*. St Louis: Mosby, 1991, p. 53.
22. Kylstra J, Lamkin JC, Runyan DK. Clinical predictors of scleral rupture after blunt ocular trauma. *Am J Ophthalmol* 1993;**115**:530–5.
23. Barr CC. Prognostic factors in corneoscleral lacerations. *Arch Ophthalmol* 1983;**101**:919–24.
24. Kennedy RH, Brubaker RF. Traumatic hyphaema in a defined population. *Am J Ophthalmol* 1988;**106**:123–30.
25. Little BC, Aylward GW. The medical management of traumatic hyphaema. *J R Soc Med* 1993;**86**:458–9.
26. Crouch ER Jr, Frenkel M. Aminocaproic acid in the treatment of traumatic hyphema. *Am J Ophthalmol* 1976;**81**:355–60.
27. Edwards WC, Layden WE. Traumatic hyphema. A report of 184 consecutive cases. *Am J Ophthalmol* 1973;**75**:110–16.
28. Milauskas AT, Fueger GF. Serious ocular complications associated with blowout fractures of the orbit. *Am J Ophthalmol* 1966;**62**:670–2.
29. Cinotti AA, Maltzman BA. Prognosis and treatment of perforating ocular injuries. *Ophthalm Surg* 1975;**6**:54–61.
30. Bressler SB, Bressler NM. Traumatic maculopathies. In: Shingleton BJ, Hersh PS, Kenyon KR, eds. *Eye Trauma*. St Louis: Mosby, 1991, pp. 187–94.
31. Cox MS, Schepens CL, Freeman HM. Retinal detachment due to ocular contusion. *Arch Ophthalmol* 1966;**76**:678–85.
32. De Villiers JC, Sevel D. Intracranial complications of transorbital stab wounds. *Br J Ophthalmol* 1975;**59**:52–6.
33. Rhee DJ, Pyfer MF, eds. *The Wills Eye Manual*, 3rd edn. Philadelphia: Lippincott, Williams & Wilkins, 1999, pp. 19–22.

34. Roper-Hall MJ. *Eye Emergencies*. Edinburgh: Churchill Livingstone, 1987, p. 88.

35. Pfister R. Chemical injuries of the eye. *Ophthalmology* 1983;**90**:1246–53.

36. Roper-Hall MJ. Review of 555 cases of intra-ocular foreign body with special reference to prognosis. *Br J Ophthalmol* 1954;**38**:65–98.

37. Percival SPB. A decade of intraocular foreign bodies. *Br J Ophthalmol* 1972;**56**:454–61.

38. Abelson MB. The final points of corneal abrasion management. *Rev Ophthalmol* 1995;February:111–12.

39. Esmaeli B, Elner S, Schork MA, Elner VM. Visual outcome and ocular survival after penetrating trauma. *Ophthalmology* 1995;**102**:393–400.

40. Committee on Trauma of the American College of Surgeons. Prophylaxis against tetanus in wound management. *Bull Am Coll Surg* 1984;**69**:22–3.

41. Friendly DS. Ocular manifestations of physical child abuse. *Trans Am Acad Ophthalmol Otolaryngol* 1971;**75**:318–32.

42. Jensen AD, Smith RE, Olson MI. Ocular clues to child abuse. *J Pediatr Ophthalmol* 1971;**8**:270–2.

43. Harley RD. Ocular manifestations of child abuse. *J Pediatr Ophthalmol Strabismus* 1980;**17**:5013–28.

44. Frisen L. Swelling of the optic nerve head: a staging scheme. *J Neurol Neurosurg Psychiatry* 1982;**45**:13–18.

45. Leigh RJ, Zee DS. Diagnosis of peripheral oculomotor palsies and strabismus. In: *The Neurology of Eye Movements*. Philadelphia: FA Davis Co., 1991, p. 331.

46. Lessell S. Indirect optic nerve trauma. *Arch Ophthalmol* 1989;**107**:382–6.

47. Fraunfelder FT, Morgan RL, Yunis AA. Blood dyscrasias and topical ophthalmic chloramphenicol. *Am J Ophthalmol* 1993;**115**:812–13.

48. Doona M, Walsh JB. Use of chloramphenicol as topical eye medication: time to cry halt? *Br Med J* 1995;**310**:1217–18.

Spinal injuries

After completing this chapter the reader will:
* understand the clinical anatomy of the spine and spinal cord
* be able to outline the initial priorities in the patient with a definite or suspected spinal injury
* understand the role of investigations in spinal injury
* understand the principles of definitive management in spinal injury.

INTRODUCTION

Acute spinal cord injury primarily affects young, otherwise healthy men (with a typical age range of 18–35 years, and a male to female ratio of 3:1). The annual incidence of acute spinal cord injury in the UK is approximately 10–15 per million population.[1,2] The permanent paralysis experienced by these 800 or so patients a year leads to major disability, a shorter life expectancy and significant economic costs. Road traffic collisions (RTCs) and falls from heights account for the majority of patients (approximately 40% and 20%, respectively), but sports and leisure activities such as gymnastics, rugby, horse riding, skiing and diving into shallow water are also associated with spinal cord injury.[3] Many patients with spinal injury have other life-threatening injuries, and these may take precedence over the spinal injury in the initial phases of management. However, consideration should be given to immobilization of the spine while resuscitation is in progress.

> In the multiply injured patient, the spine should be immobilized while the primary survey and resuscitation are ongoing.

Advances in the management of spinal cord-injured patients have resulted in an improvement in overall survival and quality of life. Nonetheless, there is still scope to reduce the consequences of secondary injury and further neurological deterioration in the acute phase.[3,4]

> The priority in the management of spinal injury is to minimize secondary mechanical or physiological insults to the spinal cord.

CLINICAL ANATOMY

The bony spine or vertebral column

The vertebral column consists of 33 vertebrae, but only the upper 24 (seven cervical, 12 thoracic and five lumbar) articulate (Figure 12.1). The five sacral and four coccygeal vertebrae are fused to form the sacrum and coccyx respectively. The vertebral column is most vulnerable to injury at the cervicothoracic, thoracolumbar and, less commonly, lumbosacral junctions. These are transition zones in terms of mobility and curvature. The thoracic vertebrae are relatively immobile compared with the cervical and lumbar vertebrae because of the alignment of the facet joints and attachment to the thoracic cage.[5] The sacral vertebrae are relatively fixed within the bony pelvis.

The stability of the spinal column depends primarily on the integrity of the ligaments and intervertebral discs connecting the vertebrae. When assessing the injured spine, the concept of stability is important, as it refers to the ability of the vertebral column to withstand further stress without further deformity or neurological damage. Stability can be determined by considering all the bony and ligamentous elements of the spinal column in three vertical regions or columns. The anterior column comprises the anterior longitudinal ligaments, the anterior part of the

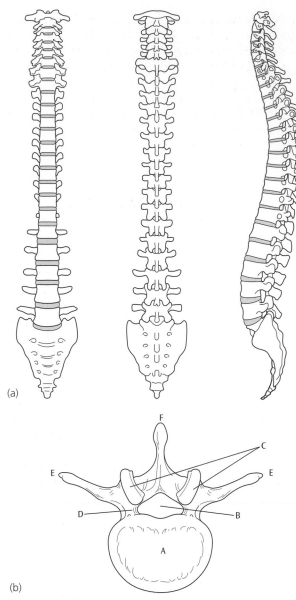

(a)

(b)

Figure 12.1 (a) The vertebral column viewed anteriorly, posteriorly and laterally. (b) The anatomy of a typical vertebra with a dense bony body (A), behind which the spinal foramen (B) carries the spinal cord. The medially facing facet joints (C) articulate withthe vertebra above. There is a laterally placed pedicle (D) from which the transverse processes (E) arise for muscular attachments. There is a posterior spinous process (F).

annular ligament and the anterior half of the vertebral body. The posterior column comprises the ligamentum flavum, supraspinous, interspinous, intertransverse and capsular ligaments (together referred to as the posterior ligament complex) along with the neural arch, pedicles and spinous processes of the vertebrae. The middle column consists of the posterior longitudinal ligament, the posterior part of the annular ligament and the posterior wall of the vertebral bodies. Instability occurs when the middle column along with either the anterior or posterior columns is injured to the extent that ligamentous or bony integrity is lost. When this occurs, the entire vertebral

column should be considered unstable. It is important to appreciate that instability may be purely ligamentous.[3]

> The stability of the spine is dependent on the integrity of the anterior, middle and posterior columns. If two of these are injured, then the spine is potentially unstable and any movement may damage the cord.

The spinal cord

The spinal cord extends from the foramen magnum, through the spinal canal to terminate between T12 and L3 (usually the lower margin of the L1 vertebral body). Below this level, the canal contains the lumbar, sacral and coccygeal spinal nerves (the cauda equina). Between the bony canal and the spinal cord is a potential space which contains extradural fat and blood vessels. The space varies along the length of the spine, and is narrowest in the thoracic area. Fractures of the thoracic spine are thus frequently complicated by spinal cord injury.[6] In contrast, there is a large potential space at the level of C1 behind the odontoid peg, and bony injuries in this area may not involve the cord.

The spinal cord is divided into 31 segments each with a pair of anterior (motor) and dorsal (sensory) spinal nerve roots. On each side, the anterior and dorsal nerve roots combine to form the spinal nerves as they exit from the vertebral column. Each segmental nerve root supplies motor innervation to specific muscle groups (myotomes) and sensory innervation to a specific area of skin (dermatome). By testing sensory modalities and motor functions, it is possible to localize any neurological abnormality to specific spinal levels. The neurological level of injury is the lowest (most caudal) segmental level with normal sensory and motor function. A patient with a C5 level exhibits, by definition, abnormal motor and sensory function from C6 down. It is important to remember that the spinal cord segments do not correspond to the vertebral levels.

> The neurological level of injury is the lowest (most caudal) segmental level with normal sensory and motor function.

The spinal cord is organized into paired bundles of nerve fibres or 'tracts' that carry motor (descending) and sensory (ascending) information (Figure 12.2). These tracts are specifically organized anatomically within the cord. The most important are the corticospinal and spinothalamic tracts and the dorsal or posterior columns. Within the tracts, the more centrally situated fibres innervate more proximal areas of the body (e.g. the arms) and the more lateral fibres innervate the distal areas (e.g. sacrum). The corticospinal tracts carry descending motor fibres and are

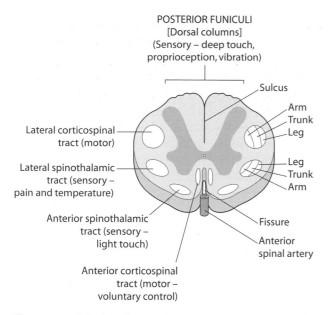

POSTERIOR FUNICULI
[Dorsal columns]
(Sensory – deep touch,
proprioception, vibration)

Sulcus

Arm
Trunk
Leg

Lateral corticospinal
tract (motor)

Lateral spinothalamic
tract (sensory –
pain and temperature)

Leg
Trunk
Arm

Anterior spinothalamic
tract (sensory –
light touch)

Fissure

Anterior
spinal artery

Anterior corticospinal
tract (motor –
voluntary control)

Figure 12.2 Spinal cord anatomy.

located anteriorly within the cord. These tracts decussate (cross the midline) in the medulla before descending into the spinal cord. Injuries to the corticospinal tracts therefore produce signs on the same side (ipsilateral) as the injury. The dorsal columns carry ascending sensory fibres and are located posteriorly in the cord. They transmit light touch, proprioception and vibration sense. As they ascend through the medulla, the dorsal columns also decussate. Signs following injury are therefore also ipsilateral. The spinothalamic tracts lie in two areas: the lateral spinothalamic tracts transmit pain and temperature, while the anterior spinothalamic tracts transmit light touch. In contrast to the corticospinal tracts and dorsal columns, the anterior and lateral spinothalamic tracts usually decussate within three spinal segments (or two vertebral bodies' height) of their entry to the spinal cord. Injuries therefore tend to affect sensation on the opposite (contralateral) side. These anatomical and functional differences are important in determining both the level and the nature of cord injury.[3]

Sympathetic autonomic nervous system fibres exit from the spinal cord between C7 and L1, while parasympathetic pathways exit between S2 and S4. Progressively higher spinal cord lesions cause increasing degrees of autonomic dysfunction. Severe autonomic dysfunction, resulting in hypotension, relative bradycardia, peripheral vasodilatation and hypothermia, causes neurogenic shock (see Neurogenic shock, p. 139).

The spinal cord is supplied with blood by three longitudinal vessels: one anterior spinal artery and two posterior spinal arteries. The anterior spinal artery runs down the midline in the anterior median fissure of the cord. It supplies the anterior two-thirds of the cord along its whole length. The two posterior spinal arteries primarily supply the posterior third of the cord, and frequently anastomose with each other and the anterior spinal artery. Ischaemic injury to the cord may be caused by arterial occlusion

secondary to trauma or a period of profound hypotension. Although the principal watershed area of the spinal cord is the mid-thoracic region, at any given level of the spinal cord, the central cord is also a watershed area. Thus, ischaemic injury can produce a variety of clinical syndromes depending on the vessels involved, the segmental level and the degree of damage in watershed areas. A vascular injury may also cause ischaemia which extends to several segments higher than the initial injury.

PATHOPHYSIOLOGY OF SPINAL INJURY

Mechanism

Combinations of abnormal flexion, extension, rotation and compression will injure the spine in predictable ways. Extension or flexion with rotation is the main cause of injury in the cervical spine, whereas compression with flexion or rotation is the main mechanism of injury in the thoracic and lumbar spine. Although minor degrees of injury may cause significant damage in patients with pre-existing spondylosis, an abnormally narrow spinal canal or instability from diseases such as rheumatoid arthritis, the mechanisms are broadly the same. Whatever the mechanism, approximately 14% of all spinal injuries will result in cord damage.[7] Of these, 40% occur in the cervical region, 10% in the thoracic area, 35% at the thoracolumbar junction and 3% in the lumbar region.

FLEXION

Hyperflexion injuries are typically caused by flexion about an axis anterior to the vertebral bodies. In countries where lap-type seat belts are used (rather than three-point belts), hyperflexion injuries in RTCs are common. Other causes of flexion injuries include rapid deceleration in the flexed position, falls on the back of the head with flexion of the neck, diving and contact sports such as rugby. Anterior column compression and, more importantly, posterior ligament complex distraction occur. The typical bony lesion associated with this mechanism is a horizontal fracture extending through the body, pedicle and posterior elements of the vertebra (Chance fracture). Pure hyperflexion injuries in the cervical vertebrae are less common because flexion is limited by the chin abutting the chest. Extreme cervical hyperflexion can fracture the anterior superior corner of the inferior vertebrae (teardrop fracture) and rupture the posterior ligaments. This unstable injury is usually found in the C5/6 region. The odontoid peg of C2 may also be fractured by sudden severe flexion.

FLEXION WITH ROTATION

The combination of hyperflexion with rotation is much more likely to produce significant injury to the cervical and thoracic spine than other mechanisms. Between 50% and 80% of all cervical spine injuries and most thoracolumbar injuries are caused by this mechanism. Such injuries often follow RTCs or direct trauma. There is significant disruption of the posterior ligament complex and the posterior column. The facet joints, lamina, transverse processes and vertebral bodies may fracture. In the cervical region the relatively flat facet joints may dislocate, without causing a fracture. The spinous processes of C6/7 can also be avulsed by the interspinous ligaments (the clay-shoveller's fracture). With greater shearing forces, all the intervertebral ligaments may tear and the upper vertebral body can be displaced relative to the one below.

EXTENSION

Hyperextension injuries tend to be found only in the cervical and lumbar region. Hyperextension damages the anterior column, and an avulsion fracture of the anterior inferior aspect of the vertebral body may be seen. The posterior aspect of the vertebral body may also be crushed, with a risk of retropulsion of bony fragments or intervertebral disc into the vertebral canal. A special type of hyperextension fracture occurs through the pedicles of C2 following hyperextension with distraction or compression (the hangman's fracture). This may occur with judicial hanging (rather than conventional suicide attempts, which usually result in asphyxiation) or striking the chin on a steering wheel in a collision.

ROTATION

Rotation rarely occurs in isolation. Whether associated with flexion or extension, these forces primarily injure the posterior ligament complex and are frequently associated with instability. There may be an associated facet joint dislocation.

COMPRESSION

Wedge fractures are the most common type of fracture of the lumbar and thoracic vertebral bodies and are usually stable because the posterior ligaments remain intact. They result from forward or lateral flexion around an axis which passes through the intervertebral disc. If the force was sufficient to compress the anterior vertebral body to half the height of the posterior vertebral body, the posterior ligaments must also be considered to be damaged and the injury regarded as unstable. If the direction of force is such that lateral flexion occurs, there will be a compression fracture of the lateral part of the vertebral column. An axial stress that causes both the anterior and middle columns to fail is referred to as a burst fracture. In these injuries, retropulsion of the posterior vertebral wall or intervertebral disc into the canal places the cord at risk.

A specific compression fracture is the Jefferson's fracture of C1 (the atlas). If a weight falls on the head or the patient lands on the head after a fall or strikes the top of the head, the atlas will be compressed between the occipital condyles and C2 (the axis). The lamina and pedicles are fractured and, in addition, the transverse ligament holding the odontoid peg in position can be torn. The transverse ligament prevents posterior excursion of the odontoid peg. The skull and C1 may then slide forward on C2. Despite this, significant displacement must occur before the odontoid impinges on the cord (the anterior third of the spinal canal of the atlas is occupied by the odontoid peg, the posterior third is occupied by the spinal cord and the middle third is occupied by areolar tissue).

Primary neurological damage

Primary cord injury results from mechanical disruption of neural elements. There is a transient or permanent reduction in spinal canal volume by bone fragments, haematoma or soft tissue, with direct impingement on the spinal cord. Penetrating injuries may also cause direct injury. Primary spinal cord injury without radiological abnormality (SCIWORA) occurs in children who are less than 8 years old. The unique hypermobility and ligamentous laxity of the paediatric bony cervical and thoracic spine predisposes to SCIWORA.[8] It has been reported in 20–36% of children with traumatic myelopathy. The most common mechanism is flexion/extension injury, but others, such as axial loading, rotation, lateral bending and distraction, have been described. However, SCIWORA is now almost a misnomer as magnetic resonance imaging (MRI scanning) will reveal many of the abnormalities of spinal ligaments, discs and the cord itself that were undetected previously. Injuries associated with SCIWORA tend to be stable injuries and are often treated non-surgically with prolonged immobilization. Regardless of mechanism, the primary cord injury causes pericapillary haemorrhages that coalesce and enlarge, particularly in the grey matter. Infarction of grey matter and early white matter oedema are evident within 4 hours of experimental blunt injury. Eight hours after injury, there is global infarction at the injured level, and only at this point does necrosis of white matter and paralysis below the level of the lesion become irreversible. The necrosis and central haemorrhages subsequently enlarge to occupy one or two levels above and below the point of primary impact.[9] The extent of this primary neurological damage depends on the spinal level of the injury.

Secondary neurological damage

Major contributing factors to neurological injury are secondary insults occurring in the minutes and hours following injury. Secondary damage leads to interstitial and intracellular oedema, which may further compromise any reduction in spinal perfusion. As this oedema spreads, neurones are compressed and further clinical deterioration can result. With high spinal injuries, this process can lead to respiratory failure. Even when a complete transverse myelopathy is evident immediately after injury, some secondary damage will occur which is avoidable. The common causes of secondary injury to the spinal cord are:

- hypoxia;
- hypoperfusion;
- further mechanical disturbance of the spine.

Although there is little evidence that mishandling of patients is a common cause of secondary mechanical injury, neurological damage can result from malpositioning of the spine in uninjured patients,[10] so extreme caution should be exercised in moving and positioning patients with proven or potential spinal injury.

HYPOXIA

Hypoxia can result from head or chest injuries in the multiply injured patient, and attention should be paid to optimizing oxygenation and ventilation in all trauma patients.

Spinal injury itself can directly impair ventilation or lead to respiratory failure (Table 12.1). There is a direct relationship between the level of cord injury and the degree of respiratory dysfunction. With lesions above C5, there is weakness or paralysis of the diaphragm, vital capacity is reduced to 10–20% of normal and coughing is weak and ineffective. Thus, patients with lesions above C5 will usually require mechanical ventilation. Patients with high thoracic cord injuries (T2–T4) have vital capacities at 30–50% of normal and a weak cough. With descent to lower cord injuries, respiratory function improves, and at T11 respiratory dysfunction is minimal, vital capacity is essentially normal and coughing is strong.[11] To reduce secondary hypoxic damage, impairment in ventilation must be recognized and normal oxygenation and ventilation must be maintained.

> Optimization of oxygenation and ventilation will prevent secondary injury from hypoxia.

Table 12.1 Respiratory failure in spinal cord injury

Intercostal muscle and phrenic nerve paralysis
Atelectasis secondary to decreased vital capacity
Ventilation–perfusion mismatch from sympathectomy/adrenergic blockade
Increased work of breathing (because compliance is decreased)
Decreased coughing with inability to expectorate (with risk of atelectasis and pneumonia)
Muscle fatigue

HYPOPERFUSION

The early phases of primary injury are associated with reduced regional blood flow from direct capillary damage. Further, secondary hypoperfusion may result from either systemic hypotension owing to bleeding elsewhere or a failure of autoregulation. Without autoregulation, a fall in mean arterial pressure will result in a reduction in spinal perfusion. Conversely, if the pressure is increased too much, then a spinal haemorrhagic infarct or haematoma could develop. Secondary damage from hypoperfusion is reduced by early recognition and treatment of hypoxia, hypovolaemia and neurogenic shock.

> Early recognition and treatment of shock will prevent secondary injury from hypoperfusion.

Neurogenic shock

In acute spinal cord injury, shock may be neurogenic, haemorrhagic, or both. Following injuries at or above T6, there is significant loss of the sympathetic autonomic (adrenergic) outflow. Consequently vasomotor tone is reduced and, if the lesion is high enough, sympathetic innervation of the heart is lost. This loss of sympathetic tone results in hypotension and also enhances vagal reflexes, causing profound bradycardia. The triad of hypotension, bradycardia and peripheral vasodilatation resulting from the interruption of sympathetic nervous system control is termed neurogenic shock. It is important to consider this cause of shock in the patient with spinal injuries, although spinal injuries are frequently associated with other major injuries, and hypovolaemia must be excluded before attributing persistent hypotension to neurogenic shock. Hypotension associated with injury below the level of T6, and hypotension in the presence of a spinal fracture alone, with no neurological deficit, are invariably caused by a haemorrhage. To complicate matters, patients with injury above T6 may not show the classical physical findings associated with haemorrhage (tachycardia and peripheral vasoconstriction). Thus, neurogenic shock may mask the normal response to hypovolaemia resulting from other injuries, and the two may coexist.

> Neurogenic shock = hypotension + bradycardia + peripheral vasodilatation.

Spinal shock

For each mechanism of injury described above, there may be complete or incomplete (partial) cord injury. The distinction between complete and incomplete cord injury cannot, however, be made until the patient has recovered from spinal shock. Spinal shock is defined as the complete loss of all neurological function, including reflexes, rectal tone and autonomic control, below the level of spinal cord injury. Spinal shock is unrelated to hypovolaemia or neurogenic shock. It usually involves a period of 24–72 hours of complete loss of sensory, motor and segmental reflex activity with flaccid paralysis and areflexia below the level of the injury. Despite this profound paralysis, areas of the cord are still capable of a full recovery.

> Spinal shock is a neurological, not a cardiovascular, condition.

Within the spinal cord, sacral fibres are positioned more laterally than corresponding fibres from other regions of the body. Spinal injuries (particularly anterior and central) that primarily affect the midline of the spinal cord may not affect the sacral fibres. This results in 'sacral sparing' in which sensation is retained over the sacral and perineal area. Preservation of sacral function may indicate an incomplete cord lesion. However, definitive characterization of the nature of the injury cannot occur until spinal shock has resolved. This is usually indicated by return of reflex activity below the level of injury.

> Complete and incomplete cord injury cannot be distinguished in the presence of spinal shock.

ASSESSMENT AND MANAGEMENT OF PATIENTS WITH SPINAL INJURY

The possibility of spinal injury should be considered in all trauma patients.[12] Common reasons for missing significant spinal injuries include failing to consider injuries in patients who are either unconscious, intoxicated or have pre-existing risk factors (such as arthritis), failing to examine patients adequately, and errors in the interpretation of radiographs.[13–16]

Primary survey

CONTROL OF CATASROPHIC EXTERNAL HAEMORRHAGE

Obviously, any life-threatening external haemorrhage must be immediately controlled before the primary survey is continued. In the majority of cases this will have been carried out before the patient arrives at hospital.

AIRWAY WITH CERVICAL SPINE CONTROL AND BREATHING

During assessment of airway, breathing and circulation, efforts must be made to protect the spinal cord from potential secondary mechanical and physiological injury. Prevention of secondary mechanical injury is achieved by early immobilization of the whole spine. Thereafter, further evaluation of the spine can be safely deferred until immediately life-threatening conditions have been assessed and resuscitation is under way.

The priority in trauma patients is to maintain oxygenation through a patent airway, which may necessitate airway opening manoeuvres such as a jaw thrust, use of suction or basic adjuncts, and ultimately securing a definitive airway in the form of an endotracheal tube. High-flow oxygen should be administered, and ventilation supported as necessary. In conscious patients with signs of a high spinal cord injury (for example, weakness in arms and legs, neurogenic shock or diaphragmatic breathing), early intubation and ventilation should be considered, with indications including CO_2 retention and poor respiratory effort with a low vital capacity. Intubation is not contraindicated in the presence of spinal injury. The ideal technique is fibreoptic intubation with cervical spine control. However, there is little evidence that a properly performed orotracheal intubation with manual in-line stabilization (MILS) will cause further cervical spine injury.[17,18] Oral suction, laryngoscopy and intubation may precipitate severe bradycardia from unopposed vagal stimulation in patients with autonomic disruption from cervical or high thoracic spinal cord injury, so atropine should be immediately available.

During this phase of assessment, the spine should be protected initially by MILS, followed by three-point immobilization with rigid collar, blocks and tape or straps. During this initial phase, the whole spine must be maintained in neutral alignment after gentle controlled movement to a neutral position if this is necessary. Attempts to bring the head into neutral alignment against palpable resistance or if the patient complains of pain should be abandoned and the head immobilized as it is found. The rest of the spine should be immobilized during extrication and transfer using an extrication device or scoop stretcher. The majority of trauma patients will have been immobilized during the pre-hospital phase.[19] The adequacy of immobilization and the position of cervical collars, head blocks and other extrication devices should be checked on arrival at the emergency department. Patients who are agitated and moving around should not have their cervical spine immobilized in isolation. Long spine boards should be removed as soon as possible, usually as part of the log-roll, decreasing the risk of pressure sore development in the spinally injured.

> Do not leave patients on long spine (extrication) boards: remove them during the log-roll. If the patient has sustained a significant head injury, the neck should be immobilized using a spinal board, head blocks and tape without a cervical collar in order to avoid significant rises in intracranial pressure.

CIRCULATION

Persistent signs of shock must not be attributed to spinal cord injury until haemorrhage has been excluded. Almost 80% of patients with spinal cord injury have multiple injuries.[20] The most common sources of occult haemorrhage are:

- chest injuries (often associated with thoracic spine fractures);
- intra-abdominal haemorrhage;
- retroperitoneal haemorrhage;
- pelvic fractures;
- multiple or open long-bone fractures.

Clinical signs of intra-abdominal haemorrhage may be even more difficult to detect in a patient with spinal injuries. Referred shoulder tip pain may be the only indication of intra-abdominal injury, and further abdominal investigation [focused assessment with sonography for trauma (FAST), diagnostic peritoneal lavage or computed tomography (CT)] is essential to exclude intra-abdominal bleeding. Urgent control of continuing bleeding is required to reduce the risks of hypoperfusion and secondary nerve damage.

If occult sources of haemorrhage have been excluded, initial treatment of neurogenic shock involves cautious fluid resuscitation. The therapeutic goals for neurogenic shock are adequate perfusion with a systolic blood pressure of 90–100 mmHg (acceptable for patients with complete cord lesions), a heart rate of 60–100 beats/min, urine output above 30 mL/h and normothermia.

THE LOG-ROLL

A log-roll should be performed as part of the secondary survey. This allows assessment of the back and spinal column and the removal of the long spine board if one is present. Before the log-roll is commenced, MILS should be instituted before blocks and straps are removed. The collar can also be removed at this stage to check the neck for any deformity, tenderness, bogginess or spasm. To examine the remainder of the vertebral column, the patient must be 'log-rolled'. This technique requires at least five people. One person, the team leader, is responsible for maintaining the in-line stabilization of the head and neck and coordination of the log-roll. A second person holds the patient's shoulder with one hand and places the other hand on the pelvis. The third person holds the pelvis with one hand and places the other hand under the patient's opposite thigh. The fourth person places both arms under the opposite lower leg and supports it during the roll. The fifth person is responsible for examining the back, conducting a rectal and perineal examination, observing pressure areas and clearing debris. Further staff will be needed to assist with the removal of a long spine board. The team leader must give clear audible instructions and indicate in advance what these will be. For example: 'We are going to roll ninety degrees to the patient's left. The instruction will be ready, brace, roll. We will roll on the R of roll.'

The examination of the back includes looking for evidence of bruising or swelling, palpation over the spinous processes for deformity, swelling, wounds or increased tenderness down the whole length of the spine. Local tenderness at any point should be used to guide radiographic examination. Examination of the perineum should identify sacral sparing, assess anal tone by digital rectal examination and check for the presence of priapism (a sustained penile erection secondary to spinal injury). Once the log-roll is completed, the patient can be rolled back to the supine position using similar instructions as before.

Patients with an altered level of consciousness or other distracting injuries may not have any features on examination of the back to suggest spinal injury, and may be unable to cooperate with neurological examination. Other signs which suggest spinal injury in these patients are listed in Table 12.2. These patients will require spinal immobilization until they regain full consciousness, at which time further neurological assessment should take place.

Secondary survey

The secondary survey involves a head-to-toe examination including top, bottom, left, right, back and front. In conscious patients this includes a focused history to establish pre-existing medical conditions, the mechanism of injury and the presence of back or neck pain, limb weakness and sensory disturbance. Most conscious patients with spinal injury will complain of pain in the region of the injury, although this is less reliable in patients with an altered level of consciousness or multiple injuries.[21–24] The patient should then be asked to move each limb in turn, provided that there is no pain or discomfort in the limb or spinal column. In addition, direct questions should be asked regarding absent or abnormal sensation in the limbs or trunk. The spectrum of symptoms and signs associated with incomplete cord lesions is so varied that any sensory or motor symptoms should be taken seriously. At this stage, a more thorough

Table 12.2 Signs of spinal injury in the unconscious patient

Diaphragmatic breathing
Neurogenic shock (hypotension and bradycardia)
Flaccid areflexia (spinal shock)
Flexed posture of the upper limbs (loss of extensor innervation distal to C5)
Response to pain above the clavicles only
Priapism (the erection may be incomplete)

Table 12.3 Segmental values for dermatomes and myotomes

Segment	Representative dermatomes	Representative myotomes
C5	Sensation over deltoid	Deltoid muscle
C6	Sensation over thumb	Wrist extensors
C7	Sensation over middle finger	Elbow extensors
C8	Sensation over little finger	Middle finger flexors
T1	Sensation over inner aspect of elbow	Little finger abduction
T4	Sensation around nipple	–
T8	Sensation over xiphisternum	–
T10	Sensation around umbilicus	–
T12	Sensation around symphysis	–
L1	Sensation in inguinal region	–
L2	Sensation on anterior upper thigh	Hip flexors
L3	Sensation on anterior mid-thigh	Knee extensors
L4	Sensation on medial aspect of leg	Ankle dorsiflexors
L5	Sensation between first and second toes	Long toe extensors
S1	Sensation on lateral border of foot	Ankle plantar flexors
S3	Sensation over ischial tuberosity	–
S4/5	Sensation around perineum	–

neurological examination should be carried out. Each dermatome should be tested for sensitivity to a sterile pin or similar stimulus (pain) and cotton wool (light touch). Coordination, tone, power and deep tendon reflexes must then be tested and any asymmetry noted. The root values of dermatomes and myotomes must be known in order to interpret the findings (Table 12.3). Assessment of power should be standardized to allow comparison over time and between limbs (Table 12.4).

The aim of the neurological examination is to determine the level and nature of the lesion, document the deficit and identify the need for emergency treatment. Injuries above C5 cause quadriplegia and respiratory failure. At C4 and C5 the deltoid, supraspinatus and infraspinatus are weak or movement is absent, and at C5 and C6 the biceps are also weak or movement is absent. Injuries at C7 cause weakness or loss of use of the triceps, wrist extensors and forearm pronators. Injuries at T1 and below cause paraplegia; the precise level can be determined from the level of sensory loss. Injuries from T10 down can cause a cauda equina syndrome. The cauda equina includes the terminal spinal cord and the spinal roots from T12 to S5. Acute compression may cause bilateral leg pain, flaccid paralysis and retention of urine. Pain in the sacral dermatomes may also be present. A burst fracture of L1 is a typical cause of acute cauda equina syndrome.

By the end of the secondary survey, there should be a clear indication of the presence and immediate consequences of any spinal injury. The patient should also have a nasogastric tube and urinary catheter *in situ*. These help to prevent bladder and gastrointestinal distension developing after spinal injury. Urinary catheterization must be performed under strictly aseptic conditions in order to reduce the incidence of infection.

Incomplete cord injury

A complex situation can arise in which there is an incomplete cord injury. In general, it is not possible to determine the precise nature of the injury in the acute phase, and inappropriate attempts to do so may distract from more immediate clinical priorities. However, any motor or sensory sparing revealed by meticulous examination in the acute phase may have enormous prognostic value.[25] There are three principal patterns of incomplete cord injury which can sometimes be recognized – anterior, central, and lateral cord syndromes.

- An anterior cord syndrome results from direct mechanical compression of the anterior cord or obstruction of the anterior spinal artery. It affects the spinothalamic and corticospinal tracts, resulting in variable loss of motor function (corticospinal tracts) and impaired pain/temperature sensation (spinothalamic tracts). There is preservation of light touch, proprioception and vibration sense (dorsal columns).
- Central cord syndromes are produced by brief compression of the cervical cord and disruption of the central grey matter. They usually occur in patients with an already narrow spinal canal, either congenitally or

Table 12.4 Muscle power

0 = no flicker of movement
1 = a flicker of contraction, but no movement
2 = movement, but not against gravity
3 = movement against gravity
4 = movement against resistance
5 = normal power

from cervical spondylosis. There is weakness of the arms, often with pin-prick loss over the arms and shoulders, and relative sparing of leg power and sensation on the trunk and legs. Abnormality of bladder function and dysaesthesias in the upper extremities (burning hands or arms) are common. There is usually sacral sparing. This pattern is a result of the anatomical arrangement of fibres within the cord. The more centrally situated fibres supply the arms and these are therefore the most affected by central lesions in the cervical cord.

- Penetrating trauma may cause a lateral cord syndrome (Brown-Séquard syndrome). All sensory and motor modalities are disrupted on the side of the wound at the level of the lesion. Below this level, however, there is ipsilateral loss of muscle power and tone, proprioception, vibration sense and motor function with contralateral loss of pain and temperature sensation.

RADIOGRAPHY

Fully conscious patients who are not under the influence of alcohol or drugs and who have no neck pain or tenderness, no abnormal neurological symptoms or signs and no major distracting injuries do not require cervical spine radiographs.[26] Under these circumstances the spine can be cleared clinically.

Patients with symptoms or signs, altered consciousness, intoxication or major distracting injuries require three cervical spine radiographs: a lateral to include the top of the T1 vertebral body; a long anteroposterior (AP) view; and an open-mouth AP view to show the C1/C2 articulation.[21,22,27–30] The combination of these three views has a high sensitivity for spinal injury,[31] although injuries may still be missed.[32] All radiographs should be interpreted using the ABCDS system (Table 12.5). The interpretation of all three standard cervical spine radiographs is summarized in Table 12.6.[33,34]

Given that up to one-quarter of patients with spinal injury have damage at more than one level, it is usually necessary to obtain further radiographs once resuscitation is complete. Combinations of cervical and thoracic fractures or thoracic and lumbar fractures are most common.[35] In conscious patients, these should be guided by symptoms and signs, but additional films typically include AP and lateral thoracic or lumbar spine radiographs. All five lumbar vertebrae should be clearly visible along with the lumbosacral junction and the thoracic vertebrae under investigation. The alignment can be

Table 12.5 The ABCDS system of radiographic interpretation

Adequacy and alignment
Bones
Cartilage and joints
Disc space
Soft tissue

Table 12.6 Interpretation of cervical spine radiographs

Lateral view
Top of T1 must be visible
The three longitudinal arcs should be maintained
The vertebral bodies should be of uniform height
The odontoid peg should be intact and closely applied to C2

Anteroposterior view
Spinous processes should be in a straight line and equally spaced

Open-mouth view
Base of the odontoid peg is intact
Lateral margins of C1 and C2 align
Spaces on either side of the odontoid peg are equal

assessed on lateral films using the three lines described for the cervical spine. These change from kyphotic to lordotic at the T1/L1 junction. In the lumbar region, a line running through the facet joints should also trace out a smooth curve, although this is difficult to see in the thoracic region because of the overlying ribs. On the AP views, vertical alignment of the spinous processes should also be checked. In addition, the distance between the two lateral borders of the vertebra, the pedicles and the facet joints increases progressively down the vertebral column. Malalignment may indicate a unifacet dislocation or a fracture of the lateral articular surface. In these cases, the spinous process tends to rotate towards the side of the injury.

The intervertebral discs should be similar and even throughout, and their height usually increases progressively down the spine to L4/L5. Commonly, the disc at L5/S1 is narrower than that at L4/L5, and is associated with dense sclerosis of the underlying cortical surfaces and marginal osteophytes. The soft-tissue shadows around the vertebral column may be the only clue to an underlying bony or ligamental injury. Soft-tissue changes on AP films following fractures of the upper thoracic vertebrae can mimic a ruptured thoracic aorta, as paravertebral soft-tissue swelling is difficult to distinguish from mediastinal enlargement. The interpretation of thoracic and lumbar spine radiographs are summarized in Table 12.7.

Table 12.7 Interpretation of thoracic and lumbar spine radiographs

Lateral views
The three longitudinal arcs should be maintained
The vertebral bodies should be of uniform height
Loss of height or wedging should be sought
Normal posterior concavity of vertebral bodies maintained

Anteroposterior views
Spinous processes should be in a straight line and equally spaced
Soft-tissue paraspinal line does not bulge
The vertebral bodies should be of uniform height
Distance between pedicles shows normal slight widening

Computed tomography

Computed tomography scanning has become the mainstay for definitive imaging of vertebral column injuries. Middle and posterior column fractures can be clearly visualized,[36] although fractures, subluxations and dislocations that parallel the plane of the scan (typically involving the odontoid peg, facets or pedicles) may be better visualized on plain films as they can be missed by CT.[37] There is evidence that routine imaging of the upper cervical spine in patients undergoing CT for head injury will reveal abnormalities not detected on the plain film,[38] and CT of the cervical spine is standard in patients who are intubated and ventilated prior to CT of the head.

Magnetic resonance imaging

Magnetic resonance imaging (MRI) is ideal for imaging the contents of the spinal canal and detecting ligamentous and intervertebral disc damage,[39] as well as vascular injury. It will also identify extradural spinal haematomas and spinal cord haemorrhage, contusion and oedema.[40,41] Sagittal T2-weighted images are regarded as most useful in defining ligamentous injury. However, MRI scanning is currently suitable only for haemodynamically stable patients and is therefore unlikely to be of use in the resuscitation phase of dealing with a patient with multiple injuries.

Flexion/extension views

Conscious patients who have well-localized, severe central neck pain but no neurological or radiographic abnormalities may have an unstable ligamentous injury.[42,43] Such injuries are much more common in the cervical spine. If there is any suggestion of abnormality on the plain films, CT should be undertaken before flexion/extension views.[44] Flexion views of the cervical spine may be useful in demonstrating any instability; these are achieved by asking the patient to flex his or her neck voluntarily during exposure, after which the film should be examined for evidence of subluxation. Flexion/extension views are much less commonly used now that CT and MRI scanning have become widespread.

EMERGENCY TREATMENT

The aim of emergency treatment in spinal injury is to reduce secondary injury, improve motor function and sensation and reduce the extent of permanent paralysis. This should concentrate on minimizing secondary physiological and mechanical injury by optimizing oxygenation, ventilation and perfusion, maintaining spinal immobilization, and in some cases surgical decompression.

Steroids

One of the most controversial areas in the management of spinal cord injury is the use of steroids. There has been much debate over the last two decades as a result of limited evidence from the three US National Acute Spinal Cord Injury studies (NASCIS), which investigated the use of methylprednisolone in acute spinal cord injury.[45–49] Initial reports of improved outcome in certain subgroups of patients were a result of post hoc analysis, which has led to methodological criticism. Further studies have provided no evidence of benefit.[50] Indeed, there is mounting evidence that adverse event rates are higher with the use of steroids, including sepsis, incidence of pulmonary embolism, pancreatitis and gastrointestinal haemorrhage.

This has led to statements being issued by several international organizations including the British Association of Spinal Surgeons, and there seems to be agreement that, when the current evidence is considered, there is no role for the use of steroids in the management of acute spinal cord injury.

Surgery

Although open wounds require surgical exploration, the timing of surgery in patients who have sustained a closed acute spinal cord injury remains controversial.[51] Surgically remediable and potentially reversible cord compression owing to dislocation of a vertebral body or displaced bone fragments must be treated urgently. Decompression within 2 hours may allow some recovery of spinal cord function. However, even stable injuries can be associated with significant cord compression and may benefit from decompression. Early decompression is also advocated for incomplete lesions, especially if the limbs are becoming progressively weaker. Detailed clinical and radiological evaluation will usually be required in order to make informed treatment decisions.

DEFINITIVE CARE

Although some fractures heal with immobilization and time (usually 2–3 months), many patients with complex vertebral fractures will require closed or open reduction and internal fixation to ensure stability. This is usually undertaken by neurosurgeons or orthopaedic surgeons with a specialist interest in spinal surgery. Skull traction may be required in the interim, or may be used as definitive treatment. Manipulative reduction in experienced hands can result in dramatic improvement.[52] When spinal cord injury is present, the patient should be discussed with, and preferably managed by, a specialist spinal injuries unit. If this requires transfer, the patient should be fully resuscitated and accompanied by appropriately trained staff to maintain immobilization and manage any complications (such as respiratory failure).

Obtain early specialist advice.

SUMMARY

The management of suspected spinal cord injury involves early immobilization of the whole spine and the institution of measures to prevent secondary injury from hypoxia, hypoperfusion or further mechanical disturbance. Early ventilation and management of neurogenic shock are the key elements of resuscitation specific to spinal injuries. All spinal injuries should be considered unstable and incomplete until proven otherwise. Careful and informed neurological assessment, together with appropriate plain radiography, will identify the majority of spinal injuries. Early surgical decompression should be considered. Imaging using computed tomography and magnetic resonance imaging may be required to define the extent and nature of the injury. Definitive care is best undertaken in specialist multidisciplinary units, and may involve further operative stabilization of the spine.

REFERENCES

1. Swain A. Trauma to the spine and spinal cord. In: Skinner D, Swain A, Peyton R, Robertson C, eds. *Cambridge Textbook of Accident and Emergency Medicine*. Cambridge: Cambridge University Press, 1997, pp. 510–32.

2. Leggate JRS, Driscoll PA, Gwinnutt CL, Sweeby CA. Trauma of the spine and spinal cord. In: Driscoll P, Skinner D, eds. *Trauma Care: Beyond the Resuscitation Room*. London: BMJ Books, 1998, pp. 135–55.

3. Grundy D, Swain A. *ABC of Spinal Cord Injury*, 3rd edn. London: BMJ Books; 1996.

4. Toscano J. Prevention of neurological deterioration before admission to a spinal cord injury unit. *Paraplegia* 1988;26:143–50.

5. Savitsky E, Votey S. Emergency approach to acute thoracolumbar spine injury. *J Emerg Med* 1997;15:49–60.

6. Burt AA. Thoracolumbar spinal injuries: clinical assessment of the spinal cord injured patient. *Curr Orthop* 1988;2:210–13.

7. Riggins RS, Kraus JF. The risks of neurologic damage with fractures of the vertebrae. *J Trauma* 1977;17:126–33.

8. Kriss VM, Kriss TC. SCIWORA Spinal Cord Injury Without Radiographic Abnormality in infants and children. *Clin Pediatr* 1996;35:119–24.

9. Janssen L, Hansebout RR. Pathogenesis of spinal cord injury and newer treatments: a review. *Spine* 1989;14:23–32.

10. Merli GJ, Staas WE Jr. Acute transverse myelopathy: association with body position. *Arch Phys Med Rehabil* 1985; 66: 325–8.

11. Ali J, Qi W. Pulmonary function and posture in traumatic quadriplegia. *J Trauma* 1995;39:334–7.

12. Cohn SM, Lyle WG, Linden CH, *et al.* Exclusion of cervical spine injury: a prospective study. *J Trauma* 1991;31:570–4.

13. Ravichandran G, Silver JR. Missed injuries of the spinal cord. *BMJ* 1982;284:953–6.

14. Reid DC, Henderson R, Saboe L. Etiology and clinical course of missed spine fractures. *J Trauma* 1987;27:980–6.

15. Gerritis BD, Petersen EU, Mabry J, *et al.* Delayed diagnosis of cervical spine injuries *J Trauma* 1991;31:1622–6.

16. Davis JW, Phraener DL, Hoyt DB, *et al.* The etiology of missed cervical spine injuries. *J Trauma* 1993;34:342–6.

17. Majernick TG, Bieniek R, Houston JB, Hughes HG. Cervical spine movement during oro-tracheal intubation. *Ann Emerg Med* 1986;15:417–20.

18. Mcleod ADM, Calder I. Spinal cord injury and direct laryngoscopy – the legend lives on. *Br J Anaesth* 2000;84:705–9.

19. Faculty of Pre-hospital Care of the Royal College of Surgeons of Edinburgh and Joint Royal Colleges Ambulance Service Liaison Committee. Joint position statement on spinal immobilization and extrication. *Prehosp Immediate Care* 1998;2:168–72.

20. Burney RE, Maio RF, Maynard F, Karunas R. Incidence, characteristics and outcome of spinal cord injury at trauma centers in North America. *Arch Surg* 1993;128:596–9.

21. Ringenberg BJ, Fischer AK, Urdaneta LF, Midthun MA. Rational ordering of cervical spine radiographs following trauma. *Ann Emerg Med* 1988;17:792–6.

22. Ross SE, O'Malley KF, de Long WG, Born CT, Schwab CW. Clinical predictors of unstable cervical spine injury in the multiply injured patient. *Injury* 1992;23:317–19.

23. Roberge RJ, Wears RC. Evaluation of neck discomfort, neck tenderness and neurological deficits as indicators for radiography in blunt trauma. *J Emerg Med* 1992;10:539–44.

24. Cooper C, Dunham M, Rodriquez A. Falls and major injuries are risk factors for thoracolumbar fractures: cognitive impairment and multiple injuries impede the detection of back pain and tenderness. *J Trauma* 1995;38:692–6.

25. Folman Y, Masri W. Spinal cord injury: prognostic indicators. *Injury* 1989;20:92–3.

26. Hoffman JR, Mower WR, Wolfson AB, Todd KH, Zucker MI. Validity of a set of clinical criteria to rule out injury to the cervical spine in patients with blunt trauma. National Emergency X-Radiography Utilisation Study Group. *N Engl J Med* 2000;343:94–9.

27. Hoffman JR, Schriger DL, Mower W, Luo JS, Zucker M. Low risk criteria for cervical radiography in blunt trauma: a prospective study. *Ann Emerg Med* 1992;21:1454–60.

28.   Ross SE, Schwab CW, Eriberto TD, Delong WG, Born CT. Clearing the cervical spine: initial radiologic evaluation. *J Trauma* 1987;27:1055–60.

29.   MacDonald RL, Schwartz ML, Mirich D, Sharkey PW, Nelson WR. Diagnosis of cervical spine injury in motor vehicle crash victims: how many X-rays are enough? *J Trauma* 1990;**30**:392–7.

30.   West OC, Anbari MM, Pilgram TK, Wilson AJ. Acute cervical spine trauma: diagnostic performance of single-view versus three-view radiographic screening. *Radiology* 1997;**204**:819–23.

31.   Streitweser DR, Knopp R, Wales LR, Williams JL, Tonnemacher K. Accuracy of standard radiographic views in detecting cervical spine fractures. *Ann Emerg Med* 1993;**12**:538–42.

32.   Woodring JH, Lee C. Limitations of cervical radiography in the evaluation of acute cervical trauma. *J Trauma* 1993;**34**:32–9.

33.   Kathol MH. Cervical spine trauma. What is new? *Radiol Clin North Am* 1997;**35**:507–32.

34.   Raby N, Berman L, de Lacey G. *Accident and Emergency Radiology: A Survival Guide.* London: WB Saunders, 1995.

35.   Keenan TL, Antony J, Benson DR. Non-contiguous spinal fractures. *J Trauma* 1990;**30**:489–91.

36.   Borock EC, Grabram SG, Jacobs LM, Murphy MA. A prospective analysis of a two year experience using computer tomography as an adjunct for cervical spine clearance. *J Trauma* 1991;**31**:1001–6.

37.   Woodring JH, Lee CL. The role and limitations of computerised tomography scanning in the evaluation of cervical trauma. *J Trauma* 1992;**33**:698–708.

38.   Kirshenbaum KJ, Nadimpalli SR, Fantus R, Cavallino RP. Unsuspected upper cervical spine fractures associated with significant head trauma: role of CT. *J Emerg Med* 1990;**8**:183–98.

39.   Benzel EC, Hart BL, Ball PA, *et al.* Magnetic resonance imaging for the evaluation of patients with occult cervical spine injuries. *J Neurosurg* 1996;**85**:824–9.

40.   Flanders A, Schaefer D, Doan H, *et al.* Acute cervical spine trauma: correlation of MR findings with degree of neurological deficit. *Radiology* 1990;**177**:25–33.

41.   Johnson G. Early imaging of spinal trauma. *Trauma* 1999;**1**:227–34.

42.   Wilberger JE, Maroon JC. Occult post-traumatic cervical ligamentous instability. *J Spinal Disord* 1990;**3**:156–61.

43.   Lewis LM, Docherty M, Ruoff BE, *et al.* Flexion/extension views in the evaluation of cervical spine injuries. *Ann Emerg Med* 1991;**20**:117–21.

44.   Clancy MJ. Clearing the cervical spine of adult victims of trauma. *J Accid Emerg Med* 1999;**16**:208–14.

45.   Bracken MB, Shepard MJ, Hellenbrand KG, *et al.* Methylprednisolone and neurological function 1 year after spinal cord injury. Results of the National Acute Spinal Cord Injury Study. *J Neurosurg* 1985;**63**:704–13.

46.   Bracken MB, Shepard MJ, Collins WF, *et al.* Methylprednisolone or naloxone in the treatment of acute spinal cord injury. Results of the second National Acute Spinal Cord Injury Study. *N Engl J Med* 1990;**322**:1405–11.

47.   Bracken MB, Shepard MJ, Collins WF, *et al.* Methylprednisolone or naloxone treatment after acute spinal cord injury: 1 year follow up data. Results of the second National Acute Spinal Cord Injury Study. *J Neurosurg* 1992;**76**:23–31.

48.   Bracken MB, Shepard MJ, Holford TR, *et al.* Administration of methylprednisolone for 24 or 48 hours or tirilazad mesylate for 48 hours in the treatment of acute spinal cord injury. Results of the third National Acute Spinal Cord Injury randomized controlled trial. *JAMA* 1997;**277**:1597–604.

49.   Bracken MB, Shepard MJ, Holford TR, *et al.* Methylprednisolone or tirilazad mesylate administration after acute spinal cord injury: 1-year follow up. Results of the third National Acute Spinal Cord Injury randomized controlled trial. *J Neurosurg* 1998;**89**:699–706.

50.   Pointillart V, Petitjean ME, Wiart L, *et al.* Pharmacological therapy of spinal cord injury during the acute phase. *Spinal Cord* 2000;**38**:71–6.

51.   Tator CH, Fehlings MG, Thorpe K, Taylor W. Current use and timing of spinal surgery for management of acute spinal injury in North America: results of a retrospective multicentre study. *J Neurosurg* 1999;**91**:12–18.

52.   Duke RFN, Spreadbury TH. Closed manipulation leading to immediate recovery from cervical spine dislocation with paraplegia. *Lancet* 1981;**2**:577–8.

Abdominal trauma

OBJECTIVES

After completing this chapter the reader will:
- be aware of anatomy and pathophysiology relevant to abdominal injury
- be able to discuss the initial evaluation and management of abdominal injury
- be able to establish a system for the investigation of abdominal injury
- be able to examine prioritization issues involving the abdomen in multisystem injury
- be able to outline the techniques utilized in both non-operative and operative management of abdominal injury.

INTRODUCTION

In the UK approximately 20% of all trauma deaths are attributable at least in part to injuries arising within the abdomen and pelvis.[1] Early deaths are usually because of exsanguinating haemorrhage and sepsis, and late deaths are usually due to multiple system organ dysfunction, often as a consequence of intestinal injury. The costs of treatment of these injuries are high because of the extensive use of operative and intensive care facilities. Advances in technology such as laparoscopy, computed tomography and bedside ultrasound scanning as well as an increased appreciation of the significance of the physiological derangement associated with severe abdominal injury have led to changes in the resuscitation, investigation and surgical management of abdominal trauma. Abdominal injury frequently occurs as part of the picture of multiple injury, and therefore prioritization issues become paramount in its management.

ANATOMY

The abdominal cavity extends from the level of the fifth intercostal space on full expiration to the inguinal ligaments inferiorly and between the two anterior axillary lines. The flank encompasses the area between the anterior and posterior axillary lines with the back lying posterior to this, where its thick musculature may offer some protection against penetrating injury. The peritoneal and retroperitoneal compartments lie internally, with the upper abdominal viscera lying under the lower ribs in the intrathoracic abdomen which may be injured in thoracic trauma.[2] The retroperitoneal viscera are distributed in four zones of relevance when deciding upon surgical intervention for retroperitoneal injury. The central zone contains the aorta, vena cava, pancreas and duodenum. The left and right lateral zones contain the kidneys, adrenals, ureters and colon. The pelvic zone contains the pelvic vessels together with parts of the bladder and rectum.

MECHANISM OF INJURY

Blunt trauma

Blunt trauma remains the most common cause of abdominal injury in the UK and most commonly occurs as a result of a road traffic collision (RTC). It is frequently associated with multisystem injury, making abdominal evaluation difficult and presenting problems in the prioritization of investigation and management. Injuries may be produced by crushing such as the direct impact of a steering wheel, when abdominal contents that are relatively immobile by virtue of peritoneal attachments (for example the liver, spleen and kidney) are most at risk; massive haemorrhage may ensue. Abdominal compression can raise intra-abdominal pressure acutely, resulting in rupture of hollow viscera or of the diaphragm.

Deceleration and rotational forces that impinge on the intra-abdominal organs, especially at the interface between mobile and fixed structures, result in tearing or shearing of both hollow organ viscera and major vessels in the retroperitoneum. Pelvic fractures are frequently associated with urethral and urinary bladder injuries and with injuries to the pelvic vessels.[3] Bony fragments from pelvic fractures may also act as secondary missiles causing penetrating injury. Lumbar vertebral fractures (Chance fractures) are associated with intra-abdominal injuries in one-third of cases in adults and half of paediatric cases. Transverse process factures are frequently found in association with cases of renal injury and horizontal vertebral body fractures are associated with pancreaticoduodenal and small bowel injuries.[4]

> The mechanism of injury and associated distant injuries may suggest an increased likelihood of abdominal trauma.

Penetrating trauma

Penetrating trauma from stabbings far exceeds that from gunshot injury in the UK, and the injury is confined to the wound track. Only half of abdominal stabbings will penetrate the peritoneum, and less than half will significantly injure the underlying organs. Abdominal gunshot wounds almost always injure the viscera, but the degree of damage is a function of the level of energy transferred and the physical characteristics of the incident tissues. The pathophysiology of ballistic injury is discussed further in Chapter 18, but suffice it to say here that, in general, handguns produce low-energy-transfer wounds with minimal cavitation whereas rifles and close range shotguns (<5 m) produce high-energy-transfer wounds with marked cavitation and contamination. The tissue destruction may be significant.

Blast injury

The effects of blast are commonly divided into four categories, all of which may be considered as special forms of other pathophysiologies such as blunt, penetrating or thermal trauma. Primary abdominal blast injury is uncommon except in underwater explosions. Blast injury is considered fully in Chapter 19.

CLINICAL PRESENTATION

The clinical presentation of abdominal trauma can vary widely from haemodynamic stability with absent abdominal signs through frank peritonism to complete

cardiovascular collapse requiring resuscitative laparotomy. The mechanism of injury should suggest the likelihood of intra-abdominal pathology. Clinical signs of peritonitis may be absent early on, be dismissed as being abdominal wall related, be overlooked because of other distracting injuries or be difficult to elicit owing to the patient's conscious level. The patient's haemodynamic status and the initial response to fluid must also be assessed and will influence investigation and management.

> Injury above and below the abdomen should generate a high index of suspicion of abdominal injury.

IMMEDIATE ASSESSMENT AND RESUSCITATION

Early surgical referral is essential for cases in which abdominal injury is suspected, particularly in polytrauma, and a senior member of the surgical team should be part of the trauma team. Features of the history of particular relevance to abdominal trauma include the speed of the RTC, the use of seat belts and airbags, the nature of the weapon in penetrating injury and the distance from which a gun was fired, if known. Initial priorities should follow standard assessment protocols and the abdomen must be initially assessed in the circulation and haemorrhage control phase of the primary survey ('C') as the abdomen may conceal significant haemorrhage without external signs. The abdominal assessment comprises a full clinical examination of the abdomen, flanks and back for bruising, penetrating wounds and distension, followed by palpation of the abdominal quadrants to elicit tenderness and/or peritonism and percussion for subtle signs of tenderness. Auscultation in the busy emergency department adds little to the evaluation. Abdominal wall bruising in the pattern of the restraining seat belt in RTC patients should be noted. Rectal examination is essential, and vaginal examination should be considered depending on the nature of the injuries. The rectal examination may elicit reduced tone from spinal cord injury, bleeding from lower gastrointestinal trauma, bony penetration in pelvic fracture and a high-riding prostate associated with pelvic fracture, an indicator of potential urethral injury. Clinical assessment may be augmented early on by ultrasound scanning in the form of a FAST scan (see Focused abdominal sonography for trauma, p. 150). Vaginal bleeding should be identified and a gynaecological opinion sought.

Maintenance of urine output is an easy and reliable indicator of adequate tissue perfusion and, thus, these patients should be catheterized after a digital rectal examination has excluded any significant pelvic injury. The catheter should be placed urethrally unless there are markers of potential urethral injury (Table 13.1), in which

Table 13.1 Indicators of urethral trauma

Blood at the urinary meatus
High-riding prostate
Scrotal or perineal haematoma
The presence of significant pelvic fracture without the above signs should raise suspicion and precautionary measures should be considered

case the options are urethrography to exclude urethral injury, a urological opinion, a single gentle attempt at urethral catheterization or placement of a suprapubic catheter – all are justifiable depending on local practice and facilities. A nasogastric tube will decompress the stomach, relieve acute gastric distension and provide evidence of upper gastrointestinal bleeding. Oral insertion of a Ryle's tube is sometimes necessary if there is significant facial or base of skull trauma, or if it is impossible to insert a tube via the nose. Both nasogastric tube and urinary catheter insertion are prerequisites to performance of diagnostic peritoneal lavage (DPL).

In trauma patients who are bleeding, limiting fluid resuscitation to the level of maintenance of a radial pulse (~80 mmHg) is likely to confer a survival advantage, especially in penetrating abdominal trauma,[5] as the chances of disrupting a fragile nascent clot at the site of injury are reduced, as are the consequences of dilutional coagulopathy. If there is a significant head injury component of the polytrauma victim or evacuation to definitive surgery is delayed beyond 2 hours, then the deleterious metabolic consequences of prolonged under-resuscitation should be considered and resuscitation to normotension considered in the light of the likely risk of exsanguination.[6]

The questions to be answered following abdominal trauma are simple: Have the intra-abdominal organs been injured? Does the patient need a laparotomy? If so, how quickly? And a fourth question that has been added recently: Does the patient need damage control surgery? The answers to these questions may be obvious. The shocked patient with a gunshot wound to the abdomen mandates immediate laparotomy without further investigation; in the grossly shocked patient this may necessitate transfer to the operating room during the course of the primary survey for resuscitative laparotomy. In many cases, however, things are not that clear-cut and there will be a need for adjunct investigations to help decide whether surgical intervention is needed. Both the clinical evaluation and ultrasound assessment may need to be repeated.

> Resuscitation is not a substitute for timely surgical control of haemorrhage.

INVESTIGATIONS

Clinical examination in abdominal trauma is neither sensitive nor specific for intra-abdominal injury, even in experienced hands, and it therefore presents the surgeon with a diagnostic dilemma. The abdomen is often not the only injured area, raising questions about whether the abdomen or a remote injury should be managed first. Certain situations or findings suggest a high likelihood of abdominal injury and are indications for investigation (Table 13.2). In addition, conventional physical examination of the abdomen may not be appropriate, as neurological injury, paraplegia, intoxication or distracting pain at a nearby site may lead to confusion in the evaluation of the patient. These situations call for the use of additional investigation to aid the surgeon's decision-making process.

Various investigations have been suggested as optimal; each has its advantages and limitations, and no single investigation is ideal in all circumstances; often a combination of tests will be most appropriate to allow an informed decision to be made regarding whether to act conservatively or to proceed to a laparotomy.

Diagnostic peritoneal lavage

Diagnostic peritoneal lavage has been the 'gold standard' for the investigation of blunt abdominal injury for more than 30 years,[7] with a 97.3% accuracy with false-positive and false-negative rates of only 1.4% and 1.3% respectively,[8] using lavage counts of 100 000 red cells per mm^3 and 500 white cells per mm^3. The most frequent criticism of this technique is the rate of non-therapeutic laparotomy performed after a positive cell count. This is a consequence of the balance between false-negative results and oversensitivity, and is variously estimated at 10–15%. Unfortunately, DPL does not allow conservative management in the presence of blood in the abdominal cavity. Computed tomography (CT) may be used as an adjunct in the stable patient, although if DPL is performed first the presence of lavage fluid and air may limit interpretation of the scan, as it may any subsequent ultrasound scan. The value of DPL in penetrating trauma remains controversial because of its unacceptably low sensitivity and specificity if 'blunt' lavage count criteria are used; lower lavage cell counts of between 5000 and 10 000 red cells per mm^3 have been used to attain a false-negative

Table 13.2 Indications for investigation of blunt abdominal injury

High index of suspicion from the mechanism of injury
Injuries above and below the diaphragm
Clinical signs of abdominal injury
Seat belt sign, bruising of the abdominal wall

rate of 5%.[9] Diagnostic peritoneal lavage is being used less frequently owing to the rise in popularity of other modes of investigation, such as FAST and CT,[10] but it remains an important investigative modality, especially in the absence of these more high-technology modalities. The technique of DPL is described in Box 13.1.

The presence of scarring from previous abdominal surgery, especially a lower midline incision, will make DPL more difficult and reduce the chances of a diagnostic result. In these circumstances DPL should be performed only by the surgeon who will be making the decision on whether a laparotomy is required. Complications of DPL include gut perforation, haemorrhage and infection. A DPL is contraindicated only by the presence of an indication for laparotomy; relative contraindications include pregnancy, childhood and previous abdominal surgery.

Focused abdominal sonography for trauma

Kristensen et al.[11] first reported the use of ultrasound in the investigation of abdominal trauma in 1971. Since then the technique has become widely accepted in Europe. More recently, in America, Grace Rozycki and colleagues have developed the focused abdominal sonography for trauma (FAST) technique – a standard approach to abdominal trauma ultrasound that involves imaging a limited number of ultrasound windows to detect fluid. It is important to understand that FAST is designed solely to detect free fluid, not visceral injury, and may therefore be performed by non-radiologists. Ultrasound of the viscera by a suitably trained radiologist is a separate entity and is often not available in a timely fashion to aid the assessment of the traumatized abdomen. The four FAST stations are as follows:

- *Subxiphoid.* The transducer is angled upward and slightly to the left shoulder to identify haemopericardium. If poor views are obtained, consider the transverse left intercostal position in the third or fourth interspace.
- *Right upper quadrant.* Place the transducer in the final intercostal space in anterior axillary line with a slightly oblique posterior orientation to image the liver and right kidney. Fluid accumulates in Morrison's pouch between the two.
- *Left upper quadrant.* Place the transducer far posteriorly in a low intercostal space (generally two spaces higher than on the right) and angle the probe anteriorly to visualize the left kidney, spleen and the space between the two where fluid accumulates. The left subdiaphragmatic space and lower thorax (for pleural effusion/haemothorax) may also be visualized.
- *Pelvic.* The probe is placed transversely suprapubically to identify the bladder and then turned 90° to demonstrate fluid behind the bladder. If the bladder is empty, saline may be instilled via a urinary catheter to provide an acoustic window.

A collected review of nearly 5000 patients[12] (in whom FAST was performed by a surgeon rather than a radiologist) demonstrated a sensitivity of 93.4%, a specificity of 98.7% and an accuracy of 97.5% for haemoperitoneum. The FAST technique can be successfully performed by radiologists, accident and emergency staff or surgeons as long as they have been adequately trained and maintain a sufficient level of experience. Fluid is most commonly detected in the right upper quadrant and correlates well with the presence of hepatic, splenic and retroperitoneal injuries.[13]

The application of FAST is more limited in penetrating trauma as the volume of blood that can be reliably detected restricts the sensitivity. The minimum detectable volume is approximately 100 mL, and in one study the mean volume of fluid needed for detection was 619 mL.[14] A small volume of free fluid in the pelvis of women of reproductive years is now regarded as a physiological normal finding.[15] Ultrasound can be used as a screening tool in the resuscitation room and, if positive, can be followed in the stable patient by CT scanning to determine organ-specific injuries. Rapid trauma ultrasound screening of the abdomen has also been shown to have a major role in multiple casualty incidents.[16,17]

Ultrasound is fast, non-invasive and, with the advent of hand-held machines, portable. It is, however, operator

---

Box 13.1 The techniques for diagnostic peritoneal lavage

The open technique

- Urinary catheter and nasogastric tube placement are mandatory prior to DPL.
- Aseptic preparation of the subumbilical midline with local anaesthetic infiltration.
- Sharp dissection through skin, subcutaneous fat and linea alba to peritoneum.
- Open peritoneum between clips.
- Infuse 1 litre of warmed saline (20 mL/kg if used in children) using a sterile giving set directed into the pelvis.
- Place the saline bag below the patient and collect the lavage return
- Send samples for laboratory analysis (microscopy, amylase, cell counts and Gram stain).

The Seldinger technique

- The preparation (catheter, nasogastric and asepsis) is identical to the open technique.
- The needle is introduced into the abdomen angled towards the pelvis and exchanged for a lavage tube over a guide-wire using the Seldinger technique. Infusion of fluid and collection of samples is as for the open technique.

dependent and limited by factors such as surgical emphysema and obesity.

Computed tomography

In the patient that is cardiovascularly stable, CT is the investigation of choice for assessment of the injured abdomen. The standard trauma CT scan with a modern multidetector scanner can be completed in a single breath hold, and should include intravenous contrast. The addition of oral (or nasogastric) and rectal contrast (the triple-contrast scan) increases the detection rate of gastrointestinal injury.[18] Owing to difficulties in assessing in which cavity the abnormality lies, scans should image from the root of the neck to pubic symphysis and pelvis, to visualize the whole of the thorax and abdomen. However, in the haemodynamically unstable patient, the CT scanner must be avoided and another investigative modality used to assess the cause of the instability.

The organ specificity and ability to grade injuries offered by CT has advanced the cause of conservative management; nevertheless, this decision should be made in conjunction with clinical parameters. In addition, CT has the advantage of visualizing the retroperitoneal structures. However, in common with DPL and FAST, the diaphragm is poorly imaged by CT.

Laparoscopy

Diagnostic laparoscopy (DL) in trauma is an investigation with an evolving role, although the evidence suggests that it forms a useful part of the evaluation of abdominal trauma – especially where conservative management of penetrating trauma is practised. Ahmed et al.[19] used DL to assess all penetrating wounds in stable patients who would normally be assessed by laparotomy. In 33% of cases there was no peritoneal penetration; in 29% there was peritoneal penetration alone, requiring no further surgery; in 38% there was peritoneal penetration with visceral injuries requiring no further surgery, such as non-bleeding injuries to the liver, omentum or mesentery with good haemostasis; and in only 23% was open laparotomy required for surgical treatment of the injury. Other investigators have found similar outcomes for DL in penetrating injuries and have demonstrated a reduced hospital stay as a result of avoiding laparotomy.[20,21] A DL has a sensitivity of 100% for the identification of peritoneal penetration,[22] and therefore is valuable for evaluating penetration in abdominal stab wounds and tangential gunshot wounds.[23] Laparoscopy is also the most effective investigation for diagnosing diaphragmatic injury.[24] The laparoscopic ports should be sited away from the entry wound as using the wound as an entry portal may restart bleeding.

Studies have shown DL to be 97% accurate[25] in blunt abdominal trauma, but its use in this scenario is limited by

time, cost and the need for a general anaesthetic, and it is hampered by the presence of peritoneal blood. A small study from the USA describes emergency department laparoscopy in 13 patients with stab wounds and two patients with tangential gunshot wounds using local anaesthetic and sedation. It allowed 10 patients, including the two gunshot cases, to be discharged directly from the emergency room,[26] suggesting that the role of laparoscopy may be expanding.

Wound exploration

Wound exploration is an imprecise technique and has an accuracy of only 55%, with up to 88% false-positive results.[27] When performed, it must be carried out in the operating theatre by a surgeon as a formal procedure under appropriate anaesthesia with consent to proceed to a laparotomy. The wound should be extended if necessary and penetration of the peritoneum identified or excluded. Haemostasis can then be obtained and laparotomy carried out or the wound closed in an appropriate manner. This procedure is not recommended as a routine but may be useful in combination with DL in experienced hands.

Choice of investigation in abdominal trauma

There needs to be a high index of suspicion for abdominal injury in all cases of multiple trauma. The key issue in the choice of investigation for blunt abdominal trauma is the cardiovascular stability of the patient. Patients who are unstable with unequivocal abdominal signs require a laparotomy, not investigation. The dilemma arises in multisystem injury when the abdomen is only one of the potential sources for the cardiovascular instability. In this situation a rapid bedside test is required – local resources and experience will dictate whether DPL or FAST is the primary choice. In the haemodynamically stable patient, the appropriate choice of study is CT scan, which provides organ specificity and allows the option of conservative management of solid organ injury where appropriate.

In patients with penetrating trauma, the choice of investigation again depends upon the stability of the patient, but also upon the experience of the surgeon and facilities of the unit. If conservative management of penetrating trauma is being considered, then CT is the investigation of choice, accompanied by frequent clinical reassessment of the patient. In patients with stab wounds and suspected peritoneal penetration, laparoscopy and wound exploration may be employed in lieu of laparotomy, with evidence of peritoneal penetration as the end-point. Most institutions still employ a policy of obligatory laparotomy for abdominal gunshot wounds, as the incidence of organ injury following gunshot wounds is over 90%,[9] although high-volume units have reported the successful non-operative management of abdominal

Table 13.3 Summary of investigations for suspected intra-abdominal injury

Haemodynamically unstable patients with signs of intra-abdominal injury require surgery

Haemodynamically unstable patients with uncertainty about the abdomen require rapid abdominal evaluation (DPL or ultrasound)

Haemodynamically stable patients with other severe injuries should have rapid evaluation to exclude covert abdominal injuries (DPL or ultrasound)

In the presence of minor associated injuries, a haemodynamically normal patient with a clinically equivocal abdomen requires CT evaluation

Haemodynamically stable patients with abdominal signs should have CT, allowing non-operative management if appropriate

CT, computed tomography; DPL, diagnostic peritoneal lavage.

gunshot wounds in over one-third of cases.[28] In less experienced units, mandatory laparotomy remains safe and acceptable – the only exceptions being the stable patient in whom the track of the missile appears tangential and peritoneal penetration is unlikely, or in whom the injury is thoracoabdominal and assessment is required to determine whether the injury is wholly thoracic. In these instances, laparoscopy in theatre with the patient prepared for laparotomy is reasonable. Table 13.3 summarizes the choice of investigations.

AREAS OF DIAGNOSTIC DIFFICULTY IN STABLE PATIENTS

The areas discussed below present diagnostic difficulty only in the stable patient – the unstable patient should be investigated by laparotomy.

Diaphragm

The diagnosis of diaphragm injury remains elusive to non-invasive modalities. An initial chest radiograph with an *in situ* nasogastric tube evident in the chest may confirm the diagnosis. The investigation of choice in the stable patient where there is clinical suspicion, or where there are equivocal chest radiograph appearances, is DL.

Renal tract

Intravenous urography (IVU) has been replaced by CT as the investigation of choice in renal injury. It allows an assessment to be made of both function and anatomical disruption of the kidneys. A one-shot IVU is still useful in the resuscitation room or operating theatre to determine the presence of renal injury and establish the presence of

two functioning kidneys. A completely shattered kidney or pedicular avulsion necessitates nephrectomy irrespective of the contralateral kidney. The cystogram remains the investigation of choice for suspected bladder disruption, and gentle urethrography may be performed where there is a suspicion of a urethral tear.

Pancreas

Serum amylase has little value in the initial evaluation of pancreatic injury as it has a positive predictive value of only 10% and a negative predictive value of 95%,[29] although a rising level over time on repeated measurement occurs in just under half of patients with pancreatic injuries. Elevated serum lipase levels are a reasonable indicator of a pancreatic contusion (values in the hundreds) or major duct injury (values in the thousands). However, the absence of an elevated lipase level does not exclude either injury.[30] Contrast spiral CT is probably the best investigation and has a sensitivity of 85%, although CT scans early in the investigation may miss injuries to the pancreas (Figure 13.1). Endoscopic retrograde cholangiopancreatography may be of value in a number of select cases.

Stab wounds to the flank, back and buttocks

The evaluation of penetration in these injuries is difficult as the muscles of the back are thick and penetration of retroperitoneal organs may not present with abdominal signs. Contrast CT (including rectal contrast) is the most sensitive investigation. It must be assumed that injuries to the buttocks penetrate the abdominal cavity; therefore appropriate investigation of the abdomen should be

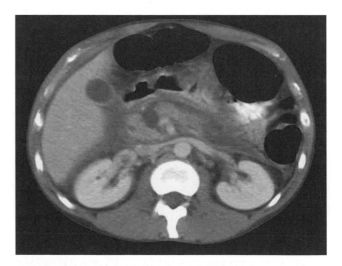

Figure 13.1 Computed tomography (CT) scan of the abdomen showing almost complete transection of the pancreatic neck. This scan was taken 4 days afer blunt abdominal trauma. The initial CT scan on presentation was normal.

carried out as well as digital rectal and sigmoidoscopic examination for blood. Water-soluble contrast studies may be used to further investigate potential rectal injuries in the otherwise stable patient.

CRITICAL DECISION-MAKING AND PRIORITIZATION IN MULTISYSTEM INJURY

Although abdominal injury may at times present in isolation, in the UK, where blunt trauma predominates, such injury is frequently found as part of the picture of multiple trauma. Prioritization of the investigations in this situation has already been discussed; however, it is clear that prioritization of the management of injuries must occur to provide the best outcome for the injured patient. Firm leadership of the resuscitation team is paramount in order to organize the competing surgical responses in multiple-injury scenarios. Contention may arise in patients with abdominal injuries and coexisting head injury, pelvic injury or multiple fractures.

Patients who have sustained both head and abdominal injury, as frequently occurs in RTCs, may present resuscitation, investigation and management dilemmas. The policy of hypotensive resuscitation is not appropriate in this scenario, as attention must be paid to maintaining the cerebral perfusion pressure. Prioritization of investigation and management is difficult and depends upon the severity of the injuries. An exsanguinating abdominal injury demands a laparotomy to control bleeding before assessment of the head injury. However, this must be a damage control laparotomy to save life and stabilize the patient prior to further investigation and appropriate management. When the patient is more stable, trauma CT from head to symphysis pubis is the appropriate investigation, and treatment is then directed towards the most life-threatening injuries first. These decisions are judgements made from experience of trauma management.

The fractured, open-book pelvis is a major source of blood loss in the trauma patient[31] and, in the scenario in which there is concomitant abdominal and pelvic injury, prioritization of management must occur. Laparotomy before stabilization of the pelvis will potentially open the pelvic haematoma and allow free bleeding; thus, the rapid application of an external fixator to stabilize the pelvis either in the resuscitation room or in theatre immediately before laparotomy is the appropriate response, taking care to site the pelvic fixator so as to least interfere with the conduct of the laparotomy. If pelvic haemorrhage is the major concern, then angiography and embolization are preferable to laparotomy. Laparotomy takes priority over other orthopaedic injuries, which may be splinted temporarily in the resuscitation room. Occasionally it may be appropriate to place external fixators at the same time as laparotomy. If angioembolisation is not available prior to laparotomy then extraperitoneal pelvic packing may limit pelvic haemorrhage.

SURGICAL STRATEGIES

Non-operative management of solid-organ injury

Selective non-operative management (SNOM) of both adult and paediatric patients with solid-organ injury from blunt abdominal trauma is now well established[32,33] and is based on the widespread use of CT in stable patients. Patients managed non-operatively have great potential for rapid deterioration. As a consequence, they must be monitored closely for haemodynamic instability, fluid and transfusion requirements in a high-dependency unit or intensive care unit, where signs of early deterioration can be detected and surgical intervention undertaken rapidly if required. They should be repeatedly re-examined, preferably by the same senior clinician, to detect subtle changes in abdominal signs. This implies that the patient must be available for repeated assessment, and thus patients who are undergoing lengthy operations for other reasons, such as definitive management of limb injuries, are not candidates for SNOM. The increasing accuracy of rapidly acquired multislice CT imaging allows grading of solid organ injury according to the American Association for the Surgery of Trauma system.[34] Patients with grade I–III liver, spleen and kidney injuries are all suitable for SNOM with or without the addition of interventional radiology to arrest haemorrhage. The criteria for SNOM are listed in Table 13.4. Haemodynamic instability, marked or worsening abdominal signs or high-grade injury on CT remain indications for laparotomy. Although it is still uncommon in the UK, SNOM of penetrating abdominal trauma is widely practised in the USA and South Africa (see Global perspectives, p. 156). In these institutions, peritoneal violation alone is no longer an indication for laparotomy, and so eviscerated omentum and small bowel can be safely cleaned and returned to the abdomen, avoiding laparotomy. In less experienced hands, laparotomy for penetrating trauma that violates the peritoneum remains reasonable.

Non-operative management may be appropriate in up to 50% of adults with isolated blunt liver injuries, and has a 50–80% success rate.[33] It has also been shown to be successful in 93%[35] of less severe injuries in blunt splenic trauma. Thirty-eight per cent of abdominal gunshot

Table 13.4 Indications for non-operative management of solid organ injury

Appropriate injuries (grades I–III) of solid organs on computed tomography
Minimal physical signs
Cardiovascular stability with a requirement of less than 2 units of blood acutely
High-dependency or intensive care facilities available
Patient available for repeated examination

wounds were successfully managed conservatively in one series from Los Angeles – the rate of success was twice as high for posterior wounds as for those with anterior entry points.[28]

Trauma laparotomy

Following the decision to operate, broad-spectrum antibiotics should be given immediately, together with the preoperative placement of a nasogastric tube and urinary catheter if they are not already in place. Further antibiotics should be given if there has been contamination of the peritoneum by bowel contents. Body temperature must be maintained by the use of warm air blankets and warmed intravenous fluids. The entire abdomen, thorax and groins are prepared and draped to allow extension of the laparotomy into junctional areas. The abdomen is opened by a full-length midline incision. Consideration should be given to the collection of autologous blood and retransfusion where possible – this is not contraindicated by enteric contamination.[36] Two suckers are used to evacuate intraperitoneal haematoma and 'four-quadrant' packing is placed above and below the liver, and in the left upper quadrant, both paracolic gutters and the pelvis. These packs are then removed sequentially starting in the quadrant judged least likely to be the cause of the major haemorrhage. Sites of bleeding are controlled temporarily, as the most serious bleeding may remain undiscovered. When all packs are removed and all bleeding sources controlled, definitive control of haemorrhage may be attempted – or a damage control strategy adopted. Enteric contamination is similarly controlled temporarily before definitive or damage control surgery continues. Injuries should be dealt with in order of their degree of lethality (major vessels, solid organ haemorrhage, mesenteric and hollow organ haemorrhage and, finally, contamination). There is no role for the removal of retained foreign bodies or weapons anywhere but in theatre at laparotomy, under direct vision and with control of potential haemorrhage or contamination.

Retroperitoneal haematoma

The management of retroperitoneal haematomas found at trauma laparotomy is guided by their anatomical location and thus likely underlying pathology. Central haematomas should always be explored to exclude injuries to the great vessels, pancreas and duodenum. Lateral haematomas should be left unopened unless expanding or the patient is hypotensive with no other injuries. Pelvic haematomas should not be explored. An expanding pelvic haematoma should be packed and angiography undertaken with a view to subsequent embolization of the vessel injury as surgical exploration frequently leads to uncontrollable and potentially fatal blood loss.

Damage control

The majority of patients who undergo laparotomy for abdominal injury can tolerate definitive vascular and organ repair at the initial operation. However, up to 10% of patients with multiple trauma are so physiologically deranged by the 'bloody vicious triad of trauma' – hypothermia (<34°C), acidosis (pH <7.2) and coagulopathy, which act synergistically – that the time taken for definitive initial surgery allows the metabolic consequences to become irreversible.[37] A survival advantage has been demonstrated in this group of patients using a limited 'damage control' procedure compared with a definitive primary operation.[38]

Damage control surgery is an abbreviated laparotomy (<1 hour) to obtain temporary control of haemorrhage and contamination before temporary abdominal wall closure, transfer to the intensive care unit and the restitution of normal physiology (temperature, acid–base balance and clotting). Major vessel haemorrhage is shunted and minor vessels ligated. Solid organ haemorrhage is packed.[39] Bowel injury is isolated by clamps, tapes or stapling. Pancreaticobiliary injury is drained. Abdominal closure can be by running nylon suture to skin alone, multiple towel clips, a Bogota bag or an Opsite® sandwich. Once physiologically stable, the patient can be returned to theatre for definitive repair of injuries and abdominal closure 24–48 hours later.

ABDOMINAL COMPARTMENT SYNDROME

Abdominal compartment syndrome (ACS) is typified by an acute rise in intra-abdominal pressure accompanied by evidence of end-organ dysfunction. Common causes include situations requiring aggressive high-volume fluid resuscitation such as pancreatitis, burns, major trauma or bowel obstruction as well as laparotomy closure under tension. Clearly, trauma laparotomy victims are at high risk of this complication. The intra-abdominal hypertension splints the diaphragm limiting respiration and gas exchange resulting in a rising $PaCO_2$ and falling PaO_2 – ventilatory pressures increase dramatically. Inferior vena caval compression results in reduced venous return and decreased cardiac output. Direct renal artery and splanchnic arterial compression induces mesenteric ischaemia and renal dysfunction, resulting in acidosis and oliguria. These features in the face of an apparently well-filled patient in the context of a trauma laparotomy should suggest ACS. The abdominal pressure can be measured by connecting a transducer to the urinary catheter with the bladder filled with 100–250 mL of saline – the normal value is below 8 mmHg. Pressures over 25 mmHg strongly suggest the diagnosis of ACS. Treatment is in most cases decompression of the abdomen by relaparotomy. The abdomen is managed with a temporary closure method as detailed above. The mortality of ACS is approximately 50%.[40]

INTERVENTIONAL RADIOLOGY

Angiography is an important diagnostic adjunct in trauma as it allows the accurate diagnosis of bleeding and provides therapeutic options in both surgical and non-operative management. In abdominal trauma, interventional radiological techniques have been widely accepted in the diagnosis and management of haemorrhage from complex pelvic fractures. Where closure of an open-book pelvic fracture with an external fixator has failed to control bleeding, it is appropriate to proceed to angiography and embolization of the bleeding vessels.[41] Interventional radiology techniques can also be successfully employed as an adjunct to non-operative management of solid organ injury[28] by demonstrating haemorrhage, followed by control using coil embolization of the bleeding vessels. In addition they can be used as an additional means of haemorrhage control after laparotomy if complete haemostasis has not been obtainable.[42]

Case scenario

A 47-year-old man is accosted by a gang of youths in the street who jostle past him. He feels a sharp pain in his left side and becomes short of breath, falling to the ground in pain. He is taken by ambulance to the nearest emergency department. He is maintaining his own airway and has a Glasgow Coma Scale (GCS) score of 15. His respiratory rate is 33 breaths per minute, his pulse is 105 beats per minute and oxygen saturation on pulse oximetry is 93% on room air. He is bleeding from a wound on his left side/flank.

What is your initial management?
Initial management is according to <C>ABCDE protocols concentrating on airway, breathing and circulation initially. He is maintaining his own airway but a left-sided flank wound and tachypnoea may suggest a thoracic injury. He requires high-flow oxygen pending assessment of his breathing and chest radiography, wide-bore venous cannulation and withdrawal of blood for cross-match as well as baseline bloods. He should be given intravenous analgesia if in pain. Examination reveals what appears to be a stab wound in the lateral aspect of his left upper quadrant. Some fat, potentially omentum, is poking through.

What are your concerns and what imaging is appropriate?
The patient appears to have sustained a penetrating abdominal stab wound in an area where the posterior thorax is also at risk and he needs a pneumothorax to be excluded by chest radiography; thereafter the choice is between wound exploration, FAST scanning, CT scanning or transfer to the operating theatre.

A chest radiograph shows a poor inspiratory effort but no clear-cut chest problem. He is haemodynamically stable and you opt for a CT scan as no-one is qualified to perform a FAST scan. The scan shows free fluid and free air predominantly in the left upper quadrant; his liver and spleen are intact. No comment is made upon the state of the diaphragm but the radiology registrar wonders whether he does indeed have a small pneumothorax.

What are you going to do now?
Free fluid and air in the absence of solid visceral injury in this setting are highly suggestive of gastrointestinal perforation; in such circumstances conservative management is inappropriate and emergency laparotomy should be arranged. If there were no thought of gastrointestinal injury then diagnostic laparoscopy could be considered to assess the diaphragm. As he will be ventilated during his general anaesthetic, a prophylactic tube thoracostomy should be inserted on the left side prior to administration of general anaesthetic. Through an upper midline incision, a stab wound of the splenic flexure of colon with an associated mesenteric haematoma in the area are discovered. There is a small penetrating injury of the diaphragm. The diaphragmatic injury is closed directly and the splenic flexure is mobilized to the midline and inspected. If there is no impairment of the blood supply then direct suture repair is permissible – concerns over the blood supply from the mesenteric injury should prompt consideration of resection with immediate anastomosis. This is performed and he makes an uneventful recovery, leaving hospital on day 6.

SUMMARY

Abdominal injury presents in the emergency department in many different ways, and a high index of suspicion for abdominal injury must be maintained in all trauma patients. Haemodynamic stability remains the overriding factor when deciding on the investigation of the injured abdomen. Cardiovascular instability in the face of abdominal trauma remains an indication for urgent laparotomy. In the stable patient, computed tomography is the investigation of choice but may need to be supplemented with other imaging modalities. Selective non-operative management of many blunt injuries is now widely practised but requires repeated close assessment of the patient; a similar approach has been successful in penetrating trauma in units receiving large volumes of such injuries. In the UK, surgeons should maintain a low threshold for laparotomy in penetrating abdominal trauma. Pelvic fractures are best treated by stabilization and angiographic embolization of the bleeding points rather than surgery, which is often catastrophic. In the physiologically exhausted patient, definitive repair of all injuries at initial laparotomy will increase mortality and morbidity – a damage control approach should be adopted.

GLOBAL PERSPECTIVES

Despite the high levels of gun crime in the USA and South Africa, road traffic accidents are still the leading cause of abdominal injury in those countries, and all the management issues described above are as relevant there as they are in the UK. The striking difference is the experience that many US and South African centres have developed in managing penetrating torso trauma – in the USA it is largely gunshot wounds whereas in South Africa stabbings are more common. Centres such as the LA County Trauma room see over 5000 penetrating torso injuries per year and are staffed by a team of dedicated trauma attending surgeons – in this context conservative management of penetrating injury is much easier to perform as the continuity of experienced care is available in contrast to most areas of the UK. Velmahos et al.[28] reported a series of 1856 abdominal gunshot wounds collected over an 8-year period – 38% were successfully managed non-operatively; 80 patients initially selected for non-operative management proceeded to laparotomy, one-quarter of which were non-therapeutic. Only five patients suffered complications attributable to a delay in surgery, but none died. According to the authors, the rate of unnecessary laparotomies fell from 47% to 14%, resulting in 3500 saved hospital bed days and a cost saving of $9 million. Where the facilities and experience are available there is much to commend selective non-operative management of abdominal trauma, even from gunshot wounds. Where either is lacking, careful and timely laparotomy remains appropriate management.

REFERENCES

1.   Office of National Statistics. *Mortality Statistics: Cause.* London: Her Majesty's Stationery Office, 2004.

2.   Deane S, Gunning K, Hodgetts T, Sugrue M, Turner L. *Trauma Rules*, 2nd edn. London: BMJ Books, 2006.

3.   Demetriades D, Karaiskakis M, Toutouzas K, *et al.* Pelvic fractures: epidemiology and predictors of associated abdominal injuries and outcomes. *J Am Coll Surg* 2002;**195**:1–10.

4.   Rabinovici R, Ovadia P, Mathiak G, Abdullah F. Abdominal injuries associated with lumbar spine fractures in blunt trauma. *Injury* 1999;**30**:471–4.

5.   Bickell WH, Wall MJ, Jr, Pepe PE, *et al.* Immediate versus delayed fluid resuscitation for hypotensive patients with penetrating torso injuries. *N Engl J Med* 1994;**331**:1105–9.

6.   Parry C, Garner J, Bird J, Watts S, Kirkman E. Reduced survival time with prolonged hypotensive versus normotensive resuscitation. *Br J Surg* 2005;**92**(Suppl.1):112.

7.   Root HD, Hauser CW, McKinley CR, Lafave JW, Mendiola RP, Jr. Diagnostic peritoneal lavage. *Surgery* 1965;**57**:633–7.

8.   Powell DC, Bivins BA, Bell RM. Diagnostic peritoneal lavage. *Surg Gynecol Obstet* 1982;**155**:257–64.

9.   Moore EE, Moore JB, Van Duzer-Moore S, Thompson JS. Mandatory laparotomy for gunshot wounds penetrating the abdomen. *Am J Surg* 1980;**140**:847–50.

10.   Smith J, Caldwell E, D'Amours S, Jalaludin B, Sugrue M. Abdominal trauma: a disease in evolution. *Aust N Z J Surg* 2005;**75**:790–4.

11.   Kristensen JK, Buemann B, Kuhl E. Ultrasonic scanning in the diagnosis of splenic haematomas. *Acta Chir Scand* 1971;**137**:653–7.

12.   Rozycki GS, Shackford SR. Ultrasound, what every trauma surgeon should know. *J Trauma* 1996;**40**:1–4.

13.   Rozycki GS, Ochsner MG, Feliciano DV, *et al.* Early detection of hemoperitoneum by ultrasound examination of the right upper quadrant: a multicenter study. *J Trauma* 1998;**45**:878–83.

14.   Branney SW, Wolfe RE, Moore EE, *et al.* Quantitative sensitivity of ultrasound in detecting free intraperitoneal fluid. *J Trauma* 1996;**40**:1052–4.

15.   Sirlin CB, Casola G, Brown MA, *et al.* US of blunt abdominal trauma: importance of free pelvic fluid in women of reproductive age. *Radiology* 2001;**219**:229–35.

16.   Miletic D, Fuckar Z, Mraovic B, Dimec D, Mozetic V. Ultrasonography in the evaluation of hemoperitoneum in war casualties. *Mil Med* 1999;**164**:600–2.

17.   Sarkisian AE, Khondkarian RA, Amirbekian NM, *et al.* Sonographic screening of mass casualties for abdominal and renal injuries following the 1988 Armenian earthquake. *J Trauma* 1991;**31**:247–50.

18.   Shanmuganathan K, Mirvis SE, Chin WC, Killeen KL, Scalea TM. Triple-contrast helical CT in penetrating torso trauma: a prospective study to determine peritoneal violation and the need for laparotomy. *AJR Am J Roentgenol* 2001;**177**:1247–56.

19.   Ahmed N, Whelan J, Brownlee J, Chari V, Chung R. The contribution of laparoscopy in evaluation of penetrating abdominal wounds. *J Am Coll Surg* 2005;**201**:213–16.

20.   Mahajna A, Mitkal S, Bahuth H, Krausz MM. Diagnostic laparoscopy for penetrating injuries in the thoracoabdominal region. *Surg Endosc* 2004;**18**:1485–7.

21.   Chelly MR, Major K, Spivak J, *et al.* The value of laparoscopy in management of abdominal trauma. *Am Surg* 2003;**69**:957–60.

22.   Zantut LF, Ivatury RR, Smith RS, *et al.* Diagnostic and therapeutic laparoscopy for penetrating abdominal trauma: a multicenter experience. *J Trauma* 1997;**42**:825–9; discussion 829–31.

23.   Sosa JL, Sims D, Martin L, Zeppa R. Laparoscopic evaluation of tangential abdominal gunshot wounds. *Arch Surg* 1992;**127**:109–10.

24.   Friese RS, Coln CE, Gentilello LM. Laparoscopy is sufficient to exclude occult diaphragm injury after penetrating abdominal trauma. *J Trauma* 2005;**58**:789–92.

25.   Leppaniemi AK, Elliott DC. The role of laparoscopy in blunt abdominal trauma. *Ann Med* 1996;**28**:483–9.

26.   Weinberg JA, Magnotti LJ, Edwards NM, *et al.* Awake laparoscopy for the evaluation of equivocal penetrating abdominal wounds. *Injury* 2007;**38**:60–4.

27.   Oreskovich MR, Carrico CJ. Stab wounds of the anterior abdomen. Analysis of a management plan using local wound exploration and quantitative peritoneal lavage. *Ann Surg* 1983;**198**:411–19.

28   Velmahos GC, Demetriades D, Toutouzas KG, *et al.* Selective non-operative management in 1856 patients with abdominal gunshot wounds: should routine laparotomy still be standard of care? *Ann Surg* 2001;**234**:395–403.

29.   Jurkovich GJ. Injury to the duodenum and pancreas. In: Feliciano DV, Moore EE, Mattox K, eds. *Trauma*, 3rd edn. Stamford, CT: Appleton & Lange, 1996, pp. 573–94.

30.   Nadler EP, Gardner M, Schall LC, Lynch JM, Ford HR. Management of blunt pancreatic injury in children. *J Trauma* 1999;**47**:1098–103.

31.   Dalal SA, Burgess AR, Siegel JH, *et al.* Pelvic fracture in multiple trauma: classification by mechanism is key to pattern of organ injury, resuscitative requirements, and outcome. *J Trauma* 1989;**29**:981–1000.

32.   Ozturk H, Dokucu AI, Onen A, *et al.* Non-operative management of isolated solid organ injuries due to blunt abdominal trauma in children: a fifteen year experience. *Eur J Paediatr Surg* 2004;**14**:29–34.

33.   Carrillo EH, Platz A, Miller FB, Richardson JD, Polk HC, Jr. Non-operative management of blunt hepatic trauma. *Br J Surg* 1998;**85**:461–8.

34.   Moore EE, Shackford SR, Pachter HL, *et al.* Organ injury scaling: spleen, liver and kidney. *J Trauma* 1989;**29**:1664–6.

35.   Smith JS Jr, Wengrovitz MA, DeLong BS. Prospective validation of criteria, including age, for safe, nonsurgical management of the ruptured spleen. *J Trauma* 1992;**33**:363–8.

36   Bowley DM, Barker P, Boffard KD. Intraoperative blood salvage in penetrating abdominal trauma: a randomised, controlled trial. *World J Surg* 2006;**30**:1074–80.

37.   Hirshberg A, Walden R. Damage control for abdominal trauma. *Surg Clin North Am* 1997;**77**:813–20.

38.   Rotondo MF, Schwab CW, McGonigal MD, *et al.* 'Damage control': an approach for improved survival in exsanguinating penetrating abdominal injury. *J Trauma* 1993;**35**:375–82; discussion 382–3.

39.   Morris JA, Jr, Eddy VA, Rutherford EJ. The trauma celiotomy: the evolving concepts of damage control. *Curr Probl Surg* 1996;**33**:611–700.

40.   Moore AF, Hargest R, Martin M, Delicata RJ. Intra-abdominal hypertension and the abdominal compartment syndrome. *Br J Surg* 2004;**91**:1102–10.

41.   Velmahos GC, Chahwan S, Falabella A, Hanks SE, Demetriades D. Angiographic embolization for intraperitoneal and retroperitoneal injuries. *World J Surg* 2000;**24**:539–45.

42.   Velmahos GC, Demetriades D, Chahwan S, *et al.* Angiographic embolization for arrest of bleeding after penetrating trauma to the abdomen. *Am J Surg* 1999;**178**:367–73.

Musculoskeletal trauma

After completing this chapter the reader will:
* be able to describe types and mechanisms of musculoskeletal injuries, excluding spinal injury
* be able to provide guidance for initial life- and limb-saving management

* be able to discuss subsequent management and its effect on outcome.

INTRODUCTION

Limb injuries are common, accounting for 70–80% of all emergency department attendances and a similar proportion of war casualties in conflict.[1,2] Although usually not life-threatening, even relatively minor limb injuries may account for significant long-term morbidity, especially if these are overlooked or overshadowed by major trauma elsewhere.[3] Limbs are vulnerable to blunt and penetrating trauma and the pattern of injury can be partly explained by the anatomy.

LIMB ANATOMY

Figure 14.1 illustrates the general anatomy of a limb. A central bone strut is surrounded by soft tissue consisting predominantly of muscle with its fascial sheath, and skin. Vessels and nerves are small and generally well protected and thus relatively rarely injured. If an injury is severe enough to cause bone fracture, soft-tissue damage *will* have occurred and may be of greater overall significance. Limbs have a high volume and surface area, and fluid loss from wounds and burns may be considerable.

ANATOMY OF THE PELVIS

Pelvic bone is highly vascular and bleeds readily if fractured. The shape and strength of the pelvis mean that considerable energy is required to fracture it and the associated soft-tissue injury may be profound. The large vessels that pass in

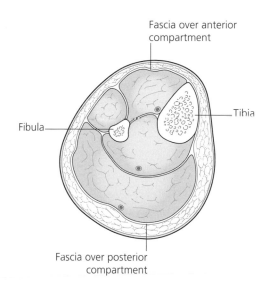

Figure 14.1 Cross-section of the leg at mid-calf level. Tissues vulnerable to trauma include skin, fascia, muscle, blood vessel, nerve and bone.

front of the sacrum are liable to be torn by distracting pelvic injury such as 'open-book' fractures, when the symphysis pubis is opened and the sacroiliac joint widened (Figure 14.2). There is a large potential space for bleeding in the pelvis and, if not stabilized, pelvic fractures may continue to bleed preventing effective resuscitation.[4]

TYPES OF INJURY

Limb injury in the UK is usually a result of blunt trauma.

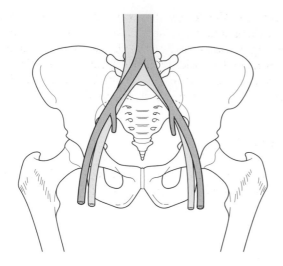

Figure 14.2 View of the pelvis showing vessels close to the sacroiliac region. These are vulnerable if the posterior pelvic ring is fractured.

Blunt trauma

SPORT

Sport provides the greatest number of limb injuries that present to the emergency department, although the majority are not severe. Common injuries include joint sprains, ligament or meniscal injuries to the knee and minor closed fractures. Although inconvenient and painful, these injuries are rarely associated with major morbidity even though the overall cost to society is high because of their frequency.

ROAD TRAFFIC

Collision causes some of the most severe limb injuries, when a pedestrian is struck by a car bumper, even when the car speed is not particularly high.[5,6] These injuries usually include a high-energy open fracture of one or both tibiae and there may be associated life-threatening trauma. Occupants of cars are now much better protected but, ironically, as high-speed crashes become more survivable, the patients with severe limb injuries who now survive to present to hospital may have complex multiple fractures.

FALLS

The elderly fall regularly, and proximal femoral fractures are exceedingly common. Falls from a height are rare and are often attempted suicides. Although industrial falls are now very rare, DIY enthusiasts falling off ladders are less so. Typical injuries include os calcis, tibial plateau and compressed spinal fractures.

Penetrating trauma

In civilian practice, all gunshot wounds are becoming increasingly common. In conflict, limb injuries as a result of gunshot or fragment wounds are more frequent, as individual ballistic protection has markedly reduced the incidence of penetrating torso injury. Low-energy-transfer penetrating limb injuries in civilian life are common in societies that permit individual handgun possession and are generally benign.[7] Most soft-tissue wounds are not severe and the fracture can be managed by the same principles as for a closed injury. High-energy-transfer wounds due to rifle bullets or close-range shotgun blasts are much more severe and require full debridement. Fragment wounds from bomb blast injuries may be multiple and are often contaminated, needing extensive exploration and wound toilet. Stab wounds to limbs are of concern only if named blood vessels are damaged.

INITIAL MANAGEMENT OF THE PATIENT WITH LIMB INJURY

Clearly, the survival of the patient takes precedence over treatment of the limb injury, and in severe trauma cases the limb damage may warrant a low treatment priority. Alternatively, a visually dramatic limb injury may distract from the associated, occult, life-threatening trauma.

Management of the whole patient

In the majority of cases, casualties have only one injury to a single limb and, in practice, dealing with 'the tibia in cubicle 6' or 'the wrist in minors' becomes the norm. It is vital, however, that, when circumstances dictate, <C>ABCDE principles are followed for the initial assessment and management of patients with polytrauma. Limb injuries that may be immediately life-threatening include major pelvic disruption, multiple long-bone fractures with occult haemorrhage or frank bleeding and traumatic amputations.

Control of bleeding is usually the most common reason for early intervention in limb injury and may occur under <C>. A proximal penetrating limb wound may bleed profusely, but sensibly applied pressure and elevation are usually sufficient to arrest haemorrhage. Very proximal injuries, particularly to the femoral triangle region, may need substantial pressure, sometimes with a fist in the groin, which cannot be removed until the patient is in theatre.

PRE-HOSPITAL

There is little other than basic wound dressing and splintage that can be effectively achieved in the pre-hospital setting. Rough alignment of the limb is sensible and practical, and inflatable or gutter splints are sufficient to rest the limb for transit. Traction splintage may be applied if available and will not unduly delay transfer. A patient with an unstable pelvic injury is best managed by splinting the legs together and applying a pelvic splint.

TRANSPORT

If pre-hospital time is short, elegant splintage is unnecessary but, if prolonged, splintage will not only be much more comfortable for the patient, but may also significantly reduce blood loss. Most patients with polytrauma will be on a spine board; this helps provide a base for the lower limbs, but if injured these must be adequately protected from further injury, particularly, for example, the inadvertent catching of a foot in a doorway. During transport, footwear can be loosened or removed, and this may be a good opportunity to record neurovascular status.

> Splintage of limb injuries decreases bleeding and is more comfortable for the transported patient.

Management of the limb

Once in hospital, assuming that the airway is protected, breathing is supported and the patient's general condition stabilized, attention can be directed towards the limb injury. Where possible, the whole of the affected extremity should be exposed for inspection. Skin wounds should be photographed and documented, obvious misalignment identified and neurovascular status assessed. Each limb segment is passively moved looking for pain, swelling and crepitus; where appropriate, the clinically injured area can then be radiographed.

> Orthopaedic examination: look–feel–move–radiograph.[8]

Haemorrhage

Exsanguinating external haemorrhage should be immediately controlled as part of <C>. Pressure and elevation is often all that is required, but other techniques, including tourniquets and topical haemostatic agents, are described in Chapter 5. Otherwise, bleeding from limb wounds can wait until the airway and chest have been effectively assessed and managed (A and B). Less serious external haemorrhage should be controlled with a pressure dressing and elevation. Betadine-soaked gauze applied to the wound, and held in place with crepe bandages is effective for most bleeding wounds. Circumferential crepe bandaging should be applied firmly starting distally and progressing proximally.

Wounds should not be explored in the emergency department and blind application of artery forceps to bleeding arteries is never indicated. Traumatic amputations or partial limb avulsions can be difficult to dress effectively without the use of a tourniquet. If absolutely essential, a tourniquet is acceptable for short periods.

Alignment

Prompt realignment of a fractured and deformed extremity has the following immediate benefits:

- reduces pain;
- restores vascular supply;
- reduces damage to soft tissues;
- reduces bleeding;
- permits adequate splinting;
- decreases the incidence of fat embolism.

It is a general rule that, to restore a limb to its normal length, rotation and alignment will do no harm. Care must be taken but, providing the patient is warned, has adequate pain relief and traction is applied sensibly, restoration is generally easy. For a typical tibial fracture with an externally rotated foot, the sequence of events should be:

- Ensure adequate analgesia (e.g. i.v. application of morphine).
- Grasp the foot in two hands, leaning backwards to apply traction progressively, and lift off trolley.
- Slowly internally rotate the distal part of leg until the patella and hallux are both pointing upwards.
- An assistant applies a dressing to the wound, and a plaster of Paris back slab.
- Maintain traction until plaster provides firm support.

If, during this procedure with an open fracture, the previously exposed bone ends reduce into the wound, this is not of concern. The fracture will be undergoing full debridement within hours and any possible contamination will be dealt with then. It is better that the limb alignment is restored for the reasons detailed.

Neurovascular status

Significant vascular injury occurs in 3% of limb fractures, whilst neurological injury is less common.[9] It is, however, vital to recognize vascular damage promptly, as the results of repair or reconstruction are poor after a delay of 6 hours from the time of injury. Profuse bleeding from a wound overlying a main vessel is obvious, but arterial injuries may contract and stop bleeding spontaneously. Poor distal perfusion must be specifically looked for and distal pulses assessed, using a Doppler probe if necessary. Intimal damage, following a knee dislocation for example, may be subtle and become clinically manifest only after a delay of some hours. If vascular injury is suspected and clinical signs are equivocal, percutaneous arteriography may be required.[10] Arterial duplex and CT arteriography are potential alternatives.

Nerve injury is not usually amenable to immediate repair, but accurate recording of sensation and muscle power early in the assessment of the limb is essential, particularly if definitely normal, as any subsequent change can be determined more accurately.

Analgesia/anaesthesia

Pain control is vital for humanitarian and practical reasons. A comfortable patient will not thrash around, endangering him- or herself and others, breathing will be more controlled and bleeding will be reduced. Oral medication is impractical and will not be absorbed. Intravenous titration of opiates, usually morphine, is effective and safe and is unlikely to result in respiratory depression in a patient with significant pain. Intramuscular drugs, however, may not be as effective, and a large bolus dose may result because circulatory collapse is reversed during resuscitation, washing the intramuscular drug into the circulation.

Local anaesthetic nerve blocks are safe and effective and may facilitate application of splintage, such as Sager or Thomas splints for a fractured femur. A femoral nerve block can be administered safely by non-anaesthetists, as described in Chapter 21, and should markedly reduce pain in the distribution of the femoral nerve for 4–6 hours. Other nerve blocks can be easily learnt from anaesthetic texts.

Antibiotics

Open fractures require immediate antibiotic therapy with the first dose to be given as soon as it is practicable.[11,12] Current UK practice is subject to review as a result of an association between cephalosporin use and *Clostridium difficile* infection. A reasonable initial regimen is flucloxacillin 500 mg, gentamicin (dose is dependent on a number of factors including age and renal function) with the addition of metronidazole 500 mg in severely contaminated wounds. The patient's antitetanus status should be established and managed appropriately.

MANAGEMENT OF SPECIFIC INJURIES

Wounds

In addition to haemorrhage control, skin and soft-tissue wounds require careful assessment and management. Any obvious contaminating material should be removed when the wound is inspected, although significant foreign bodies should be left in place until they can be removed in the operating theatre. Inappropriate attempts to do so in the emergency department may cause significant haemorrhage, which can, on occasion, be life-threatening. Gentle irrigation with normal saline may be helpful, but most substantial wounds will require formal exploration in the operating theatre. Photographs should be taken; digital cameras/camera phones provide plentiful images.

Wounds should be lightly packed with dry gauze; there is no place for forcing reams of ribbon gauze into the wound cavity as this may cause damage and be difficult to remove. Open fractures should be dressed with betadine-soaked dressings to reduce bacterial count. Further gauze pads can be added as required and crepe bandages applied to hold the dressing firmly in place.[13] Definitive wound management is usually undertaken in theatre under general anaesthetic. The principles of wound debridement are shown in Table 14.1.

Degloving skin wounds, in which the deep blood supply to the skin is avulsed from the underlying fascia, are difficult to assess as the skin may appear well perfused at first; if there is doubt, it is best to preserve skin of uncertain viability and undertake a second debridement 24–36 hours later. The management of burns is discussed elsewhere in the manual.

Fractures

The general principles of the treatment of limb and pelvic fractures are discussed.

PELVIS

Pubic rami fractures in the elderly are common as a result of osteoporosis and do not lead to significant haemorrhage. For a young person's pelvic ring to be broken, considerable

Table 14.1 Principles of wound debridement

Principle	Method
Preserve skin	Excise only devitalized skin edges
Avoid tension	Perform fasciotomy
Remove all foreign material	Expose whole wound and palpate all areas
Debride dead muscle	Excise all muscle that does not contract, capillary bleed, have colour or have a consistency that appears normal
Leave wound open	Delayed closure, skin graft

energy transfer is needed, and the associated soft-tissue damage is much more marked. Haemorrhage is the major problem, and it is often not immediately obvious, becoming so only after attempts to resuscitate the patient are ineffective. Fractures that displace the hemipelvis laterally, superiorly or both are most commonly associated with major bleeding from the iliac vessels. These injuries may require early external fixation with an anterior frame to hold the pelvis steady, preventing movement between the fragments and allowing tamponade of the soft tissue. In addition, an interventional radiologist may be able to identify and embolize bleeding arterial vessels.[10]

Pelvic fractures may be associated with penetration of the rectum or vagina, and associated bladder and urethral injuries are seen in roughly 5% of cases. Urinary and faecal diversion procedures will be necessary in these cases and mortality is increased significantly. The features of pelvic fractures are summarized in Table 14.2.

LIMB FRACTURES

Extremity injuries that have a fracture are best managed according to the principle that fractures are soft-tissue injuries complicated by a bony trauma. This is particularly true for tibial fractures. The tibia is not completely surrounded by muscle and the subcutaneous border is commonly where open fractures will emerge, stripping away what little soft-tissue attachment the bone has. Bone derives virtually all its blood supply from the overlying soft tissue, so the tibia is particularly prone to healing problems. It is essential that the management of all limb fractures attempts to minimize further disruption of the blood supply to the fracture fragments – it is only with a viable blood supply that healing can occur.

> A fracture is a soft-tissue injury complicated by a break in a bone.

Restoration of length, rotation and alignment are the long-term aims of limb fracture treatment but, in the early stages, rotation and alignment are most important in order to remove the tension from vessels and nerves involved in the zone of injury. Partial venous obstruction may lead to congestion and compartment syndrome, arterial

compression to ischaemia and nerve compression to permanent dysfunction.

Open fractures must be debrided within 6 hours.[6,14] This prevents exponential bacterial growth converting contamination into infection. The wound is extended and fascia opened. Devitalized bone fragments are removed as they will not heal and will act as foreign material. The tissues are irrigated, preferably with copious warm saline lavage. Bone ends and the medullary canals of both main fragments are cleaned of debris and contaminated haematoma. Reduction is usually easy as the wound is open, and fixation is with an intramedullary nail, a plate or an external fixation device. The original skin wound is not closed, but the surgically performed extensions can be closed at this stage. The principles of open fracture management are outlined in Table 14.3.

DISLOCATIONS

All dislocated joints must be reduced to prevent secondary damage and restore function. Most dislocations are obvious and reduction is easily achieved such as for the shoulder or proximal interphalangeal joints. Some, for example the hip, are difficult to reduce and require a general anaesthetic. Particular problems with individual joint dislocations are detailed in Table 14.4.

COMPARTMENT SYNDROME[15,16]

The consequences of failing to diagnose and treat compartment syndromes are disastrous. In an injured

Table 14.2 Features and management principles of pelvic fractures

Feature	Management
Unstable fracture pattern	Splintage, binder, external fixation
Haemorrhage	Appropriate resuscitation, consider embolization
Rectal injury	Colostomy
Bladder injury	Urinary diversion
Urethral rupture	Catheter (?suprapubic)

Table 14.3 Principles of open fracture initial surgery

Extend wound to allow full inspection and palpation
Perform fasciotomy if required
Remove foreign material and devitalized bone
Irrigate with pulsed lavage
Complete reduction and fixation
Ensure delayed closure

Table 14.4 Specific problems of joint dislocations

Joint	Problem
Hip	Avascular necrosis – minimized if reduction is carried out within 4–6 hours
	Acetabular lip fracture
Knee	Vascular injury, common peroneal nerve injury, major ligament disruption
Ankle	Chondral damage
Subtalar joint	Often missed, talar avascular necrosis
Midfoot (Lisfranc)	Often missed, permanent pain
Elbow	Medial ligament injury causing chronic instability
Wrist	May be missed

extremity, tissue pressure is likely to rise. Venous congestion, arterial compromise, relative ischaemia and contusion all predispose to raised interstitial pressures. In unrestricted soft tissues, this rise in pressure is accommodated by swelling and expansion, tending to reduce tissue pressure towards normal. If a fascial envelope surrounding a limb compartment restricts expansion, then a steady rise in tissue pressure ensues, which in turn increases relative ischaemia by restricting both venous outflow and arterial inflow to the injured area. A vicious spiral of pressure rises is set in place, leading ultimately to critical ischaemia and tissue death. It is particularly common in the lower limb (Figure 14.3).

The clinical features of compartment syndrome are:

- increasing pain – worse than can be anticipated, despite adequate splintage and analgesia;
- severe pain on passively moving the toes or fingers, causing their tendons to move within the affected compartment;
- late neurovascular compromise with sensory alteration distally (note: pulses may be preserved despite compartment death).

If a compartment syndrome is suspected, these clinical features are very often strongly positive. It is essential to ensure that casts and dressings are not too tight on the limb and, if there is doubt, a repeat assessment in 15–30 minutes will often ensure the diagnosis is confirmed. In a patient who is not responsive to pain, sedated or ventilated in the intensive care unit (ICU), compartment pressures can be assessed accurately using arterial pressure transducers passed into the anterior compartment below the knee, or with proprietary compartment pressure monitors. A pressure rise towards mean arterial pressure, rather than a specific pressure value, is indicative of compartment syndrome.[17]

> If a compartment syndrome is suspected, it should be treated as such.

Treatment consists of surgical decompression. All four compartments below the knee should be widely opened.

Thigh compartment syndrome is rare and requires decompression of the anterior and posterior compartments via a lateral approach. Flexor compartment syndrome in the forearm can be decompressed using a Henry anterior approach and carpal tunnel decompression.

The onset of compartment syndrome is usually slow and insidious, often after the patient is stabilized and frequently following an operative intervention. A high index of suspicion in these cases is vital, and repeated returns to the beside may be needed to establish the diagnosis. Once the condition is confirmed, treatment is technically easy and always effective, providing critical ischaemic change has not occurred. In the event of a delayed diagnosis (onset >6 hours), surgery should be avoided if possible as infection will be inevitable and amputation highly likely.

AMPUTATION

Amputations from trauma are rare and tend to raise management dilemmas, particularly if they are incomplete. Dressing a true complete traumatic amputation is usually easy, but, when there is residual soft-tissue bridging between the two parts of the limb, circumferential dressings and splintage may be difficult. If there is clearly just a thread of skin between the stump and the distal part, this should be divided and the amputation completed prior to dressing.

PRESERVATION SURGERY

The decision to attempt reconstruction of a severely mangled extremity may be exceedingly difficult. Modern techniques make most surgery possible in the right centre, but the outcome may be so poor that early amputation would have been preferable. Various scores have been devised to aid with decision-making in these circumstances,[18] but in general the indications for amputation of, for example, a below-the-knee injury with major vascular compromise, rather than attempted salvage, are:

- division of the posterior tibial nerve;
- massive skin loss;
- severe life-threatening associated injuries;
- pre-existing systemic illness.

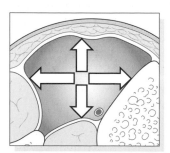
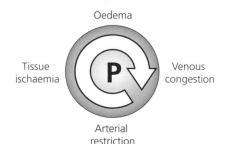

Figure 14.3 Limb cross-section with increasing pressure vicious circle.

In practice, the tendency is to attempt preservation initially and make a firm decision regarding amputation at the second-look procedure. It is important to include two senior surgeons in the decision-making process, preferably after discussion with the patient. Dissatisfaction with the attempts at limb reconstruction may ultimately lead to amputation, and this is rarely as satisfactory as if the amputation was undertaken early.

REPLANTATION

The technical feasibility of replanting traumatically amputated parts can allow excellent functional and aesthetic recovery after devastating injury. Successful replantation relies on having a well-resuscitated patient, a viable part and surgical expertise. It is important to remember that the first priority in managing amputated parts is to manage the person from whom the part was amputated. The <C>ABCDE approach must be used. Good first aid and vascular spasm may have reduced the bleeding, while compensatory mechanisms may be maintaining the blood pressure. A careful assessment of the circulatory state must be made to avoid underestimating the degree of hypovolaemia.

Management of these injuries is often hampered by a mental fixation on the part rather than the person. The patient is likely to be in significant distress, and adequate intravenous analgesia should be administered early. Associated injuries should not be overlooked, and a full and thorough secondary survey must be performed. It is essential that radiography be carried out on both the residual stump and the part. Replantation surgery draws heavily on operating theatre resources. The reimplantation team should be informed as early as possible, thus maximizing the time available to organize the necessary facilities.

Management of the amputated part aims to reduce the warm ischaemia time. Urgent transfer of the patient and the part must be organized unless the patient is already in a specialist centre. The temperature of the part should be lowered as much as possible, without allowing it to freeze. This is best achieved by taking the following steps:

- gross contamination is gently removed, but damage caused by rubbing is avoided;
- the part is covered in a single layer of damp (not dripping-wet) gauze;
- the covered part is placed in a plastic bag and the bag is sealed;
- the sealed bag is placed in a container of water/ice mix.

The amputated part should never be allowed to come into direct contact with ice as this will cause frostbite.

Digits have little muscle volume and are more tolerant of warm ischaemia. Surgical techniques continue to improve, and crushed or avulsed tissue may be salvageable. Similarly, if the part cannot be implanted, effective use may be made of undamaged skin. It is inappropriate for the non-expert to deny the patient possible replantation based on time since injury or mechanism of injury. Expert surgical advice should always be sought.

> All potentially replantable limbs or limb parts should be discussed as early as possible with the replantation centre.

General measures

OXYGENATION

Maintenance of the patient's overall condition may have a profound effect on wound healing following limb injury. Adequate perfusion of the tissues with satisfactory oxygenation and correction of acidosis is vital. As with all trauma patients, supplementary oxygen should be given by facemask as soon as possible and, even if the patient is not intubated, extra oxygen should be provided throughout the acute phase of the injury.

WOUND HANDLING

Details of the initial surgery and how wounds should be addressed have been covered already. Once the initial surgery has been completed, planning for the second and subsequent operations must be undertaken. A well-dressed wound that has been adequately debrided, in a resuscitated patient, can be left undisturbed for 48–72 hours. For that period, gauze dressings will absorb wound exudate and blood, keeping the wound surface clean and moist. If fluids soak through the dressings, further layers should be added rather than attempting removal. Beyond this time, the dressings will become heavily contaminated and infection in the wound may be apparent.

Therefore, it is prudent to take the patient back to theatre at 48–72 hours after the initial debridement. At this time any further muscle death will have declared itself and this tissue can be removed. Conversely, if the wound is clean and the skin edges healthy, it is safe to close it, or apply a split-skin graft, at this operation. If there is doubt about the condition of the soft tissues, further irrigation and, if necessary, excision of non-viable tissue can be performed, with the wound again being dressed and left open as before. Sometimes these serial debridements may have to continue on several occasions before the wound can be deemed healthy. Although it is safe to continue to perform repeated wound washouts, the chances of achieving a delayed *primary* closure become less over time, and skin grafting or other plastic surgical manoeuvres may become necessary.

DEEP VENOUS THROMBOSIS/FAT EMBOLUS

Venous thromboembolism (VTE) is a complication of all trauma, limb trauma in particular. Pelvic and femoral fractures are particularly likely to cause VTE and the prolonged bed rest of the multiply injured patient predisposes to the condition. Prophylaxis for VTE is essential (Table 14.5).

Fat embolism syndrome involves globules of fat and other debris passing from the injured limbs into the pulmonary circulation and beyond. It is characterized by difficulties with maintaining oxygen saturation, an acute confusional state, petechial haemorrhages and fat in the urine.[19] Preventative measures include early stabilization of fractures and possibly avoiding intrameduallary fixation techniques and use of bone cement.[20] The treatment is to support respiratory function and anticoagulate the patient when it is safe to do so.

SUBSEQUENT MANAGEMENT AND OUTCOME

Often the initial treatment of the injury will be the definitive management and no further operations are required. In the event of multiple trauma, however, it is usually not possible or safe to attend to every injury on the first intervention. If the patient is haemodynamically unstable, coagulopathic and acidotic, it is prudent to spend as little time on the operating table as possible, consistent with stabilizing the important injuries. This 'damage control' approach to polytrauma is associated with increased survival rates and with limb injury, generally meaning that there is rapid debridement of wounds and placement of external fixation devices to stabilize the major fractures with a view to replacing the fixators with internal fixation after a period of resuscitation in the ICU.[21] This approach is safe and does not compromise fracture and wound outcomes.

Table 14.5 Prophylaxis for venous thromboembolism after trauma

Acute phase	Recovery
Correction of hypovolaemia	Antiembolism stockings/calf
Use of colloids such as dextrans	pumps
Early stabilization of fractures	Early mobilization where
Antiembolism stockings	possible
Pneumatic calf pumps	Low-molecular-weight heparin/
	warfarin

Soft-tissue management

It cannot be overstressed that musculoskeletal injuries are defined and governed predominantly by the state of the soft tissues, and the ultimate outcome will be determined mainly by how well these heal. Patients produce differing degrees of scar tissue, and scar and joint capsule contractures may negate the successful results of bone-healing measures.

DEBRIDEMENT

Although repeat debridement may be necessary, removal of too much soft tissue can produce problems with healing. Where possible, tendons should not be excised as they will often survive despite suboptimal perfusion. Nerves must be preserved and covered with muscle or fascia. All joints should have an attempt made at capsular closure and must be covered with soft tissue. Bone stripped of periosteum is unlikely to provide a satisfactory bed for a skin graft and should be covered with muscle.

WOUND CLOSURE AND COVERAGE

An unclosed wound can heal only by secondary intention. Until a wound is 'clean, closed and dry' options for any secondary surgery, such as bone grafting, will be limited. Open wounds are metabolically uneconomical, and the acute phase of the injury is incomplete until skin coverage is achieved. The reconstructive ladder (Table 14.6) describes the options for wound closure in ascending order of complexity.

Early mobilization and physiotherapy reduce wound contracture development. Avoidance of common contractures is important and measures to reduce this risk in the lower limb include:

- maintaining the ankle at 90° after a tibial fracture with a resting splint or cast, even if the tibia is fixed;
- avoiding knee flexion contracture by using an extension splint and by avoiding resting the knee on pillows;
- encouraging the patient to lie prone following transfemoral amputation.

Table 14.6 Techniques for wound closure

Technique	Comments
Primary closure	Unsafe for potentially contaminated wounds or open fractures (except hands)
Delayed primary closure	At 48–72 hours post injury. Ideal if wound is clean and can be closed without tension
Split-skin graft	Good coverage if meshed. Not for bare cortical bone. Cosmetic issues
Suction dressing	Excellent for cases in which healing by secondary intention is acceptable. Very prolonged
Local flap	Fasciocutaneous etc. A plastic surgeon is usually required
Free flap	Plastics only

Fracture management

INITIAL FIXATION

The relative merits of fixation over traction and what type of fixation to use are beyond the scope of this manual. In general, however, most open fractures will now be treated with some form of fixation: either with an external frame or an internal device. This allows rigid fixation, access to soft-tissue wounds and early joint movement. Intra-articular fractures will be fixed to promote accurate primary healing without callus formation and to reduce the risk of arthrosis. Multiply injured patients have better outcomes and survival following operative fixation of fractures.[22,23] Non-surgical management of closed fractures still has a role and avoids the risk of infection in an otherwise uncontaminated area. Upper limb injuries, in particular, will still often only require simple measures to allow satisfactory healing.

BONE-HEALING MEASURES

Delayed or non-union of fractures causes significant morbidity following limb injury. Prolonged pain, loss of function, disuse syndrome and depression are all important sequelae, and every effort must be made to encourage fracture union as rapidly as possible. The causes of delayed union are summarized in Table 14.7.

In the event of slow fracture healing, general measures such as stopping smoking will help. Surgical manoeuvres such as bone grafting or exchanging the intramedullary nail may be necessary. In extreme cases, bone ends may be non-viable and may need to be excised and the limb shortened to allow healing to commence. Limb-lengthening techniques can then be employed to restore the correct length.

Return to function

The sole aim of treatment of musculoskeletal trauma, beyond preservation of life, is to allow restoration of limb function. The purpose of the upper limb is to position the hand in space, and that of the lower limb is to allow ambulation. Limb injury outcome is measured by functional return but most attention is still drawn to initial treatment.

Table 14.7 Causes of delayed union of fractures

Local factors	General factors
Poor blood supply to fracture especially the distal tibia	Poor nutritional status
	Cigarette smoking
Instability (with excessive movement)	Prolonged use of non-steroidal anti-inflammatory drugs
Reinjury	

Physiotherapy

This should begin immediately following the first intervention, be it surgery or bed rest. Maintenance of lung function is vital and can be enhanced with breathing exercises. Non-injured parts must be kept active, especially if the patient is paralysed and ventilated, and daily passive movement of all joints is ideal. If long-bone fractures have been rigidly fixed, physiotherapy including continuous passive motion can begin almost immediately; as soon as patients can sit up, they can sit out of bed. If there is one intact lower extremity (including the pelvis), the patient can stand with assistance and transfer in and out of bed. Most fractures in the lower limb will be sufficiently healed to start protected weight bearing after 6 weeks.

Upper limb physiotherapy is vital, and fine movements of the hand and fingers will be restored much more effectively if intervention is prompt. In the event of nerve injury needing delayed repair or reconstruction, the ultimate result will be very positively influenced by early passive physiotherapy to maintain the mobility of the small joints in the wrist and hand while the nerve supply to the muscles that move those joints is interrupted.

Occupational therapy to maintain and restore complex movements and functional activity is often vital to good outcomes, and long-term rehabilitation units concentrate on this.

Psychology

It is common for trauma victims to pass through several episodes of mood alteration. The elation of surviving a major injury is followed by depression owing to pain, immobility, loss of function and concerns about the future. To the patient the healing process often seems very prolonged, even if the doctors and therapists believe that the patient's recovery is going well. It is vital to maintain patients' optimism and to engage their enthusiasm for doing their exercises etc., some of which may be difficult and painful. Outpatient visits are very important and should be regarded as important milestones, often with substantive objective measures of progress such as radiographs showing good callus formation at the fracture site.

Often the victims of trauma will be seeking compensation. It is important that their recovery does not become affected by concerns about subsequent financial payments.

> A good outcome far outweighs the compensation for a poor one.

Rehabilitation

In an ideal system, all patients with substantial injuries should pass from hospital to a dedicated rehabilitation facility in order to maximize their potential for recovery. In practice, this may be limited to those who have suffered spinal or head injuries or those with amputations. The majority of limb-injured patients will undertake rehabilitation in conjunction with their local hospital's physiotherapy department, and it is vital that health services provide satisfactory funding for this. Motivated patients will often positively contribute to their recovery by joining a gym or going to the local swimming pool to practise hydrotherapy.

Patients and carers alike should be aware that most musculoskeletal injuries will continue to show improvement for up to 18 months following trauma, and every effort should be made to maximize recovery during this period.

Delayed reconstruction

The most common long-term sequela following limb trauma is joint arthrosis. Osteoarthritis of the hip, knee and ankle is likely to follow intra-articular fractures of these joints, although the incidence of osteoarthritis is reduced if near-anatomical reduction of the fracture is achieved and maintained. Good results of hip replacement are now universally expected, with knee replacement being slightly less predictable. Ankle replacement is still largely experimental, and ankle osteoarthritis, if severe, will result in fusion. In the upper limb, shoulder and elbow replacement generally provides better pain relief than function.

Although rare with modern techniques, lower limb misalignment following fracture is a potential source of delayed complications due to abnormal stresses being place through the joints. Corrective osteotomy before secondary changes occur is worthwhile in selected cases.

Case scenario

A 54-year-old woman was the driver in a high-speed, head-on car collision. She was wearing a seat belt and the airbag deployed. She suffered no apparent head or chest injuries but had obvious open fractures of both femurs, open fractures of the right patella, right tibia, left humerus and right os calcis and also had a right middle finger extensor tendon laceration. There were multiple cutaneous lacerations.

Outline appropriate pre-hospital interventions
The open wounds were dressed with gauze. Both lower limbs were rested in gutter splints, a hard cervical collar was applied *in situ* and the patient was immobilized on a spine board. She was cannulated and was receiving i.v. fluids and supplemental oxygen on arrival at the accident and emergency department. She had received i.v. opiate analgesia.

Aside from the standard <C>ABCDE approach, what else should the emergency department do?
A Sager splint was applied to both lower limbs. Resuscitation continued, as did the ongoing assessment of injuries. Trauma room radiographs showed a C2 burst fracture (Figure 14.4a), an intact pelvic ring but a fractured right femoral shaft (Figure 14.4b) and a segmental left humeral fracture (Figure 14.4c). Prophylactic antibiotics were administered and the patient's tetanus status was found to be up

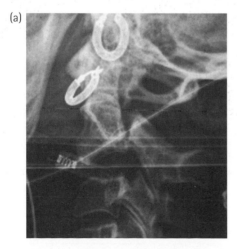

(a)

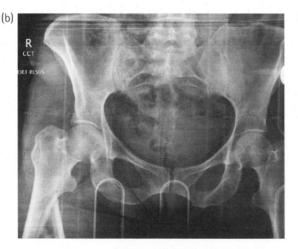

(b)

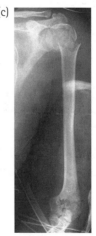

(c)

Figure 14.4 Initial radiographs. (a) C2 burst fracture. (b) Intact pelvis with right femoral fracture. (c) Segmental fracture of the left humerus.

to date. In view of ongoing hypotension and right upper quadrant and shoulder tip pain, a focused assessment with sonography for trauma (FAST) scan of the abdomen was performed, disclosing significant free fluid in the right upper quadrant and suggesting a hepatic laceration.

What surgical management is appropriate? Is conservative management of the hepatic injury indicated?

In the presence of severe polytrauma requiring potentially prolonged general anaesthesia, a damage control approach is appropriate. In this case the liver was packed to control bleeding and peritoneal contamination dealt with. Under the same general anaesthetic, damage control orthopaedic techniques were applied. Both legs were placed in traction on the operating table while laparotomy was undertaken and all the leg wounds debrided and irrigated. Both legs had across-the-knee external fixators applied spanning fractures with two pins in each segment (Figure 14.5). Because of the high risk of compartment syndrome following the right tibial fracture, right calf, four-compartment fasciotomies

were performed and left open. The upper limb wounds were debrided and irrigated. A plaster of Paris back slab was used to immobilize the left humerus fractures.

What happened next?

At 48 hours, all wounds were inspected and redebrided as necessary. The external fixator on the right tibia was exchanged for an intramedullary nail and the patellar tendon reattached to a lower pole on that side. The medial right calf fasciotomy wound was closed, as was the upper limb wound, both of which were clean and healthy. At this point, the right hand extensor tendon was repaired and a halo frame applied for the C2 burst fracture. At this point attempts at further definitive surgery are likely to worsen the patient's physiological status and this was therefore deferred. At about day 5, both femurs were plated or nailed (a distal femoral nail was used in addition to plating on the right in this patient). Unclosed wounds, such as the right foot, were skin grafted and any remaining fasciotomy wounds closed. At 8 days post injury, the proximal and distal left humerus fractures were plated (Figure 14. 6).

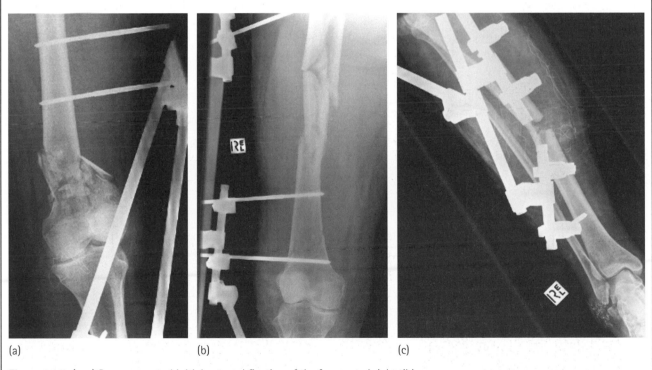

(a)   (b)   (c)

Figure 14.5 (a–c) Damage control initial external fixation of the femurs and right tibia.

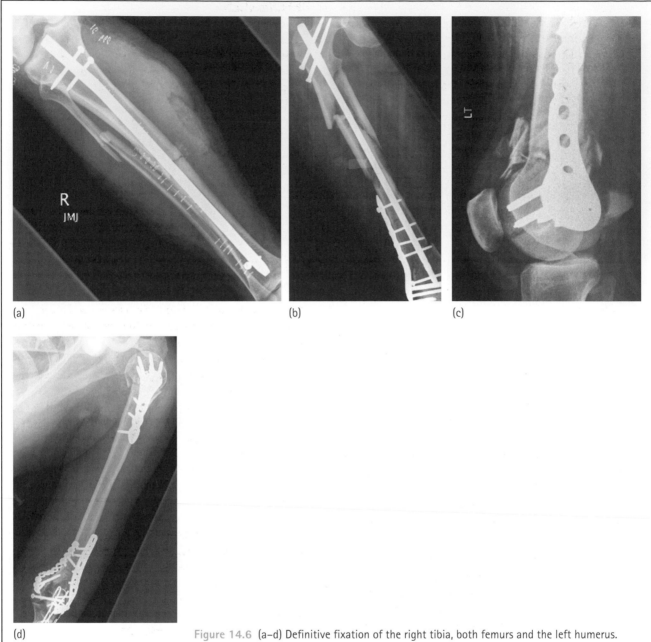

(a)

(b)

(c)

(d)

Figure 14.6 (a–d) Definitive fixation of the right tibia, both femurs and the left humerus.

SUMMARY

Limb injuries are generally isolated and uncomplicated. When they are suffered in association with multiple system trauma, they may be the cause of prolonged morbidity and disability, despite being rarely life-threatening at the outset. Assessment of limb trauma should be rapid and accurate once life-threatening injuries have been either excluded or treated.

Although definitive surgical management of isolated injuries will usually be undertaken as soon as possible, damage control surgery to rapidly debride wounds and stabilize long-bone and pelvic fractures may be life saving, allowing resuscitation to continue over the initial 24–48 hours following injury. Delayed, definitive, orthopaedic reconstruction can then be undertaken with much less risk to the patient.

GLOBAL PERSPECTIVES

Limb injuries are common in any area of the world, but their causation may differ with location. In most countries, motor vehicle accidents are responsible for the majority of serious limb injuries. Sporting activity may account for a large proportion of less serious injuries.

In areas of low-intensity warfare, there are many cases of limb injury due to landmine explosion or detonation of previously unexploded ordnance, such as cluster munitions. These are frequently crippling injuries, commonly with traumatic amputation and often affecting children.

Possession of firearms by a significant proportion of a country's population leads to a higher incidence of gunshot wounds in peacetime, and a significant proportion of limb trauma in the USA is due to handgun bullet wounds.

Clearly, medical systems and individuals will need to be organized and trained to deal with the type of trauma most commonly encountered. It is unusual for a UK orthopaedic surgeon to have to manage a gunshot wound or landmine injury; it would be inappropriate to expect that surgeon to operate in, for example, a Red Cross hospital in Pakistan close to the Afghan border without undergoing additional training.

REFERENCES

1. Coupland RM. *War Wounds of Limbs: Surgical Management.* Oxford: Butterworth-Heinemann Ltd, 1993.
2. Rowley DI. *War Wounds With Fractures: a Guide to Surgical Management.* Geneva: International Committee of the Red Cross, 1996.
3. Kenzora JE, Burgess AR. The neglected foot and ankle in polytrauma. *Adv Orthop Surg* 1983;7:89–98.
4. Dalal SA, Burgess AR, Siegel JH, *et al.* Pelvic fracture in multiple trauma: classification by mechanism is key to pattern of organ injury, resuscitative requirements, and outcome. *J Trauma* 1989;29:981–1002.
5. Caudle RJ, Stern PJ. Severe open fractures of the tibia. *J Bone Joint Surg Am* 1987;69:801–7.
6. Gustilo RB, Merkow RL, Templeman D. The management of open fractures. *J Bone Joint Surg Am* 1990;72:299–304.
7. Bowyer GW, Rossiter ND. Management of gunshot wounds to limbs. *J Bone Joint Surg Br* 1997;79:1031–6.
8. Apley AG, Solomon L, eds. Principles of fractures. In: *Apley's System of Orthopedics and Fractures,* 6th edn. London: Butterworths, 1982, pp. 333–68.
9. Gustilo RB, Anderson JT. Prevention of infection in the management of one thousand and twenty five open fractures of long bones. *J Bone Joint Surg Am* 1976;58:453–8.
10. Raby N, Berman L, de Lacey G. *Accident and Emergency Radiology: a Survival Guide.* London: WB Saunders Co., 1995.
11. Court-Brown CM, McQueen MM, Quaba AAR. *Management of Open Fractures.* London: Martin Dunitz, 1996.
12. Mellor SG, Easmon CSF, Sanford JP. Wound contamination and antibiotics. In: Ryan JM, Rich NM, Dale RF, Morgans BT, Cooper GJ, eds. *Ballistic Trauma.* London: Edward Arnold, 1997, pp. 61–71.
13. Bowyer GW, Ryan JM, Kaufmann CR, Ochsner MG. General principles of wound management. In: Ryan JM, Rich N, Dale R, Morgans B, Cooper GJ, eds. *Ballistic Trauma.* London: Edward Arnold, 1997, pp. 105–19.
14. Esterhai JL, Jr, Queenan J. Management of soft tissue wounds associated with type III open fractures. [Review]. *Orthop Clin North Am* 1991;22:427–32.
15. Elliott KGB, Johnstone AJ. Diagnosing acute compartment syndrome. *J Bone Joint Surg Br* 2003;85:625–32.
16. McQueen MM, Christie J, Court Brown CM. Acute compartment syndrome in tibial diaphyseal fractures. *J Bone Joint Surg Br* 1996;78:95–8.
17. McQueen MM, Court-Brown CM. Compartment monitoring in tibial fractures. The pressure threshold for decompression. *J Bone Joint Surg Br* 1996;78:99–104.
18. Bosse MJ, MacKenzie EJ, Kellam JF, *et al.* A prospective evaluation of the clinical utility of the lower-extremity injury-severity scores. *J Bone Joint Surg Am* 2001;83:3–14.
19. Fabian TC. Unravelling the fat embolism syndrome. *N Engl J Med* 1993;329:961–3.
20. Pape H-C, Auf'm'Kolk M, Paffrath T, *et al.* Primary intramedullary femur fixation in multiple trauma patients with associated lung contusion – a cause of posttraumatic ARDS? *J Trauma* 1993;34:540–8.

21. Giannoudis PV. Surgical priorities in damage control in polytrauma. *J Bone Joint Surg Br* 2003;**85**;478–83.

22. Bone LB, Johnson KD, Weigelt J, Scheinberg R. Early versus delayed stabilization of femoral fractures. A prospective randomized study. *J Bone Joint Surg Am* 1989;**71**:336–40.

23. Schatzker J, Tile M. *The Rationale of Operative Fracture Care*, 2nd edn. Berlin: Springer, 1996.

Injuries in children

OBJECTIVES

After reading this chapter the reader will:
- be able to highlight differences in trauma care between children and adults
- be able to provide an overall introduction to the increasingly evidence-based subject of paediatric trauma care
- be able to offer an approach to the severely injured child, based on the accepted system adopted in adult trauma
- assessment, focusing on the key differences between children and adults
- understand the importance of considering non-accidental injury in the differential diagnosis of paediatric trauma.

INTRODUCTION

In the UK each year, 2 million children are taken to emergency departments following injuries and 100 000 are admitted to hospital. Accidents causing injuries are currently the second leading cause of death in children in the UK.

Children are not small adults and when physicians manage major injury in children it can be stressful. This is because of differences in drug and fluid calculations, different equipment sizes, communication difficulties with very young children, developmental, physiological and anatomical differences specific to children as well as any personal emotional impact of seeing severely injured children. Unless they are parents themselves, many clinicians find dealing with small children to be an alien environment.

Many children who are injured have minor injuries; injury severity forms a continuum and there is no precise cut-off point between 'minor' and 'major' trauma. Victims of major trauma may have life- or limb-threatening injuries as well as minor fractures or soft-tissue injuries. Physicians managing trauma in children therefore require a broad knowledge base and skill set.

An awareness that not all injuries are caused through accidents is also important. Health care professionals should have a detailed working knowledge of child protection protocols and strategies when managing any suspected non-accidental injury (NAI).

In 2003 there were 215 childhood deaths in the UK from injury compared with over a thousand in 1979. Rates of death from injury fell from 11.1/100 000 children in the 1981 census to 4.0/100 000 in the 2001 census. This decrease is largely a result of injury prevention strategies supported by changes in legislation. Injury prevention education is a key component in the management of injured children. Socioeconomic inequalities do persist and rates of injury and death remain relatively high in children from families with a lower and poorer socioeconomic classification.[1]

Expert hospital care is also contributing to the decline in the injury death rate in young people. Between 1989 and 1995 there was a substantial decline in the probability of death among children admitted to hospital after severe injury: a 16% per year reduction. As health care professionals become increasingly expert at the delivery of trauma care to children it is hoped that more young lives will be saved in the future in the UK.

INITIAL ASSESSMENT

Management of paediatric trauma should start before the child arrives in the resuscitation room. Trauma teams should be alerted and mobilized to attend urgently. The presence of a paediatrician is vital. The age of the child is usually known to the pre-hospital teams, and if this is communicated to the hospital trauma team then equipment and drugs can be prepared before the child arrives. The following calculations are helpful:

- Weight (kg) = (age + 4) × 2.
- Endotracheal tube diameter (mm) = (age/4) + 4.

- Endotracheal tube length (cm) from mouth = (age/2) + 12.
- Crystalloid bolus = 10 mL/kg.
- Volume of blood replacement = 10 mL/kg.
- Dose of adrenaline = 0.1 mL/kg of 1:10 000.
- Dose of morphine = 0.2 mg kg.

These formulae should be prominently displayed in the resuscitation room, and all equipment and drugs must be prepared and readily available. A trauma team leader must be identified, and care should follow a structured approach in a calm environment with clear and precise instruction from the appointed team leader. Documentation is important, and someone should be detailed to make clinical records. A named carer should make early contact with the child's parents or carers and should update them regularly and counsel them appropriately. Physical contact between them and the child should be encouraged and parents should be allowed to remain close by unless they choose not to.

PRIMARY SURVEY

As with adult trauma management the primary survey focuses on the <C>ABCDE priorities and is followed by a detailed secondary survey.

Catastrophic haemorrhage control

This is rarely of concern in paediatric trauma although the principles of control of life-threatening bleeding remain the same.

Airway

The assessment of airway patency is a priority in the acutely injured child. Airway compromise is a major cause of death in this age group. For each patient the following should be asked:

- Is the patient breathing?
- Is the airway patent?
- Is ventilation adequate?
- Do I have all the necessary and age appropriate equipment?

If there is concern regarding airway compromise, follow the initial management procedure: jaw thrust, suction, 100% oxygen through a non-rebreathing facemask and calling for immediate help. If airway obstruction does not respond to initial management, then two choices of airway adjuncts are available: oropharyngeal or nasopharyngeal airways.

The oropharyngeal airway is sized from the central incisors to the angle of the jaw with the concave side upwards. The procedure is usually tolerated in the poorly responsive patient, but the risk of inducing vomiting should be remembered and suction must be available. In children, a tongue depressor is used and it is guided in with the concave side upwards. There is no rotation, as there is in adults, in order to avoid causing damage to the soft tissues of the palate.

The nasopharyngeal airway should be used with care in patients with fractures of the anterior base of the skull and complex maxillofacial fractures, or if there is a difficult or aberrant congenital nasal anatomy. However, if a nasopharyngeal airway is the only immediate way of providing a patent airway pending more complex techniques, even in the presence of a possible skull fracture, one should be carefully inserted. It is sized from the tip of the nose to the tragus of the ear and is useful in responsive patients. It is also often better tolerated in this group than the oropharyngeal airway. The technique for its insertion includes lubricating the airway and inserting it along the base of the nose (not angled upwards). The diameter is such that it should not cause any blanching of the alae nasi.

Airway sizing:
- Oropharyngeal airway – central incisors to the angle of the jaw.
- Nasopharyngeal airway – tip of the nose to the tragus.

The child's condition should improve. If it does not, an advanced airway technique may be indicated. Specific indications for intubation include:

- inability to protect the airway which is not relieved by simple measures;
- the need for positive-pressure ventilation;
- airway burns or inhalational injuries;
- severe head injury with a Glasgow Coma Scale (GCS) score less than 8;
- major maxillofacial injury;
- apnoea, cardiac arrest or severe shock.

Whenever possible, tracheal intubation should be performed by a competent practitioner, such as a paediatric anaesthetist or paediatric emergency physician, experienced and practised in advanced airway techniques in children. A potentially difficult airway should be expected in patients with certain conditions, such as juvenile idiopathic arthritis (abnormal mouth opening and poor temporomandibular joint function), trisomy 21 (cervical spine abnormalities) and Pierre Robin syndrome (micrognathia). Craniofacial anomalies, burns to the airway and facial fractures may also make intubation difficult.

There are several major differences between the paediatric and adult airway, which are detailed in Table 15.1. The Mallampati classification of assessment of airway anatomy and difficulty of intubation has been adopted

Table 15.1 Differences between the paediatric and adult airway

Tongue	Larger in relation to the oral cavity
Epiglottis	Short and stubby, U-shaped, protrudes and angled over laryngeal inlet which makes control with the laryngoscope more difficult
Hyoid bone	Not calcified in infants
Larynx	Higher (C3–C4) and more anterior in infants than in adults (C5–C6). Also angled at right angles, in relation to floor of mouth, and is funnel shaped in children
Thyroid	Not calcified in infants
Cricoid	Cone shaped, narrowest part of the airway, therefore consider using uncuffed tubes in a patient less than 8 years old
Trachea	Deviates posteriorly

from adult anaesthetic practice but has not been validated in children. It is more useful in the child older than 9 years.

RAPID-SEQUENCE INDUCTION

The indication for rapid-sequence induction (RSI) is the need for the rapid securing of an airway in the presence of a full stomach. This is by fast, uninterrupted injection of a predetermined dose of anaesthetic agent followed by a fast-acting muscle relaxant. Tracheal intubation with cricoid pressure (except in infants) is then achieved. The techniques of RSI are outlined in Chapter 4 and are as applicable to children as to adults, although the drug dosages will need to be calculated taking into account the patient's size. Failure to establish a definitive airway through intubation is rare (2 per 100 000 intubations) but may occasionally be an indication to perform a needle cricothyroidotomy. Formal cricothyroidotomy can be performed in the adolescent.

INJURIES TO THE AIRWAY

Blunt laryngotracheal trauma accounts for 80–90% of paediatric airway injuries.[2] Most airway injuries in children are in boys; the mean patient age is 10 years and major causes are bicycle crashes, road traffic collisions (RTCs), seat belt injuries and airbag injuries. Penetrating injuries are very uncommon in children.

Signs and symptoms of airway injury include stridor, hoarseness, aphonia, cough, haemoptysis, neck tenderness, subcutaneous emphysema and cyanosis. Soft-tissue neck films and chest radiographs may reveal additional information, for example soft-tissue oedema, fractures or subcutaneous emphysema. Infant cartilage is not ossified so some of the injuries, such as a fractured hyoid, cannot be assessed radiologically.

The paediatric larynx is relatively protected by its position at the level of C3–C4, where it is shielded by the mandible and its cartilaginous pliability, limiting the risk of fracture. In the stable patient, flexible endoscopy and computed tomography (CT) are useful diagnostic adjuncts. Endoscopy is performed by the ear, nose and throat team and should be discussed with them in the first instance.

> In the unstable patient with airway compromise, airway protection is the priority.

Cervical spine control

There is no national guideline or consensus for clearance of the cervical spine in children after trauma. Establishment of local protocols for the management of suspected cervical spine injuries results in decreased time to accomplish clearance and fewer missed injuries.[3] Compared with adults, cervical spine injury is uncommon in children. Of all children injured, only 1–2% will have a significant cervical spine injury.

The early assessment and stabilization of the paediatric cervical spine is often challenging because of communication difficulties, difficulty in accurate clinical examination and the unsuitability of immobilization devices for the very young child.[4] As an improvised device, babies can be effectively immobilized in a lower limb box splint.

When deciding whether to immobilize a child's neck, clinical judgement and common sense should be applied. A suitably sized hard collar with head blocks either side of the patient and tapes and straps is the gold standard. This may be difficult to apply and poorly tolerated in children under the age of 3 years. Immobilization can be extremely upsetting for some children, and particularly restless and agitated children can do more harm during movement when the body pivots about the immobilized neck than if they were left without immobilization. Using age-appropriate distraction therapy and adequate explanations and reassurance to the parents and the child may help in this difficult and stressful situation. Allowing movement with a collar on will provide some protection and may be the *only* realistic option in the very agitated child. A hard collar will allow up to 60° flexion and extension and will offer some protection if used alone if the child refuses to be strapped or held down. Another person, such as the parent, holding the head in line with the rest of the body in the neutral position again may be the *only* technique available to immobilize the cervical spine.

MECHANISM OF INJURY

Sports injuries, RTCs and falls from heights are the most common causes of cervical spine injury. In the case of RTCs, spine injury is commonly seen in pedestrians who are hit by a car and in passengers in high-speed impacts. Rarer causes are diving accidents, non-accidental injuries and birth-related injuries in neonates. It is important to note that there is some under-representation in hospital audits on cervical spine injuries in children because many of the high-speed cervical spine injuries will cause death at the scene of the accident.

WHO SHOULD BE IMMOBILIZED IN THE PRE-HOSPITAL ENVIRONMENT?

The following are indications for pre-hospital cervical spine immobilization in children:

* an unconscious patient with a history of possible trauma;
* a conscious patient with multiple trauma, a significant injury above the clavicle, neurological deficit or neck pain with limitation of movement;
* a mechanism of injury that may suggest spinal injury, for example a pedestrian or cyclist hit by a car, a passenger in a car that has collided at high speed or a patient who has had a fall or severe electric shock.

Patients meeting these criteria should arrive in the trauma room with cervical spine immobilization in place. Prolonged immobilization for more than 1 hour must be avoided.

IS A RADIOGRAPH INDICATED FOR ALL PAEDIATRIC PATIENTS?

It is standard practice to receive immobilized patients in the resuscitation room, and it is the trauma team's role to distinguish who has or has not sustained a significant cervical spine injury. The Nexus Study[5] attempted to define who should undergo cervical spine imaging by identifying criteria associated with a low probability of cervical spine injury. Of the 3065 patients under 18 in the subset analysis in the Nexus Study, 30 had spinal cord injuries (four were aged less than 8 years). It could be argued that these numbers were too small to be able to conclude that the

Nexus criteria can be applied confidently to children. However, the authors concluded that, in principle, and with caution, the Nexus criteria may be applied when dealing with children. The five preconditions (all of which must be present) for considering *not* investigating with a plain radiograph are no neurological deficit, no spinal tenderness, a fully alert child, no intoxication, and no distracting injury. This protocol has a 99% sensitivity and a 99.8% negative predictive value for ruling out injury. In children under 10 years, an anteroposterior and lateral radiograph should be requested; an odontoid view can be added for children over 10 years old.

INTERPRETATION OF THE PLAIN RADIOGRAPH

Cervical spine injury is rare in children under 8 years. The lower cervical spine is the most common site of cervical spine injury in all injured children, and fractures are the most common type of injury.[6]

When interpreting the paediatric cervical spine radiograph, it is important to be aware of key anatomical differences compared with adults. This can also help to explain some of the different patterns of injury in children.

* The facet joints are more horizontal, enabling greater translational movement during extension and flexion.
* The spinal ligaments and joint capsules have greater elasticity and therefore allow more movement. Absent uncinate processes and weak neck muscles cause greater mobility.

Overall, the paediatric cervical spine is much more elastic than that of adults.

The fulcrum changes with age. In young children, the pivot, and therefore greatest movement, occurs at C2–C3, from 5 to 6 years old it is at C3–C4, and by adolescence it moves to the adult level of C5–C6. Therefore, younger children are prone to higher cervical spine injuries than older children. Other variations may be considered using an ABC sequence (Table 15.2).

It is important to note that confidently clearing the cervical spine radiologically in children is difficult. Accurate history-taking and communication is hard in the very young, and there are many normal variants when interpreting the plain radiographs. Cervical spine injuries

Table 15.2 Variations on the paediatric cervical spine plain radiograph

Alignment	Superior and inferior facet joints are congruous
	Absent lordosis is common
	Pseudosubluxation is common
	(24% at the C2–C3 level and 14% at the C3–C4 level)
Bones	Anterior wedging of the vertebral bodies
	Unfused synchondroses
	Incomplete ossification and fractures may not be detected radiologically
Cartilage/soft tissues	Normal preodontoid space is up to 5 mm in children

are rare in children, and therefore physicians may rarely look at these films. The advice of a paediatric radiologist, if available, is particularly helpful. If adequate views cannot be obtained using standard techniques, then consideration should be given to obtaining oblique views or CT scanning. However, in children under 10, CT should be employed only in exceptional circumstances because of possible risks associated with radiation exposure, particularly to the thyroid gland.

SPECIFIC FRACTURES

Jefferson fracture

This is a burst fracture of C1 secondary to axial loading of occipital condyles onto the lateral masses of C2. It is generally immediately stable because the bony fragments tend not to impinge on the spinal cord but, once diagnosed, neck immobility to prevent secondary harm is imperative. By definition, an overlap of 1 mm of C1 on C2 is required to make the diagnosis in children.

Hangman's fracture

It is important not to mistake the hangman's fracture for pseudosubluxation. It is a spondylolisthesis secondary to fracture of C2 and it may lead to anterior subluxation of C2 on C3 with resultant cord damage.

Atlantoaxial subluxation

This may be seen in 15% of children with trisomy 21 (Down's syndrome) as a normal variant. In the setting of trauma it may be a result of transverse ligament rupture or more commonly due to a fractured dens. Neurological symptoms are seen when the preodontoid space exceeds 7–10 mm (up to 5 mm is normal).

Cervical distraction

This injury is usually incompatible with life.

Vertebral compression, tear drop fractures, burst fractures

These are caused by compression.

Facet dislocation

A flexion/rotation stress may produce this injury. Unilateral facet dislocation may be associated with less than 50% displacement of one vertebral body on another. If there is more than 50% displacement, then bilateral facet dislocation has occurred.

SPINAL CORD INJURY WITHOUT OBVIOUS RADIOLOGICAL ABNORMALITY

Spinal cord injury without obvious radiological abnormality (SCIWORA) is, by definition, *objective signs of myelopathy in the absence of ligamentous or bony injury on plain radiography or CT*. It is more common in children than in adults.[7] It most commonly affects children under the age of 8 years and is a consequence of the greater elasticity of the paediatric vertebral column in this age group. Its incidence is reported to be 10–20% of all paediatric spinal cord injuries. More information is provided in Chapter 12.

Breathing

This is assessed by looking, listening and feeling. All injured patients should receive oxygen at 15 L/min by facemask. The following assessments should be done:

- the working of breathing, such as recession, respiratory rate and accessory muscle use;
- the effectiveness of the breathing, such as oxygen saturation and chest expansion;
- the effects of any inadequate respiration, for example mental state and heart rate.

If respiratory efforts are inadequate, ventilation should be assisted using a bag–valve–mask apparatus. The chest must then be examined looking for obvious injury, tracheal position and abnormal movements, palpating for crepitus and auscultating for normal and abnormal breath sounds. There is a higher incidence of tension pneumothorax in paediatric patients with major trauma than in comparable adults because of the more mobile mediastinum, and this needs to be excluded urgently. If detected, immediate needle thoracocentesis should be performed using a 16G cannula inserted into the second intercostal space in the midclavicular line, followed by insertion of a chest drain. If this has been excluded and breathing remains inadequate, then the use of intubation and positive-pressure ventilation should be considered.

Circulation

The early signs of shock are non-specific as children have an enormous capacity to compensate for hypovolaemia because of their excellent physiological reserve. It may therefore be difficult to recognize *early* circulatory compromise in children. Assessment of the child's circulatory state is performed by observing:

- pulse rate;
- skin colour;
- capillary refill time (skin over the sternum is pressed for 5 seconds and the refill time should be less than 2 seconds);
- blood pressure – normal systolic blood pressure is 80+ (age in years × 2);
- heart rate (see Table 15.3);
- effects of an inadequate circulation such as on mental state and respiratory rate (it is important to remember that tachycardia is non-specific and may be caused by pain or fear).

Table 15.3 Heart rate in children

Age (years)	Normal heart rate range (beats/min)
<1	110–160
2–5	95–140
5–12	80–120
>12	60–100

All severely injured children should have i.v. access via a peripheral vein. Ideally, this should be in the antecubital fossa bilaterally with the largest cannula that is practicable. Veins on the hands and feet are also suitable. This may be technically difficult to perform, especially in the chubby toddler. Rather than making repeated unsuccessful attempts, the inexperienced should seek help whilst accessible undamaged veins remain. Once i.v. access is gained, blood should be checked for bedside glucose, cross-matching and standard haematological and chemistry profiles.

If peripheral venous access is not possible, then intraosseous access should be considered. This technique is usually used up to the age of 6 years but can also be performed on older children if necessary. The two most common sites are the anterior tibia, 1 cm below and medial to the tibial tuberosity, and the anterolateral femur, 2 cm above the lateral condyle.

Alternative forms of vascular access include cannulation of the femoral vein using a Seldinger technique, peripheral cut-down at the long saphenous vein or cannulation of the external jugular vein. Cannulation of the subclavian or internal jugular veins should be attempted only as a last resort as this is often a difficult procedure and complications are not uncommon. It may require an expert such as a paediatric intensivist to do this. The initial fluid bolus should be 10 mL/kg of crystalloid. If there is hypoglycaemia, this should be treated with 5 mL/kg of 10% dextrose.

Table 15.4 Glasgow Coma Scale

Eye-opening	4	Spontaneously
	3	To speech
	2	To pain
	1	No response to stimulation
Best verbal response	5	Orientated
	4	Confused
	3	Inappropriate
	2	Incomprehensible sounds
	1	No sounds
Best motor response	6	Obeys commands
	5	Localizes
	4	Normal flexion to pain
	3	Abnormal flexion to pain
	2	Extension to pain
	1	No response to pain

The initial fluid bolus should be repeated, if signs of shock persist. If there is inadequate response, despite repeated boluses, then blood should be administered (10 mL/kg). Ideally this should be cross-matched, but if cross-matched blood is not available, type-specific or O-negative blood should be used.

Disability

A rapid assessment of the neurological status is made using either the AVPU (alert, voice, pain, unresponsive) method or the GCS (Table 15.4). A modified version of the GCS is used in children under the age of 5 years (Table 15.5). The response to pain is best determined by squeezing one ear lobe hard and observing the best response to that stimulus. Also, importantly, the pupillary reflexes and posture of the child should be observed.

Exposure

Because of their greater body surface area, children are at greater risk of hypothermia than adults and they must be exposed for examination for the minimum amount of time in order to avoid excessive heat loss (as well as to avoid distress).

SECONDARY SURVEY

On completion of the primary survey, and once any immediately life-threatening injuries have been identified and treated, a secondary survey is completed which entails a detailed head-to-toe examination.

REGIONAL ANATOMICAL INJURY

Head injury

Head injury is one of the most common childhood injuries. It accounts for 500 000 childhood attendances at

Table 15.5 Modified verbal component of the Glasgow Coma Scale for children under 5 years

Best verbal response	5	Smiles, interacts well, follows objects, orientates to sounds	
		Crying	Interacts
	4	Consolable	Inappropriate
	3	Inconsistently consolable	Moaning
	2	Inconsolable	Irritable
	1	No response	No response

emergency departments in the UK each year with an incidence of 4000 per 100 000 and a death rate of 5.3 per 100 000.[8] Ninety-six per cent of head-injured children have a GCS score of 15, 3.5% have a GCS score of 9–14 and 0.5% have a GCS score of less than 8. Head injury is the most common cause of death in children aged between 1 and 15 years with an annual incidence of 5 per 100 000. It accounts for 15% of deaths in the 1–15 year age range and 25% of deaths in the 5–15 years group. It is also one of the main causes of long-term disability after trauma.

A leading cause of severe head injury and death in children are RTCs. Falls are the second most common cause of fatal head injury. Non-accidental injury makes up a proportion of those children who suffer a head injury, especially in the very young. It is important to record the mechanism of injury because infants suffering NAI and older children who are involved in RTCs tend to have more extensive injuries than from other causes.

PATHOPHYSIOLOGY

The initial injury gives rise to primary damage such as diffuse axonal injury and cortical contusions. This is largely dependent on the forces and type of injury involved. Primary damage is best modified by prevention through public health, accident prevention and legal measures including compulsory use of rear seat belts, cycle helmets, playground design and 'at-risk' registers for the most vulnerable children.

Secondary brain injury occurs after the initial trauma and may be a result of intracranial features such as haematoma, brain swelling, oedema or extracranial features such as hypoxia, hypoventilation, hypotension, hypoglycaemia and hypothermia. The common feature of secondary brain injury no matter what the aetiology is a decrease in the delivery of oxygen and nutrients below that required for optimal neuronal function and may be prevented by meticulous attention to the details of the primary and secondary survey.

PRIMARY SURVEY

Attention to the airway and cervical spine, breathing and circulation is critical in the head-injured child.

SECONDARY SURVEY

A meticulous examination of the child's head is required, looking specifically for evidence of bruising, wounds, lacerations, abrasions and boggy swellings as well as areas of tenderness that may indicate underlying fractures. Any lacerations should be *carefully* examined in order to exclude a depressed facture. Signs of basal skull fractures should be excluded by checking for periorbital bruising, haemotympanum, bruising over the mastoid process and cerebrospinal fluid and blood leakage from the nasopharynx and ears. In infants, the tension of the anterior fontanelle should be assessed. The fundi should be examined in all children with head injury, especially in the setting of NAI, and specific findings are pathognomonic in the shaken baby syndrome. If suspected, this examination must be performed by an ophthalmologist as bilateral retinal haemorrhages strongly suggest NAI. If the child is under 5 years old, the modified version of the GCS should be used. Assessment of cranial nerves, peripheral nerves, motor function, posture and pupils may be possible only by observation alone, especially in the very young. The examination of the child's head circumference as a baseline measurement is important, especially in infants.

RADIOLOGICAL IMAGING

A skull radiograph is predominantly indicated in those under 1 year of age because:

- They are more difficult to clinically assess than the older child.
- Infants have a higher incidence of skull fracture than older children.
- They are at higher risk of NAI and a skull radiograph is useful at screening for fractures associated with NAI in the under-1-year-old.[9]
- There is an increased incidence of asymptomatic intracranial injury.
- It is important to detect fractures in this age group owing to an increased risk of complications, e.g. growing skull fracture.

In the older child, evidence does not exist to demonstrate that the presence or absence of skull fracture can reliably predict or exclude intracranial injury.[10] It has been shown that 5% of children with mild head injury and no fracture on plain radiography demonstrate isolated intracranial injury on CT scanning. The clinical significance of 'missed' intracranial injury in this group remains unclear, but 1–3% of patients require neurosurgery. This implies that missed intracranial injury from mild head injury can have clinical consequences.

The Royal College of Radiologists has suggested the following criteria for CT scanning:

- full consciousness (GCS score of 15 out of 15) but with other features such as severe and persistent headache, nausea and vomiting, irritability or altered behaviour, a seizure;
- new focal neurological signs that are not getting worse;
- a deteriorating level of consciousness or progressive focal neurological signs;
- confusion or drowsiness, GCS score of 13 or 14 followed by failure to improve within 4 hours of clinical observation;
- GCS score of 12 or less, i.e. the patient opens the eyes only to pain or does not converse.

The very young may not be able to tolerate this investigation. Some children may need to be sedated before a CT can be performed, but the priority is always patient safety and stabilization.

MANAGEMENT OF MINOR HEAD INJURIES

By definition, these children have a GCS score of 15. They account for the *majority* of children who present with a head injury to an emergency department. After an appropriate history and examination, many of these children will require no further treatment other than, for example, simple scalp suturing and the provision of written advice. The child should be admitted for observation if there are any of the following concerns:

* possible NAI;
* absence of a responsible adult to care for the child;
* pre-existing neurological problems making assessment difficult;
* a long distance between home and the nearest medical facility.

If none of these risk factors is noted, children can be safely discharged with verbal and written head injury instructions given to a responsible parent or carer. This should give information about how to care for the post-head-injured child and when specifically to return to the nearest emergency department if the patient's condition deteriorates.

Despite the high frequency of childhood minor head trauma, a highly accurate or reliable clinical scoring system for deciding which children are at significant risk from traumatic brain injury does not exist. Each year about half of all head-injured children in the USA[11] undergo CT scanning, of whom about 85% have minor head injuries; only 4–8% of these show traumatic brain injury, and of these only about 5% require operative intervention, suggesting that current CT scanning practice, in the USA at least, is too liberal.[12–14]

If a child is alert and orientated with a GCS score of 15 but with features of confusion or drowsiness, abnormal behaviour, persisting nausea or vomiting, seizures, focal neurological signs or a suspicion of NAI, he or she should be admitted for observation.

> The child with confusion or drowsiness, abnormal behaviour, persisting nausea or vomiting, seizures, focal neurological signs or a suspicion of NAI should be observed, and therefore admitted.

MANAGEMENT OF SEVERE HEAD INJURIES

Children with severe head injury include those with impaired consciousness and focal neurological signs. The initial management of these seriously injured children begins in the primary survey by maintaining adequate ventilation and circulation to prevent secondary brain damage. If a child's consciousness level deteriorates, it is vital to reassess ABC. Once the child has been satisfactorily stabilized, it should be assumed that the deteriorating GCS score is a result of secondary injury from increased intracranial pressure (ICP) and steps must be taken to reduce it. Unfortunately, there is no clear consensus as to the optimal approach.

Surgery is indicated only for the evacuation of intracranial mass lesions causing significant midline shift or for the placement of ICP monitoring. An osmotic agent, be it mannitol or hypertonic saline, can help to offload cerebral oedema – at least in the short term – and hypertonic saline has been shown to decrease intensive care unit stay and reduce complications in children with a severe head injury. Formal hyperventilation to reduce the vasoconstricting effect of carbon dioxide is offset by the increased ICP generated by the increased blood flow – ventilation to low normal $PaCO_2$ levels is appropriate. Nursing the ventilated child in the 30° head-up position helps to reduce ICP. Treatment in a specialist paediatric trauma centre has been shown to improve outcome. There is no evidence that barbiturates, calcium channel blockers or steroids improve the outcome of severe paediatric head injury.[15]

Chest injury

Chest injuries are the second leading cause of death in paediatric major trauma; most are from blunt trauma. Infants and toddlers are more commonly the victims of blunt trauma secondary to RTCs or abusive injuries.[16] School-age children are injured because of transport-related mechanisms such as bicycles, scooters and skateboards. Teenagers are more likely to be injured in high-energy RTCs after risk-taking adventures. Chest injuries may present as isolated injuries, such as rib fractures, haemothorax or pneumothorax, or they may present as one feature of polytrauma.

ANATOMY AND PHYSIOLOGY OF CHEST INJURIES

Infants and children have more pliable chest walls than adults and a more mobile mediastinum. They are also more likely to hyperventilate after traumatic injury secondary to pain and fear, resulting in more air swallowing and gastric dilatation with subsequent diaphragmatic splinting. As a result, the patterns of injury in children are different from those in adults. For example, the thoracic rib cage can be compressed more in children, resulting in underlying pulmonary injury without overlying evidence of rib fracture. Children are able to haemodynamically compensate to a remarkable degree despite significant blood loss, and haemodynamic compromise will present later in patients with haemothorax, tension pneumothorax and large flail segments. It may be a *preterminal sign*. Rare injuries such as great vessel injury or cardiac trauma may remain undiagnosed because of this physiological compensation. Circulatory compromise is heralded by tachycardia long before hypotension because cardiac output in children is largely determined by heart rate and contractility; therefore, stroke volume is largely fixed in children.

> Circulatory compromise is a late sign in children and may not present until the child is in a preterminal condition.

PNEUMOTHORAX

Approximately one-third of paediatric chest injuries result in pneumothorax. Simple pneumothorax is generally asymptomatic, therefore screening chest radiographs are important in the primary survey. All traumatic pneumothoraces require tube thoracostomy because of their propensity to cause later cardiopulmonary compromise.

TENSION PNEUMOTHORAX

Tension pneumothorax is a life-threatening condition and, as in adults, needle or tube thoracostomy should be carried out immediately on diagnosis. The diagnosis may be detected clinically through tracheal deviation, unilateral absent breath sounds and a hyper-resonant chest. Treatment should be initiated before obtaining a chest radiograph. Other conditions may *mimic* tension pneumothorax, including haemorrhage, pneumothorax, cardiac tamponade and a pulmonary embolism.

HAEMOTHORAX

Penetrating injuries to the chest and injury to intrathoracic vessels or lung may cause a haemothorax. Rib fractures can lacerate intercostal arteries or veins and, more rarely, the aorta or vena cava may be disrupted, causing a haemothorax. In the child, each hemithorax is able to hold 40% of the child's circulating blood volume, so large bleeds can be fatal. Plain radiographs do not allow for a reliable estimation of the volume of blood: CT is much better. The treatment is emergency tube thoracostomy after establishment of adequate intravenous access. Early drainage of blood will give an indication of the blood loss and also helps prevent late complications, such as secondary empyema, sepsis and fibrous scarring.

PULMONARY CONTUSION

Pulmonary contusions are the most common thoracic injuries in children and, owing to the child's chest wall elasticity, may occur in the absence of an overlying rib fracture. Contusion may manifest as an area of consolidation on the radiograph, but radiographic signs may lag behind clinical signs. However, the resultant ventilation–perfusion mismatch will decrease compliance, cause hypoventilation and lead to hypoxia in the injured child. The clinical course will therefore depend on the extent of the injury, and mechanical ventilation may be necessary in up to 35% of children with pulmonary contusion. Fluid restriction, supplemental oxygen, pain control and the avoidance of prolonged immobilization or general anaesthetic all contribute to the management of this condition.

TRAUMATIC ASPHYXIA

Traumatic asphyxia occurs primarily in younger children with more pliable chest walls. It results from a sudden severe crushing blow to the chest when the glottis is closed and the sudden raised intrathoracic pressure forces blood into the head and arms, producing classical petechial haemorrhages, commonly in the distribution of the superior vena cava. Rarely, children may present with neurological deficits and coma owing to cerebral oedema, but most cases of traumatic asphyxia are less severe.

RIB FRACTURES

Rib fractures are rare in the paediatric patient, and their presence will be associated with severe underlying chest injury. If they occur in children less than 12 months of age, the possibility of NAI needs to be considered as well as osteogenesis imperfecta or rickets. A first rib or posterior rib fracture is highly suspicious of child abuse. If a rib fracture is detected, the emergency physician should be alerted to the possibility of associated injuries such as pneumothorax, haemothorax or major vascular injury. Multiple rib fractures are a marker of severe injury and are associated with high mortality rates. The management of rib fractures is supportive. The goal is to provide oxygenation and pain relief in order to prevent atelectasis and secondary pneumonia.

FLAIL CHEST

A flail chest is a rare finding in children, but if present it will cause significant respiratory compromise because of the effects on respiration by paradoxical movement of the flail segments.

OESOPHAGEAL RUPTURE

Oesophageal rupture results from blunt or penetrating trauma. Blunt injury is caused by sudden passage of gastric contents into the oesophagus, resulting in a linear tear in the distal oesophagus near the gastro-oesophageal junction. Penetrating injury to the oesophagus is much rarer in the UK. Oesophageal ruptures result in mediastinitis and spillage of oesophageal contents into the pleural space. On the plain radiograph, mediastinal and subcutaneous surgical emphysema are suggestive of the diagnosis. Intravenous antibiotics should be commenced if the diagnosis is suspected along with consideration of tube drainage of the chest. Further treatment may include surgery, such as thoracotomy, drainage of the mediastinum and primary repair of the oesophagus.

TRACHEOBRONCHIAL DISRUPTION

Tracheobronchial disruption injuries are unusual in children but they can be fatal. The rarity of the injury is probably a result of the greater flexibility and mobility of the paediatric mediastinum.

CARDIAC CONTUSION

This is also rare in children. It may present as chest pain or unexplained hypotension and arrhythmia. Elevated cardiac enzymes may be found and 12-lead electrocardiography (ECG) may show ST ischaemic changes, premature beats, sinus tachycardia or atrial arrhythmia. The presence of a sternal fracture has been suggested as a marker for myocardial contusion, therefore observation for 24–48 hours is recommended if such a fracture is detected. It is, however, rare for children who present initially haemodynamically stable and in sinus rhythm to develop subsequent cardiac arrhythmia or cardiac failure. Significant haemodynamic changes should prompt the early use of echocardiography to evaluate the extent of cardiac injury.

PERICARDIAL TAMPONADE/CARDIAC RUPTURE

Pericardial tamponade (or cardiac rupture) is potentially life-threatening. It may present as the classic Beck's triad (muffled heart sounds, distended neck veins and hypotension), but more commonly these findings are absent and the chest radiograph and ECG may be normal. If the diagnosis is suspected, cardiac ultrasound is the definitive test. Cardiac rupture is very rare in the paediatric trauma patient and, if it occurs, it is associated with a very high mortality rate.

DIAPHRAGMATIC INJURY

Blunt diaphragmatic rupture involves the left hemidiaphragm in two-thirds of patients. The radiographic signs of this injury are high-riding diaphragm, abnormal contour of the diaphragm and overlap of abdominal visceral shadows in the chest. If a nasogastric tube has been inserted, this may be seen to sit in the gastric bubble within the chest. This injury may go unrecognized and may not be detected for weeks or even years.

Abdominal injury

The abdomen is the third most common site of injury in children. The intra-abdominal organs are more vulnerable in children than in adults. Blunt injury is more common than penetrating injury in the UK. Most paediatric abdominal injury is managed non-operatively, and surgery is unusual.[17,18] Specific areas should be examined and the following should be noted:

- areas of tenderness or pain;
- rebound tenderness, suggesting peritoneal irritation;
- areas of rigidity, suggesting peritonitis.

RADIOLOGICAL STUDIES

Plain abdominal radiographs usually add little to the trauma evaluation and adjunctive imaging is usually a choice between CT or focused assessment with sonography in trauma (FAST) scanning. Diagnostic peritoneal lavage is technically feasible in children but not recommended as its high sensitivity for even minor intra-abdominal injury precludes the use of a selective non-operative approach to the injured child.

The radiological study of choice for evaluating the stable patient with intra-abdominal injury is CT. In one series of children undergoing CT following blunt abdominal trauma, 96% of hollow viscus injuries requiring laparotomy were identified and all solid organ injuries were identified by CT scanning. The main disadvantages are that the child often needs to be removed from the resuscitation area in order to complete the test and the requirement for conscious sedation needs to be considered.

In many centres, FAST scanning is now available and is a specific modality for detecting intra-abdominal injury. It is weaker than CT at 'ruling out' injury, and a negative scan can be considered unreliable. The main advantages are that it is quick to perform, non-invasive and easily repeated without the need to move the child or use conscious sedation. It can identify children who may require laparotomy early on in their trauma management. There is an emerging evidence base for the use of FAST scanning in children.

Urinalysis is useful for ruling out the presence of blood in the urinary tract after blunt abdominal trauma, and a urine bag may be useful in younger children; urinary catheterization solely to collect a specimen for analysis is inappropriate.

SPLEEN

The spleen is the most commonly injured intra-abdominal organ in children with blunt abdominal trauma. Most children with this injury are haemodynamically stable and they are commonly managed non-operatively. If laparotomy is undertaken, the aim is to preserve the spleen and its important cellular and humeral immune function.

Most splenic injury is secondary to blunt injury in RTCs. More rarely, infectious mononucleosis may predispose to splenic rupture in the presence of relatively minor trauma. Grading of the splenic injury is enabled by CT but despite this many splenic ruptures have a delayed diagnosis.[19]

LIVER

This is the second most common solid organ to be injured in blunt trauma but the most common in penetrating trauma. Damage to the liver is the most common lethal injury in blunt abdominal trauma in children. These injuries can be more serious than splenic injury and are more likely to rebleed post-operatively. The decision to operate is usually taken on the basis of whether or not haemodynamic compromise responds to resuscitative measures.

RENAL

In non-penetrative trauma, renal damage often results from deceleration in a RTC. Most renal injuries are found in association with other injuries, especially splenic injury in left renal trauma. Abdominal CT is the investigation of choice. Only 10% will require surgery.

GASTROINTESTINAL

Gastrointestinal injury is difficult to diagnose in children and is relatively uncommon as only 5% of children with abdominal trauma will have a bowel injury. The most common site is the jejunum. A delay in diagnosis is common, and the injury may be detected only when signs of peritonism become apparent. A useful sign is the presence of abdominal ecchymosis, which is associated with a 50% chance of small bowel injury. Early physical examination and radiological studies are normal, but close monitoring is important to detect late presentations or delayed perforations.

PANCREAS

Only 3% of abdominal injuries are pancreatic injuries. The classical paediatric case is the youngster who is thrown onto the handlebars of his or her bicycle after an abrupt stop. Traumatic pancreatitis is a difficult diagnosis to make and is commonly diagnosed late. Both CT and serum amylase may be normal in early injury. The pancreas is a retroperitoneal organ, and therefore relatively few signs may be present on an abdominal examination. Treatment is defined by the degree of ductal disruption, with minor ductal injury being managed conservatively whereas major duct disruption requires surgery.

BLADDER INJURY

Bladder rupture and contusion is heralded by gross haematuria and lower abdominal pain. Other features include inability to void, especially after bladder catheterization. Ten per cent of patients with pelvic fractures have an associated bladder injury. A urethrogram performed in the resuscitation room will aid diagnosis.

Paediatric burns

Burn injuries rank third amongst injury-related deaths in children, and paediatric patients have one of the highest mortality rates associated with burn injury. Most are a result of accidents, but certain patterns of burns may suggest intentional harm.[20]

Thermal burns are the most common type, such as scalds from hot liquids or contact burns from flames and hot surfaces. The type of injury is age dependent, with the toddler age group more commonly suffering scalds and having the highest incidence of hospitalization. School-age children are more likely to suffer burns from flames. Adolescents are more commonly burnt through risk-taking behaviour.

As with adults, burns are classified by depth and extent – they may be partial or full thickness, with partial-thickness burns being further subclassified as epidermal, superficial dermal, mid-dermal or deep dermal burns. Epidermal burns are erythematous and extremely painful but without blistering. These heal over several days without scarring, and management is focused on symptom control with adequate analgesia. Superficial partial-thickness burns involve some destruction of the dermis and are painful, red and blistered. Healing occurs with minimal scarring by 10 days. Deep partial-thickness burns involve more than 50% of the dermis (by depth) and the nerve fibres may be destroyed; as a result, they may be relatively anaesthetic. These take 2–3 weeks to heal and scarring will often develop. Where the burn is full thickness, destruction of the nerves results in anaesthesia, but a ring of surrounding partial-thickness burn is almost invariably present and is intensely painful. Full-thickness burns are potentially life-threatening.[20]

Burns are also classified according to their extent. The Lund and Browder chart may be used to determine the percentage surface area burn for children of various ages. Superficial burns are not counted in the calculation. Alternatively, the child's palm equals 1% of body surface area.

The priority is assessment of the ABCs followed by focusing on any circumferential burns as these may require early emergent escharotomy. The cause of the burn should be ascertained and any clothing that is burning or exposed to chemicals should be removed or cooled to stop the burning process. The overall health of the child should be noted, including immunization status. Early analgesia is extremely important, and this should not be delayed. Intravenous opiates are commonly used, especially during the application of dressings. Baseline blood tests and a chest radiograph should be ordered, including assessment of carbon monoxide and possible cyanide levels if the child has been involved in a house fire. Airway compromise should be anticipated and early intubation should be performed if there are perioral or perinasal burns, stridor, burnt eyelashes and eyebrows or hoarse voice. Supraglottic airway oedema results from direct thermal injury but lower airway irritation may occur, especially following inhalation of toxins and smoke, and a chemical pneumonitis may present later. The clinical signs should be anticipated over the first 24 hours of management.

Intravenous access should be obtained early and fluid resuscitation requirements calculated and started. Urine output calculated through catheterization may facilitate this. A urinary output of 2 mL/kg/h for infants, 1 mL/kg/h for children and 0.5 mL/kg/h for adolescents are considered normal urine outputs. The Parkland formula can also be used for children with greater than 15% body surface area (BSA) burns:

$$4 \, mL \times weight \, (kg) \times BSA \, (\%): ½ \, over \, first \, 8 \, hours \, and \, the \, rest \, over \, the \, next \, 16 \, hours[21]$$

The excellent physiological reserve of children means that signs of cardiovascular collapse may occur late; therefore, regular assessment of pulse rate, capillary refill and blood pressure is important.

Minor burn pain can be managed with non-steroidal anti-inflammatory drugs, but more extensive burns will require opiates. Covering a burn and protecting it from air flow is an important part of therapy and is sometimes neglected until late in the child's management. A dressing that covers but is transparent is most useful as it allows reinspection of the wound without removing the dressing. Covering the burn will help protect from secondary infection. Partial-thickness and deep-thickness burns are at risk from later infection, and tetanus immunization should be offered in the unimmunized child.

Superficial burns are the most common type and therefore most childhood burns can be managed in the emergency department outpatient setting. Any child with a burn >5% BSA should be referred to a regional burns centre. If there are any suspicions of NAI, then these should be documented and the concerns relayed to the burns unit for further investigation.

Electrical burns are less common. More harm is caused by alternating than by direct current as this causes muscle tetany and an inability to let go of the electrical apparatus causing the burn. The main source for low-voltage injury is from household electrical equipment, and high-voltage injury is found more commonly in adolescents through risk-taking behaviour or, extremely rarely, from lightning strikes. Any current that passes across the chest may be associated with cardiac arrhythmias and any that passes through the head may cause seizures. The cutaneous manifestations include mottled cyanotic skin, arc or contact burns. Assessment of underlying structures is vital with consideration of deeper burns and compartment syndrome. A baseline myoglobin level, renal function and ECG are performed in most instances. If there are burns to deeper structures such as underlying muscle, then this should be managed by a burns centre. It should be noted that burns to the oral cavity from biting electrical cord can be complicated 2–3 weeks later by bleeding from the labial artery after the eschar separates.

Acid burns result in coagulation necrosis, which limits the depth of the burn, whereas alkali burns are deeper and more penetrative. The priority is to stop the burning process by removing all contaminated clothing followed by copious irrigation for 30 minutes with saline. The pH can be checked after irrigation. Hydrofluoric acid should be treated with calcium gluconate topical gel or injection but expert advice should be sought. Hypocalcaemia secondary to absorption of hydrofluoric acid may occur and can cause muscle tetany and ventricular arrhythmia.

MINOR INJURY IN CHILDREN

Injury severity in children forms a continuum and there is no precise cut-off point to distinguish major from minor trauma, but minor trauma is much more common than major injury in the paediatric population.

Assessment of minor injuries

To maximize success in assessing any injury, it is important to have a child-friendly and age-appropriate approach.[22] Useful tips are to:

- Examine the child on the parent's lap.
- Get down to the level of the child.
- Use distraction or imagery.
- Comment on toys, smile and avoid quick movements.
- Handle the child and the injured area gently and deal with pain by early analgesia or splinting.
- Give only two choices when asking children to choose and make requests as simple as possible.

Wound management

The child's need for analgesia and for sedation must be assessed and decisions must be taken regarding how the wound will be anaesthetized and subsequently closed as well as any other treatments that will be needed, such as splinting, tetanus prophylaxis or antibiotics.

HOW TO GIVE A PAINLESS INJECTION OF LOCAL ANAESTHETIC

This is important because, if it is done well, the child's trust will not be lost. If it is done badly, the child will become frightened and uncooperative. Do not use cold local anaesthetic straight from the fridge and try to warm it by keeping it in your pocket for 10 minutes. Inject the anaesthetic slowly, using the smallest (27G) and longest needle available to avoid multiple puncture sites. Inject into the wound edges and very slowly in order not to stretch the skin, which is the main source of pain. Give a good field block around the edges of the wound and allow sufficient time (5 minutes) for the local anaesthetic to take effect. Use nerve blocks where possible.

Wound preparation

Wounds should be pressure irrigated before closure. Normal saline via an 18G nozzle in the ratio of 50 mL per 1 cm of wound should be used. Detergent containing antiseptics may be harmful to tissue and soaking with iodine does not alter infection rates. Any obviously non-viable tissue should be debrided from the wound edges and any hair kept away from the edges of wounds by using antibiotic cream to flatten the hair. Clipping is not generally recommended. Eyebrows should not be shaved as regrowth may be unpredictable. When closing the wound, the minimum tension should be applied to close and evert the wound edges. Primary closure of facial wounds may be attempted within 24 hours of injury, other wounds should be closed within 12 hours.[23]

How to make procedures go smoothly with children

It is important to be organized and well prepared, to give reassurance and to build rapport with the child. Being friendly and confident will help, and using parents as an ally by keeping them in the room is important. Local anaesthetic should not be drawn up or instruments prepared in front of the patient as this will cause fear and anxiety.

If the child becomes uncooperative, the assistance of a play therapist can be extremely helpful. Using distraction therapy and guided imagery, such as asking a child to imagine being on holiday, may well gain the child's trust and cooperation again. The use of conscious sedation should be considered in selected patients.

Specific injuries

SOFT-TISSUE BRUISING

It is important to consider the pattern of bruising and whether it is consistent with the history of trauma, for example bruising is common on the shins in toddlers. The possibility of NAI should always be considered, especially with certain types of injuries such as pinch marks and linear bruises across the buttocks, which may be caused by the child being struck.

ABRASIONS

Abrasions should be washed with clean tap water or saline. Any foreign body or foreign material should be removed by gentle scrubbing in order to prevent tattooing. Topical anaesthesia, such as lidocaine gel or EMLA cream, may be useful in order to facilitate the scrubbing process. Abrasions should be covered with a non-stick dressing and heavily contaminated wounds should be reviewed within 48 hours in order to monitor for infection.

LACERATIONS AND INCISED WOUNDS

Lacerations are caused by blunt force tearing tissues. Incised wounds are caused by sharp objects cutting the skin. Assessment of the neurovascular status and underlying structures is imperative. The possibility of an underlying fracture must also be considered.

Closure techniques

TISSUE ADHESIVES

The cosmetic result for a wound closed with tissue adhesive is the same as for wound closure achieved with sutures, staples or adhesives strips. However, because of the weaker tensile strength of glues they can be used only on low-tensile, immobile wounds less than 3 cm in length. There is a slight increase in the incidence of wound dehiscence, but all other wound complications are the same.

ADHESIVE STRIPS

These are useful in wounds that are relatively small and superficial, in an area that does not undergo much skin movement or tension and for aligning small flaps of skin over the back of a wound. The patient or his or her parents should be asked to keep the wound dry for 72 hours. There should be sufficient space between each adhesive strip to allow drainage of fluid from the wound.

SUTURES

As absorbable sutures have higher reactivity and therefore produce an inflammatory reaction, there may be concern about poorer cosmetic appearance, although this is unsupported by evidence. However, many clinicians do not use these type of sutures on facial wounds. They are useful for intraoral and lip lacerations. Elsewhere the use of non-absorbable sutures is recommended.

ALTERNATIVE TO SUTURES

Staples are useful for injuries to the scalp and if using only one staple then local anaesthetic may be contraindicated. It is important to remember that the ability to explore and irrigate these wounds may be reduced because the wounds are not being anesthetized.[24]

MUSCULOSKELETAL TRAUMA

Fractures in children

Fractures are common in children, and the plasticity of children's bones means that they may be incomplete. Certain unique fractures are common in children, for example greenstick fractures and bowing fractures. The Salter–Harris classification of fractures is also limited to children (Figure 15.1). There are also ossification centres that must be differentiated from fractures on plain radiographs. A number of radiological variants (for example, pseudosubluxation) can also be confused with true injury.

Falls are the most common cause of injury resulting in a fracture. If a child presents clinically with swelling, deformity and bony point tenderness then a fracture is highly likely.

As has been mentioned before, minor injury is sometimes difficult to distinguish from major injury. However, it could be defined as a type of injury that might be expected to heal without major medical intervention. Table 15.6 lists the common fractures seen in children, with a description of management in an emergency department and the criteria for referral to orthopaedic services for more definitive treatment.[25]

> Forearm fractures in toddlers must be treated in an above-elbow cast – a below-elbow cast will be removed by the child.

Compartment syndrome

Pallor, paralysis and pain out of proportion to the injury are the cardinal late signs. Early compartment syndromes may be difficult to diagnose. The lower leg and forearm are the most common sites. If the diagnosis is suspected, then measurement of fascial compartment pressures should not be delayed as urgent fasciotomy may be required. Immediate orthopaedic opinion is mandatory.

Vascular and neurological injury

Vascular compromise may be relieved by fracture reduction and limb immobilization. Neurological assessment can be hard in the young, frightened child but any concerns should be clearly documented and early referral for specialist opinion should be considered.

PSYCHOLOGICAL CARE

Children and adults involved in a traumatic episode, even in the absence of physical injury, are at risk of psychological injuries. The commonest psychological disorder associated with trauma is post-traumatic stress disorder (PTSD), which is seen in all ages. The horrific sounds, disturbing visual scenes and other sensory inputs of a catastrophe can invoke fear, terror and, above all, a sense of helplessness; these factors predispose to the development of PTSD. Between 15% and 30% of children involved in RTCs may develop PTSD or severe traffic-related fears.

Unconsciousness with its consequent amnesia, while being a marker for possible brain injury, protects against PTSD as psychological mechanisms are not operational. Post-traumatic stress disorder may be preventable by protecting uninjured children from witnessing severe injuries, particularly if accompanying an injured parent, and by helping them to make sense of the event.

Other psychological sequelae, which occur after traumatic events, include:

- phobias (particularly of cars and roads);
- separation anxiety disorders (especially in young children);
- increased propensity to risk-taking (especially in adolescents, which renders them vulnerable to further accidents);
- depression, especially if there is bereavement associated with the traumatic event.

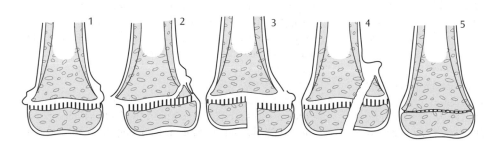

Figure 15.1 Salter–Harris classification of physeal injuries.

Table 15.6 Common fractures that can be managed in the emergency department

Fracture location	Emergent treatment	Criteria for immediate referral to orthopaedic surgeon
Clavicle	A broad arm sling for 3–4 weeks is provided. Adequate analgesia should be provided and it is recommended that the patient does not participate in contact sports for at least 6 weeks. A lump will develop at the fracture site which will be visible for 1 year. Follow-up radiography is not always necessary	Skin tenting, involvement of the acromioclavicular joint or brachial plexus injury
Surgical neck of humerus	Manage with a sling for 3 weeks if undisplaced	Displacement or marked angulation
Shaft of humerus	Collar and cuff or with U-shaped slab to reduce movement and minimize pain if undisplaced. Check the integrity of the radial nerve	Transverse, displaced or comminuted fractures
Supracondylar fracture of humerus	Collar and cuff or back slab with the elbow flexed to 110° for 4 weeks if undisplaced. The integrity of the radial artery, radial nerve, median nerve and ulnar nerve should be checked	Angulation >20°, displacement >50% or comminution
Shaft of radius and/or ulna	Above elbow cast if less than 20° angulation	Open fractures or displacement or angulation >20°
Distal radius	Short arm/above elbow cast for 2–4 weeks for Torus fractures (depends on age of child)	Open fractures or displacement or angulation >20°
Hand fractures	Neighbour strapping, volar slab or ulna gutter splint for undisplaced fifth metacarpal fractures	Rotation or angulation >20° (second metacarpal); >30° (third metacarpal); >40° (fourth metacarpal); >50° (fifth metacarpal)
Tibial fracture	Suspect a spiral fracture in any toddler who is non-weight bearing after an injury. Above-knee plaster for proximal or mid-shaft fractures and below-knee plaster for distal fractures. For the 'toddler's fracture' (undisplaced spiral fracture distal tibia) allow as much weight bearing as the child allows, especially if the pain is minimal. If there is pain at rest or nocturnal pain, it may be helpful to fit a below-knee plaster for 2–3 weeks	Displacement or angulation
Metatarsal fractures	Lower leg plaster slab for 4 weeks. Elevation for the immediate few days may help to minimize swelling	

Prevention of psychological injury

Practitioners treating children in the immediate aftermath of a traumatic event can contribute to the prevention of acute and long-term psychological problems by:

- keeping young children with a familiar figure. If it is necessary to separate the children from this person (for example, owing to the parents' own injuries) they must be cared for by one person until the arrival of a familiar figure.
- protecting the children from distressing sights, sounds, smells and other sensory inputs. Children should not see mutilating or bloody wounds, especially if these belong to a parent, and the cries of the injured should not be audible to children. The advent of audio-visually

separated paediatric emergency department areas from the general emergency department areas may help in this respect.

- ensuring that children have received adequate sedation and analgesia. This is especially important in those children who are clearly distressed or who need to have a potentially painful procedure carried out.
- taking time to explain to the child what is going to happen, and why. Careful explanation of one's actions directed towards the child's level of comprehension is imperative, irrespective of the underlying problem. It is important to avoid remarks such as 'You have been lucky, you could have been killed', as this increases death anxiety.
- giving advice and help to parents and other carers. Parents should be advised about the features to look out for, and told that further expert help is available. The

Child Accident Prevention Trust publishes very useful literature including a helpful pamphlet, which should be given to parents, entitled *Getting over an Accident. Advice for Parents and Carers.*

> Steps to diminish psychological injury:
> - Keep young children with a familiar figure.
> - Protect them from distressing sights, sounds, smells and other sensory inputs.
> - Ensure that children have received adequate sedation and analgesia.
> - Take time to explain to the children what you are doing, and why.
> - Give advice and help to parents and other carers.

Early treatment

Psychological sequelae are common – particularly in young children – and irrespective of the extent of injuries, as childrens' emotional immaturity can magnify their fears and concerns over the event. An assessment made 6 weeks after the incident should be made to look for symptoms of PTSD and other psychological disturbances. Referral can be made to expert help such as a clinical child psychologist or child psychiatrist accordingly.

PROCEDURAL SEDATION AND ANALGESIA IN CHILDREN

Procedural sedation and analgesia is *the use of sedative, dissociative and analgesic drugs to relieve suffering when attempting to perform diagnostic or therapeutic procedures.* It is increasingly performed by non-anaesthetists and is being driven by the recognition that procedures in children sometimes *do* need to be performed outside of the operating theatre, as well as by the arrival of newer and safer drugs and monitoring technology, and expanded practitioner skills in those physicians who manage acutely injured children.[26]

Pharmacology

The combination of fentanyl and midazolam is a common regimen for use in children with a strong safety profile, providing both drugs are titrated to effect. Fentanyl is a strong analgesic that has no anxiolytic or amnesic properties; its effects are rapid and last for up to 40 minutes. Importantly, adverse effects can be reversed with the opioid antagonist naloxone. Midazolam is the most common benzodiazepine used for procedural sedation and its effects last for up to 60 minutes. Usefully, it can be administered using a variety of routes – intramuscular, intravenous, rectal or intranasal. As many as 15% of

children will have paradoxical reactions, such as crying, agitation and combativeness, and this should be monitored for and parents informed of this potential before the drug is administered. Respiratory depression is the most common side-effect and should be monitored.

Ketamine produces a state of cortical dissociation that allows procedures to be done more consistently than with any other procedural sedative. It provides analgesia, sedation and amnesia whilst preserving the protective airway reflexes. It may be administered intramuscularly or intravenously.

Nitrous oxide provides mild sedation and analgesia as well as anxiolysis. It has an excellent safety profile and is self-administered through a demand valve mask. For this reason, however, it is unlikely to be suitable for the very young child.

Who can practise procedural sedation in children?

Non-anaesthetists who practise sedation in children must be competent in the following areas:

- basic and advanced airway management;
- resuscitation;
- vascular access in children;
- pharmacology of the drugs used.

The definition of 'competence' in these areas is open to discussion, but it is important that physicians involved in procedural sedation do not step outside their own level of skill and expertise. Safety should always be paramount.

CHILD PROTECTION AND NON-ACCIDENTAL INJURY

When managing children with injuries the possibility of a non-accidental cause must be considered. Checklists incorporated into local practice have been found to increase awareness by being a reminder of the possibility, improving documentation and increasing referral rates for further investigation.[27,28] A checklist may remind the physician to ask:

- Has there been a delay in seeking medical attention for the injury?
- Is the history of injury consistent each time?
- Are there any other unexplained injuries?
- Is there 'normal' interaction between carer and child?

Abuse may present in other forms than intentional injury, including neglect, sexual abuse and emotional abuse or a combination. It may occur in certain specific situations such as in the setting of domestic violence, in the children of parents who have mental health issues, and in children with drug-abusing parents. Compulsory intervention in family life will be justified if significant harm has been done to a child or if the child is considered to be at significant risk.

Recognition of intentional harm

Non-accidental injury is a spectrum of trauma from minor injury to murder. Certain injury patterns make NAI more likely, especially when taken in context with the developmental age of the child. Immobile children rarely bruise. Slap marks, bruising on the buttocks and lower back, chest and abdomen, mastoid and lower jaw and pinch marks are specifically linked to NAI. Accidental bruising is more common over bony prominences and is found in mobile, active children. Grip marks and bruising to the perineum may be associated with sexual abuse. If investigating bruising, a family history of coagulation disorders should be sought and blood tests for inherited clotting abnormality should be ordered, such as for von Willebrand disease. Sometimes consultation with a paediatric haematologist may be required. Attempts to age bruises are unreliable[29] and should not be attempted.

Bites are always inflicted injuries. The pattern needs to be recorded and human bites may be distinguished from animal bites by pattern recognition.

Non-accidental head injury is the most common form of severe NAI, and 95% of such injuries occur below the age of 1. Inflicted traumatic brain injury is not an uncommon injury in children, especially in those aged less than 1.[30] The mortality is up to 30%. It is also a cause for long-term neurodisability. Presenting symptoms and signs of shaken baby syndrome are often non-specific, and so health care professionals must have an index of suspicion when infants and children present with neurological and respiratory symptoms.[31] This is important because, if a diagnosis of intentional harm is missed, a repeat and more severe injury may occur.[32]

The consequences of head injury include skull fractures, bilateral retinal haemorrhages, subdural haemorrhage, cervical cord damage, and direct brain injury with contusions and hypoxic ischaemic injury. Investigation must include a skull radiograph (if below age 1), a CT head scan and skeletal survey, as well as a septic screen to rule out meningitis where appropriate. Ultrasound imaging of the head is unreliable for detecting traumatic bleeds. Eye examination by an experienced ophthalmologist should also be performed as bilateral retinal haemorrhage strongly suggests NAI. If a child presents with a subdural haematoma and little or no history of trauma then that child must be investigated for suspected child abuse.[33]

Rib fractures require significant force and are highly specific for child abuse. Non-accidental rib fractures tend to be posterior and result from gripping during shaking. Rib fractures may be of varying ages when detected. Fractures require significant force and, if found, must be consistent with the developmental age. Eighty per cent of abused children with fractures are less than 18 months old.

A spiral fracture of the humerus, femoral fractures in non-mobile children and metaphyseal fractures are all associated with NAI. If a child aged less than 15 months presents with a humerus fracture or an infant presents with rib fractures, then child abuse should be considered.[34,35] The differential diagnosis of fracture includes osteogenesis imperfecta, osteopenia, birth injury and unwitnessed accidental injury. If NAI is suspected, a skeletal survey should be performed if a child is less than 2 years old in order to detect occult fractures.

A deliberate blow to the abdomen can result in injury to a solid organ or hollow viscus. A ruptured duodenum is notoriously difficult to diagnose and abdominal wall bruising is not only rare but is also usually a late sign.[36]

Intentional burns may present as well-circumscribed, deep-crater cigarette burns, when the differential diagnosis includes local skin infection such as impetigo. Scalds from liquids thrown, especially on the face, or carpet burns from a child being dragged may also be found with NAI. Immersion burns that are bilateral without splash marks and with a clear immersion line on the feet and bilaterally on the buttocks and hands are also specific for NAI. When determining whether or not a burn is accidental, the child's developmental capabilities must be considered and not just his or her age.[37]

Severe NAI may present in a *medical* way. Presentations may include poor feeding, lethargy, unresponsiveness, irritability, diarrhoea and vomiting.

Management of suspected child abuse

In the severely injured, the priority is attention to the primary survey and adequate resuscitation. The child's safety comes first and assessment must be performed in an objective, non-accusatory and non-judgemental manner. Documentation must be thorough, legible and contemporaneous. Age-appropriate consent and confidentiality should be respected throughout.

Early on, the NAI is often only a 'concern' and much more detailed information will need to be obtained after management has focused on resuscitation and medical intervention. Information should be shared and the named paediatrician for child protection must be involved early on in the child's management. The concerns should be discussed with the child's carers or parents unless it is judged that this could potentially put the child at greater risk of harm. Consultation should be wide and may include social services and the police, although this will usually be undertaken by the paediatricians after admission. The police should be called immediately if a dead or severely injured child has been found or allegations of rape have occurred. Children should be admitted to hospital if there is a need for ongoing care or if a place of safety is needed. In summary, a multidisciplinary approach involving many members of the area 'Safeguarding Children' team is required including involvement of the police, social services, general practitioner and health visitor.

Willingness to consider NAI may depend upon personal physician bias. Physicians should assess the likelihood of NAI on objective criteria. Bias is known to cloud judgement and can cause errors.[38]

INJURY PREVENTION

Children have an insatiable urge to discover and explore. Their development, especially in the early years, is rapid and children of all ages learn by taking risks. In their early years, prevention of harm is focused on allowing a child to explore in a safe environment protected from unnecessary harm. Later, risk reduction is focused on everyday risks, such as traffic awareness, and parental and teacher education, as well as safety measures brought about through legislation.

Injuries should not be seen in isolation but viewed in the context of the child's development, family dynamics, overall mental and physical health and child social circumstances. The poorest children in society are five times more likely to die from injury, 15 times more likely to die in a house fire and five times more likely to die as a pedestrian. Boys are twice as likely to be injured as girls.

Changes in legislation and changes in design and engineering can have an important influence on injury prevention. Programmes known to be effective include:

- smoke alarm programmes;
- education campaigns on burn and scald prevention;
- educational interventions aimed at children and parents to prevent poisoning;
- skills training for child pedestrians.

An episode or consultation by a physician treating an acute injury is a time to promote injury prevention and behaviour change. This is when parents are known to be most receptive to that information.

Case scenario

A 2-month-old boy is brought to the emergency department with the story that he rolled off a table onto the floor. His stepfather states that no adult was present when the incident occurred. On examination, the child is distressed and screams when his left arm is touched. There are no other apparent injuries.

What are your concerns?
A 2-month-old child cannot roll over and fall off a table, although otherwise sensible parents do occasionally put their children in situations which could put them at risk when such manoeuvres are possible. An isolated arm injury would be relatively unusual in this situation if the mechanism of injury were indeed true.

What else do you want to know?
A careful assessment of any previous medical problems with the child and a detailed obstetric history is important. Was the child premature? Is the child well or does he or she have any specific problems. Is the child behaving and developing normally? Are there any other siblings and what are the domestic circumstances? Is the child on the at-risk register? Has the baby been brought to the emergency department before?

What investigations would you carry out initially?
A skull radiograph and radiographs of the arm should be performed.

The skull radiograph is normal, the arm film shows a spiral fracture of the humerus. What are your concerns?
The mechanism of injury described is a highly unlikely one for a spiral fracture of the humerus, which is more likely to have been caused by rough or aggressive handling.

What do you do next?
This child should be admitted for a formal paediatric assessment as well as joint care with the orthopaedic surgeons for the fracture. Further investigations will be necessary including detailed interviews with the parents.

SUMMARY

Injury severity in children forms a continuum with no clear cut-off point to distinguish major from minor trauma. All health care providers dealing with injuries in children should have the knowledge and skills to deal with both. Life-threatening major trauma in children is rare in the UK. Health care providers managing the severely injured child can find it stressful because of the unfamiliarity of the problem and the emotionally draining and highly charged environment. Adherence to the main principles of trauma management coupled with knowledge about the specific differences in anatomy and physiology and injury patterns of children enables excellent management of paediatric trauma to be achieved.

Accidents are the most common cause for injuries in children in the UK. However, an awareness that intentional harm may also be a cause of a child's injury is important, and all physicians managing paediatric trauma should be aware of the principles and management of non-accidental injury. Promotion of injury prevention through education, changes in design and engineering, and legislation is vital if the trend for falling annual death rates from paediatric trauma is to continue in the UK.

REFERENCES

1. Edwards P, Roberts I, Green J, Lutchmun. Deaths from injury in children and employment status in family: analysis and trends in class specific death rates. *BMJ* 2006;**333**:119–25,

2. Mandell DL. Traumatic emergencies involving the pediatric airway. *Clin Pediatr Emerg Med* 2005;**6**:41–8.

3. Anderson RCE, Kan P, Hansen KW, Brockmeyer DL. Cervical spine clearance after trauma in children. *Neurosurg Focus* 2006;**20**:e3.

4. McCall T, Fassett D, Brockmeyer D. Cervical spine trauma in children: a review. *Neurosurg Focus* 2006;**20**:e5.

5. Hoffman JR, Mower WR, Wolfson AB. Validity of a set of clinical criteria to rule out injury to the cervical spine in patients with blunt trauma. *N Engl J Med* 2000;**343**:94–9.

6. Viccellio P, Simon H, Pressman BD, *et al.* A prospective multicenter study of cervical spine injury in children. *Pediatrics* 2001;**108**:e20.

7. Slack SE, Clancy MJ. Clearing the cervical spine of paediatric trauma patients. *Emerg Med J* 2004;**21**:189–93.

8. Marcovitch H. Managing head injury in children. *BMJ* 2006;**333**:455–6.

9. Browning JG, Reed MJ, Wilkinson AG, Beattie T. Imaging infants with head injury: effect of a change in policy. *Emerg Med J* 2005;**22**:33–6.

10. Munro A, Maconochie I. Skull fracture and intracranial injury in children. *Emerg Med J* 2001;**18**:467–8.

11. Greenes SG, Schutzman SA. Clinical indicators of intracranial injury in head injured infants. *Pediatrics* 1999;**104**:861–7.

12. Geijerstam JL, Oredsson S, Britton M. Medical outcome after immediate computed tomography or admission for observation in patients with mild head injury: randomised controlled trial. *BMJ* 2006;**333**:465–77.

13. Munro A, Maconochie I. Indications for head CT in children with mild head injury. *Emerg Med J* 2001;**18**:469–70.

14. Dunning J, Batchelor J, Stratford-Smith P, *et al.* A meta-analysis of variables that predict significant intracranial injury in minor head injury. *Arch Dis Child* 2004;**89**:653–9.

15. Goodwin V, Evans RJ. The management of children with head injuries. *Curr Pediatr* 2001;**11**:420–32.

16. Pitetti R, Walker S. Life-threatening chest injuries in children. *Clin Pediatr Emerg Med* 2005;**6**:16–22.

17. Potoka DA, Saladino RA. Blunt abdominal trauma in the pediatric patient. *Clin Pediatr Emerg Med* 2005;**6**:23–31.

18. Rothrock SG, Green SM, Morgan R. Abdominal trauma in infants and children: prompt identification and early management of serious and life-threatening injuries. Part I. Injury patterns and assessment. *Pediatr Emerg Care* 2000;**16**:106–15.

19. Rothrock SG, Green SM, Morgan R. Abdominal trauma in infants and children: prompt identification and early management of serious and life-threatening injuries. Part II.

Specific injuries and ED management. *Pediatr Emerg Care* 2000;**16**:189–95.

20. Klein KL, Herndon DV. Burns. *Pediatr Rev* 2004;**25**:411–17.

21. Reed J, Pomerantz W. Emergency management of pediatric burns. *Pediatr Emerg Care* 2005;**21**:118–29.

22. Quaba O. A users guide for reducing the pain of local anaesthetic administration. *Emerg Med J* 2005;**22**:188–9.

23. Young SJ, Barnett PLJ, Oakley EA. Bruising, abrasions and lacerations: minor injuries in children I. *Med J Aust* 2005; **182**:588–92.

24. Kanegaye JT. A rational approach to the outpatient management of lacerations in pediatric patients. *Curr Probl Pediatr* 1998;**28**:210–34.

25. Young SJ, Barnett PLJ, Oakley EA. Fractures and minor head injuries: minor injuries in children II. *Med J Aust* 2005;**182**:644–648.

26. Krauss B, Green S. Procedural sedation and analgesia in children. *Lancet* 2006;**367**:766–80.

27. Benger RB, Pearce VP. Simple intervention to improve detection of child abuse in emergency departments. *BMJ* 2002;**324**:780–2.

28. Resmiye O, Kerri LB, Charles J. Fractures in young children: are physicians in the emergency department and orthopedic clinics adequately screening for possible abuse? *Pediatr Emerg Care* 2003;**19**:148–53.

29. Barber MA, Sibert JR. Physical child abuse: challenges and pitfalls in the diagnosis. *Curr Paediatr* 2001;**11**:480–5.

30. King WJ, MacKay M, Sirnick A. Shaken baby syndrome in Canada: clinical characteristics and outcomes of hospital cases. *Can Med Assoc J* 2003;**168**:155–9.

31. Keenan HT, Runyan DK, Marshall SW. A population based study of inflicted traumatic brain injury in young children. *JAMA* 2003;**290**:621–6.

32. Jenny C, Hymel KP, Ritzen A. Analysis of missed cases of abusive head trauma. *JAMA* 1999:**281**;621–6.

33. Feldman KW, Bethel R, Shugerman RP. The cause of infants and toddler subdural haemorrhage: a prospective study. *Pediatrics* 2001;**108**:636–46.

34. Strait RT, Siegel RM, Shapiro RA. Humeral fractures without obvious etiologies in children less than 3 years of age: when is it abuse? *Pediatrics* 1995;**96**:667–71.

35. Bulloch B, Schubert CJ, Brophy PD. Cause and clinical characteristics of rib fractures in infants. *Pediatrics* 2000;**105**:e48.

36. Gaines BA, Shultz BS, Morrison K. Duodenal injuries in children: beware of child abuse. *J Pediatr Surg* 2004;**39**:600–2.

37. Allasio D, Fischer H. Immersion scald burns and the ability of young children to climb into a bathtub. *Pediatrics* 2005;**115**:1419–21.

38. Lane WG, Rubin DM, Monteith R. Racial differences in the evaluation of pediatric fractures for physical abuse. *JAMA* 2002;**288**:1603–9.

16

Trauma in women

OBJECTIVES

After reading this chapter the reader will:
- understand the physiological and anatomical changes that occur in women during pregnancy
- recognize the mechanisms of injuries in pregnant women and the implications for both woman and fetus
- understand the required adaptations to trauma management in the pregnant patient
- recognize when to involve obstetricians, gynaecologists and neonatologists in the management of pregnant women.

INTRODUCTION

When considering the female trauma victim, the majority of management is the same as in men. This chapter examines those instances in which the pattern of injury or treatment is necessarily different, the most common of which is the pregnant trauma patient, and the possibility of this must be considered in any women of reproductive age. The physiological changes associated with pregnancy will impact upon the maternal response to injury and must be considered during management, in addition to the anatomical considerations of a pregnant uterus and fetus. A multidisciplinary approach that adds obstetricians and neonatologists to the standard trauma team must be considered in order to ensure the best outcome for both mother and fetus. This chapter also addresses non-obstetric female trauma, including domestic violence and genital mutilation, but the management of sexual assault and rape[1] is beyond its scope.

EPIDEMIOLOGY

Trauma remains one of the most common causes of death associated with pregnancy. In the 2000–2003 Confidential Enquiry into Maternal and Child Health (CEMACH), 19 of the 391 deaths (5%) were a result of trauma, either accidental or non-accidental[2] – 11 women were murdered by their partners. It has been reported that 6–7% of all pregnant women experience some sort of physical trauma.[3]

ANATOMICAL CHANGES OF PREGNANCY

For the first 12 weeks of pregnancy the uterus is protected within the bony pelvis. During the second and third trimesters it becomes an increasingly large intra-abdominal organ, displacing the other viscera laterally. This may provide some protection to the mother, but leaves the uterus and fetus vulnerable (Figure 16.1). As the uterus increases in size, the initially thick musculature

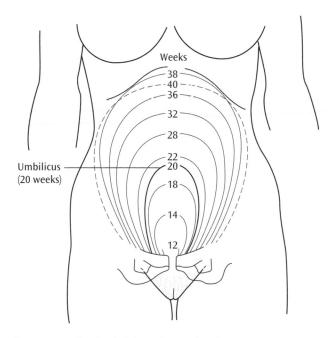

Figure 16.1 Uterine height and gestational age.

thins and the relative volume of amniotic fluid decreases, providing less protection for the intrauterine fetus. The placenta is inelastic and usually attaches high up in the uterine fundus anteriorly; its lack of elasticity renders it susceptible to shearing forces such as occur in blunt abdominal trauma, which may lead to occult haemorrhage or complete placental abruption.

PHYSIOLOGICAL CHANGES IN PREGNANCY

The changes of pregnancy will affect most maternal physiological systems and impinge on most facets of the primary and secondary trauma survey. During pregnancy there is a decrease in gastrointestinal motility, prolonged gastric emptying and relaxation of the lower oesophageal sphincter, all of which significantly increase the risk of aspiration if the consciousness level is altered.

Oxygen consumption is markedly increased due to the increasing demands of the uterus, placenta and fetus as well as the mother, whose basal metabolic rate also rises. This is met by a marked increase in minute ventilation secondary to a rise in tidal volume of up to 40% and a progesterone-mediated increase in respiratory rate. The functional respiratory capacity (FRC) decreases by as much as a quarter as a result of the enlarging uterus impinging on the diaphragm, which may be elevated by up to 4 cm above the normal level. The decrease in FRC and increase in oxygen demand predisposes the mother to rapid decreases in SaO_2 during periods of hypoventilation. The increased minute ventilation leads to a compensated respiratory alkalosis with increased renal excretion of bicarbonate – the maternal $PaCO_2$ may be as low as 4.0 kPa at full term. When there is lack of maternal CO_2 exchange from maternal trauma-induced hypoventilation, the development of fetomaternal acidosis is rapid, may occur when the $PaCO_2$ is still only 5.3 kPa and limits the effectiveness of resuscitation.

Maternal blood volume increases by 11% as early as 7 weeks into gestation and continues to rise until 32 weeks' gestation – by full term, plasma volume is 45–50% greater than in the non-pregnant individual. Red cell mass also increases but to a lesser extent than the increase in plasma volume, resulting in a physiological anaemia of pregnancy. There are also minor changes in the levels of white blood cells, plasma proteins and clotting factors throughout gestation, but none is of significance in the trauma setting. Uterine blood flow, and therefore cardiac output, increases throughout pregnancy to a maximum during the third trimester, at which stage 10% of cardiac output is to the uterus. Potential uterine blood flow is therefore maximal and during low-flow hypoxic conditions can respond only by vasoconstriction in the uteroplacental bed, compromising the fetus. In the second half of pregnancy, the gravid uterus impinges on the aorta, vena cava and pelvic vessels, especially when supine, leading to a significant decline in venous return and a fall in cardiac output.

In view of these changes, significant maternal blood loss of up to 1.5 litres can occur with minimal clinical signs of shock in the mother, but the consequent shunting of blood from the fetoplacental unit to the mother can easily result in fetal hypovolaemic shock in the face of apparent maternal normovolaemia. Conversely, signs of fetal distress may be an early indicator of maternal haemorrhage.

> Clinical signs of shock may be a late occurrence in the pregnant trauma patient – fetal distress may be the first clinical sign.

Severe pre-eclampsia and eclampsia are serious complications of late pregnancy and threaten the life of both the mother and fetus. The presentation of either with decreased consciousness level or fitting may be confused with traumatic head injury, especially if the woman is found collapsed. The presence of hypertension, oedema and proteinuria alongside neurological signs should raise the suspicion of an eclamptic episode and obstetric help must be summoned.

MECHANISMS OF INJURY

Pregnant women may be subject to any of the mechanisms of injury that afflict the non-pregnant population, but the peculiar anatomical and physiological changes of pregnancy alter the impact of the injuries sustained, as well as potentially injuring the fetus.

Blunt impact

Road traffic collisions (RTCs) still predominate among blunt impact trauma patients, and deaths from head and intra-abdominal injury are the leading cause of non-obstetric mortality. Invariably this also results in fetal death; maternal death remains the most common cause of fetal death, followed by placental abruption. Falls, non-penetrating blows and physical abuse are mechanisms of injury that may seem outwardly trivial, with minimal maternal injury, but can have lethal consequences for the fetus owing to placental disruption.[4]

The abdominal wall musculature, the pregnant uterus and amniotic fluid all afford some protection to both mother and fetus by absorbing applied forces. However, acceleration, deceleration and shearing forces or direct blows applied to the abdominal wall in later pregnancy may result in placental abruption, with or without disseminated intravascular coagulation, uterine rupture and direct injury to the fetus.[5]

Many of the predictable maternal injuries from blunt trauma, such as head injuries or limb fractures, are not affected by being pregnant. The physiological effects of pregnancy on the renal system, including renal enlargement and ureteric dilatation can lead to unsuspected damage – haematuria in pregnancy is not normal and requires investigation to exclude renal tract injury. The pelvic organs in pregnant women are hypervascular, and trauma to the vagina and surrounding tissues can result in a rapid, significant and unexpected haemorrhage.

In the 2004 CEMACH report, 23 unnatural, coincidental deaths were reported. Eight resulted from RTCs, of which seven were in the antenatal period. Four of the women who died were not wearing a seat belt, two of whom suffered uterine rupture. Those whose lives could have been saved by wearing a seat belt were *young girls or others with marked features of social exclusion*. A survey of pregnant women's knowledge and use of seat belts showed that 98% wore seat belts as a front passenger but only 68% wore them in the back of the car.[6] In the same study, only 48% of pregnant women identified the correct positioning of seat belts in pregnancy, and only 37% had received instruction regarding the correct placement of seat belts during pregnancy.

Recommendations for the use of seat belts in pregnancy were repeated in the 2004 CEMACH report. All pregnant women should be given the advice about the correct use of seat belts as soon as pregnancy is confirmed, *above and below the bump, not over it*.

The evidence for the benefit of airbag deployment to the pregnant woman and her fetus is conflicting. One study described three patients in whom airbag deployment did not increase the risk of pregnancy-related injuries;[7] however, two case studies[7,8] have suggested an increased risk of placental abruption or uterine rupture. A recent retrospective review of 30 pregnant women between 20 and 37 weeks' gestation involved in an RTC in which airbags were deployed concluded that placental abruption does not occur frequently. One-quarter of the women (either drivers or passengers) were not wearing seat belts.[9]

Uterine rupture is associated with a high fetal mortality rate. It usually occurs as a result of either rapid deceleration or direct compression injuries and is usually associated with other organ injury,[10] although the degree of force needed to rupture the uterus in women who have had previous caesarean sections (particularly through the classical midline approach) is much reduced. If associated with rupture of membranes, the fetus will enter the peritoneal cavity and there is the potential for massive haemorrhage, both concealed and vaginally. The patient complains of excruciating abdominal pain and contractions cease; the abdomen is commonly rigid with rebound tenderness – alternatively the patient may have little pain but fetal parts may be palpable through the abdominal wall.

Placental abruption can occur in up to 5% of patients with minor injuries and as many as 50% of women with severe injuries with a fetal mortality of up to 60%.[11] Symptoms of placental abruption include abdominal pain, uterine tenderness, premature labour and vaginal bleeding. Occasionally an abruption can cause very few of these symptoms, and it is important to ensure adequate fetal monitoring. In the event of minor trauma, significant abruption may not become apparent until 24–48 hours later. Fetal monitoring should be considered in these cases[12,13] and ultrasound scanning is diagnostic. Delayed diagnosis of abruption is associated with maternal disseminated intravascular coagulation.

Penetrating injury

Penetrating injury of pregnant women is rare in UK, where the usual pattern of injury is from stabbing or penetration of objects in RTCs, or following falls. Stab wounds and low-energy-transfer missile wounds result in laceration and crushing in the direct path of the missile or penetrating blade and the outcome is determined by the nature of the structures penetrated. During the first trimester, patterns of injury in the pregnant and non-pregnant woman are similar, provided that the injury track does not extend into the pelvis. In later pregnancy the uterus acts as a shield for the mother, but the fetus is at particular risk. Injury to maternal organs following peritoneal breach was reported to be as low as 20% in one series.[14] If the penetrating missile hits the uterus, the uterine musculature and the amniotic fluid effectively retard its progress, absorbing much of the transferred energy and reducing wounding potential, with the outcome for the fetus being determined by the nature of the structures injured. Penetration of the umbilical cord or placenta may result in abruption and haemorrhage, which may result in the death of both the mother and child.

High-energy-transfer missile injury is rare in peacetime, but is a noted feature of war, terrorism and armed conflict.[15] Although this form of injury in pregnancy is fortunately extremely rare, intra-abdominal high energy transfer in late pregnancy is likely to be lethal for both mother and fetus. It is apparent that some of these intrauterine gunshot wounds are self-inflicted in an attempt to induce abortion or are a further marker of domestic violence. If the fetus is dead, surgical evacuation is unnecessary and the need for laparotomy is based on the treatment of other injuries.

Burn injury

Burn injury in the first trimester differs little from a similar injury in the non-pregnant patient. Beyond the first trimester, an increasing percentage of maternal cardiac output is diverted to the uteroplacental circulation, reducing maternal compensation in the face of sudden loss of circulating volume. Maternal mortality rises sharply with the extent of the burn. Burn injuries of less than 30% body surface area (BSA) appear to have little effect on maternal or fetal survival, provided that management is optimal and is delivered with assistance from teams from both obstetric and burn units. When injury exceeds 50% of BSA, maternal death is certain unless the fetus is delivered.[16] Delay not only poses a grave risk to the mother but also exposes the fetus to increasing risk because of maternal hypoxia and hypovolaemia. In late pregnancy, if burns are 50% of BSA or greater, urgent delivery should be considered as time does not improve fetal outcome. If burns are less than 30% of BSA, prognosis is good and delivery may be delayed depending on gestation and fetal well-being.

Electrical burn injury is rare in pregnancy, but poses a unique risk of fetal electrocution because of the low resistance offered by the uterus and amniotic fluid. Electrical burn injury in pregnancy should prompt emergency admission to a critical care environment for continuous fetal monitoring by Doppler ultrasound. Even if the fetus survives electrocution, long-term monitoring is required to detect fetal growth retardation and oligohydramnios. Decisions regarding delivery will depend on gestational age and fetal well-being. At full term or when the fetus has died, delivery should occur as soon as the patient is stable either by induction of labour or caesarean section if necessary.

ASSESSMENT AND EARLY MANAGEMENT

Unsurprisingly, the assessment and early management of the pregnant trauma victim is based on the standard approach outlined in Chapter 4 with modifications to take account of the physiological and anatomical changes already described. The overriding consideration remains, in general, the welfare of the mother, with the welfare of the fetus being best assured by the well-being of the mother.

The primary survey

<C>

Catastrophic external haemorrhage from associated injuries must be controlled (Chapter 5).

A WITH CERVICAL SPINE CONTROL

In view of the increased risks of aspiration from decreased gastrointestinal motility and reduced oesophageal sphincter tone, aggressive airway management is key and early consideration of endotracheal intubation with a cuffed tube is warranted. Orofacial swelling may obscure the landmarks necessary for a surgical airway.

B

If ventilation is necessary, then account must be taken of the physiological hyperventilation of pregnancy, and chest

drains, if necessary, should be inserted one intercostal space higher than normal to avoid the raised diaphragms displaced by the gravid uterus.

C

If a patient is noticeably pregnant, from about 20 weeks' gestation, resuscitation will be aided by reducing the aortocaval compression. This is achieved by manual displacement of the uterus to the left, left lateral tilt of the table or spinal board or wedge elevation under the right hip.

> Always relieve aortocaval compression.

A tilt of between 15° and 30° prevents aortocaval compression and reduces the detrimental effect on cardiac compression if this becomes necessary, which will already be less effective as the pressure of the enlarged uterus on the diaphragm reduces forward blood flow. As well as the standard blood tests, a sample should be drawn for the Kleihauer–Betke test, which will detect the presence of fetal erythrocytes in the maternal blood – a positive test in a rhesus-negative woman suggests that the mother is at risk of rhesus isoimmunization. Anti-D immunoglobulin should always be given to rhesus-negative mothers sustaining abdominal trauma. As the fetoplacental unit may autotransfuse the mother, disguising the normal signs of severe haemorrhage, the practice of hypotensive resuscitation is not recommended – these women should be fluid resuscitated to normotension.

> Hypotensive resuscitation is contraindicated in pregnancy.

Secondary survey

The secondary survey differs from that in the non-pregnant female only in respect of the abdominal examination. Ideally it should be performed by both a general surgeon and an obstetrician. Aside from the standard assessment of abdominal trauma, the examination should estimate uterine size and therefore gestation, attempt to discern whether the uterus is intact, the placenta is still attached and if there are signs indicative of serious obstetric injury (Table 16.1). The presence of any of these signs demands urgent obstetric consultation if an obstetrician is not present in the trauma team. In most of these instances the abdominal assessment should be augmented by digital and speculum vaginal examination – this too should ideally be deferred to the obstetrician, if available, as injudicious manipulation can precipitate catastrophic haemorrhage from concealed placenta praevia.

Table 16.1 Signs of serious obstetric injury

Uterine contractions
Tetanic contractions with vaginal bleeding
Asymptomatic vaginal bleeding
Leakage of amniotic fluid
Abdominal pain and/or tenderness
Abnormal fetal heart activity
Dilatation of the os
Cervical effacement

Table 16.2 Signs of fetal distress or decompensation

Bradycardia of <100 beats/min or abnormal fetal baseline
    heart rate
Repeated decelerations unrelated to uterine contractions
Absence of acceleration in response to fetal movements
Increasing uterine activity
Positive Kleihauer–Betke test – although not an acute sign

Doppler ultrasound should be used to detect the fetal heart rate, which is normally a regular 120–160 beat/min – bradycardia below 100 beats/min indicates fetal distress. Markers of potential fetal distress (Table 16.2) should prompt an obstetric opinion.

Adjunctive investigations, such as focused assessment with sonography for trauma (FAST) scanning, plain radiology and diagnostic peritoneal lavage (DPL), should not be deferred because of pregnancy, although DPL is more difficult in the pregnant abdomen and a supraumbilical or lateral lavage site should be identified. In trauma, the benefits of radiographs far outweigh any potential risks to the fetus.

> Perform radiography if needed.

Surgical intervention

If laparotomy is indicated for abdominal trauma, the presence of a gravid uterus should not delay this, nor should it alter the procedures undertaken. Operative intervention is recommended in all cases of penetrating injury in the pregnant woman.[17] At laparotomy, the uterus must be carefully assessed for evidence of penetration and the viability of the fetus assessed. Evidence of uterine penetration is widely regarded as an indication for immediate caesarean section. Prior to 28 weeks, it may be possible to delay the delivery of the fetus if the uterus does not compromise any other surgical intervention. At these early gestations the chances of fetal survival need to be weighed against need for delivery. In patients with uterine rupture, evacuation of the uterine contents with primary repair is best, but emergency caesarean hysterectomy may be required if laceration is extensive with involvement of parametrial vessels and structures.

Perimortem and post-mortem caesarean section

The need to carry out peri- or post-mortem caesarean section is extremely rare. In cardiopulmonary arrest due to traumatic haemorrhagic shock, delivery of a viable fetus should be initiated within 4 minutes of cardiac arrest with the fetus delivered at 5 minutes. The main aim is to optimize maternal rather than fetal survival; however, the long-term outcome for fetuses is better if they are delivered earlier.

Once a decision has been made to perform perimortem caesarean section, time is of the essence and the procedure should be performed by the most experienced surgeon available, ideally an obstetrician. The technique is that of the classical caesarean section using a long midline longitudinal incision aided by the natural diastasis of the recti abdomini in late pregnancy to access the uterus through a bloodless field. A longitudinal incision is made through the uterus, enabling the fetus to be delivered. Delivery of the placenta and repair of the uterus depends on the outcome of the resuscitation – if the mother survives, the uterus should be closed in three layers to aid haemostasis.

NON-OBSTETRIC TRAUMA IN WOMEN

Non-obstetric trauma, although uncommon, is reported.[18] Common causes include falls astride handlebars etc., consensual sexual intercourse, sexual assault and injudicious insertion of a wide variety of objects into the genital tract. The genital tract may also be injured in association with penetrating and blunt high-energy pelvic trauma.

Vulval injury

Falls astride a rigid object may result in contusion or laceration. Closed injuries can usually be managed conservatively, but it may be necessary to drain extensive haematomas. Lacerations are managed in the usual way, with control of haemorrhage being by direct pressure, followed by direct repair in an operating theatre.

Vaginal injury

Tears to the hymen may occur following first coitus, resulting in brisk bleeding. Rarely, tears to the hymen extend posteriorly into the perineum and anal sphincter. These injuries require assessment under general anaesthesia in an operating theatre. Vaginal lacerations result from the insertion of a variety of objects, and may be situated in any part of the vaginal tract. Careful examination under anaesthesia is usually indicated to determine accurately the extent of injury. On rare occasions, injury may extend into the peritoneal cavity, necessitating laparotomy. Clinical decision-making is in no way different from other cases in which the peritoneum has been breached.

Injury to the non-pregnant uterus

Blunt uterine injury in this context is rare and almost never occurs in isolation. The most common mechanism is high-energy pelvic disruption. Penetrating injury is rare in European practice, and may result from stab injury or penetration by bullets or fragments.

Female genital mutilation

The UK is a multicultural society, and female genital mutilation (FGM), previously confined to other areas of the world, is now almost certainly practised here. The World Health Organization defines female genital mutilation as *all procedures involving partial or total removal of the external female genitalia or other injury to the female genital organs whether for cultural, religious or other non-therapeutic reasons.* Encompassed in FGM is a wide variety of mutilating genital procedures, ranging from minimalist cutting to extensive surgical excision of large portions of the female external genitalia.[19] As many of these procedures are practised in a clandestine way, patients with complications may present to emergency departments. In managing such conditions, the possibility of injury must first be considered. Early complications are haemorrhage and damage to adjacent organs such as the bladder and bowel. Short-term complications include acute urinary retention, secondary haemorrhage and other manifestations of sepsis. Longer term complications include scarring with resulting stenosis of the introitus, dysuria and menstrual problems. The patient is likely to be a young or adolescent girl.

Domestic violence

Domestic violence is defined as the intentional abuse inflicted on one partner by another in an intimate relationship. It can be physical, psychological or sexual. In heterosexual relationships women are the victims in 90% of cases. Domestic violence often starts or escalates during pregnancy, and rates of domestic violence in pregnancy of 0.9–20% have been reported; CEMACH 2000–2002 reported 11 women murdered by their partners during or soon after pregnancy.[2] During pregnancy, injuries are often to the pregnant abdomen, genitals or breasts, and are often hidden by clothing.

Victims of domestic violence often present late, some time after the injury was incurred; in addition, the mechanism of injury often does not fit the extent of the injury and the partner often attends and refuses to leave the patient and frequently answers questions. Multiple attendances in the accident and emergency department with minor complaints is also common.

A greater awareness of the possibility of domestic violence when assessing patients and a familiarity of the injury patterns associated with abuse may aid in its detection. These are listed in Table 16.3.

In cases of suspected domestic violence it is essential to ensure careful documentation of the patient's statements and clear diagrams or photographs for illustration as they may be required if legal action is taken. Child protection issues must be considered with appropriate referrals to social services if concerns regarding the unborn child or existing children are highlighted.

Table 16.3 Indicators of possible domestic violence

Patterned injuries (injuries that show the imprint of objects used)
Injuries to the arms, especially defensive bruises along the ulnar border
Injuries to the genitals and breasts
Injury to the abdomen during pregnancy, vaginal bleeding and threatened abortion
Periorbital haematoma
Nasal fracture
Perforated tympanic membrane
Fractured mandible
Burns from cigarettes, electrical appliances, friction and arson
Occult presentations (masked by drug/alcohol abuse or psychiatric problems)

Case scenario

A 27-year-old female car passenger is involved in an RTC. She is 35 weeks' pregnant and wearing a seat belt. Her husband, the driver, was killed. She is brought to the emergency department by ambulance on a spinal board with cervical spine immobilization *in situ*. She is unresponsive on arrival with a pulse of 130 beats/min, blood pressure 60/– mmHg, respiratory rate of 30 breaths per minute and oxygen saturations of 91% on 15 litres of oxygen. She has suffered obvious facial injuries with blood around her mouth and her breathing is noisy and laboured.

What should the emergency department response be?

She fulfils the criteria for a trauma call and this should be instituted; in addition the on-call obstetricians and neonatologists should be summoned urgently.

What are the key features of her primary survey?

<C>
There is no external haemorrhage.

A
Her facial injuries and noisy breathing suggest impending airway obstruction. The resuscitation trolley should be tilted head down to help prevent aspiration, given the relaxation of the gastro-oesophageal sphincter and raised intra-abdominal pressure from the pregnancy, and she should be intubated using rapid-sequence induction techniques.

B
Her tachycardia, tachypnoea, hypotension and hypoxia suggest significant chest pathology. She has tracheal deviation to the right and is hyper-resonant over the left hemithorax. She undergoes immediate needle decompression of her left tension pneumothorax and insertion of a left-sided chest drain. Her oxygen saturations improve to 96% on 4 litres and her respiratory rate slows to 22 breaths per minute; her pulse slows to 120 beats/min.

C
She is significantly hypotensive despite relief of the tension pneumothorax and ongoing concealed haemorrhage is the likely cause. She has two 14G cannulae inserted, baseline bloods, urgent cross-match and a Kleihauer–Betke test taken. Fluid resuscitation is commenced and the use of O-negative blood is considered. Brief abdominal examination reveals a tender uterus and profuse vaginal bleeding. She requires resuscitative laparotomy and is transferred immediately to theatre for a midline laparotomy by the general surgeons and obstetricians.

On induction of general anaesthesia the patient suffers a cardiac arrest. As well as advanced life support, what other measures may help maternal survival?

The fetus needs to be delivered immediately. Through a midline laparotomy and upper midline uterine incision the fetus is delivered within 4 minutes of arrest and handed over to the neonatologists for resuscitation. At this stage, attention can turn to haemorrhage control from the placental abruption that is now evident. Surgical control at this stage may included an emergency hysterectomy.

SUMMARY

Managing trauma in women uses the same basic principles as for men. The possibility of pregnancy must always be considered. During resuscitation of the pregnant woman the key points are:

- The mother is the priority.
- Occult maternal blood loss may occur – fetal distress may be the first clinical sign.
- Aortocaval compression must be relieved.
- Hypotensive resuscitation is contraindicated.
- Radiographic examinations should be performed as clinically indicated.
- Delivery may be necessary to aid resuscitation and further management.
- Multidisciplinary team involvement including obstetricians and neonatologists is essential.

GLOBAL PERSPECTIVES

Although pregnancy is a natural phenomenon the world over, patterns of injury, cultural norms and access to health care are not.

Although road traffic collisions remain the most common cause of fetal trauma death across the world, 6% of such fetal deaths in the USA are from gunshot wounds;[20] UK literature contains no cases of uterine gunshot wounds at all. Awwad et al.[15] have reported the largest series of uterine gunshot wounds, 14 in total, collected during the 16 years of civil war in Lebanon from 1975 – only two of the women died, neither solely attributable to the abdominal injuries, but half the fetuses died.

The World Health Organization estimates that between 100 and 140 million women have been subjected to genital mutilation and that worldwide approximately 2 million girls each year are so mutilated. This is almost entirely on the African continent and it is of note that the practice is not restricted to any individual religious group; it appears to be a cultural practice.

REFERENCES

1.   Dalton M. *Forensic Gynaecology*. London: RCOG Press, 2004.
2.   *Confidential Enquiry into Maternal and Child Health 2000–2003*. London: RCOG Press, 2004.
3.   Vaizey CJ. Trauma in pregnancy. *Br J Surg* 1994;**81**:1406–15.
4.   Farmer DL, Adzick NS, Cromblehome WR, *et al*. Fetal trauma: relation to maternal injury. *J Pediatr Surg* 1990;**25**:711–14.
5.   Ali J, Yeo A, Gana TJ, McLellan BA. Predictors of foetal mortality in pregnant trauma patients. *J Trauma* 1997;**42**:782–5.
6.   Johnson H, Pring DW. Car seat belts in pregnancy: the practice and knowledge of pregnant women remain causes for concern. *Br J Obstet Gynaecol* 2000;**107**:644–7.
7.   Sims C, Boardman C, Fuller S. Airbag deployment following a motor vehicle accident in pregnancy. *Obstet Gynecol* 1996;**88**:726.
8.   Schultze P, Stamm C, Roger J. Placental abruption and fetal death with airbag deployment in a motor vehicle accident. *Obstet Gynecol* 1998;**92**:71.
9.   Metz TD, Abbott JT. Uterine trauma in pregnancy after motor vehicle crashes with airbag deployment: a 30-case series. *J Trauma* 2006;**61**:658–61.
10.   Stauffer DM. The trauma patient who is pregnant. *J Emerg Nurs* 1986;**12**:89–93.
11.   Henderson SO, Mallon WK. Trauma in pregnancy. *Emerg Clin North Am* 1998;**16**:209–28.
12.   Doan-Wiggens L. *Trauma in Pregnancy*. In: Benrubi GI, ed. *Obstetric and Gynaecological Emergencies*. Philadelphia: Lippincott, 1994, pp. 57–76.
13.   Higgens SD, Garite TJ. Late abruption placentae in trauma patients: implications for monitoring. *Obstet Gynecol* 1984;**63**(Suppl.):10S.
14.   Lavin JP, Scott Polsky S. Abdominal trauma during pregnancy. *Clin Perinatol* 1983;**10**:423–37.
15.   Awwad JT, Azar GB, Seoud MA, Mroueh AM, Karam KS. High-velocity penetrating wounds of the gravid uterus: review of 16 years of civil war. *Obstet Gynecol* 1994;**83**:259–64.
16.   Matthews RN. Obstetric implications of burns in pregnancy. *Br J Obstet Gynaecol* 1982;**89**:603–9.
17.   Higgins SD. Trauma in pregnancy. *J Perinatol* 1988;**8**:288–92.
18.   Sill PR. Non-obstetric genital tract trauma in Port Moresby, Papua New Guinea. *Aust N Z J Obstet Gynaecol* 1987;**27**:164–5.
19.   Khaled MA, Cox C. Female genital mutilation. *Trauma* 2000;**2**:161–7.
20.   Weiss HB, Songer TJ, Fabio A. Fetal deaths related to maternal injury. *JAMA* 2001;**286**:1863–8.

Trauma in the elderly

OBJECTIVES

After completing this chapter the reader will:
- understand the anatomical and physiological changes that occur in the elderly
- understand the factors that make the elderly vulnerable to injury
- recognize the mechanisms of injury and injury patterns common in elderly patients
- appreciate the interaction of pre-existing medical problems and prescription medications with traumatic injuries in elderly patients
- understand the principles of management in elderly patients and how this may differ from younger adults
- recognize and understand the implications of violence against elderly patients

INTRODUCTION

The assessment and management of injuries is especially challenging in elderly patients. Compared with younger patients, the elderly are more likely to sustain more serious injuries in any given accident and have a higher mortality.[1] Census data in 2001 demonstrated that for the first time there are more people in the UK over the age of 60 years than under the age of 16 years.[2] The so-called 'demographic time bomb' of an increasingly elderly population is common to most developed countries (Figures 17.1 and 17.2).

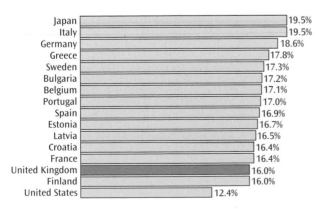

Figure 17.1 The world's 15 'oldest' countries and the UK. The percentage of population aged 65 or over. (Reproduced from *The World Population Data Sheet* courtesy of the Population Reference Bureau, Washington, DC.)

Elderly patients with equivalent Injury Severity Scores (ISS) are more likely to require admission, will spend longer in hospital and are more likely to die as a result of their injuries[3] than are younger patients. The mechanism and spectrum of injury differs in the elderly. In the over-75-year-olds falls are overwhelmingly the leading cause of death,[4] and at least 40% of falls are associated with medical factors.[5]

Anatomical and physiological changes associated with ageing attenuate the normal compensatory mechanisms that constitute the body's response to trauma. This is further complicated by the interaction of co-morbid pathology and prescription medications.

Despite the challenges of trauma care in the elderly, appropriate, early, management is rewarding and leads to increased survival without loss of quality of life or independence.[6]

EPIDEMIOLOGY

In the past 50 years the population of the UK has aged considerably. Although the proportion aged under 16 years has decreased from 24% to 20%, the population aged over 60 years has increased from 16% to 21%. The ageing of the population reflects longer life expectancy because of improvements to living standards and health care. There has been a big increase in people aged 85 and over – who now number over 1.1 million (1.9% of the population).[2] The impact of this changing demographic on emergency

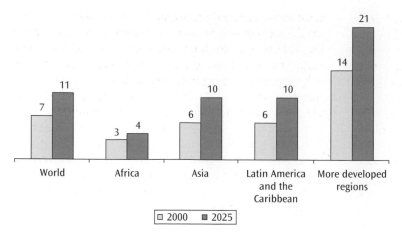

Figure 17.2 Trends in ageing by world region. Percentage of the population aged over 65 (courtesy of the Population Reference Bureau, Washington, DC).

department attendance has been reported by a number of authors.[7,8] George et al.[7] demonstrated a 198% increase in patients over 70 years old attending a district general hospital in Oxford, with a staggering 671% increase in patients aged over 90 years. Patients older than 70 years were 4.9 times more likely to require admission, and their average length of stay was 6.9 times longer[7] than that of younger patients. Similarly, the outcome of domestic accidents in the elderly is relatively poor. In the UK, 12–13% of all domestic accidents were in the over-65 age group but this age group accounted for at least 70% of domestic deaths.[9] Trauma is the fifth leading cause of death in people aged over 65 years. However, it is likely that published figures underestimate the true incidence of death as a result of trauma (Table 17.1). Patients may be certified as dying as a result of a complication (such as pneumonia) that was a consequence of the traumatic insult rather than the initial injury.

The spectrum of mechanism of injury differs in older people. As people age they are more likely to suffer a fall, such that in patients over the age of 75 falls represent the leading cause of accidental death. Precipitating factors include hazards within the home (poor lighting, loose rugs, etc.), poor mobility, failing eyesight, multiple coexisting medical problems and drug-induced side-effects.[10,11] Fire is the second most common cause of accidental death in the elderly.[12] Burns in older patients are associated with a high fatality rate and are often a result of scalds. Injuries tend to be more significant as a result of a combination of relative immobility and age-related

atrophic changes in the skin.[13] The elderly are especially vulnerable as pedestrians in road traffic collisions (RTCs), given that they may have reduced mobility and response times.[3] As drivers, they may have impaired skills or may suffer the acute effects of a medical condition while driving. Preusser et al.[14] demonstrated that drivers between the ages of 65 and 69 years were 1.29 times more likely to be involved in a fatal RTC than a cohort of 40- to 49-year-olds. This figure rises to a 3.74 times relative risk in over-85-year-olds. A study of RTCs in which elderly people were found to be at fault highlights the significant contribution of medical conditions.[15] In another study, elderly diabetic patients were shown to be 2.6 times more likely to suffer an accident than non-diabetic control subjects.[16]

The elderly are vulnerable to injury whether in their own homes or outside. Relative social isolation and poor housing compounds the risk of injury (Table 17.2). Equally, non-accidental injury (NAI) at the hands of family or carers is increasingly recognized in high-risk elderly patients.[17]

SPECIFIC INJURY PATTERNS

Head injury

As in all age groups, the majority of older patients who die as a result of multisystem trauma have a serious head injury. The incidence of central nervous system injury is twice as high in non-survivors as in survivors, and severe head injury is second only to shock as an independent

Table 17.1 Common causes of traumatic death in the elderly

Falls
Fire
Road traffic collisions – pedestrians
Road traffic collisions – drivers
Non-accidental injury
Non-accidental injury of elderly people by family and carers is a more recently recognized cause of injury[17]

Table 17.2 Factors increasing the risk of injury in the elderly

Poor housing
Social isolation
Low income
Reduced functional capacity
Dependency on others

predictor of death in elderly patients.[18] Compared with younger patients, intracranial haematomas tend to be more common and larger in the elderly. Brain weight decreases by approximately 10% by 70 years of age. This process of cerebral atrophy leads to stretching of bridging veins, increasing the risk of subdural haemorrhage. The dura becomes tightly adherent to the skull, therefore extradural haematomas are less common. Even minor head injury may be poorly tolerated in the elderly. The resulting impairment may lead to loss of independence, thus prolonging hospital stay.

In a survey of 527 patients with intracranial haemorrhage, Munro et al.[19] found that patients over the age of 65 years waited longer for CT scanning and were less likely to be transferred to a neurosurgical centre. Age appeared to be the main predictor of the decision to transfer, rather than clinical status and pre-morbid disease or functional capacity. Once transferred there was no difference in rates of intervention. The need for early imaging and intervention in the elderly has been emphasized by a number of authors. Good outcomes from surgery in elderly patients rely on intervention before coma or pupillary dilatation occurs.[20,21]

Cervical spine injury

Although more common in younger patients, the elderly are vulnerable to cervical spine injury as degenerative changes make the neck less flexible and able to withstand trauma. Cervical spine injuries are commonly missed in the elderly, and radiographs may be difficult to interpret. Complete or incomplete spinal cord injuries are poorly tolerated by the elderly, and the resulting immobility may lead to fatal complications. A particular problem is cervical cord injury as a result of a hyperextension injury. A central cord syndrome is commonly caused by a simple fall: degenerative changes reduce the diameter of the spinal canal and hyperextension results in compression on the cervical cord between anterior cervical osteophytes and inward buckling of the posterior ligamentum flavum or a cervical disc. The patients present with greater weakness of the arms than the legs with a variable and inconsistent sensory loss in the upper limbs. There is often evidence of frontal head injury. It is often misdiagnosed because radiographs of the cervical spine are usually normal and the complex neurological signs are not recognized.[22]

Chest injury

The elderly are at increased risk of significant morbidity and mortality from thoracic trauma. Although older patients are more likely to present with evidence of respiratory or cardiovascular compromise, a high index of suspicion is required when assessing elderly patients. The aorta and great vessels are relatively inelastic, making

transection or aneurysm formation more likely. Reduced cardiovascular and respiratory reserve make the elderly less able to tolerate lung injury or pneumothorax. The chest wall and bony thorax is less elastic, making the elderly prone to fractures. Sternal fractures in seat belt wearers involved in RTCs are six times more common in older patients.[3] Similarly, multiple rib fractures and flail segments are more common. Even a relatively minor thoracic injury may prove disastrous in older patients as the respiratory system has reduced reserve. Even without a bony injury, chest wall pain may lead to hypoventilation and failure to clear secretions predisposing to the development of pneumonia.

Abdominal injury

Blunt abdominal trauma of sufficient force to cause intra-abdominal injury has a mortality rate almost five times higher in the elderly than in younger patients.[23] Assessment may be difficult given that peritonitis may be more difficult to detect and that hypovolaemic shock, if present, is less likely be a result of intra-abdominal bleeding than in the young.[24] Although the elderly tolerate emergency surgery less well and are vulnerable to postoperative complications, early treatment is associated with better outcomes.[25]

Pelvic injury

Pelvic fractures presenting with haemodynamic instability are associated with high morbidity and mortality. Fatality rates of up to 50% are reported, rising to 90% for open fractures.[26] Complex pelvic fractures are associated with high energy transfer, such as in RTCs, but, more commonly, a simple fall will result in a pubic rami fracture. The aim of management in this case is early mobilization with analgesia, with the aim of avoiding the complications of immobility.[27]

Skeletal limb injuries

A combination of increased falls and decreased bone density make fractures common in the elderly. Even a minor fracture may lead to temporary loss of independence and hospital admission. The aims of treatment should include rapid mobilization to promote an early return to normal activities.

Injuries to the upper limbs are often seen in mobile patients. Neck of humerus fractures account for 5–10% of all joint and bone injuries. Similarly, acute glenohumeral dislocation is increasingly common with age; this injury is twice as common in women as in men. Rotator cuff injuries are also more common in the elderly than in the young. There is a sharp increase in the incidence of Colles fractures in women between the ages of 45 and 60 years: as many as 95 per 100 000. A large proportion of these patients are found to have decreased bone density.

The most common lower limb injury is fracture of the femoral neck. The incidence rises with age from 1 in 1000 at age 55 years to 30 in 1000, in women, and 15 in 1000, in men, at age 85 years. For many frail patients this injury proves life-threatening. Death rates vary from 10% to 40% at 6 months. Indicators of poor survival include the presence of dementia, postoperative chest infection, neoplasia, wound infections and increasing age.

Burns

Slow reaction times, poor mobility and age-related trophic skin changes predispose the elderly to deeper burns. The elderly have higher mortality rates for a burn of any size, but older patients are particularly vulnerable to burns of large surface area. Baux's formula predicts that the mortality is equal to age plus the percentage surface area of the burn.[1] As such, a lower threshold to hospital treatment should be applied to the elderly. Equally, several authors have suggested that, given that elderly patients with 70% burns or greater do not survive, this should be considered when weighing up how aggressive therapy should be.[13]

Intentional violence (elder abuse)

Elder abuse may be physical, sexual or emotional and is increasingly recognized when dealing with injuries in older patients. Its true extent is not known but it may be as common as child abuse.[28] Abuse could be defined as the wilful infliction of injury, confinement, intimidation or neglect by family members or carers. Signs may be subtle and by its nature many cases go unreported.

> Consider non-accidental injury in the elderly.

ASSESSMENT AND MANAGEMENT OF THE ELDERLY PATIENT

The interaction of co-morbid pathology and decreased functional reserve makes assessing the injured elderly patient difficult. Ageing is associated with decreased functional reserve and a reduced ability to cope with physiological stress. This affects all organ systems to a variable extent and may influence survival following injury. Co-morbid pathology has been identified in large surveys of trauma outcome data. Chronic lung disease, ischaemic heart disease, chronic liver disease, coagulopathies and diabetes are all associated with poor outcome.[29]

Control of catastrophic external haemorrhage

Where present, catastrophic external haemorrhage should be controlled by the methods outlined in Chapter 5.

Airway with cervical spine control

Airway maintenance may be complicated by poor dentition, microsomia and relative macroglossia. Similarly, nasopharyngeal structures may be friable and diseased. Mouth opening may be limited by arthritis of the temporomandibular joints. Arthritis of the cervical spine makes the elderly particularly vulnerable to injury and fixed deformity owing to spondylosis may make protection and positioning challenging. Degenerative changes and calcification of laryngeal structures increases the risk of airway compromise from direct injury to the neck.[28]

Supplemental oxygen should be administered as soon as possible. Early endotracheal intubation by a skilled operative should be considered given the likely limitation in cardiovascular and respiratory reserve.

> Careful assessment and anticipation of a difficult airway is required in elderly patients.

Breathing

Assessment of breathing may be complicated by a reduction in respiratory reserve associated with restrictive and obstructive lung pathology. An elderly patient may therefore tolerate a chest injury less well. Similarly, pre-existing lung disease may make the interpretation of chest radiographs and analysis of arterial blood gases more difficult. Impending respiratory failure may not be appreciated in these patients owing to failure to recognize the increase in effort of breathing and poor respiratory reserve.

Supplemental oxygen should not be withheld because of concerns regarding the possibility of carbon dioxide retention. The patient should be monitored closely, preferably by end-tidal CO_2 or by serial blood gas monitoring. Adequate pain control and close observation with early intervention is required.

> Closely monitor and observe the elderly following chest injury. Intervene early with intubation and ventilation.

Circulation

Changes in myocardial contractility reduce cardiac reserve and impair responses to blood loss. Hypovolaemia may be poorly tolerated by patients with longstanding hypertension and ischaemic heart disease. Medications may impair a normal response to hypovolaemia. Beta-blockers and calcium antagonists may abolish the body's ability to mount a compensatory tachycardia or may reduce peripheral vasoconstriction. A decline in renal function may also impair the ability to cope with haemodynamic disturbance. Failure to recognize and institute early treatment for circulatory insufficiency may lead to increased risk of multiple organ failure.

Management should be targeted at avoiding delays in definitive treatment. Early use of invasive monitoring may help reduce the frequency of unrecognized hypoperfusion and the risk of multiple organ failure. Assessment of abdominal trauma on clinical grounds alone may miss significant pathology. Abdominal ultrasound is a rapid means of establishing the presence of abnormal fluid collections within the abdomen but CT will better image abdominal injuries and will demonstrate retroperitoneal bleeding. The risk of non-operative management of blunt solid organ trauma may be greater than the risk of early surgery in the elderly.

> Consider invasive monitoring. Avoid delays in definitive treatment.

Disability

Assessing head injury in the elderly may be complicated by pre-existing cognitive deficits or acute confusional states. Decline in visual and auditory acuity may further complicate assessment. Equally, physical signs, such as confusion owing to head injury, may be attributed to non-traumatic causes. The elderly are vulnerable to spinal injuries as a result of degenerative changes in intervertebral discs, interspinal ligaments and paraspinal muscles. Similarly, degeneration of the facet joints may lead to spinal stenosis. Osteoporosis with vertebral collapse may lead to kyphosis, making spinal immobilization and protection difficult.[28]

Early CT scanning following significant head injury with early neurosurgical intervention is the key to

---

Case scenario

An 84-year-old man with a known history of chronic obstructive pulmonary disease (COPD) is brought into the emergency department having fallen in his nursing home and banged his left chest area. Initial observations are a pulse of 88 beats/min, a respiratory rate of 30 breaths per minute and a systolic blood pressure of 110 mmHg. He is clearly in pain.

Outline your initial management
In the absence of catastrophic haemorrhage his airway becomes the first priority. He is talking, albeit in gasps, and is maintaining his airway. He has tender ribs on the left side with contusions and the suspicion of a flail segment. There is markedly reduced air entry on the left side and dullness to percussion at the base. He requires an urgent chest radiograph, supplemental high-flow oxygen by facemask and arterial blood gases to assess oxygenation. He requires large-bore venous access and blood drawing for routine biochemistry and full blood count estimation. An i.v. fluid infusion commences. Examination of the rest of the patient reveals numerous bruises of different ages.

The chest radiograph confirms a left-sided flail segment and a large basal haemorthorax. His PaO_2 is 6.5 on 15 litres. What are your next priorities?
He needs analgesia to enable him to breathe without pain. He needs the haemothorax drained and consideration of an invasive ventilatory strategy as he will have an extremely poor respiratory reserve, especially with his history of COPD.

The on-call intensivist is invited to review him. Discuss his likely choices
Standard opioid analgesia may reduce the man's respiratory effort and may make matters worse so an alternative analgesic strategy is needed. Intercostal nerve blocks would be ideal in this situation. The next decision is what respiratory support strategy would be appropriate. In many cases, intubation and ventilation is appropriate as the elderly tire quickly and decompensate rapidly. This patient has a history of severe COPD so it is unlikely that he would be a good candidate for intubation and ventilation as there would be a high risk of him not weaning from the ventilator. In this situation, institution of non-invasive ventilation or continuous positive airway pressure (CPAP) would be a good alternative. It may also be appropriate to set limits on his treatment after discussion with him and his family so that the level of respiratory support would not be escalated beyond CPAP. Once settled with good analgesia from the nerve blocks he should have a basal chest drain inserted by the least traumatic method, which would probably be a Seldinger technique, avoiding the flail segment if possible. He will need aggressive physiotherapy to try to help him clear his secretions aided by nebulized β_2 agonists.

What is his likely outcome?
Unfortunately, elderly patients with severe chest injury and co-morbid chest conditions do not do well and the likelihood that the patient will not survive is high.

management in the elderly. A high index of suspicion should be maintained with regards to spinal injury.

> Consider head injury as a cause of confusion in the elderly.

Exposure and environment

A number of factors, including cold exposure, impaired responses, the effects of systemic disease and medications, reduce the ability of some elderly patients to maintain their core body temperature.[30] The true incidence of accidental 'urban' hypothermia is unknown, but the elderly represent nearly half of hypothermia admissions.[31] Hypothermia may be the cause of deterioration resulting in injury; equally, it may be as a result of a fall or medical condition. Rewarming is associated with cardiovascular instability and increased mortality.

The injured elderly patient should be protected from hypothermia. If there is evidence of pre-existing hypothermia, the possibility of underlying pathology, such as sepsis, pancreatitis or hypothyroidism, should be considered. Rewarming should be cautious with a target rate of no more than 1°C per hour.

SUMMARY

Improvements in the management of trauma in the elderly have been demonstrated over the last 30 years. Age-specific mortality from accidental falls decreased by 63.5% in the USA between 1962 and 1988.[27] Despite evidence that early investigation and management can lead to increased survival and functional recovery, there is evidence that treatment may be withheld simply on the grounds of age.[19]

The ageing population will bring challenges to health care providers. The provision of appropriate trauma care with an understanding of the need for aggressive resuscitation and monitoring of elderly patients as well as knowledge of the ageing process and appreciation of injury patterns commonly seen in the elderly are necessary for improved outcome.

REFERENCES

1.   Hughes G. Trauma in elderly. In: Skinner D, Swain A, Peyton R, Robertson C, eds. *Cambridge Textbook of Accident and Emergency Medicine*. Cambridge: Cambridge University Press, 1997.

2.   http://www.statistics.gov.uk/census2001/demographic_uk.asp (accessed 20 October 2006).

3.   McCoy GF, Johnstone RA, Duthie RB. Injury to the elderly in road traffic accidents. *J Trauma* 1989;**29**:494–7.

4.   Waters E, Cliff K. Accidents will happen. *Nurs Mirror* 1981;**153**:46–7.

5.   Poyner B Hughes N. *Home and Leisure Accident Research: Personal Factors*. London: Department of Trade and Industry, 1990.

6.   DeMaria EJ, Kenney PT, Merriam MA. Aggressive trauma care benefits the elderly. *J Trauma* 1987;**27**:1200–6.

7.   George G, Jell C, Todd BS. Effect of population ageing on emergency department speed and efficiency: a historical perspective from a district general hospital in the UK. *Emerg Med J* 2006;**23**:379–83.

8.   Wass A, Zoltie N. Changing patterns in accident and emergency attenders. *J Accid Emerg Med* 1996;**13**:269–71.

9.   Poyner B. *Home and Leisure Accident Research – the Elderly*. London: Department of Trade and Industry, 1986.

10.   Livesley B. Reducing home accidents in elderly people. *BMJ* 1992;**305**:2–3.

11.   Close JCT, Hooper R, Glucksman E, Jackson SHJ, Swift CG. Predictors of falls in a high risk population: results from the prevention of falls in the elderly trial (PROFET). *Emerg Med J* 2003;**20**:421–5

12.   Elder AT, Squires T, Bussutil A. Fire fatalities in elderly people. *Age Ageing* 1996;**25**:214–16.

13.   Anous MM, Haimbach DM. Causes of death and predictors in burned patients more than 60 years of age. *J Trauma* 1986;**26**:135–9.

14.   Preusser DF, Williams AF, Ferguson SA, Ulmer RG, Weinstein HB. Fatal crash risk for older drivers at intersections. *Accid Anal Prev* 1998;**30**:151–9

15.   Rehm CG, Ross E. Elderly drivers involved in road crashes: a profile. *Am Surg* 1995;**61**:435–7.

16.   Koepsell TD, Wolf ME, McCloskey L, *et al.* Medical conditions and motor vehicle collision injuries in older adults. *J Am Geriatr Soc* 1994;**42**:695–700.

17.   Bennett G, Kingston P, Penhale B. *Dimensions of Elder Abuse*. London: Macmillan, 1997.

18.   Oreskovich MR, Howard JD, Copass MK. Geriatric trauma: injury patterns and outcome. *J Trauma* 1984;**24**:565–9.

19.   Munro PT, Smith RD, Parke TRJ. Effect of patients' age on management of acute intracranial haematoma: prospective national study. *BMJ* 2002;**325**:1001

20.   Rozelle CJ, Wofford JL, Branch CL. Predictors of mortality in older patients with subdural hematoma. *J Am Geriatr Soc* 1995;**43**:240–4.

21.   Seelig JM, Becker DP, Miller JD, *et al.* Traumatic acute subdural hematoma; major mortality reduction in comatose patients treated within four hours. *N Engl J Med* 1981;**304**:1511–18.

22.   Johnston RA. Management of old people with neck trauma. *BMJ* 1989;**299**:633–4.

23.   Finelli FC, Jonsson J, Champion HR, Morelli S, Fouty WJ. A case control study for major trauma in geriatric patients. *J Trauma* 1989:**29**:541–8.

24.   Pedowitz RA, Shackford SR. Non-cavitary hemorrhage producing shock in trauma patients: incidence and severity. *J Trauma* 1989;**29**:219–22.

25.   Sutherland FR, Temple WJ, Snodgrass T, Huchcroft SA. Predicting the outcome of exploratory laparotomy in ICU patients with sepsis or organ failure. *J Trauma* *1989*;**29**:152–7.

26.   Mucha P, Farnell MB. Analysis of pelvic fracture management. *J Trauma* 1984;**24**:379–86.

27.   Grimley Evans J, Franklin Williams T, Lynn Beattie B, Michel J-P, Wilcock GK. Injuries in the elderly. In: *Oxford Textbook of Geriatric Medicine*, 2nd edn. Oxford: Oxford University Press, 2003.

28.   American College of Surgeons. *Advanced Trauma Life Support Manual*. Chicago: American College of Surgeons, 2004.

29.   Bernadini B, Meiecke C, Pagani M, *et al*. Comorbidity and adverse clinical events in the rehabilitation of older adults after hip fracture. *J Am Geriatr Soc* 1995;**43**:894–8.

30.   Pedley DK, Paterson B, Morrison W. Hypothermia in elderly patients attending an accident and emergency department. *Scot Med J* 2002;**47**:10–11.

31.   Mills GL. Accidental hypothermia in the elderly. *Br J Hosp Med* 1973;**2**:691–9.

18

Gunshot injuries

After reading this chapter the reader will:
- understand the basic scientific principles of ballistic wounding
- be able to outline basic protocols for the treatment of gunshot wounds.

INTRODUCTION

Wounds caused by guns occur throughout the world. In the developed world, criminal acts increasingly involve the use of firearms, and we are now more than ever in the midst of an epidemic of firearm-related injuries. Wounds which were once rare outside military conflict are now regularly seen in the UK. In 2003, the General Medical Council published *Reporting Gun Shot Wounds. Guidance for Doctors in Accident and Emergency Departments* in response to this growing problem.

BALLISTIC FEATURES OF GUNSHOT WOUNDING

The science of ballistics addresses the aspects of missile and bullet flight and relates these to the potential for injury. When a bullet strikes tissue, it will impart some of its kinetic energy into it; the more energy it loses to the tissue, the greater the damage that will be caused. The available energy for a bullet, or indeed any other missile, is given by the following formula, where m = mass and v = velocity:

$$\text{Kinetic energy (KE)} = \tfrac{1}{2}mv^2$$

Therefore, if a bullet does not exit the body after striking it, the energy available for damaging tissue is the total kinetic energy of the missile. If the missile passes through the body, slowing as it goes from its entry velocity (v_i) to its exit velocity (v_e) the energy available to cause damage is:

$$\text{Available energy} = \tfrac{1}{2}m(v_i^2 - v_e^2)$$

From this it follows that it is theoretically possible for a missile to pass straight through a body with minimal slowing and minimal tissue damage. It is also clear that the more a bullet slows, and the more rapidly it slows, the more effective it will be in causing injury. The factors that influence the wounding capacity of projectiles are:

- available energy;
- tissue factors;
- missile features;
- aerodynamics of the missile.

Available energy

Bullets are somewhat arbitrarily divided into high-energy and low-energy missiles. In general, handguns, such as pistols and revolvers, fire low-energy bullets and rifles (long-barrelled weapons) fire high-energy bullets. These were formerly referred to as low- and high-velocity missiles, but it should be clear from the discussion above that the injuring potential of a missile is related to the amount of energy transferred rather than simply the velocity. The key clinical distinction is that low-energy rounds produce tissue damage effectively confined to the track of the missile whereas the passage of a high-energy round is associated with the phenomenon of *cavitation*.

When a high-energy round passes through tissue, it generates a shock wave which pushes tissues away from the missile track, creating a temporary cavity many times the diameter of the missile. As this cavity expands, dirt, clothing and bacteria are drawn in by the subatmospheric pressure, remaining as contaminants after the passage of the missile and the collapse of the cavity. The result is a major wound associated with tissue contamination and damage often at a considerable distance from the actual wound track. In some cases, the shock wave is sufficiently strong to fracture bone at a distance from the track of the missile, although such fractures tend to be less complex than those associated with direct missile strike of missile on bone.

Tissue factors

A number of tissue factors affect the injury potential of a bullet. Even a low-energy transfer wound to the heart is likely to be fatal, whereas a high-energy transfer wound to the leg is entirely survivable with good medical care. Similarly, ballistic injuries to other essential organs, such as the brain, are associated with a poor prognosis. Because the amount of tissue damage is related to the slowing of the bullet, it is also apparent that denser tissues, which offer a greater degree of retardation to the missile, will sustain more significant injuries than less dense ones. Thus, a bullet may pass through an air-containing organ, such as the lung, with minimal slowing and little damage or through the denser liver with rapid slowing, considerable energy loss and massive tissue destruction. The damage to the liver and all other encapsulated organs is exacerbated by the inelasticity of its capsule, preventing acceleration of tissue away from the missile.

When a bullet strikes bone, it may fragment and will dump its energy almost instantaneously, producing a massively comminuted compound fracture. In addition, energized bone fragments will then act as secondary missiles, causing further tissue damage. Fractures caused by the close proximity of a high-energy round are characteristically less dramatic than those caused by direct bone strike.

Missile features

Bullets may be designed or modified to increase tissue damage on impact. A sharp-nosed bullet will have a smaller presenting area than a snub-nosed bullet. Military bullets have a metal casing around a lead core (a 'full metal jacket') in order to reduce the chance of them fragmenting; some other bullets are designed to break up on impact, dramatically increasing the energy transfer. Bullets can also be designed to increase tissue damage by incorporating a soft or hollow tip that expands on impact. The most notorious of these was the bullet manufactured for the British in the Indian village of Dum Dum. Military use of these bullets is banned under international law, although they are used by law enforcement agencies to maximize the chance of killing a criminal whilst minimizing the chance of collateral injury due to a bullet passing through its intended victim.

Aerodynamics of the bullet

Bullets do not fly straight through the air, but undergo a series of movements, of which the most significant is 'yaw' (Figure 18.1). Yaw is oscillation of the bullet about its long axis. Depending on the position at the time of impact, the bullet may strike tissue travelling forwards or side on, increasing its cross-sectional area and energy loss on impact. Once the bullet enters tissue, the greater density of the medium through which it is travelling causes it to become completely unstable and its yaw becomes *tumbling* as it rotates through 360° about its long axis. As a result of this tumbling, its rate of slowing is enormously increased and the potential tissue damage magnified. Tumbling may put sufficient strain on the bullet to cause it to fragment, further increasing the tissue damage. It is because of tumbling that, where complete penetration occurs, the exit wound tends to be larger than the entrance wound.

WEAPON TYPES

Some information about the likely magnitude of injury can be gained from a knowledge of the type of weapon involved, although what follows is intended as a guide only.

> The first rule in the management of ballistic injury is to treat the wound, not the weapon.

It is essential not to anticipate likely injuries either in terms of magnitude or which cavities or organs are involved, but to treat the injuries exactly as they are found, dealing with life-threatening problems first.

Handguns

The most common types of these weapons fire a bullet with a diameter of 9 mm and have a muzzle velocity of

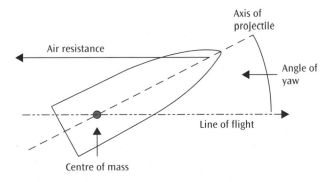

Figure 18.1 Movements of a missile in flight. In terms of wounding potential, the most significant is yaw.

around 1000 feet per second. As such, they are low-energy weapons, producing only a small temporary cavity, injury being essentially confined to the bullet track. Magnum handguns fire bullets which have an extra gunpowder charge to increase their velocity and available energy – the available kinetic energy at the muzzle of a .44 magnum handgun round is three-quarters of that of an AK47 assault rifle.

Shotguns

The bore of a shotgun is the internal diameter of its barrel and is derived from the days when muskets fired single lead balls. An eight-bore shotgun has the same bore as a 2-ounce lead ball as 8×2 oz = 16 oz or 1 lb; a 12-bore shotgun has a bore the same as a 1.33-oz lead ball since $12 \times 1.33 = 16$ oz or 1 lb. However, modern shotguns fire cartridges containing many small lead pellets rather than a single ball. The diameter of these pellets can vary from 1 mm ('birdshot') to 10 mm ('buckshot'). Once fired, the pellets disperse in a cone-shaped pattern. The degree and rapidity of dispersion is proportional to the size and number of pellets as well as the diameter of the shotgun barrel at the muzzle. Owing to their aerodynamics, the velocity of individual pellets will attenuate over short distances, even in air. Furthermore, the conical dispersion leads to a rapid decline in the number of pellets that will hit a particular target as range increases. These two factors lead to the weapon being virtually ineffective at ranges over 50 m. At close range, however, the shotgun can create very severe patterns of injury, effectively equivalent to being hit by a single projectile of the total mass of the pellets. Although each pellet may be travelling only at low velocity, the combined effect of multiple pellets is a formidable destructive force, shredding tissues and causing massive disruption. Shortening the length of the barrel ('sawn-off shotgun') increases the velocity and energy of the pellets as they leave the muzzle and at short range significantly increases the wounding potential. Shotguns with a barrel less than 24 inches in length are prohibited in the UK.

Military 'assault' rifles

Probably the most common of these weapons worldwide is the AK47, of which there are an estimated 125 million in circulation. Military rifles use a bullet of 7.62 mm diameter and 3 mm length that leaves the weapon at a speed of around 900 m/s. The British military version is the modified SA80 (A2), which fires a 5.56-mm round. In all assault weapons, rifling of the barrel sets the bullet spinning, which, combined with the increased velocity, leads to greater accuracy at long range. Weapons of this kind are in widespread use among terrorist organizations.

The much greater kinetic energy of these bullets leads to a much bigger temporary cavity than seen in low-muzzle-velocity weapons. As described above, the subatmospheric pressure in the cavity will suck in clothing and other debris from outside the wound, causing contamination. The shock front of accelerating tissue, propagating away from the point of impact, causes stretching and tearing of the tissues, cellular disruption and microvascular injury. The margin of tissue around the cavity, termed the *zone of extravasation*, is full of haemorrhage, has little tendency to further bleeding and, if muscle, shows no tendency to contract when stimulated. This tissue is non-viable and will become a culture medium for infection if left in place. The shock wave itself can cause fracture of bone and intimal disruption of major vessels.

TREATMENT OF BALLISTIC INJURY

All wounds are caused by the transfer of energy to tissues. Ballistic wounds are no different. Problems associated with the management of gunshot wounds arise more from unfamiliarity than from any other factor.

> The second rule of managing ballistic injury is do not speculate about the nature of wounds.

There is absolutely no point in speculating whether wounds are entry wounds or exit wounds. It is true that *in general* exit wounds are larger than entry wounds, but this is affected by many factors and is of no clinical help in patient management. In particular, close-range shotgun wounds and wounds caused by weapons held very close to the skin will cause large entrance wounds.

In addition, in many cases, there will be no exit wound since the bullet has remained inside the body; alternatively, there may be several exit wounds where the bullet has fragmented or even where segments of energized bone have acted as secondary fragments. However, the main reason for avoiding speculation is that it does not help in the management of the patient and may lead to errors, as well as wasting valuable time.

Resuscitation

The initial measures in the treatment of gunshot wounds are similar to those for any severe injury. First, a primary survey is carried out with resuscitation of the patient, addressing life-threatening conditions according to <C>ABCDE priorities.

CONTROL OF EXSANGUINATING HAEMORRHAGE

Severe external exsanguinating haemorrhage is relatively rare in gunshot wounds, but, if it occurs, it must be controlled. Simple dressing and pressure may be adequate, otherwise the techniques described in Chapter 5 should be employed.

AIRWAY

The airway is managed using the stepped approach beginning with simple measures. High-flow oxygen is essential. In most cases advanced airway manoeuvres will be required only in preparation for surgery.

BREATHING

Open pneumothorax should be treated with an Asherman seal followed by placement of a chest drain and replacement of the seal with an occlusive dressing. Under no circumstances should an intercostal drain be placed through a wound. Pneumothorax and haemothorax owing to ballistic injury are treated in the same manner as those owing to any other cause.

CIRCULATION

Fluids should be administered according to the principles described in Chapter 8. Abdominal tenderness should be sought and excluded. If there is any possibility of abdominal involvement, FAST (focused abdominal sonography for trauma) is the initial investigation of choice.

DISABILITY

An immediate AVPU (alert, voice, pain, unresponsive) evaluation should be followed by a formal Glasgow Coma Scale score.

EXPOSURE

A detailed head-to-toe examination is essential in order to exclude missed wounds. Particular attention should be paid to the back (log-roll), buttocks, perianal area and scalp. All wounds should be carefully recorded and, ideally, photographed.

Dressings should be applied to open wounds. All victims of bullets are likely to be the subject of some form of police investigation, and as a consequence clothes should be removed carefully, taking care never to cut through holes made by bullets or other projectiles. Property should be carefully labelled, bagged individually and handed to a named individual, preferably a police officer.

For the conscious patient i.v. opiate analgesia should be administered, with the dose titrated against the level of discomfort. Femoral nerve block is useful if the femur is fractured.

Antibiotics must be given at the first opportunity. For an adult patient, benzyl penicillin (1.2 g i.v.) and flucloxacillin (1 g i.v.) is appropriate. Staphylococcal cover

is essential if there is an underlying fracture, and if there is abdominal involvement metronidazole (500 mg i.v.) should be added.

It should be remembered that the patient may not have been immunized against tetanus. As the wounds from high-energy bullets are often grossly contaminated and contain devitalized tissue, tetanus toxoid is appropriate. If there is gross contamination with soil or similar material, human antitetanus immunoglobulin should be administered.

> Rule three for the management of gunshot wounds is *anticipate* and *exclude* injury to all body cavities.

It is impossible to predict missile tracks from external study of the inflicted wounds. The key determinant of the path of a missile is the position of the patient at the time of wounding (Figure 18.2), which may not be known during resuscitation. Thus the patient with a gunshot wound to the buttock may have injuries to pelvic contents, abdomen and chest. As a result it is *imperative* that ballistic injury to all body compartments is *specifically* excluded.

Cervical spine damage is unlikely in penetrating ballistic injury outside the neck. However, chest, abdominal and pelvic radiographs are essential if there is any possibility of penetration of one or more of these cavities. Radiographs of the injured body parts will be required but can wait until immediately life-threatening injuries have been identified and treated. Fractures should be splinted using either traction splintage or plaster of Paris as appropriate. For injuries involving the limbs, the distal neurovascular status should be assessed and recorded.

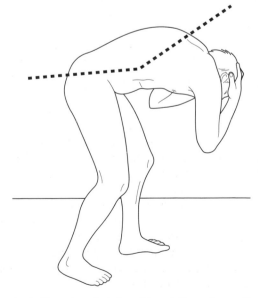

Figure 18.2 Wound track and position at time of wounding.

DEFINITIVE MANAGEMENT

All bullet wounds will require surgical exploration and debridement; discussion with a surgeon is therefore a vital part of the initial assessment and management of these patients.

Wound debridement and excision is a surgical procedure involving removal from the wound of any dead and contaminated tissue which, if left, would become a medium for infection. It is most relevant to high-energy-transfer bullet wounds with large cavities and considerable amounts of dead tissue and contamination. In wound excision, all dead and contaminated tissue as well as foreign material should be excised. In the case of low-energy-transfer wounds, because of the minimal cavitation and zone of extravasation, the debridement will generally be less extensive, and in certain circumstances and experienced hands these wounds can be managed without surgery. When surgery is performed, delayed closure is appropriate in order to reduce the risk of infection and damage resulting from tissue swelling. Fasciotomy is often necessary as part of the initial surgical management of ballistic limb injuries.

The definitive management of ballistic fractures is complex and varies with anatomical region. Specialist advice is necessary. In general, immobilization in plaster of Paris or external fixation are preferred to immediate internal fixation because of the risks of infection. External fixation is likely to be necessary in order to maintain bone length or integrity in highly comminuted fractures. Internal fixation may be performed as a secondary procedure once the initial risk of infection has lessened.

Abdominal gunshot wounds have traditionally been managed by mandatory laparotomy, but several centres with a heavy workload of such injuries have recently successfully employed a policy of selective non-operative management in up to 30% of abdominal gunshot wounds. It remains the province of the experienced trauma surgeon, whereas laparotomy remains a safe and acceptable practice for those less experienced: it is discussed fully in Chapter 13.

Case scenario

A 22-year-old man is brought to the emergency department by the police following a shooting incident. He is cooperative but complaining of pain in his left thigh. Examination reveals a single wound on the outer aspect of his thigh. He is speaking clearly and his respiratory rate is 24 breaths per minute, with no obvious abnormality on chest examination. His abdomen is tender. He is haemodynamically stable with a pulse of 104 beats/min.

What imaging would you order?
He requires chest and pelvic radiographs as part of the trauma series workup as well as a plain radiograph of the injured thigh to exclude femoral fracture and to identify any retained bullet fragments. In addition, there should be a high index of suspicion of intra-abdominal injury in the face of abdominal signs following gunshot wounding; thus, his abdomen needs to be imaged. In the emergency department this is most effectively done by FAST scanning if available. If no-one is FAST trained then, assuming haemodynamic stability, an abdominal computed tomography scan should be requested.

A chest radiograph shows gas under the diaphragm and FAST shows free fluid in the abdomen. The pelvic radiograph shows a comminuted fracture of the ileum, and the radiograph of the left femur shows a fracture of the upper shaft with massive comminution (Figure 18.3).

What are your management priorities?
The immediate priority is treating his intra-abdominal injuries, which in the UK equates to mandatory laparotomy. Thereafter, his limb injuries may be debrided and fixation applied to stabilize the fractures.

He underwent laparotomy and wound exploration where two penetrating wounds of the small bowel were identified and repaired without resection or stoma. The bullet was removed from the right lower quadrant. The pelvic wound was debrided and non-viable tissue removed. The left thigh was explored and non-viable tissue and bone removed and a thigh fasciotomy performed. The femoral fracture was managed by immobilization in a splint with traction.

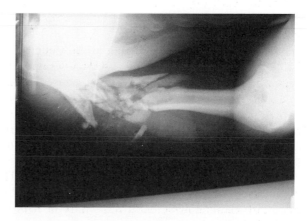

Figure 18.3 Radiograph of a high-energy ballistic fracture of the femur.

SUMMARY

Gunshot wounds are a potential source of severe injury. Some understanding of ballistics can help in the assessment of these injuries, and also assist in determining the surgical strategy necessary for their care. Three rules should always be followed:

- Treat the wound not the weapon.
- Do not speculate about the nature of wounds.
- Anticipate and exclude or treat injury to all body cavities.

Injuries to the chest are treated in the conventional manner and those to the abdomen by laparotomy. Bullet wound tracks are treated by laying open and excision of dead and non-viable tissue. This is likely to be a more radical procedure with high-energy-than low-energy-transfer wounds.

Fractures are treated by immediate stabilization followed by appropriate surgery. In general, external fixation is preferred to internal fixation, which may be appropriate as a delayed procedure.

Treatment according to basic principles following the pattern described for all the victims of trauma will lead to the best possible clinical outcome.

FURTHER READING

Mahoney PF, Ryan JM, Brooks AJ, Schwab CW, eds. *Ballistic Trauma: a Practical Guide*, 2nd edn. New York: Springer, 2005.

GLOBAL PERSPECTIVES

Recent figures for deaths and injuries from gunshot wounds are given in Table 1. Fortunately, compared to countries like the USA and parts of Africa and Asia, UK death rates from gunshot remain low at 0.1 per 100,000 deaths. Recent figures suggest that there are 200,000 deaths per year from firearms in non-conflict situations – 28,000 in the USA alone, with a further 300,000 deaths per year in conflict situations world wide. There are at least 688,000,000 small arms and light weapons in existence and of these, 230,000,000 are in the USA – 98% in private civilian hands

19

Blast injury

OBJECTIVES

After completing this chapter the reader will:
- be able to explain the physics and pathophysiology of blast effects
- be able to identify primary blast injury
- be able to undertake emergency treatment of blast injury and recognize the differences between it and 'ordinary' trauma.

INTRODUCTION

The upsurge in terrorist activity around the world has brought the spectre of blast injury to a host of countries which previously had seemed immune to the violence that has plagued the UK and Israel for decades – such atrocities have now occurred in Kenya, Tanzania, the Yemen and Spain, to name but four. This chapter explains the physics of explosions and the pathophysiology of blast injury, before outlining the diagnosis and treatment of the injuries that result, so that clinicians who have previously been unfamiliar with this area of trauma medicine may be prepared and able to deal with an influx of blast casualties when the unexpected terrorist atrocity occurs near them.

CLASSIFICATION OF BLAST INJURY

Blast injury research came of age during the Second World War and it is the classification outlined by Zuckerman[1] in 1940 that is still used to describe blast injuries (Table 19.1). Many of the features of secondary, tertiary and quaternary blast will be familiar to clinicians, but primary blast effects have until recently remained largely unknown in civilian practice, and these will be the main area of consideration of this chapter.

EPIDEMIOLOGY

The incidence of primary blast injury (PBI) is difficult to ascertain with certainty as it is poorly understood and far from the forefront of many clinicians' minds. It may simply

Table 19.1 Classification of blast injury

Type of injury	Mechanism of injury
Primary	Interaction of the blast wave with the body
Secondary	Fragment effects from original device or environmental debris transported by the blast wind
Tertiary	Physical displacement of a body or structural collapse onto body by effects of the blast wind
Quaternary	Other effects including psychological trauma, burns and inhalational injury

be overlooked as a potential diagnosis as its external manifestations may be subtle and often overshadowed by more obvious secondary and tertiary blast effects. Reports of primary blast injury prior to the Second World War are scarce, although stories of men dying in the First World War without external injury except the occasional trail of blood leaking from mouth or nose were later recounted.[2] Surprisingly, military data on PBI remain scarce. Only two cases are recorded from Vietnam – neither from enemy action. The Chinese reported an incidence of 0.3% among casualties of the Korean War,[3] and the Israeli campaigns in Lebanon in 1982 yielded a rate of 2.3%, although this may have been inflated by inclusion of some casualties with secondary wounding effects.[4] In the civilian context, quantification of PBI is often easier – the numbers involved are generally lower and the facilities in a civilian peacetime infrastructure aid data collection. Analysis of 828 British servicemen[5] killed or injured by explosions in Northern Ireland showed that 11% of the dead had pulmonary blast injury but no external injuries to account for their demise; however, only 2 out of 612 survivors required treatment for blast lung.

THE PHYSICS OF EXPLOSIONS

An explosion is a process that rapidly liberates large amounts of energy in the form of high-pressure shock waves in a short space of time, and thus the energy per unit time, i.e. the power, is huge, although the overall energy released may be significantly lower than slower chemical releases of energy such as combustion of carbon fuels. The energy is released by the process of detonation, which breaks down the chemical bonds within the explosive. Application of thermal energy to the explosive begins to break these bonds in an exothermic reaction, which is initially contained, generating an internal pressure in the form of a wave. This detonation wave traverses the remaining explosive almost instantaneously, rapidly liberating energy in the form of a shock wave, gaseous products and thermal energy. As the detonation wave reaches the explosive–air interface, it generates a shock (blast) wave in the surrounding air and compresses a rim of air around the ball of explosive products. The cloud of very hot, highly energized gaseous products of explosion expands far quicker than the speed of sound in air, and the rim of compressed air formed by the propagation of the detonation wave into the air remains attached to the gaseous products. As the gases expand, they rapidly cool and slow down and when their speed becomes subsonic the rim of compressed air containing the pressure pulse detaches and propagates through the atmosphere (Figure 19.1). The pressure changes of the blast wave are usually described as those at a single point over time: there is a virtually instantaneous sharp rise in air pressure surrounding the blast, rapidly attaining its peak (static) *overpressure*. As the blast wave propagates through the atmosphere, the magnitude of the pressure wave decreases rapidly in inverse proportion to the third power of the radius of its sphere of expansion. Overexpansion because of an inertial effect in air is followed by rarefaction and pressures below ambient pressure (the *underpressure*), which then returns to ambient atmospheric pressure (Figure 19.2). This 'Friedlander wave' describes the pressure changes for a free-field detonation, i.e. one without obstacles to the passage of the blast wave. In addition, passage of the blast wave accelerates the air it traverses and the mass movement of air is known as the blast wind or dynamic *overpressure* – and is different from the cloud of gaseous products arising directly from the detonation that initially forms part of the blast wave.

PATHOPHYSIOLOGY OF BLAST INJURY

Primary blast injury

Where two materials of differing densities meet, a shock wave will be both *reflected* and *coupled into* the incident target. Primary blast injury is the effect of the blast wave at the air–body interface and is most marked where the density differential is greatest such as tissue–air interfaces in the ears, lungs and gut. Solid organs including the skin are relatively resistant to energy transfer from blast, and a seriously blast-injured casualty may have no visible stigmata of injury.

An incident blast wave generates two types of energy wave on striking a human body. It is coupled into the body wall, resulting in a short-duration, low-velocity acceleration of the wall, in turn generating stress waves of high amplitude and velocity that propagate through the body at speeds greater than the speed of sound in that medium. At internal tissue density interfaces, energy is coupled across the junction, causing intense local forces over a short duration, resulting in microscopic damage rather than macroscopic lacerations. When long-duration waves interact with the body, there is gross deformation of

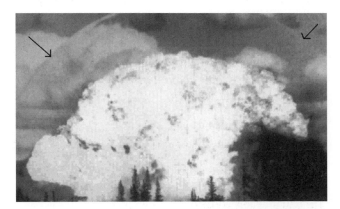

Figure 19.1 Explosion showing the blast wave detaching from the gaseous products and traversing the air as a sphere of expansion.

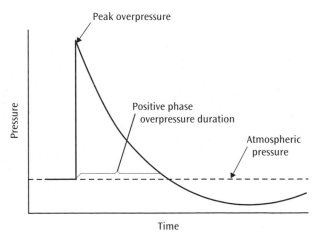

Figure 19.2 Changes in the atmospheric pressure at a fixed point over time in free-field conditions – the classical Friedlander wave.

the body wall and generation of a low-velocity, long-duration transverse shear wave. Tissues of different densities will move differentially under the influence of these waves, resulting in tearing of organs at points of attachments, such as the small bowel mesentery, and shearing of solid organs such as liver and spleen.

In addition, thoracic, but not abdominal, blast generates a reflexive triad of apnoea, hypotension and bradycardia[6] which occurs within 10 seconds of exposure but whose effects may last for several hours. These effects are almost certainly vagally mediated and appear to interfere with cardiovascular responsiveness.[7] It is likely that this triad is responsible, at least in part, for those casualties in whom immediate death supervenes after blast exposure but without any external evidence of injury.

Pulmonary PBI extends from mucosal bruising of the hypopharyngeal trachea through to disruption of the delicate alveolar septi and associated interalveolar capillaries.[8] There is haemorrhage into the alveoli and egress of air, manifest as impaired gas exchange and peribronchiolar emphysema or haemo/pneumothoraces in superficial alveoli.[9] Alveolar–venous fistulae allow air emboli into the systemic circulation, and these may be visible in the retinal arteries on fundoscopy.[10] Damage is greatest when the stress wave is concentrated in areas of reflection, such as the intercostal spaces, costophrenic angles and adjacent to the mediastinum[8,11] (Figure 19.3).

In the abdomen, the differing effects of stress and shear waves are more readily appreciable. The short-duration stress waves deposit energy at the mucosal surface of the gut, creating a mural haematoma that expands towards the serosal surface depending on the level of energy transfer – if sufficiently large, immediate perforation ensues.[12] The long-duration shear waves caused by the gross displacement of the body wall injure the fixed viscera (solid organs and retroperitoneal colon) as well as the small bowel mesentery adjacent to its points of fixation. Auditory blast injury is the most common of all primary blast effects, with the tympanic

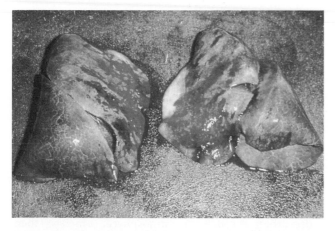

Figure 19.3 Concentration of primary blast injury in the intercostal spaces results in a striped appearance of the pulmonary haemorrhages.

membrane rupturing at low peak overpressures.[13] Middle ear ossicular dislocation and sensineural injury may also occur, but more rarely.[9] Direct cardiac blast injury is rare, as is a primary injury to the central nervous system. Cardiovascular and neurological upset is much more frequently found as a result of air embolism.[14]

> The diagnosis of primary blast injury requires a high index of suspicion.

Secondary blast injury

Secondary blast injuries are the penetrating wounds caused by the accelerated bomb casing, its contents or environmental debris. The degree and clinical significance of secondary blast injury depends on the extent of mechanical damage, the nature of the tissues involved and the level of contamination.[15] The level of mechanical damage is a function of the amount of energy transferred to the tissues, itself a function of the fragment's available kinetic energy and the degree of retardation exerted upon it by the tissues. Lung parenchyma is highly elastic and exerts little in the way of retardation, and penetrating fragments may traverse lung parenchyma depositing little kinetic energy. Conversely, the dense liver parenchyma provides a significant retarding force to a penetrating missile, increasing the level of energy transfer to the liver. Secondary blast effects differ significantly depending on the distance of the casualty from the explosion. In contrast to bullets, fragments from explosions tend to be of irregular shape, size and mass, which dissipate energy rapidly because of air resistance en route to their target – penetration is usually only superficial and the effects of cavitation limited at a distance from the blast. The fragment injuries may, however, be multiple and widespread. In contrast, closer to the site of explosion, the small fragments are highly energized and may penetrate visceral cavities, contributing significantly to the death toll.[16] It is worth remembering that gross mechanical damage, for example a large fragment wound to the buttock, does not necessarily imply significant clinical impairment, whereas minor mechanical damage, such as a penetrating eye injury, may have significant clinical impact. The recent popularity of suicide bombings introduces a further secondary blast effect – that of implantation of biological fragments of the bomber, at least one of whom has proven to be hepatitis B positive, into victims, although no cases of disease transmission have yet been recorded.[17]

Tertiary blast injury

Tertiary blast injury occurs as a result of the physical displacement of the victim by the blast wind or as a result of the effects of the blast wind on other structures, causing structural collapse and crush injury. Traditionally, traumatic amputation has been classed as a wholly tertiary effect, with the blast wind avulsing the flailing limb through a joint, akin to fast jet pilots ejecting into the slip stream. Experimental and epidemiological data now prove otherwise. Post-mortem examinations on 56 bodies with blast-induced traumatic amputations revealed only one occurring through a joint;[18] instead, the sites of predilection are the upper third of the tibia, upper and lower thirds of the femur in the lower limb, and the proximal thirds of both the arm and the forearm. The mechanism has been confirmed in an animal model to be initial fracture by coupling of the primary blast wave into the long bone with subsequent separation by the blast wind.[19] Traumatic amputation is uncommon in blast survivors, occurring in less than 1.5% of cases in one large series, for the reasons alluded to above – victims close enough to the explosion to suffer traumatic amputation are usually overcome by the other (primary and secondary) effects. Traumatic amputation in a survivor, therefore, is a marker of likely severe blast exposure.[20] Bodily displacement and subsequent impact with solid obstacles contributes to mortality through head trauma, and many late deaths occur because of this neurological injury.[21]

Quaternary blast injury

This disparate group of injuries comprises any blast effects that cannot be categorized in one of the preceding three groups. The two most common are burns and psychological injury. Some authorities include crush injury in the quaternary category. Despite the enormous amounts of thermal energy liberated by an explosion, burns are usually superficial flash burns and affect the exposed skin of face and hands (and legs in women). The psychological consequences of blast exposure are significant in those exposed and those treating the injured, as well as in the non-involved general public,[22] confirming the terrorist's *raison d'être* that the aim of terrorism is to terrorize and the old Chinese proverb 'Kill one – frighten 10 000'. Other quaternary effects are uncommon and include inhalational injury in association with burns or infectious or noxious agents dispersed by the dynamic overpressure.

Special situations

The chapter so far pertains to simple free-field detonations; however, common sense suggests that explosions can and do occur in 'non-idealized' circumstances and that these may modify the blast effects and distribution of injuries.

BLAST IN ENCLOSED SPACES

The most obvious circumstance is an explosion in an enclosed space. On detonation, the blast wave behaves as a Friedlander wave, but on encountering an obstacle, such as a wall, the blast wave is reflected and combines with the incident wave to increase the magnitude of the blast overpressure: twofold when reflected from a flat wall, by a factor of 4 when reflected from the junction of two walls and eightfold at the junction of three reflecting surfaces such as on the floor in the corner of a room. Thus, people close to a blast may be relatively unaffected by the passage of the blast wave, but people further away in areas of blast reflection may be killed by the magnified overpressure.[16]

UNDERWATER BLAST

This differs from air detonation by virtue of the transmission characteristics of water, which act to transmit the blast wave more effectively whilst retarding the passage of energized fragments; hence there is a greater incidence of PBI but decreased secondary effects in underwater blast. In addition, the 'blast wind' acts as an energized water ram, causing gross body wall distortion and shear wave generation with tearing of fixed organs such as the liver. Reflection of the blast wave at the water's surface is a reductive phenomenon, with the overpressure being least just beneath the surface and increasing with depth. This exposes the abdomen to a greater blast load with relative thoracic sparing and explains the much greater incidence of abdominal blast injury in underwater explosions.[23] Anyone in the water when an explosion is imminent should therefore float on his or her back to minimize the blast effects.

> Suspect abdominal primary blast injury in underwater blasts.

BLAST THROUGH BALLISTIC PROTECTION

There is controversy as to whether ballistic protection vests may potentially increase the incidence of pulmonary PBI, perhaps by increasing presented area or by the Kevlar layers increasing intrathoracic coupling of the blast wave. The limited evidence from experimental studies is conflicting, but overall the benefits of ballistic protection outweigh any potential negative effects in the much rarer situation of blast exposure.

ENHANCED BLAST WEAPONS

These use a primary air burst to distribute a volatile hydrocarbon through the atmosphere, which is then secondarily detonated generating a blast wave of increased duration but slightly lower peak pressure over a wide area compared with standard explosives. In contrast to conventional munitions, enhanced blast weapons (EBW) utilize the blast wave to primarily engage the target as the secondary effects are minimal. They are readily available in a variety of formats, including shoulder launched missiles, and have been used with great success in Chechnya, Afghanistan and Iraq.[24]

IMMEDIATE TREATMENT PRIORITIES

Notification of an explosion and the likelihood of blast casualties must include information regarding the location and circumstances, as this influences the distribution of injuries. Blast in an enclosed space such as a bus generates significantly greater mortality, a higher incidence of pulmonary PBI amongst survivors and a greater need for tube thoracostomy compared with open-air blast.[25] Initial assessment is carried out in a systematic manner as for any other trauma casualty, with <catastrophic haemorrhage>, airway, breathing and circulation the priorities. Where structural collapse is the predominant feature, such as in the bombing of the Alfred Murrah building in Oklahoma, a different pattern of injury can be expected, with few patients requiring ventilatory support but tertiary effects, particularly crush injuries, predominating.[26] Crush injuries, often in conjunction with haemorrhage, mandate adequate resuscitation to maintain the circulating volume and maintain a diuresis in the face of acute nephropathy from rhabdomyolysis.

Diagnosis of primary blast injury

Diagnosis of primary blast injury requires a high index of suspicion. The most accessible places to assess for PBI are the tympanic membranes. A ruptured tympanic membrane will occur in up to 90% of significant blast exposures but does not correlate with blast injury elsewhere; indeed, pulmonary PBI has been reported with intact tympanic membraness.[27] Despite this, otoscopic examination can be used as a rapid preliminary triage tool, especially when there are mass casualties. The pathophysiological effects of pulmonary blast

injury result in a recognizable constellation of signs, symptoms and radiographic appearances (Table 19.2).

> Tympanic membrane rupture is a marker of blast exposure; absence of rupture does not exclude primary blast injury.

Most authorities contend that these signs, symptoms and chest radiograph appearances are apparent at presentation,[27] although progression of the radiographic appearances over the following 48 hours followed by gradual resolution is to be expected. Alveolar haemorrhage limits gas exchange, and hypoxaemia, with or without hypercarbia, may be an early indicator of pulmonary PBI before other signs are readily apparent.[28] Abdominal blast injury may be readily apparent, with signs of peritonism from gastrointestinal perforation or bleeding from solid visceral injury mandating urgent laparotomy; it may present more insidiously, however, with delayed perforation of a mural haematoma up to 14 days after injury. Patients may also present with cramping abdominal pain, vomiting and melaena from partial obstruction by the haematomas.[29] It is notable that in the absence of peritoneal signs mandating laparotomy, no radiological or laboratory investigation is sufficiently accurate to diagnose abdominal blast injury.

De Palma et al.[28] propose a triage algorithm based upon the presence of injuries, the integrity of the eardrums and the maintenance of oxygen saturations; in addition, any casualty in whom blast injury is even fleetingly suspected should undergo plain chest radiography unless a mass casualty situation precludes it. Box 19.1 lists those people who would be suitable for discharge from the emergency department.

Treatment of primary blast injury

Pulmonary PBI resembles pulmonary contusions of other aetiologies and the basic tenets of management are similar.

Table 19.2 Clinical manifestations of pulmonary primary blast injury

Symptoms	Signs	Chest radiograph appearances
Cough – initially dry, progressing to white frothy sputum and eventually haemoptysis	Tachypnoea Cyanosis Subcutaneous emphysema	Bilateral fluffy infiltrates (butterfly wings appearance). New infiltrates after 48 hours suggest acute respiratory distress syndrome or superadded infection
Shortness of breath	Dullness to percussion	Haemo/pneumothorax
Pleuritic chest pain – typically retrosternal	Decreased breath sounds	Subcutaneous emphysema
Hoarse voice	Widespread rhonchi	Pneumomediastinum
	Retrosternal emphysema	Pneumoperitoneum
	Haemo/pneumothorax	Peribronchial emphysema
	Retinal artery emboli	

High peak inspiratory pressures are injurious to an already damaged lung and predispose to further lung injury – alveolar haemorrhage, pneumothoraces and dispersal of systemic air emboli. The ideal strategy is a high-frequency, low-tidal-volume and low-inflation-pressure regimen with permissive hypercapnia.[30] In addition, novel strategies such as nitric oxide ventilation, independent lung ventilation and extracorporeal membrane oxygenation have also been tried with variable results.[31] Fluid therapy is tailored to avoid exacerbating pulmonary oedema. The possibility of delayed pneumothorax during mechanical ventilation remains, and if prolonged general anaesthesia, air evacuation or positive end-expiratory pressure is necessary, prophylactic tube thoracostomies are recommended. The outcome from primary pulmonary blast injury, however, is excellent, with normal lung function to be expected in survivors.[32] Ruptured tympanic membranes generally need no acute intervention, and most will heal spontaneously if kept clean and dry; significant debris in the ear canal should be gently removed and antibiotic eardrops started. Patients with large perforations or perforations that have not healed should be referred for specialist opinion and potential tympanoplasty, although this is often delayed until 1 year after injury. Implantation of keratinized squamous epithelium into the middle ear is responsible for cholesteatoma formation in up to 12% of patients[33] and may occur up to 4 years after perforation, implying a need for longer term follow-up of these people. Abdominal blast injury is similar to any other blunt abdominal trauma. Large mural haematomas (>15 mm in small bowel and >20 mm in the colon) are resected as they have a significant chance of later

Case scenario

A 21-year-old plumber was fixing an industrial boiler in a factory when the system exploded with him in close proximity. The fire service recovered him from the blazing factory and, after application of first aid in the form of water cooling of the obviously burnt areas, he was blue lighted to the local emergency department 5 minutes away. On arrival in the resuscitation room he is tachypnoeic (32 breaths per minute), tachycardic (100 beats/min) and in pain. He complains of pain on inspiration and has full-thickness burns to his arms and torso. He complains of tinnitus and deafness. There are scorch marks on his face and his nasal hairs are singed. He has a number of small penetrating wounds on his body from accelerated fragments. He also complains of severe abdominal pain.

Outline his likely injuries and detail your initial management

His proximity to a large explosion suggests that he is at risk of blast injury in many forms. He is likely to have primary blast injury involving his ears (tinnitus and deafness) and lungs (pleuritic chest pain, tachycardia and tachypnoea), and the presence of abdominal pain suggests abdominal blast injury as well. He has secondary blast injuries in the form of fragment penetrating injuries. He has burns as a quaternary blast effect. Pulse oximetry reveals an oxygen saturation of 89% despite high-flow oxygen by facemask, and his work of breathing is increasing. The decision is made to intubate him (hypoxia, singed nasal hairs and scorch marks, worsening respiratory function). Arterial blood gases reveal a PaO_2 of 6.2. A chest radiograph reveals bilateral pulmonary infiltrates. His torso burns total 12% of his body surface area and are not circumferential at any site. Abdominal examination suggests widespread peritonism and a decision is made to perform computed tomography (CT) scanning. The CT scan reveals intra-abdominal free fluid and a large amount of free gas.

Describe the significance of his abdominal CT findings and your continued management. How should he be ventilated?

The abdominal CT suggests that he has a gastrointestinal perforation necessitating emergency laparotomy. This reveals three full-thickness mural haematomas, one in the descending colon of 30 mm in diameter and two small bowel lesions, one of 10 and one of 20 mm diameter. There is also a frank perforation of his terminal ileum. The perforation and the two larger haematomas should be resected – the decision on anastomosis depends on the degree of contamination and his haemodynamic stability at that stage. Throughout this he should be ventilated using a low-pressure, high-frequency strategy allowing permissive hypercapnia.

After 48 hours of ventilation he is successfully weaned from the ventilator and makes an excellent recovery. He returns to normal lung function, and long-term ear, nose and throat follow-up after his ruptured eardrums reveals no evidence of cholesteatoma.

perforation.[34] Immediate perforations may be closed directly if there is no contamination, but exteriorization or repair with proximal diversion may be safer. Rhabdomyolysis from crush injury may need renal dialysis.

Treatment of other forms of blast injury

Limbs amputated or partially severed by secondary or tertiary blast effects are rarely suited to reimplantation or salvage, and a well-planned high amputation in healthy tissue well above the level of dissemination of contamination is indicated – the stump should be left open, reinspected and delayed primary closure undertaken at 5 days or when the wound is sufficiently clean. Direct closure with antibiotic coverage is rarely indicated and usually dangerous. Secondary blast wounds in survivors are often superficial, and conservative management may be undertaken if the criteria outlined in Box 19.2[35] are met – otherwise thorough debridement is needed.

Burns should be covered to minimize heat loss and, if >15% body surface area (or 10% in children or the elderly) is affected, i.v. fluid resuscitation using a recognized burns formula should be instituted. It is interesting that almost no articles dealing with blast injury suggest any potential treatments for the psychological effects of blast exposure. Therefore, recommendations for practice are difficult, although it is worth noting that critical incident stress debriefing has not been shown to decrease psychological

morbidity in survivors or the public at large[36] and has largely been abandoned.

> **Box 19.2 Criteria for conservative management of fragment wounds[35]**
>
> - Entry/exit wound <1 cm
> - No evidence of permanent cavitation within the wound
> - No neurovascular compromise
> - No compartment syndrome
> - Stable fracture pattern
> - No signs of infection
> - Have been treated early with dressings and antibiotics

SUMMARY

The globalization of terrorism with its attendant upsurge in bombings around the globe means that knowledge of the pathophysiology, diagnosis and treatment of blast injury is no longer the sole preserve of the military medical services. Blast injury should be actively suspected in all those potentially exposed to a blast until proven otherwise. In mass casualties, otoscopic examination of the tympanic membranes may be used as a triage tool. Primary blast lung has a recognizable constellation of symptoms, signs and radiographic appearances on which to make the diagnosis – treatment is ventilatory support utilizing a low-volume/low-pressure approach. An excellent functional recovery is to be expected in survivors. Abdominal blast injury is uncommon outside of underwater blast victims but may present with peritoneal signs from perforation or haemorrhage; however, the presentation may be delayed for many days because of the role of delayed perforation of gastrointestinal mural haematomas. Auditory blast injury is common but is often of little clinical relevance except for the potential for later cholesteatoma formation.

GLOBAL PERSPECTIVES

The global threat from terrorism now means that interest in the effects of blast injury is no longer confined to doctors in Northern Ireland and Israel – the railway bombing in Madrid in 2004 killed 191 people and injured more than 2000, with an incidence of primary blast lung injury of 63% among the critically ill immediate survivors.[37] It is noteworthy, however, that, international terrorism aside, the FBI reported 17 579 bombings, 427 related deaths and 4063 injuries in the USA between 1988 and 1997,[38] a significant proportion of the deaths and injuries resulting from the bombing of the Alfred Murrah building in Oklahoma city in 1995 by a disaffected American citizen – i.e. explosions and blast injury may be 'home grown'. The other 'blast' issue that has an enormous global impact is that of landmines. Despite the worldwide ban on their use in 1997, an estimated 70 million are still dispersed throughout the world,[39] and 24 000 new deaths or injuries from landmines are reported annually.[40] Detonation by stepping on one directs the shock wave directly into the limb, causing soft-tissue destruction and fractures of the bony skeleton by stress wave coupling into the limb bones. As the distances involved are short, the flow of hot gaseous products also plays a part, and this strips the soft tissues and exerts significant torsional forces on the long bones, which may, of course, already have been fractured by the blast wave effects. The subsequent dynamic overpressure then serves to detach or partially detach the injured limb and implant environmental debris, including soil, vegetation, clothing and shattered bone spicules, for a substantial distance proximal to the level of obvious injury, precluding limb salvage in most cases and necessitating a high amputation with consequent difficulties in rehabilitation.

REFERENCES

1.   Zuckerman S. Experimental study of blast injuries to the lungs. *Lancet* 1940;**2**:219–24.

2.   Logan DB. War wounds and air raid casualties. *BMJ* 1939:864–6.

3.   Ripple GR, Phillips Y. Military explosions. In: Cooper GJ, Dudley HAF, Gann SF, Little RA, Maynard RL, eds. *Scientific Foundations of Trauma*. Oxford: Butterworth-Heinemann, 1997, pp. 247–57.

4.   Danon YL, Nili E. Triage, Primary Treatment and Evacuation: the IDF experience in Lebanon. Paper presented at: Second International Congress in Israel on Disaster Management; 16–19 September 1984. Jerusalem: Israel Defence Force.

5.   Mellor SG, Cooper GJ. Analysis of 828 servicemen killed or injured by explosion in Northern Ireland 1970–84: the Hostile Action Casualty System. *Br J Surg* 1989;**76**:1006–10.

6.   Guy RJ, Kirkman E, Watkins PE, Cooper GJ. Physiologic responses to primary blast. *J Trauma* 1998;**45**:983–7.

7.   Irwin RJ, Lerner MR, Bealer JF, Brackett DJ, Tuggle DW. Cardiopulmonary physiology of primary blast injury. *J Trauma* 1997;**43**:650–5.

8.   Chiffelle TL. Pathology of direct air blast injury. *Technical progress report on contract DA-49-146-XZ-055 Ref. No. DASA-1778*. Albuquerque, NM: Lovelace Foundation for Medical Education and Research, 1966.

9.   Horrocks CL. Blast injuries: biophysics, pathophysiology and management principles. *J R Army Med Corps* 2001;**147**:28–40.

10.   Guy RJ, Glover MA, Cripps NPJ. Primary blast injury: pathophysiology and implications for treatment. Part III. Injury to the central nervous system and the limbs. *J R Nav Med Serv* 2000;**86**:27–31.

11.   Cooper GJ, Taylor DE. Biophysics of impact injury to the chest and abdomen. *J R Army Med Corps* 1989;**135**:58–67.

12.   Goligher JC, King DP, Simmons HT. Injuries produced by blast in water. *Lancet* 1943;**2**:119–23.

13.   Kerr AG. Blast injuries to the ear. *Practitioner* 1978;**221**:677–82.

14.   Clemedson CJ, Hultman HI. Air embolism and the cause of death in blast injury. *Mil Surg* 1954;**114**:424–37.

15.   Hill PF, Edwards DP, Bowyer GW. Small fragment wounds: biophysics, pathophysiology and principles of management. *J R Army Med Corps* 2001;**147**:41–51.

16.   Cooper GJ, Maynard RL, Cross NL, Hill JF. Casualties from terrorist bombings. *J Trauma* 1983;**23**:955–67.

17.   Eshkol Z, Katz K. Injuries from biologic material of suicide bombers. *Injury* 2005;**36**:271–4.

18.   Hull JB, Bowyer GW, Cooper GJ, Crane J. Pattern of injury in those dying from traumatic amputation caused by bomb blast. *Br J Surg* 1994;**81**:1132–5.

19.   Hull JB, Cooper GJ. Pattern and mechanism of traumatic amputation by explosive blast. *J Trauma* 1996;**40**(Suppl. 3):198–205.

20.   Frykberg ER, Tepas JJ, 3rd. Terrorist bombings. Lessons learned from Belfast to Beirut. *Ann Surg* 1988;**208**:569–76.

21.   Mellor SG. The relationship of blast loading to death and injury from explosion. *World J Surg* 1992;**16**:893–8.

22.   Tucker P, Pfefferbaum B, Vincent R, Boehler SD, Nixon SJ. Oklahoma City: disaster challenges mental health and medical administrators. *J Behav Health Serv Res* 1998;**25**:93–9.

23.   Huller T, Bazini Y. Blast injuries of the chest and abdomen. *Arch Surg* 1970;**100**:24–30.

24.   Dearden P. New blast weapons. *J R Army Med Corps* 2001;**147**:80–6.

25.   Leibovici D, Gofrit ON, Stein M, *et al*. Blast injuries: bus versus open-air bombings – a comparative study of injuries in survivors of open-air versus confined-space explosions. *J Trauma* 1996;**41**:1030–5.

26.   Hogan DE, Waeckerle JF, Dire DJ, Lillebridge SR. Emergency department impact of the Oklahoma City terrorist bombing. *Ann Emerg Med* 1999;**34**:160–7.

27.   Leibovici D, Gofrit ON, Shapira SC. Eardrum perforation in explosion survivors: is it a marker of pulmonary blast injury? *Ann Emerg Med* 1999;**34**:168–72.

28.   De Palma RG, Burris DG, Champion HR, Hodgson MJ. Blast injuries. *N Engl J Med* 2005;**352**:1335–42.

29.   Mellor SG. The pathogenesis of blast injury and its management. *Br J Hosp Med* 1988;**39**:536–9.

30.   Sorkine P, Szold O, Kluger Y, *et al*. Permissive hypercapnia ventilation in patients with severe pulmonary blast trauma. *J Trauma* 1998;**45**:35–8.

31.   Pizov R, Oppenheim-Eden A, Matot I, *et al*. Blast lung injury from an explosion on a civilian bus. *Chest* 1999;**115**:165–72.

32.   Hirshberg B, Oppenheim-Eden A, Pizov R, *et al*. Recovery from blast lung injury: one-year follow-up. *Chest* 1999;**116**:1683–8.

33.   Seaman RW, Newell RC. Another etiology of middle ear cholesteatoma. *Arch Otolaryngol* 1971;**94**:440–2.

34.   Cripps NP, Cooper GJ. Risk of late perforation in intestinal contusions caused by explosive blast. *Br J Surg* 1997;**84**:1298–303.

35.   Bowyer GW. Management of small fragment wounds in modern warfare: a return to Hunterian principles? *Ann R Coll Surg Engl* 1997;**79**:175–82.

36.   van Emmerik AA, Kamphuis JH, Hulsbosch AM, Emmelkamp PM. Single session debriefing after psychological trauma: a meta-analysis. *Lancet* 2002;**360**:766–71.

37.   Gutierrez de Ceballos JP, Turegano Fuentes F, Perez Diaz D, *et al*. Casualties treated at the closest hospital in the Madrid, March 11, terrorist bombings. *Crit Care Med* 2005;**33**(Suppl. 1):107–12.

38.   Noji EK, Lee CY, Davis T, Peleg K. Investigation of Federal Bureau of Investigation bomb-related death and injury data in the United States between 1988 and 1997. *Mil Med* 2005;**170**:595–8.

39.   Injuries associated with landmines and unexploded ordnance – Afghanistan, 1997–2002. *MMWR Morb Mortal Wkly Rep* 2003;**52**:859–862.

40.   Giannou C. Antipersonnel landmines: facts, fictions, and priorities. *BMJ* 1997;**315**:1453–4.

20

Injuries due to burns and cold

OBJECTIVES

After completing this chapter the reader will:
- understand the importance of burn care in trauma management as a whole
- know a meaningful burns classification
- know a simple care pathway for all burn patients

- understand the link between pre-hospital and emergency department management
- understand the course of management thereafter
- understand the range of injuries caused by cold.

INJURIES DUE TO BURNS

Definition

A burn is an injury caused by energy transfer to the body's tissues, causing necrosis and an associated inflammatory reaction. Different forms of energy transfer cause predictable patterns of injury and the severity depends on the causative agent, time and area of contact and initial management.

Introduction

Hot water splashes from a kettle or flashback whilst lighting a barbeque are common, easily recognizable examples of minor burns. Serious burns are fortunately less common. UK emergency departments see approximately 175 000 burn patients per year, 15 000 of whom have to be admitted for more advanced care.[1] The burn victim presents difficult challenges. The unpleasant nature of the injury is exacerbated by high levels of distress in the victim, their relatives and often in staff. Burns are life-changing and potentially life-threatening injuries. As with all victims of trauma, appropriate and timely assessment, resuscitation and transfer to definitive care offer the best chance for optimal recovery.

Pathophysiology

Temperatures >40°C denature proteins and cause cellular dysfunction. Above 45°C, cellular repair mechanisms are overwhelmed and cell death occurs in about 1 hour. At 60°C necrosis and vessel thrombosis occur almost immediately.[2]

The inflammatory process associated with burn injury evolves during the 8–24 hours after the burn and can cause further local and systemic injury. There is increased capillary permeability with fluid loss from the intravascular space. The magnitude of the inflammatory response is related to the extent of the tissue injury and is most easily expressed as the percentage of the total body surface area (% TBSA) that is burnt. Superficial burns cause only erythema with no significant capillary leakage. In burns greater than approximately 20% TBSA, the inflammatory mediators affect the whole body and patients may develop a systemic inflammatory response syndrome (SIRS)[3] over several hours, with significant intravascular fluid loss and the potential for the development of hypovolaemic shock.[4] Other causes of hypovolaemia, for example from associated traumatic injuries from jumping to escape a fire, should be excluded before attributing hypovolaemia solely to the burn injury.

Burns classification

The depth of a burn dictates wound management and the need for surgery but has no bearing on first aid outside of hospital or initial resuscitative measures in the emergency department.

Classification of burn by depth is difficult to establish, even for experienced burns doctors.[5] Burns may involve the full thickness, or only part of the thickness of the skin.

Partial-thickness burns are subclassified depending on which parts of the skin are involved: epidermal, superficial dermal, mid-dermal and deep dermal burns. Burn wounds are often not homogeneous and a mixed pattern may be seen; for example, there is usually a border of intensely painful partial-thickness burn surrounding full-thickness burns, which are characteristically painless.

Communication between carers is simplified by using a classification based on burn aetiology, from which depth of burn or other sequelae can be predicted.

- *Flame burn.* The patient or part of his or her clothing has caught fire; the patient will have an area of deep burn likely to require surgery.
- *Flash burn.* Flames are seen and felt but the patient has not actually caught fire. This results most often in superficial depth burns with hair or eyebrow singeing. Although caused by high temperatures, the time exposure is short so that the resulting injury is usually not severe.
- *Scald.* Scalds often result in a mixed pattern of burn depth, with the deepest burns occurring at the point of initial contact and burns to peripheral areas being less deep. The severity of scalds depends on the temperature of the water.
- *Electrical burn.* Low voltages (<1000 volts) from domestic or DIY accidents usually result in small area(s) of deep burn. High voltages (>1000 volts) are typically associated with a 'flash' burn but the localized tissue damage is characteristically more severe, resulting in multiple systemic sequelae including renal failure and acute respiratory distress syndrome (ARDS).
- *Sunburn.* This is most often superficial but may still require fluid resuscitation depending on the area affected.
- *Chemical burns.* These are defined by whether the causative agent was acid or alkali and their severity depends on the concentration, duration of contact and the rapidity of first-aid measures. Occasionally, specific treatment with an antidote such as in hydrofluoric acid burns is required.
- *Contact burns.* These can be caused by, for example, molten metal, radiators, cigarettes, bitumen or phosphorus. The severity of the burn depends on the agent and the area and duration of contact. Specific treatment may be required, for example in the case of phosphorus burns prolonged water irrigation to remove particles of phosphorus is necessary.

Initial burn care pathway

Figure 20.1 outlines a stepwise approach to initial burn management.[6] It is a vertical pathway, but many stages may occur concurrently and clinical need may reorder the priorities. A logical <C>ABC approach is absolutely essential, although the majority of burn patients do not have injuries apart from their burn.

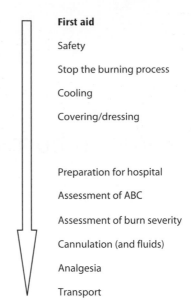

First aid

Safety

Stop the burning process

Cooling

Covering/dressing

Preparation for hospital

Assessment of ABC

Assessment of burn severity

Cannulation (and fluids)

Analgesia

Transport

Figure 20.1 A simple plan for burn patient care.

At the point of injury, the burning process should be stopped as quickly as possible by removing the patient from the source, smothering, 'drop and roll' or irrigation. Jewellery or constrictive clothing should be removed, powders or other contact agents should be brushed off and the wound should be cooled, ideally under running water for 10–20 minutes. This acts as an analgesic and decreases the inflammatory reaction associated with the injury.[7]

For smaller burns, cooling can be continued en route to hospital with the use of a cold flannel over the part or Water-Jel products, which act as a heatsink. The dressing should occlude the wound to keep it clean and cover the raw nerve endings. Clingfilm is ideal as a non-stick, temporary dressing prior to transfer.

The patient should be kept warm as hypothermia is a particular problem in patients with large-area burns and in children. Cooling should be judicious in these groups so as not to delay other actions in the care pathway or transfer to hospital. Analgesia prior to dressings may be ineffective until the wound is covered.

> At this stage, the causative agent of the burn is unimportant – simple first-aid measures performed well are the priority.

Assessment of <C>ABC is, at this stage, no different from other traumatic injuries. Initial assessment of burn severity requires knowledge of both the type and size of burn. This information is most useful to the receiving hospital but should not delay transfer. There are numerous schemes for burn size calculation, but serial halving is quick and provides satisfactory initial information (Figure 20.2). Erythema or redness should not be included in calculations; however, in reality it may be difficult to tell

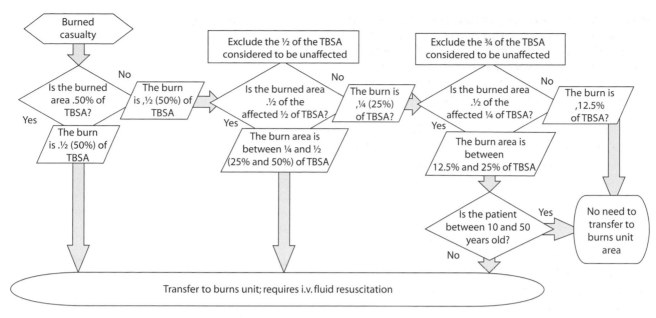

Figure 20.2 The algorithm for serial halving. TBSA, total body surface area.

the difference between simple erythema and superficial burn and it is better to overestimate burn size initially.

Cannulation outside of hospital allows early administration of i.v. analgesia and antiemetics and the commencement of i.v. crystalloid infusion. Hypovolaemia in the early stages after burn injury may signify other injuries and prompt further <C>ABC assessment. The patient should be transported to the nearest appropriate hospital, which will usually be the nearest emergency department, but in cities with more than one hospital in close proximity the hospital with the resident plastic surgery or burns service would be most appropriate, in order to allow more accurate and prompt secondary assessment and prevent needless secondary transfer.

AIRWAY/INHALATION INJURY

Inhalation injury is not a single entity, but consists of three components. Indicators of possible inhalation injury are outlined in Table 20.1.

- *True airway burns* are caused by inhalation of hot gases in the form of flame, smoke or steam. The upper airways are efficient at dissipating heat, and the larynx closes quickly. The resulting injury is thermal in nature and affects the supraglottic airway. The initial manifestation is upper airway oedema, which develops over hours and peaks between 12 and 36 hours. It requires early airway care and administration of high-flow humidified oxygen.
- *Lung injury* occurs as the inhaled products of combustion dissolve in the fluid lining the bronchial tree and alveoli. The resultant chemical injury to the lower airways leads to pulmonary failure, which is often delayed by hours or days. Lower airway injury results in difficulty in ventilation and gas exchange. Management is highly specialized and, even in the absence of a cutaneous burn, inhalational lung injury should be referred to a specialist centre.
- *Systemic intoxication* follows absorption of the products of combustion through the alveoli. The most commonly encountered substances are from carbon monoxide and cyanide, which account for the majority of deaths from fires. Death from these agents usually occurs at the scene.

Carbon Monoxide Poisoning

Carbon monoxide has a 240 times greater affinity for the haemoglobin molecule than does oxygen, which it readily displaces, inducing hypoxaemia. It also binds to the intracellular cytochrome system, causing abnormal cellular function. A carboxyhaemoglobin level <10% causes no symptoms and is commonly found in heavy

Table 20.1 Indicators of possible inhalational injury

History of exposure to fire/smoke in an enclosed space such as building or vehicle
History of exposure to a blast
Collapse, confusion or restlessness at any time
Hoarseness, cough or change of voice
Inspiratory stridor or expiratory wheeze
Obvious face burn including blisters or singed nasal hair
Soot in sputum
Inflamed oropharynx
Increased carboxyhaemaglobin levels on blood gas analysis
Deteriorating lung function

smokers. At levels above 20%, feelings of fatigue and nausea begin and higher mental functions are impaired; greater than 40% carboxyhaemoglobinaemia leads to progressive loss of neurological function, with death occurring at levels over 60%.

In the presence of carboxyhaemoglobin, pulse oximeter readings are unreliable indicators of oxygen saturation. Arterial blood gas analysis and a chest radiograph should be performed, but findings may be normal initially. The management of systemic intoxication is aimed at maximizing oxygen delivery.

> Pulse oximetry is unreliable in carbon monoxide performance.

Carboxyhaemoglobin has a half-life of 250 minutes in a patient breathing room air, but this reduces to 40 minutes when breathing 100% oxygen; thus, the highest possible oxygen concentration should be administered, which may necessitate intubation and ventilation. Dissociation of carbon monoxide from intracellular cytochromes is slower and can lead to a secondary rise in carboxyhaemoglobin levels; oxygen administration should continue for at least 24 hours. Hyperbaric oxygen treatment speeds up carbon monoxide clearance, but is not easily available and trials have not confirmed improved outcomes.[8] Steroids are of no benefit.[9]

> A burn sustained within an enclosed space is the key predictor of an inhalational injury.

Emergency department management

Burn injury assessment in the emergency department begins like any other trauma with <C>ABCDE, remembering that the burn may be an isolated finding or associated with 'escape' injuries. Any burn ≥10% TBSA should be assessed and treated in the resuscitation room. The burn wound, if adequately dressed in the pre-hospital environment, is best left covered until the primary survey is finished. The patient must be kept warm.

CATASTROPHIC HAEMORRHAGE

Catastrophic haemorrhage from associated injuries in the presence of significant burns is fortunately rare. Where it is present, conventional methods of haemorrhage control should be used before proceeding with the primary survey.

AIRWAY AND BREATHING

This concentrates on the diagnosis of any degree of inhalation injury, which allows the potential complications to be anticipated and treated appropriately. The signs and symptoms of airway oedema and pulmonary injury develop progressively over several hours and the key to diagnosis remains a high index of suspicion with frequent re-evaluation of those considered to be at risk. The main points of airway and breathing management are given in Table 20.2.

CIRCULATION

Hypovolaemic shock secondary to a burn takes some time to produce measurable physical signs; early shock in a burn victim necessitates exclusion of other causes and treatment according to the measures outlined in Chapter 8, independent of the severity of burn.

Intravenous access with two large-bore cannulae is ideal, avoiding cannulation through burnt skin if possible. Alternatives include i.v. cut-down, intraosseous infusion or central routes including the femoral vein. Blood must be sent for laboratory baseline investigations including carboxyhaemoglobin levels if inhalation injury is suspected. An initial carboxyhaemoglobin level can be established from an arterial blood gas analysis.

Fluid resuscitation of the burn wound is required for burns >10% TBSA in children and >15% in adults. The Parkland formula is the recommended UK formula for which half the calculated volume is given in the first 8 hours and the remainder in the following 16 hours:

$$\text{Volume (mL) of Hartmann's solution required in first 24 hours} = 4 \times \%\text{TBSA} \times \text{body weight (kg)}$$

The rate of fluid administration must take account of the time from injury so there is almost always a period of 'catch-up'. This formula includes the patient's weight, which if not available should be estimated. When the patient is a child, the parents may know the weight or a Broselow tape may be used; alternatively an initial fluid bolus of 20 mL/kg can be given, which can be repeated if necessary. The adequacy of resuscitation should be monitored by maintaining a urine output of at least 1 mL/kg/h for adults and children and double that for

Table 20.2 Key factors in airway and breathing treatment

All cases must receive high-concentration humidified oxygen

Any degree of upper airway obstruction mandates endotracheal intubation. Senior anaesthetic help is needed and an uncut endotracheal tube should be used as subsequent facial swelling may cause the connectors to oxygen tubing to disappear into the oropharynx

A high index of suspicion and early senior assessment will avoid the need for an emergency surgical airway

Patients with actual or suspected inhalational injury who require transfer to another hospital should be anaesthetized and intubated beforehand

toddlers. Heart rate and blood pressure are poor markers of resuscitation status in burns victims.

Deep burns, particularly following electrocution, cause the release of breakdown products of myoglobin and haemoglobin. These are excreted in the urine, turn it dark red and are deposited in the renal tubules, leading to renal failure. The initial treatment is to increase fluid resuscitation, aiming at achieving a urinary output of 2 mL/kg/h. Alkalinization of the urine and the use of mannitol can help but should be started only after consultation with the local burns centre. Regular re-evaluation is essential.

OTHER INITIAL INTERVENTIONS

Immunity against tetanus should be ensured, but in the absence of any specific indications, such as associated contaminated wounds, there is no requirement for antibiotic prophylaxis. A nasogastric tube should be considered as there is likely to be considerable gastric stasis. Adequate i.v. opiate analgesia should be administered early. The burn patient should be managed by a multidisciplinary team experienced in burn surgery, care and rehabilitation. This should ideally interface with the accident and emergency department after diagnosis and treatment of immediately life-threatening injuries.

In the absence of these other injuries early transfer to definitive care must be arranged. In the presence of other life-threatening injuries the burns specialist must be consulted so coordinated care is possible.

> Urine output is the best marker of adequacy of resuscitation in burns and urinary catheterization is essential.

Specialist management of the burn

Specialist burn assessment may be available in-house or may necessitate interhospital transfer. The patient should be reassessed using <C>ABCDE guidelines. The patient must be weighed, the size and depth of burn recalculated and the level of resuscitation and need for fluids established. The size and depth of burn will give an indication of its severity. There are three main risk factors for death following burn injury:

- age over 60 years;
- TBSA of burn over 40%;
- presence of an inhalational injury.

In major North American burn centres, the mortality rate is 0.3% if none of these factors is present, 3% if one is present, 33% if two, and 90% if all three are present.[10]

ASSESSMENT OF THE EXTENT OF THE BURN

To assess the size of a burn the patient must be completely undressed but kept warm. The size of burn is expressed as a percentage of the TBSA. There are several different ways of estimating this.

Serial Halving

The serial halving technique (Figure 20.2)[11] gives a 'rough and ready' reckoning of the size of a burn, dividing patients into those with under one-eighth, between one-eighth and one-quarter, between one-quarter and half, and over half of TBSA burns. This estimation is suited to use in the pre-hospital setting, as it allows basic management decisions to be taken regarding where to transfer the patient and the administration of i.v. fluids.

Palm = 1%

The entire palm and fingers (held adducted) of one of the *patient's* hands represent approximately 1% TBSA.

The rule of nines

The rule of nines[12] divides the body into areas representing 9% or 18% of TBSA. It is a useful rapid area assessment tool for use in adults. It is not accurate in children (especially babies and toddlers), who have bigger heads and smaller legs, and for whom *the rule of fives* can be used (Figure 20.3). It may be easier to count up the areas that are *not* burned, and take this away from the total.

Lund and Browder charts[13]

These charts break down the body into smaller pieces (Figure 20.4), allowing a more accurate assessment of burn size. There are different charts for different ages, allowing greater accuracy when assessing small children. These charts can be easily completed and faxed to the receiving burns centre.

ASSESSMENT OF THE DEPTH OF A BURN

The depth of the burn is notoriously difficult to judge, with an accuracy of only 65–80%; nevertheless, an initial assessment of burn depth is important. The classification of burn depth most commonly used by plastic surgeons is partial-thickness or full-thickness burns.

Partial-thickness burns

Partial-thickness burns do not involve the whole thickness of the skin, i.e. some viable dermis remains. Included in this category are epidermal, superficial, mid-dermal and deep dermal burns. Epidermal burns, for example sunburn, strictly are not true burns, but redness with some oedema. These burns are painful, but will heal rapidly. Superficial dermal burns involve injury to the superficial layers of the dermis. Oedema separates the dead dermis from the underlying dermis, forming blisters. The intact dermis still has a good blood and nerve supply. These

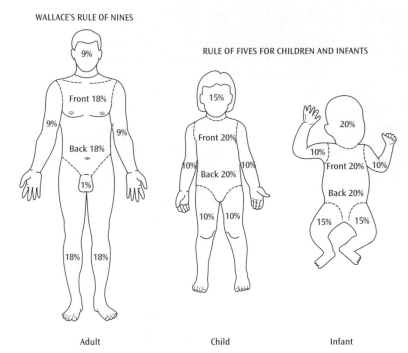

WALLACE'S RULE OF NINES

RULE OF FIVES FOR CHILDREN AND INFANTS

Adult   Child   Infant

Figure 20.3 The rules of nines and fives.

burns will blanche if touched and are very painful. Mid-dermal burns are difficult to assess clinically, even by experienced burn surgeons. The use of laser Doppler imaging can bring the accuracy of assessment up to 97%.[12] Deep dermal burns may be misleading by their 'pink' appearance, caused by the coagulated haemoglobin retained in capillaries. The majority of the dermis is injured, but with accurate and careful debridement some residual underlying dermis can be retained.

Full-Thickness Burns

In full-thickness burns, all the layers of the skin are destroyed. Healing can take place only by secondary intention, therefore surgery is indicated in all but the smallest of burns.

INITIAL DRESSINGS

After assessment of the wound, the wound should be dressed to minimize discomfort and distress and keep it clean until subsequent treatment takes place. These dressings may be the definitive treatment or be used only until surgical management of the wound commences. If the latter, the dressings are generally kept as simple and inexpensive as possible and emollient creams such as silver sulphadiazine (Flamazine™) are avoided.

Conservative management with dressings is appropriate for[14] superficial wounds that will heal by themselves within 2 weeks. Small, deeper wounds may be managed by surgery or dressings and the patient may opt for dressings with recourse to surgery if this fails. A range of dressings are available and may be coupled with the use of antibacterial agents such as Flamazine™:

- Hypafix is a contact adhesive fabric dressing that allows showering and prevents shear. It can be left on until the wound is healed or removed at 1–2 weeks.[15]
- Jelonet is non-adherent, simple and cheap. It is usually used in combination with an absorbent top layer, which needs changing every 48 hours because of accumulation of exudate.

Area	Age 0	Age 1	Age 5	Age 10	Age 15	Adult
A = ½ of head	9.5	8.5	6.5	5.5	4.5	3.5
B = ½ of one thigh	2.75	3.25	4	4.5	4.5	4.75
C = ½ of one lower leg	2.5	2.5	2.75	3	3.25	3.5

Figure 20.4 Lund and Browder chart with correction table for children.

- Mepitel is a non-adherent, silicone mesh dressing. It is more expensive than Jelonet but can be left on the wound for longer and is less painful to remove.

TIMING OF BURNS SURGERY

The decision as to whether surgery is needed, and if so when, can be complex and may be decided by the availability of staff, equipment and resources. In some centres, the burn patient may progress to early surgery in the resuscitation phase for scrubbing and cleaning of the patient and burn and early surgical techniques such as escharotomy, escharectomy, fasciotomy or burn wound excision.

ESCHAROTOMY

Burned tissue contracts as it dries out, which, combined with the tissue oedema generated by the widespread release of inflammatory mediators, can restrict the circulation to a limb or adequate ventilation of the chest. In young children, who rely on diaphragmatic movement for their ventilation, circumferential full-thickness burns to the abdomen can also cause respiratory embarrassment, seen as the need for increasing ventilatory pressures in a ventilated patient. Conventionally, this has required relieving incisions through the tight bands of burned tissues, allowing circulation to the limbs or ventilation to the chest. This is *escharotomy*.

Escharotomies are needed only if there is circulatory or ventilatory compromise, which does not usually occur until several hours after the injury, as the oedema increases – this means that it is a procedure rarely necessary outside of a specialist burns unit. It is rarely necessary for a non-specialist doctor to carry out escharotomy but, if it is, it should not be undertaken without prior discussion with the eventual receiving burns centre. Sufficient anatomical knowledge to site the escharotomy incisions avoiding superficially located nerves, such as the ulnar nerve, is essential (Figure 20.5). Escharotomy involves incisions into unburnt tissues and bleeding may be heavy. Electrocautery must be available. Appropriately equipped and resourced burns centres may proceed directly to total early burn excision, thereby eliminating the need for separate escharotomy.

EXCISION OF DEAD BURNED TISSUE

Dead burned tissue provides an almost perfect culture medium for micro-organisms and prolongs the inflammation associated with the burn. In addition, the proteins present in the slough bind nearly all topical antimicrobials used to try and prevent infection. This provides the rationale for excision of the burn wound, which should ideally be performed as early as possible to prevent invasive wound infection. Debridement should take place in a specialized centre with all necessary equipment, facilities and staff to provide the best possible

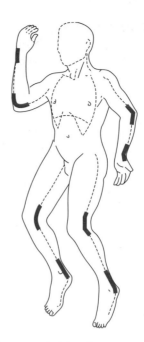

Figure 20.5 Escharatomy incision sites.

care. In children, in particular, debridement may necessitate transfer to a specialized paediatric burns centre.

The choice of which debridement method is used depends on the depth of the burn, the amount of slough and the experience of the surgeon. Very superficial burns need nothing more than gentle mechanical cleansing of loose tissue with a wet gauze swab (Box 20.1).

COVERAGE OF THE DEBRIDED WOUND

The decision as to what to cover the debrided wound with is an increasingly complex and 'hi-tech' one and a detailed description is beyond the remit of this chapter.

Skin grafting

This remains the gold standard for the reconstruction of deep dermal and full-thickness injuries. Early split-skin grafting from the patient's own unburnt skin (Figure 20.8) creates a partial-thickness skin injury that heals quickly, within 2 weeks, by secondary intention/re-epithelialization. The skin graft is tissue paper thin and, when moved to a debrided burn, the wound gains nutrition initially by diffusion from the wound base and then by ingrowth of blood vessels, which takes between 3 and 5 days. Small burn wounds can be covered with skin from readily available donor sites such as the thigh. However, large percentage TBSA burns may need repeated visits to the operating theatre, separated by time to allow donor site recovery and reuse. Skin graft coverage can be increased by meshing of the graft; however, the cosmetic appearance afterwards is not as good as with a plain sheet graft.

Box 20.1

- Tangential excision, using a Watson or Goulian knife (Figure 20.6), or a dermatome, remains the most common method to debride burns. Thin slivers of burnt tissue are removed until healthy tissue is reached. This is a fast technique, and the often significant blood loss can be reduced by the use of adrenaline infiltration and sterile tourniquets. There is a tendency to remove too much tissue, although the skin graft will still take adequately.
- *Dermabrasion* (Figure 20.7) by a rotating burr can be used to remove necrotic tissue – it is an often bloody and difficult technique.
- *Versajet™ hydrosurgery system*[16] is a new technique for debridement. It allows the removal of unhealthy tissue with the precision of dermabrasion but without the mess, and with the ease of blade excision but markedly lessened potential for excessive removal of healthy tissue. The use of the Versajet™ for surgical debridement is producing better cosmetic results following burn injury.
- *Enzymatic debridement* has been used in many parts of the world. Proteolytic and fibrinolytic enzymes, produced by bacteria, such as *Bacillus subtilis* (Travase™) or *Clostridia* species (Novuxol™), are applied to sloughy burns. Debridement spares unaffected tissue and subsequent mechanical debridement is easier. However, there are problems with bleeding, pain, wound infection and bacteraemia – in addition, the efficacy of these enzymes is reduced by the presence of commonly used antimicrobial agents, such as silver.[17] These wounds require close monitoring and potentially prophylactic topical antibiotics. Enzymatic techniques are not yet standard practice in most burns units.
- *Fascial excision*, using scalpel, cutting diathermy or harmonic (ultrasonic) scalpel, is sometimes required. This technique saves time and blood loss, but at the expense of poor cosmesis.

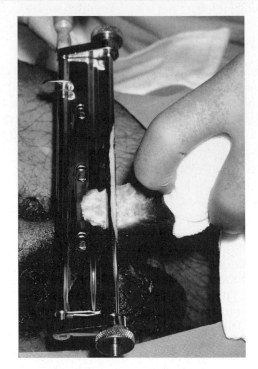

Figure 20.6 Tangential excision of a full thickness burn wound using a Watson knife.

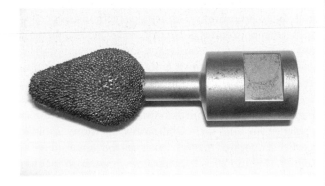

Figure 20.7 A dermabrasion burr.

Artificial skin dressings

Artificial skin dressings fall into two broad categories: temporary skin substitutes and dermal regeneration.

Temporary skin substitutes, such as Biobrane™ or Transcyte™, reduce pain scores, length of hospital stay and time to healing.[18,19] The frequency of dressing changes is also greatly reduced with the use of these dressings. They are suitable only for superficial to mid-dermal injuries. Biobrane™ is also used as a temporary wound dressing while the skin graft donor site heals, to allow reharvest, or while cultured epithelial cells are prepared.

Dermal regeneration templates, such as Integra™, can produce a better cosmetic and functional result by creating more dermis.[20] Integra™ is an 'off-the-shelf' tissue-engineered bilaminar dressing, the top silicone layer of which is removed after the underneath layer has become incorporated into the burn wound as neodermis. Like Biobrane™, Integra™ also aids in total burn wound excision and coverage when there is initially insufficient skin graft available. While the Integra™ dermal matrix is becoming integrated by the burn wound, skin graft donor sites can be reused and cultured cells prepared to place on top of the Integra™ once vascularized.

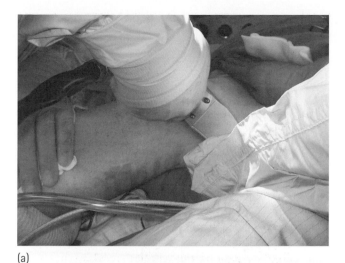

(a)

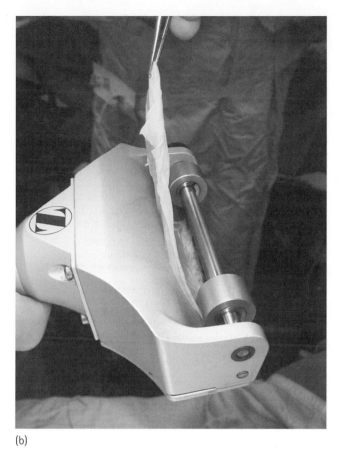

(b)

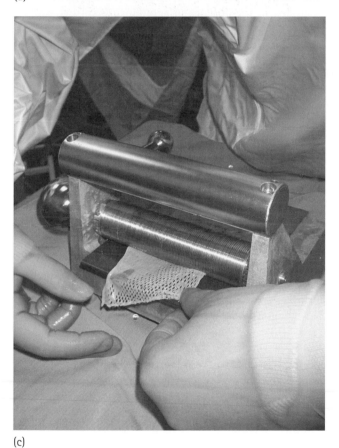

(c)

Figure 20.8   Skin graft being harvested from thigh, then meshed.

Newer developments

The use of cultured keratinocytes and non-cultured autologous keratinocyte suspensions (e.g. ReCell™) is increasing, and may remove the need for skin grafting in deep dermal burns.[21] Tissue engineering and research into embryonic and adult stem cells may one day provide an 'off-the-shelf' skin. This is likely to be a major area of research during the next 20 years.

AFTER WOUND HEALING

A burn injury can produce lifelong physical and psychological scars, which produce ongoing problems for the patient (Table 20.3). The ongoing management of these problems is outside the scope of this manual, but Table 20.4 lists some useful internet resources.

Table 20.3 Some of the ongoing problems for burns patients

Scar management including pressure garments, creams and
    sometimes further surgery to release contractures
Psychological support
Occupational therapy and physiotherapy to maximize function
Outpatient, outreach nursing support for dressings
Educational support
Different housing or change of facilities
Use of cosmetic camouflage or wigs

Table 20.4 Useful burns websites/resources

http://www.burnsurgery.com/
http://www.ilstraining.com/IDRT/idrt/brs_it_01.html
http://www.bapras.org.uk/UploadFiles/Burn%20Care%20Update%
    20-%207.pdf
http://www.who.int/violence_injury_prevention/publications/
    other_injury/en/index.html
http://www.changingfaces.co.uk/
http://www.britishburnassociation.co.uk/
http://www.emedicine.com
http://www.health.nsw.gov.au/public-health/burns/burnsmgt.pdf

INJURIES DUE TO COLD

In the UK, injuries due to cold are uncommon and, when seen, are normally associated with social deprivation or neglect. They are manifested as:

- hypothermia, the systemic effects of a reduced core temperature;
- local tissue damage.

Hypothermia

Hypothermia is defined as a reduction in the core temperature to <35°C, below which cognitive ability is reduced. Below 32°C, hypothermia is described as severe and there is cardiac irritability and progressive loss of consciousness. The normal measurable parameters of cardiac and respiratory function vary and may be difficult to elicit. The pathophysiological changes are normally reversible with rewarming.[22]

Unfortunately, hypothermia is also seen as a result of poor care of the severely injured trauma victim. The exposed unconscious patient in a cold resuscitation bay being administered unwarmed i.v. fluids has little chance of maintaining a normal core temperature. Hypothermia is an additional pathophysiological insult that impacts unfavourably on outcome.

Special low-reading thermometers need to be used when diagnosing hypothermia, and in severe cases an oesophageal probe is required.

In mild cases the patient should be kept in a warm room (30°C if possible) and all cold and wet clothes removed and replaced by warm blankets. Warmed fluids can be given by mouth or intravenously.

In severe hypothermia, an initial assessment following the <C>ABCDE approach should be performed. Invasive monitoring will be required, and the patient may be best managed in an intensive care environment. Unconscious patients require active core rewarming, and this may entail peritoneal lavage, haemodialysis or cardiopulmonary bypass – all of which should be performed only by experienced clinicians.

With a core temperature below 27°C there may be no external signs of life, yet full recovery from this situation is possible. The patient will require intubation and ventilation, and active core rewarming must be commenced. Because of cardiac irritability, unnecessary movements may trigger ventricular fibrillation, but cardiac massage must be continued in the absence of spontaneous cardiac output until the patient is warm enough for spontaneous output to return or for defibrillation to be effective. Expert management in an intensive care setting is essential.

Diagnosing death in this situation is difficult. The axiom 'not dead until warm and dead' is still valid, although due account of the circumstances surrounding the hypothermia must be taken. Resuscitative measures should continue until the core temperature is at least above 32°C or there is no rise in core temperature, despite active rewarming.

Local tissue damage

Extremities, such as the fingers, toes, nose and ears, may freeze when exposed to severe cold. The damage caused during freezing is exacerbated by a reperfusion injury on thawing, and tissue necrosis may follow. Typically, frozen skin is white and then becomes blue or purple on thawing. This is accompanied by swelling and can be extremely painful. Blistering of the skin may follow, and days later a thick carapace forms, which blackens. Eventually, sometimes after months, the carapace is shed to reveal new healthy skin underneath. In severe cases, significant amounts of tissue are lost in this process, and this can include autoamputation of entire digits.[23]

Frostnip is a minor form of frostbite in which the skin turns white and numb and which reverses on rewarming. Short-term pain and hyperaemia are the only sequelae.

If a body part is frozen, rewarming should be started as soon as possible. This is best achieved by immersion in circulating water heated to 40°C.[24] This should continue for at least 30 minutes or until thawing is complete. This process can be extremely painful, and strong analgesia will be required.[25] The subsequent management of the affected parts requires specialist care and referral should be made to a burn centre or plastic surgery unit. Avoidance of secondary infection is important, but antibiotics should be reserved for treatment rather than prophylaxis.

Case scenario

Using serial halving, estimate the area of the burn detailed in Figure 20.9
Using the serial halving technique, this burn can be seen to involve less than half of the TBSA, but more than one-quarter. This burn will need i.v. resuscitation and transfer to a burns centre.

Further assessment at the burns centre identifies this as a 38% TBSA burn and the patient weighs 78 kg on arrival at the burns centre. What are his fluid requirements for the first 24 hours from injury?
Using the Parkland formula his total volume requirements are:

$$\text{Volume (mL)} = 4 \times 38 \times 78 = 11\,856\,\text{mL}$$

This would involve infusion of approximately 6 litres in the first 8 hours after injury. In many instances, patients arrive in the burns centre having received only 1 or 2 litres in 4 hours since injury, necessitating rapid infusion of several litres in a short period of time. Another 6 litres is needed in the following 16 hours. The adequacy of this infusion rate must be assessed in light of the urine output, which must be at least 1 mL/kg/h.

In comparison, what is the TBSA shown in Figure 20.10; will this require i.v. resuscitation?
Using the serial having technique, this burn can be seen to involve less than one-eighth of the TBSA. In an otherwise fit young adult, i.v. resuscitation may not be required.

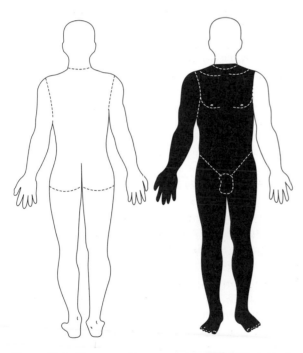

Figure 20.9 Diagrammatic representation of the extent of a patient's burn.

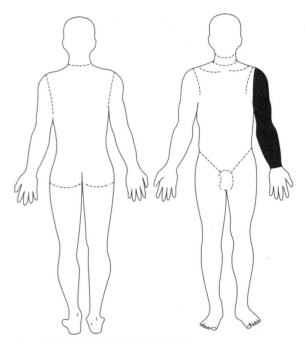

Figure 20.10 Diagrammatic representation of the extent of a patient's burn.

SUMMARY

Burns remain a common mechanism of injury in the UK and may be a result of a variety of aetiologies, although thermal burns remain the most frequent. Initial management of the burn follows the <C>ABCDE approach, recognizing that catastrophic haemorrhage is uncommon in burn victims. Cooling, analgesia and initiation of i.v. fluid replacement by a recognized formula are early priorities. Airway burns significantly increase the morbidity and mortality from a burn injury, and early recognition of the potential for airway or inhalational injury is vital. Communication with the regional burns centre is important at an early stage and is facilitated by an accurate assessment of the burnt surface area, for which age-appropriate Lund and Browder charts are ideal.

Superficial burns will heal rapidly with conservative management, but large or deep burns may need surgical intervention. Burn wound debridement has been improved by the availability of newer technologies that permit more controlled and bloodless excision of the burn wound, and similar advances in artificial skin substitutes mean that there are useful alternatives to split skin grafting when autologous skin is in short supply.

Cold injury is uncommon in the UK and is divided into hypothermia and local tissue damage, such as frostbite; gentle rewarming is the key in both situations, with the realization that extremity rewarming is extremely painful and will require good analgesic provision.

GLOBAL PERSPECTIVES

Patterns of burn injury vary according to a country's geographical and socioeconomic development. For example, flame burns from kerosene lamps are much more common in India than in the UK. Sadly, conflict also produces many burns victims from explosions and specific munitions. Many major incidents in developed countries involve multiple casualties who have multiple injuries, including burns. Triage of burns patients need not be specifically different from triage sieve or sort; however, remember impending airway compromise in the inhalation injury.[26–28] The facility for burns patient management varies across the world so that patient survival with large percentage burns will be possible only in well-funded centres or by transfer of patients to these centres.[29] It is the UK standard that burns of over 10% TBSA in children or 15% TBSA in adults receive i.v. fluid resuscitation, but in the developing world no-one with a burn under 25% TBSA would be given anything other than oral fluids.

REFERENCES

1. http://www.bapras.org.uk/cms_cat/161/National-Burn-Care-Review.htm.
2. Moritz AR, Henriquez FC. Studies of thermal injury. II. The relative importance of time and surface temperature in the causation of cutaneous burns. *Am J Pathol* 1947;**23**:695–720.
3. Arturson G. The pathophysiology of severe thermal injury. *J Burn Care Rehab* 1985;**6**:129–46.
4. Baxter CR. Fluid volume and electrolyte changes in the early post-burn period. *Clin Plast Surg* 1974;**1**:693–703.
5. Jackson DM. The diagnosis of the depth of burning. *Br J Surg* 1953;**40**:588–96.
6. Allison K, Porter K. Consensus on the pre-hospital approach to burns patient management. *Injury* 2004;**35**:734–8.
7. Jandera V, Hudson DA, deWet PM, Innes PM, Rode H. Cooling the burn wound: evaluation of different modalities. *Burns* 2000;**26**:265–70.
8. Scheinkestel CD, Bailey M, Myles PS, *et al.* Hyperbaric or normobaric oxygen for acute carbon monoxide poisoning: a randomised controlled clinical trial. *Med J Aust* 1999;**170**:203–10.
9. Levine BA, Petroff PA, Slade CL. Prospective trials of dexamethasone and aerosolized gentamicin in the treatment of inhalational injury in the burned patient. *J Trauma* 1978;**18**:188–93.
10. Ryan CM, Schoenfeld DA, Thorpe WP, *et al.* Objective estimates of the probability of death from burn injuries. *N Engl J Med* 1998;**338**:362–6.
11. Smith JJ, Malyon AD, Burge TS. A comparison of serial halving and the rule of nines as a pre-hospital assessment tool in burns. *Br J Plast Surg* 2005;**58**:957–67.
12. Pape SA, Skouras CA, Byrne PO. An audit of the use of laser Doppler imaging in the assessment of burns of intermediate depth. *Burns* 2001;**27**:233–9.
13. Lund CC, Browder NC. The estimation of areas of burns. *Surg Gynecol Obstet* 1944;**79**:532.
14. http://www.rch.org.au/burns/clinical/index.cfm?doc_id=2012.
15. Davey RB. The use of an 'adhesive contact medium' (Hypafix) for split skin graft fixation: a 12-year review. *Burns* 1997;**23**:615–19.
16. http://www.versajet.info/.
17. Hummel RP, Kautz PD, MacMillan BG, Altemeier WA. The continuing problem of sepsis following enzymatic debridement of burns. *J Trauma* 1974;**14**:572–9.
18. Barret JP, Dziewulski P, Ramzy PI, *et al.* Biobrane versus 1% silver sulfadiazine in second-degree pediatric burns. *Plast Reconstr Surg* 2000;**105**:62–5.
19. Kumar RJ, Kimble RM, Boots R, Pegg SP. Treatment of partial-thickness burns: a prospective, randomized trial using Transcyte. *ANZ J Surg* 2004;**74**:622–6.
20. Sheridan RL, Hegarty M, Tompkins RG, Burke JF. Artificial skin in massive burns – results to ten years. *Eur J Plastic Surg* 1994;**17**:91–93.
21. http://www.recell.info/hc_about.asp.
22. Riddell DI. A practical guide to cold injuries. *J R Nav Med Serv* 1986;**72**:20–5.
23. Mills WJ. Frostbite. *Alaska Med* 1983;**25**:33–8.

24. Smith DJ, Robson MC, Heggers JP. Frostbite and other cold induced injuries. In: Auerbach PS, Geehr EC, eds. *Management of Wilderness and Environmental Emergencies*. St Louis, MO: CV Mosby, 1989, pp.101–18.

25. http://www.who.int/violence_injury_prevention/publications/other_injury/en/index.html.

26. Welling L, van Harten SM, Patka P, *et al*. The cafe fire on New Year's Eve in Volendam, the Netherlands: description of events. *Burns* 2005;**31**:548–54.

27. Randic L, Carley S, Mackway-Jones K, Dunn K. Planning for major burns incidents in the UK using an accelerated Delphi technique. *Burns* 2002;**28**:405–12.

28. http://www.bapras.org.uk/UploadFiles/Burn%20Care%20Update%20-%207.pdf.

29. http://www.shrinershq.org/Hospitals/Boston/.

21

Analgesia and anaesthesia for the trauma patient

OBJECTIVES

After completing this chapter, the reader will:
- understand the specific problems of analgesia and anaesthesia in trauma patients
- understand the different modalities available for the management of trauma pain
- be able to outline the most appropriate agents for the relief of pain in trauma
- be able to identify relevant techniques for local, regional and general anaesthesia, and their complications.

INTRODUCTION

The International Association for the Study of Pain has defined pain as *an unpleasant sensory and emotional experience associated with actual or potential tissue damage or described in terms of such tissue damage.*[1]

Trauma patients will all suffer different degrees of pain, and the severity of this pain will depend not only on the nature of the injuries but also on the patients' perception of the injuries and events surrounding them as well as their emotional and psychological states,[2] and this must be taken into consideration when giving analgesia. In addition, pain should be relieved for physiological as well as compassionate reasons.

PATHOPHYSIOLOGY

Pain results in sympathetic stimulation and increases the level of circulating catecholamines. This causes peripheral vasoconstriction and tachycardia, increasing both myocardial work and afterload. This may precipitate cardiac ischaemia, especially in patients with ischaemic heart disease. Peripheral vasoconstriction diverts blood to central compartments, with the result that vascular beds such as the splanchnic circulation may suffer ischaemia. This may add to the ischaemia already induced by hypovolaemia.

Patients with painful chest and abdominal injuries are likely to avoid coughing to clear secretions from their lungs, resulting in secretion retention and possible hypostatic pneumonia.[3] However, analgesia itself may exacerbate these potential problems by causing respiratory depression. It is essential, therefore, to titrate intravenous analgesic drugs carefully in such patients,[4] and to consider methods, such as regional anaesthesia, which may avoid these complications.

ANALGESIA IN THE TRAUMA PATIENT

General considerations

Patients with multiple trauma (including head injury) will need analgesia, and this must not be withheld because of inappropriate concern that it will confuse patient assessment.

Analgesia may be provided by:

- Physical methods such as:
    - immobilization of fractures or burns dressings.
- Systemic analgesic drugs by a variety of routes and techniques (titrated boluses, simple infusion or patient-controlled infusion).
- Local anaesthetic techniques of local infiltration or regional block, which may be single-shot injection, or catheter technique for more prolonged effect.
- Psychological help by means of reassurance and explanation.

When administering analgesia, three factors should be considered:

1. the patient's condition and whether he or she has any allergies or is taking any other medications;

2. the route of drug administration, which will dictate speed of onset and duration of action;
3. the effect and side-effects of the drug, as well as potential antagonists and possible drug interactions.

Local anaesthetic blocks are useful, are often overlooked and avoid many of the risks of systemic analgesic drugs, particularly the respiratory depression that may occur with opioids. When administering systemic opioids, it is always necessary to:

- titrate the drug if given intravenously;[2]
- note the dose and time of administration;
- monitor the patient carefully;
- have naloxone available;
- have facilities for the artificial support of respiration.

Specific problems

HEAD INJURY

Patients with head injury may be restless, and/or have a reduced level of consciousness, so analgesic requirements can be difficult to assess. Some analgesic drugs have effects that are particularly dangerous in patients with a head injury:

- Opioids:
  - sedation, which complicates the assessment of level of consciousness
  - miosis, which complicates assessment of the pupils
  - respiratory depression with hypoxaemia and hypercarbia, leading to raised intracranial pressure.
- Nitrous oxide:
  - cerebral vasodilatation, which raises intracranial pressure.
- Ketamine:
  - increased cerebral blood flow and intracranial pressure.

> Give analgesia to patients with head injuries if required, but do so carefully and with appropriate monitoring.

THE 'RESTLESS' TRAUMA PATIENT

Many trauma patients are restless and distressed, and it is important to identify the cause of this before administering analgesia. Important causes of restlessness must first be excluded and treated:

- hypoxaemia;
- head injury;
- the effects of drugs or alcohol;
- a full bladder.

> Avoid analgesics in a restless patient until other treatable causes have been identified and corrected.

ROUTES OF DRUG ADMINISTRATION

Intravenous

Intravenous administration allows the drug to reach its site of action rapidly, and this is a particularly effective and controllable way of administering analgesia in the trauma patient. However, intravenous administration does not necessarily imply an immediate effect as morphine takes at least 10 minutes to achieve its peak effect because of the time taken to cross the blood–brain barrier. The optimal method of administering intravenous opioids is to use small, titrated doses. In hypovolaemic patients, the onset of action may be even slower and a lower total dose may be required. Administration by the intravenous route increases the risk of serious anaphylactic reactions and extravasation of the drug may cause a painful reaction and, in some cases, tissue necrosis.

Intramuscular and subcutaneous

These routes may be used in haemodynamically stable patients with moderate pain that is not expected to be prolonged. In patients with severe and/or prolonged pain, intravenous analgesics or a local anaesthetic technique are more appropriate. In the shocked trauma patient, absorption of the drug may be delayed because of poor peripheral circulation,[5] resulting in ineffective analgesia, and a second dose of drug may be given. When the circulation is restored, a large depot of drug is then absorbed rapidly, with the potential for overdosage. Even in haemodynamically stable patients, analgesia is often poor due to 'peak-and-trough' blood levels. This occurs because of large patient variability in dose requirements, delayed systemic absorption, and staffing issues such as delays in administration and reluctance to give repeat doses at frequent enough intervals. Intramuscular injections may also cause discomfort and local tissue reactions.

Oral

The principal disadvantage of this route is the slow absorption and delayed onset of action, which may be up to an hour after administration, exacerbated in trauma patients by delayed gastric emptying. Drugs absorbed from the gut enter the portal circulation and may be partly metabolized in the liver, reducing their efficacy. Oral administration of drugs in trauma patients has limited use, and is reserved for minor uncomplicated injuries.

Rectal and sublingual

These routes of administration allow more rapid absorption of the drug and bypass of the portal circulation; thus, more drug reaches the site of action.

Intraosseous

Drugs and fluids administered by the intraosseous route reach the circulation almost as rapidly as by the intravenous route. Many intravenous drugs used for resuscitation, analgesia and anaesthesia may also be administered by this route.[6]

Inhalation and infiltration

These are covered in the sections on nitrous oxide (p. 242) and local anaesthesia (p. 243) respectively.

> Intravenous opioid, titrated to effect, is the best method of administering analgesia to trauma patients.

SYSTEMIC ANALGESIC DRUGS

An analgesic is a drug which, in appropriate doses, relieves pain without depressing consciousness as an anaesthetic drug would. Examples include opioids, non-steroidal anti-inflammatory drugs, nitrous oxide and ketamine.

Opioids

These are drugs that are structurally related to morphine, and are either naturally occurring or synthetic.[7] They are classified by their actions on receptors for endogenous peptide neurotransmitters, enkephalins, endorphins and dynorphins. 'Opiates' are derived from the opium poppy, *Papaver somniferum*. Opioid receptors of several types are present in the brain and spinal cord, the best known being the μ, κ and δ subtypes. Opioid analgesics act as either agonists, partial agonists or antagonists at these receptors (Table 21.1).

Individual opioids vary, but have the following general side-effects:

- *Respiratory depression*: this may be severe in overdose, and the resulting hypoxaemia and hypercarbia is especially dangerous in patients with a head injury.
- *Sedation*: often advantageous, but excessive doses of opioid can lead to unconsciousness and airway compromise.
- *Hypotension*: due to vasodilatation – usually mild, but may be more severe in hypovolaemic patients. Morphine may also cause hypotension due to systemic histamine release.
- *Bradycardia*: not always seen in trauma patients due to sympathetic activation and other factors.

Table 21.1 Classification of opioid drugs, receptor types and clinical effects

	Receptor		
	μ	κ	δ
Agonists	Morphine	Pentazocine	Pentazocine
	Diamorphine		
	Pethidine		
	Fentanyl		
	Alfentanil		
	Codeine		
	Methadone		
Partial agonists	Buprenorphine	Nalbuphine	
Antagonists	Naloxone	Naloxone	
	Pentazocine		
	Nalbuphine		
Effects	Analgesia	Analgesia	Anti-analgesia, reversal of overdose
Adverse effects	Respiratory depression	Dysphoria	Dysphoria
	Sedation	Miosis	Mydriasis
	Cough suppression	Respiratory stimulation	
	Dependency	Tachycardia	
	Miosis		
	Bradycardia		
	Nausea, vomiting		

- *Nausea and vomiting*: a 'minor complication' to staff, but very unpleasant for the patient. Antiemetics are usually given with intravenous opiates.
- *Miosis*: may complicate the assessment of head injury.
- *Physical dependence*: not a problem when used for acute pain relief.

Many opioids are poorly absorbed orally due to extensive hepatic 'first-pass' metabolism. In trauma patients they are best given intravenously, and titrated to effect. High doses are often needed in severe trauma, and there is wide variability in dose requirement between patients – up to 20–30 mg of i.v. morphine may be needed in titrated doses in a fit young patient with severe injuries. The pharmacokinetics of various opioid analgesics are outlined in Table 21.2.

MORPHINE

Morphine is a widely used strong opioid, with all the side-effects listed above. A suitable intravenous starting dose is 2.5–5 mg depending on the patient's age, size and condition, with increments of 2–5 mg as required. Morphine is less lipid-soluble than some other opioids, and takes longer to penetrate the blood–brain barrier. Therefore, although some analgesia occurs within a few minutes, the peak effect is not seen for 10–15 minutes. A wheal is often seen along the track of intravenous administration due to local histamine release, although this usually resolves quickly. Systemic histamine release may contribute to mild hypotension after intravenous administration. Morphine is often used for more prolonged periods, by infusions or patient-controlled analgesia (PCA). In trauma patients with hepatic or renal dysfunction, the effect may be exaggerated by the accumulation of morphine or its metabolites after prolonged use.

DIAMORPHINE

Diamorphine (3,6-diacetyl morphine) has similar clinical effects to morphine. The effects are due to its conversion in the body to the active metabolites 6-mono-acetylmorphine (6-MAM) and morphine. Both diamorphine and 6-MAM are more lipid soluble than morphine itself. They therefore cross the blood–brain barrier more readily, leading to a more rapid onset and the requirement for a lower dose.

PETHIDINE

The actions and side-effects of pethidine are similar to those of morphine. It also has anticholinergic effects, causing a dry mouth and tachycardia. Sedation and miosis are less marked than with morphine.

FENTANYL

Fentanyl is a lipid-soluble, synthetic opioid. It has a faster onset of action than morphine when given intravenously and is shorter acting. It has similar side-effects to morphine, but causes less hypotension and does not cause histamine release. Fentanyl is commonly used in conjunction with anaesthetic induction agents to help reduce the hypertensive response to intubation, especially in patients with a head injury.

ALFENTANIL AND REMIFENTANIL

These are similar to fentanyl, but have a more rapid onset and offset of action. Remifentanil is a unique ultra-short-acting opiate, being metabolized extremely quickly by non-specific esterases. It is therefore given only by infusion. Both alfentanil and remifentanil can cause profound respiratory depression. They are used in anaesthesia and intensive care, but otherwise are of very limited use in the trauma patient.

NALBUPHINE

Nalbuphine is a partial κ agonist and μ antagonist, its advantage being that it has a ceiling level of effect. With doses over 30 mg there is no increase in analgesia, and,

Table 21.2 Pharmacokinetic characteristics of common opioid analgesics

	Initial dose	Route	Time to onset	Duration of action
Morphine	0.1 mg/kg	i.v.	10 minutes	2–4 hours
Diamorphine	0.05 mg/kg	i.v.	5 minutes	2–4 hours
Pethidine	1 mg/kg	i.v.	10 minutes	1–2 hours
Fentanyl	1–2 µg/kg	i.v.	2–5 minutes	30–60 minutes
Nalbuphine	10–30 mg	i.v.	2–3 minutes	3–4 hours
Codeine	30–60 mg	i.m or p.o.	20–30 minutes	4 hours
Tramadol	100-mg bolus, followed by 50 mg every 20 minutes to a maximum of 3 mg/kg	i.m or p.o.		

more importantly, no increased risk of respiratory depression. Nalbuphine may be administered by pre-hospital personnel, though in the emergency department the antagonist and partial agonist effects of the drug may make subsequent doses of morphine less effective. It is not recommended.

CODEINE

Codeine is a weak opioid that is better absorbed after oral administration than morphine. Approximately 10–20% of codeine is metabolized to morphine, and this is the mechanism of its effect. It is less sedating than morphine, and has minimal effects on pupillary responses. In the past it has been the opioid of choice in patients with head injury.

TRAMADOL

Tramadol is a μ-receptor agonist and also inhibits neuronal reuptake of noradrenaline and 5-hydroxytryptamine in the spinal cord. It is effective for moderate pain, and causes less respiratory depression than other opioids.[8] It may be given intravenously or orally, but may cause seizures and is associated with a high incidence of nausea. It should not be used in patients with epilepsy. Tramadol is not recommended as an analgesic for use in trauma patients.

Opioid reversal

Naloxone is an opioid antagonist, and must be available whenever opioids are used. If naloxone is used in patients who are mentally obtunded due to a possible overdose of illicit opiates, a response will not be seen unless large enough doses are used. A dose of 2 mg or more may be needed in adults, administered slowly over a few minutes. Bolus doses should be given with care, since reversal of opioids may precipitate severe pain, hypertension and seizures. If given to counteract the effects of a 'mild therapeutic excess', as little as 0.1–0.2 mg may be adequate, the ideal being to reverse respiratory depression and oversedation without causing complete reversal of analgesia. The onset of effect is 2–3 minutes, and the duration of action is 20–30 minutes. The patient should therefore be observed closely, as the opioid effects may recur once the naloxone has worn off, and repeated doses or an infusion may be necessary.

Antiemetics

Nausea and vomiting are common side-effects of opioids, and antiemetics that can be administered with opioids include:

* prochlorperazine, 12.5 mg, i.m.
* cyclizine, 50 mg, i.v. or i.m.
* metoclopramide, 10 mg, i.v. or i.m.
* ondansetron, 4–8 mg, i.v. or i.m.

Non-steroidal anti–inflammatory drugs

Non-steroidal anti-inflammatory drugs (NSAIDs) drugs act by inhibiting the cyclo-oxygenase (COX) enzyme system, reducing prostaglandin synthesis. Prostaglandins are involved in the central modulation of pain, and in the periphery sensitize nerve endings to the action of histamine and bradykinin; they are also involved in the inflammatory response. They are useful analgesics for mild to moderate pain, and can be used in combination with opioids and other drugs for more severe pain. In higher doses they act as anti-inflammatory and antipyretic drugs.[9]

Two forms of cyclo-oxygenase exist in the body:

* COX-1: involved in physiological regulation in the kidneys, gastric mucosa and platelets;
* COX-2: involved in inflammation, and produced in response to tissue damage.

Traditional NSAIDs affect both COX-1 and COX-2, but specific COX-2 inhibitors have recently become available. These are said to produce similar analgesia to non-selective NSAIDs with a reduced risk of side-effects. However, concerns have arisen about an increased risk of thrombotic events when used in patients with cardiovascular disease.[10]

A wide range of NSAIDs is available, and each doctor should be familiar with, and use, a limited number. Most NSAIDs may be administered orally, intramuscularly or rectally, though a few are available for intravenous use. Commonly used alternatives include ibuprofen (400 mg 8-hourly), diclofenac (orally, 50 mg 8-hourly, or rectally, 100 mg every 16 hours), piroxicam (sublingually, 2 mg daily) and ketorolac (10 mg i.v. initially, followed by 10–30 mg every 4 hours). Intramuscular injections of diclofenac, although available, are painful and should not be given.

The side-effects of NSAIDs vary with the individual drugs and doses, and include:

* acute renal impairment/failure;
* peptic ulceration and bleeding;
* antiplatelet effects, causing bleeding;
* bronchospasm, in patients with asthma;
* fluid retention;
* hypersensitivity.

NSAIDs are contraindicated if there is a history of renal impairment or peptic ulceration. Patients with major trauma are also at risk of bleeding due to reduced platelet aggregation and renal failure due to hypovolaemia: *these risks make NSAIDs unsuitable in the resuscitation phase of major trauma*. NSAIDs can be used safely in most asthmatic patients, as only around 10% of such individuals are susceptible to NSAID-induced bronchospasm. However, they should be avoided in patients with poorly controlled asthma and in those with a history of aspirin- or

NSAID-induced bronchospasm. The incidence of complications is significantly increased in the elderly, in whom these drugs should be used with great care.

Paracetamol

Paracetamol is an effective analgesic for mild to moderate pain, and may be given either orally or rectally. Intravenous paracetamol has recently become available[10] and may produce a more predictable effect when oral absorption is uncertain. Paracetamol acts as a central inhibitor of cyclo-oxygenase, reducing prostaglandin synthesis, and is also an effective antipyretic. It has minimal anti-inflammatory activity.

> NSAIDs and paracetamol are useful for relieving mild to moderate pain by a variety of routes.

Nitrous oxide

Nitrous oxide is a colourless, non-irritant gas, administered by inhalation. It is a potent analgesic equivalent to 15 mg of subcutaneous morphine.[11] It is not metabolized and is eliminated rapidly from the body via the lungs. By itself, nitrous oxide is not sufficiently potent to produce anaesthesia, although it is often used as part of a general anaesthetic technique together with a volatile anaesthetic agent.

Outside the operating theatre, nitrous oxide is available as Entonox, a mixture of 50% nitrous oxide with oxygen. Entonox cylinders are coloured French blue, with white shoulders. The gas is usually delivered via a demand valve, through either a facemask or a mouthpiece. The analgesic effect occurs within 45–60 seconds, is maximal after 3–4 minutes and wears off quickly when inhalation is stopped. Entonox is very useful for pain relief in short emergency procedures such as reduction of fractures and application of splints,[12] and is useful in pre-hospital care.

The features of Entonox are summarized in Table 21.3. Notably, nitrous oxide is 15 times more soluble in the plasma than nitrogen, and therefore diffuses into air-filled body cavities more rapidly than nitrogen diffuses out. Enclosed air spaces, such as the middle ear, gut, intracranial air spaces or pneumothoraces may expand, causing an increase in either pressure or volume, depending on the compliance of the space involved. Entonox should be avoided in patients with an undrained pneumothorax or head injury with aerocele as well as in those with a recent history of diving or who have recently undergone craniotomy. Nitrous oxide is also a potent cerebral vasodilator, and may increase intracranial pressure in patients with head injuries.[13]

> Entonox is an excellent analgesic for short painful procedures in trauma patients.

Ketamine

Ketamine is useful as a sole analgesic and anaesthetic agent, particularly in the pre-hospital setting and emergency department.[14] Ketamine is a derivative of phencyclidine and is unlike other anaesthetic agents. It produces a dissociative state during which patients may vocalize and move, and their eyes may remain open, but have no recall of events. In subanaesthetic doses, ketamine is a profound analgesic and also causes sympathetic stimulation that results in tachycardia and hypertension. In a patient who is hypovolaemic, this is a useful effect, as ketamine does not cause the marked hypotension seen with other anaesthetic agents. However, ketamine has a direct myocardial depressant effect, and may cause hypotension in a patient who is profoundly shocked and already maximally sympathetically stimulated. Similarly, ketamine may induce hypotension in patients with high spinal cord injuries.

Spontaneous respiration is usually well maintained with ketamine, although respiratory depression sometimes occurs. Ketamine increases muscle tone in the jaw and pharynx, so airway patency and reflexes are often preserved, and it has a bronchodilator effect.

The adverse effects of ketamine are listed in Table 21.4. In particular, it causes an increase in cerebral blood flow that results in raised intracranial pressure in patients with head injuries,[15] and increased cerebral oxygen consumption. Ketamine is therefore contraindicated in patients with head injury, although its use may be justified in certain circumstances, such as during extrication of a trapped subject from a vehicle.[16] Patients recovering from ketamine anaesthesia may also experience disturbing hallucinations, which may be prevented by coadministering a benzodiazepine and allowing the patient to recover in a darkened, quiet environment.

For anaesthesia, a dose of 1–2 mg/kg i.v. or 5–10 mg/kg i.m. is required. The onset of effect may take several minutes if given intramuscularly. For analgesia, 0.25–0.5 mg/kg i.v.

Table 21.3 Advantages and disadvantages of Entonox

Advantages	Disadvantages
Rapid onset and offset	Often causes nausea/dizziness
Moderately potent analgesia	Limits inspired oxygen to 50%
Minimal cardiovascular and respiratory depression	Expands air-containing body cavities (undrained pneumothorax, etc.)
Non-cumulative	Raises intracranial pressure
	Only suitable for short-term use

Table 21.4 Advantages and disadvantages of ketamine

Advantages	Disadvantages
Very potent analgesic/anaesthetic	Excessive salivation (may compromise airway)
Blood pressure usually maintained or increased	Hypertension/tachycardia
Respiration usually well maintained	Hypotension in severly shocked patients
Airway patency usually maintained	Increases cerebral blood flow/intracranial pressure
Bronchodilator effect	Hallucinations/'emergence delirium'
Useful in pre-hospital care	

or 1–4 mg/kg i.m. should be given. The onset is much slower, and duration of action is 10–20 minutes.

LOCAL AND REGIONAL ANAESTHESIA

Local anaesthetic techniques are extremely useful for pain relief in trauma patients.[17] Appropriately placed injections of local anaesthetics can produce excellent analgesia, without the side-effects of systemic analgesic agents. 'Regional anaesthesia' is the use of local anaesthetic drugs to block sensation from a region of the body, such as a brachial plexus block. Local anaesthetic drugs have serious side-effects and must be used with care, even by experienced personnel.

Local anaesthetic agents may be administered in the following ways:

- topically;
- by subcutaneous infiltration;
- as a peripheral nerve or plexus block;
- as a nerve plexus block;
- as a central neuraxial block (intrathecal or epidural);
- as intravenous regional anaesthesia (Bier's block).

The intrathecal ('spinal') and epidural routes are not generally suitable for use in the emergency department.

Local anaesthetic agents

A local anaesthetic is a drug that reversibly blocks the transmission of peripheral nerve impulses[18] by inhibiting the increase in sodium permeability that gives rise to the nerve action potential, thereby preventing membrane depolarization. Small unmyelinated nerves are blocked before larger myelinated ones; thus, sympathetic fibres and pain fibres are blocked before sensory and motor nerves. Local anaesthetic agents are classified as either *esters* or *amides*: the agents used most commonly in the UK (lidocaine, prilocaine and bupivacaine) are all amides.

When administering local anaesthetic agents, three important factors need to be considered:

1. potency, which is directly related to lipid solubility;
2. speed of onset;
3. duration of action, which depends on the extent of protein binding and intrinsic vasoconstriction, which limits the dissipation of the drug away from the site of action.

Most local anaesthetic agents are intrinsic vasodilators, though vasoconstrictor agents may be coadministered with them to prolong their duration of action and to limit toxicity. Preparations of local anaesthetics with adrenaline are available for this purpose.

The speed of onset and duration of effect are also influenced by the type of block being used. Local anaesthetics act more quickly when deposited close to a nerve (e.g. femoral nerve block) than when the anaesthetic has to diffuse towards the nerves, such as is the case with a plexus block or subcutaneous infiltration. The blood supply to the area also determines the duration of action and the toxicity of the agent used. Systemic absorption occurs more rapidly from areas with a greater vascularity, leading to higher plasma concentrations and a greater risk of toxicity. For example, intercostal nerve blocks have a shorter clinical effect than brachial plexus block with the same agent because of the greater vascularity of the intercostal space.

Side-effects of local anaesthetics

LOCAL ANAESTHETIC TOXICITY

Local anaesthetics act non-specifically on excitable membranes, their toxic reactions being seen predominantly in the *cardiovascular* and *central nervous* systems. These effects are due to temporary disruption of physiological function, rather than permanent tissue damage; however, even 'temporary' dysfunction of these critical organs can lead to permanent disability or death.

Toxicity is due to either:

- *absolute overdose*, in which case toxic effects occur gradually as the drug is absorbed systemically; or
- *inadvertent intravascular injection*, which is likely to lead to sudden catastrophic toxicity.

All practitioners using local anaesthesia must understand the risk of toxicity, know how to recognize and treat it, and know the maximum safe doses that can be used. The *maximum safe doses* for commonly used agents are given below, under individual drug headings:

- The maximum doses apply over a 4-hour period.
- These doses are given in mg/kg, whereas local anaesthetic drugs are available as percentage solutions. To convert, remember *a y% solution contains 10y mg/mL*, e.g. 20 mL of 1% lidocaine contains 200 mg.
- Following intravascular injection, a much smaller dose may be enough to precipitate toxicity. Intravascular injection must therefore be carefully avoided.

When *gradual* systemic absorption of a toxic dose occurs, the following progression of symptoms and signs may occur:

- perioral numbness and tingling and complaint of a metallic taste;
- visual disturbances, tinnitus, dizziness;
- slurred speech;
- tachycardia, hypertension;
- muscular twitching;
- convulsions;
- hypotension, bradycardia;
- ventricular arrhythmias;
- cardiac arrest.

In patients undergoing any local anaesthetic block, intravenous access should be established in advance. Monitoring equipment (ECG, pulse oximeter and blood pressure) and resuscitation equipment must be available. The operator should be aware of the diagnosis and treatment of toxicity reactions, and have appropriate resuscitation skills (Table 21.5).

> All practitioners using local anaesthesia must understand local anaesthetic toxicity and must know the maximum safe dose of these drugs.

HYPERSENSITIVITY

Anaphylactic and anaphylactoid reactions are uncommon but are more likely to occur with the ester-based agents, as well as

Table 21.5 Management of local anaesthetic toxicity

Advanced Life Support protocols should be followed.[19]
- Secure the airway
- Administer high-flow oxygen
- Ensure adequate ventilation

Resuscitate the circulation

Convulsions may be treated with i.v. diazepam or midazolam

Cardiac arrythmias, particularly those caused by bupivicaine, may be difficult to treat

Prolonged cardiac massage may be needed

Cardiac pacing may be required

with the preservative methylhydroxybenzoate. Genuine allergy to the amide local anaesthetic drugs is rare, and a history of 'allergy' is more often due to side-effects of vasoconstrictors or preservatives, or to a simple vasovagal reaction.

REACTIONS TO ADJUNCTS

Adrenaline may be used with local anaesthetic agents to cause vasoconstriction and prolong the action of the local block. Systemic absorption of adrenaline may cause tachycardia, cardiac arrhythmias and cardiac ischaemia. Adrenaline-containing local anaesthetics must therefore be used cautiously in patients with cardiac disease.

Adrenaline and other vasoconstrictors must be avoided in the region of end arteries, for example in the digits, nose, ears and penis, because of the risk of local ischaemia.

NERVE DAMAGE

Direct trauma to nerves with a needle and/or injection of local anaesthetic directly into a nerve can cause neurological damage. Serious nerve injury is rare, and may be due to neuropraxia, which may improve with time, but permanent injury can occur. Short-bevelled needles designed specifically for regional anaesthesia should be used where possible. A conscious patient will complain of pain and paraesthesia if the nerve is penetrated while attempting a nerve block, and the needle should be withdrawn immediately.

SIDE-EFFECTS DUE TO SITE OF INJECTION

These are due to:

- Predictable and reversible effects of local anaesthetics on adjacent nerves:
  - phrenic nerve paralysis after interscalene brachial plexus block
  - hypotension due to sympathetic block after epidural analgesia.
- Misplacement of the local anaesthetic solution:
  - intrathecal spread following attempted interscalene brachial plexus block, leading to unconsciousness and hypotension.
- Trauma to adjacent structures:
  - pneumothorax after supraclavicular brachial plexus block.

Commonly used local anaesthetics

LIDOCAINE (LIGNOCAINE)

Commonly used for subcutaneous infiltration and shorter acting blocks:

- Onset of action is 5 minutes for peripheral use, 20 minutes for plexus blocks.

- Duration of action is 60–90 minutes.
- The maximum dose is 3 mg/kg.
- The maximum dose with adrenaline is 7mg/kg.

A eutectic mixture of local anaesthetic (EMLA) is a white cream containing lidocaine 2.5% and prilocaine 2.5%, which can be applied under an occlusive dressing to provide topical analgesia of the skin. It is effective within 30–60 minutes.

PRILOCAINE

Prilocaine is commonly used for intravenous regional anaesthesia (IVRA):

- Its onset and duration of action are similar to those of lidocaine.
- The maximum dose is 5 mg/kg (3 mg/kg for Bier's block).
- The maximum dose with adrenaline is 8 mg/kg.

Prilocaine doses over 8mg/kg may cause methaemoglobinaemia, but this can be treated with methylene blue (2mg/kg).

BUPIVACAINE/LEVOBUPIVACAINE

The onset of action is 20 minutes peripherally, and 45 minutes for plexus block.

- The duration of action is up to 24 hours in plexus block.
- The maximum dose is 2 mg/kg (with or without adrenaline).

Bupivicaine is more toxic than other local anaesthetic agents and has a great affinity for cardiac muscle, thus making resuscitation more difficult. It is a mixture of two optical isomers: *levobupivacaine* is the purified L-form, which has the same maximum dose and clinical characteristics as the racemic mixture, but less potential for toxicity.

AMETHOCAINE

Amethocaine is used topically for conjunctival and corneal anaesthesia (see Chapter 11).

Local anaesthetic blocks

There are a large number of local anaesthetic blocks, and those described below are suitable for use in the emergency department.

The following general principles should always be followed when a local anaesthetic block is being used:

- The patient should be informed about the block and its side-effects, and consent should be obtained.

- A history of local anaesthetic allergy and other contraindications should be sought.
- Intravenous access must be established.
- Standard monitoring must be in place.
- Resuscitation equipment must be available.
- An aseptic technique must be used.
- Careful aspiration is performed to avoid intravascular injection.
- Injection is stopped immediately if the patient complains of pain or severe paraesthesiae.

> Resuscitation equipment must always be available when local anaesthetic blocks are performed.

FEMORAL NERVE BLOCK

This block is particularly useful for analgesia in patients with a fracture of the femoral shaft.

Anatomy

The femoral artery and vein and femoral nerve all pass behind the inguinal ligament deep to the fascia lata. The artery and vein are enclosed in a fascial sheath, with the vein being more medial. The femoral nerve lies behind and lateral to this sheath. Its position may vary between individuals, sometimes being very close to the sheath, sometimes several centimetres lateral to it. (Remember NAVY: nerve–artery–vein –Y fronts.) Just below the inguinal ligament the femoral nerve divides into several branches (Figure 21.1).

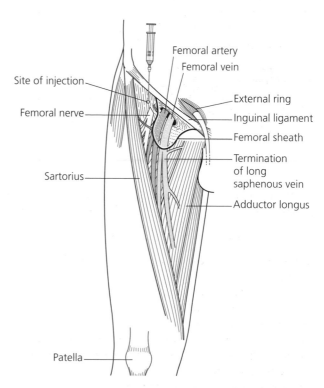

Figure 21.1 The important anatomy of the inguinal area for administration of a femoral nerve block.

Technique

A line drawn from the pubic tubercle to the anterior superior iliac spine marks the position of the inguinal ligament. The femoral artery can be palpated in the centre of this line, and the femoral nerve lies about 1 cm lateral to the artery just below the ligament. The needle is directed posteriorly and distally at a 45° angle. A 'click' may be felt as the needle pierces the fascia lata. Paraesthesia or pain may occur if the needle has penetrated the nerve, in which case the needle should be withdrawn slightly before injection in order to prevent neuronal damage. The total depth should be no more than 2.0–3.5 cm.

* Dose: 10–20 mL of 1% lidocaine or 0.25% bupivicaine.
* Onset time: 10–30 minutes.
* Duration: 4–6 hours, longer if using bupivicaine.

WRIST NERVE BLOCK

The hand distal to the palmar crease may be simply anaesthetized by blocking the terminal branches of the ulnar, median and radial nerves (Figure 21.2).

Anatomy

The ulnar nerve lies lateral to the tendon of flexor carpi ulnaris, adjacent to the ulnar artery. The median nerve lies between the tendons of palmaris longus and flexor carpi radialis. The radial nerve is posterolateral to the brachioradialis.

Technique

Three injections of local anaesthetic are required:

* directly lateral to flexor carpi ulnaris (ulnar nerve block);
* between palmaris longus and flexor carpi radialis (median nerve block);
* subcutaneous infiltration around the dorsolateral aspect of the wrist, lateral to the radial artery (block of superficial branch of radial nerve).

Dose

* A dose of 5 mL of 1% lidocaine or prilocaine can be injected at each site.
* Onset: 5–10 minutes.
* Duration: 45–60 minutes.

Blocks of the individual nerves may be considered, depending on the anatomical site of injury.

DIGITAL NERVE BLOCK

The digital nerves, two dorsal and two palmar, accompany the digital vessels. An aliquot (1–2 mL) of local anaesthetic can be injected at the base of the digit at either side to block these nerves and to anaesthetize the digit. The block is usually effective in 5–10 minutes. A finger tourniquet formed from the little finger of a surgical glove can be used, and will significantly increase the effectiveness of the block. Vasoconstrictors must be avoided as digit ischaemia will occur. It is also important to avoid injecting a large volume of anaesthetic, as the swelling may cause distal ischaemia. The digital tourniquet must be removed at the end of the procedure.

> Adrenaline-containing local anaesthetics are absolutely contraindicated in digital nerve blocks.

INTERCOSTAL NERVE BLOCKS

Intercostal nerve blocks are a useful means of providing analgesia for patients with fractured ribs.

Anatomy

The intercostal nerves run in the intercostal groove on the inferior aspect of the rib. For optimum analgesia the nerve should be blocked proximal to the origin of the lateral branch (posterior to the midaxillary line).

Technique

The patient is positioned prone, in the lateral decubitus position, or sitting and leaning forwards. The shoulders

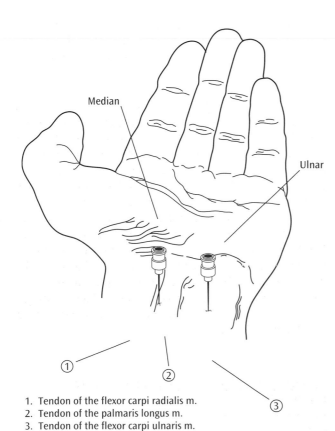

1. Tendon of the flexor carpi radialis m.
2. Tendon of the palmaris longus m.
3. Tendon of the flexor carpi ulnaris m.

Figure 21.2 Nerve blocks at the wrist.

should be abducted and the arms held forward so that the scapulae move laterally and aid access to the posterior angle of the ribs. The needle is introduced and advanced until it makes contact with the rib. The needle is then allowed to slip down off the inferior border of the rib. The needle can then be angled at 45° and advanced 0.5 cm inwards towards the intercostal nerve. The patient should be instructed to hold his or her breath during needle insertion, to avoid penetration of the pleura. Aspiration should be performed before injection to ensure that the needle is not in a blood vessel.

- Dose: 3–4 mL of 0.5% bupivicaine, with or without adrenaline, in each space.
- Onset of action: 10–20 minutes.
- Duration of action: 4–8 hours.

At least one intercostal nerve above and below the broken rib will need to be blocked in order to provide effective analgesia.

INTRAVENOUS REGIONAL ANAESTHESIA (BIER'S BLOCK)

This technique involves the injection of local anaesthetic into an exsanguinated limb, distal to a pneumatic tourniquet. Intravenous regional anaesthesia is used in the upper limb and is an effective means of providing anaesthesia for short procedures on the hand and forearm. The duration of the procedure is limited by the discomfort caused by the tourniquet, and is usually no more than 1 hour. Tourniquets should be avoided in patients with sickle cell disease or trait, Raynaud's disease or symptomatic peripheral vascular disease.

Intravenous regional anaesthesia should always be performed by two suitably qualified and experienced operators. Although a simple technique, it carries a unique risk of systemic toxicity if not performed properly, and a number of deaths associated with IVRA have been recorded.[20] These have been related to single operators, errors with the inflation and release of tourniquets and the use of bupivacaine. Bupivacaine is *contraindicated* for IVRA because of its potential for cardiac toxicity, and prilocaine is the most suitable agent.

Technique

Venous access is established in the opposite arm to the injury. A small cannula is also inserted into the back of the hand on the injured side. If this proves difficult, a cannula in the antecubital fossa is an effective alternative. The tourniquet is checked carefully before use.

The arm is then exsanguinated. Ideally, an Esmarch bandage is used, but in patients with painful forearm fractures the arm can be elevated gently and pressure applied to the brachial artery.

After exsanguination, the tourniquet is inflated to 100 mmHg above systolic arterial pressure. Prilocaine 0.5% without preservative is the anaesthetic of choice, and

should be injected slowly to prevent it being forced up the arm under the tourniquet and into the systemic circulation. The normal adult dose is 40 mL, though this may be reduced in frail, elderly patients. The patient may complain of paraesthesia almost immediately, and the skin may appear mottled. Sensory block is usually established in 10 minutes, and good muscle relaxation is obtained after 20 minutes.

A double-cuff tourniquet can be used, so that the area beneath the second (lower) cuff can be anaesthetized. This requires the upper cuff to be inflated first while the block takes effect. The lower cuff is then inflated and the upper one deflated. Errors in this sequence, however, have led to patients receiving fatal systemic boluses of local anaesthetic. A single-cuff tourniquet avoids the risk of confusion and is usually tolerated well by patients.

The tourniquet should be left inflated for *at least 20 minutes*; otherwise, once the procedure is complete, the tourniquet can be released and the patient observed closely for signs of local anaesthetic toxicity. Observation should continue for at least 2 hours. Systemic toxicity may occur if the tourniquet is released too soon.

> Intravenous regional anaesthesia is a two-operator technique.

HAEMATOMA BLOCK

Haematoma block is most commonly used for fractures of the wrist. Local anaesthetic is introduced directly into the area of the fracture and its surrounding haematoma.

Technique

The first step is familiarization with the anatomy of the fracture by careful study of the radiographs and comparison with the surface anatomy. The skin over the fracture site is cleaned thoroughly. Using a 21G needle, up to 20 mL of 1% lidocaine is then introduced into the area of the fracture. Before injection, location of the tip of the needle within the haematoma is confirmed by aspiration of blood.

Haematoma block is not suitable for fractures over 24 hours old, and analgesia is often not as good as with IVRA. Many failures of haematoma blocks could, however, be avoided by waiting until the block can be demonstrated to be effective by gentle movement of the wrist before attempting manipulation. The technique theoretically converts a closed into an open fracture, with possible infection risk.

SEDATION TECHNIQUES FOR TRAUMA PATIENTS

Sedation is a state somewhere along a line which has an awake, conscious patient in full control of the airway at one end, and a fully anaesthetized patient with no airway control at the other end. There is no fixed dividing line between these two states, and excessive sedation can easily become more akin to a general anaesthetic. The definition of sedation is a state in which *verbal contact* with the patient can be maintained.

There is large patient variability in dose requirements depending on the patient's age, weight and pathophysiological status, and 'standard' doses should be used only as a guide. An ideally sedated patient will be calm and drowsy but capable of responding to the operator's voice and of obeying commands. Some sedative agents also provide a degree of amnesia, with the result that the patient may not recall what has occurred while under sedation.

Indications for sedation in trauma patients

Patients with relatively minor trauma who are to undergo minor procedures in the emergency department may benefit from sedation.[21]

Contraindications to sedation in trauma patients include:

- altered level of consciousness due to head injury, drugs or alcohol;
- haemodynamic instability;
- a full stomach.

Restlessness due to pain, hypoxia or a full bladder is not an indication for sedation. The cause of the restlessness should be identified and treated. However, some patients who were previously cooperative may become disorientated and agitated under the effect of sedation.

Sedative drugs may precipitate respiratory depression or apnoea, loss of airway control and aspiration. When undertaking a procedure under sedation, the following is recommended:

- The patient should be fasted for at least 4 hours.
- A full explanation of the procedure should be given, and consent obtained.
- Two doctors should be present, one to administer sedation and monitor the patient and one to perform the procedure. Qualified assistance for both must be available.
- The patient should be appropriately monitored (ECG, pulse oximeter and non-invasive blood pressure).
- Intravenous access should be secured before starting sedation, and oxygen given.
- The patient should be on a tilting trolley, with resuscitation equipment available.
- If the patient is to go home after the procedure, he or she should be escorted home and someone should remain with the patient, preferably overnight.
- Patients should be advised not to drive or perform complicated tasks until the sedative effects have completely worn off.

Drugs used for sedation

BENZODIAZEPINES

These drugs are used widely as sedatives, as they produce anxiolysis and retrograde amnesia. Their main side-effect is respiratory depression. They are *not* analgesics, and therefore for painful procedures an appropriate nerve block or small dose of analgesic will be required.

Midazolam

Midazolam is a water-soluble benzodiazepine that may be administered by intravenous injection. It has a half-life of 2.5 hours, and recovery is rapid. The safest way to administer midazolam is to dilute the drug to a 1 mg/mL solution and titrate it in 1.0 mg aliquots. Elderly patients may require as little as 1–2 mg, but it may take several minutes to be effective. It is important to wait a few minutes after each small bolus in order to avoid overdose and respiratory depression. The duration of action of midazolam is also prolonged in elderly patients. A young fit patient, on the other hand, may require up to 10 mg of midazolam.

Diazepam

Diazepam is often used for sedation. This drug is not particularly water soluble, and the intravenous preparation is an emulsion (Diazemuls). This should be titrated to reach the appropriate level of sedation. Diazepam has a long half-life, and it may take several hours for its effects to wear off, particularly in the elderly. Diazepam may also be administered orally or rectally as a 5–10 mg dose.

Flumazenil

Flumazenil is a short-acting benzodiazepine antagonist and may be used to reverse the effects of benzodiazepines. It is given in a dose of 200 µg i.v. over 15 seconds, then 100 µg every 60 seconds until effective. The maximum total dose is 1 mg.

The duration of action of flumazenil is about 20 minutes, and therefore if a patient has had a large dose of benzodiazepine the effects of flumazenil may wear off, allowing the patient to become resedated. Flumazenil may cause seizures in epileptic patients. Nausea, vomiting, flushing, agitation and transient increases in heart rate and blood pressure may occur.

OPIOIDS

Opioids may be administered together with benzodiazepines to provide analgesia during sedation. Morphine or pethidine is often used, and should be titrated as small intravenous boluses. Opioids and benzodiazepines both cause respiratory depression, and when given together their effects are additive. Patients – especially the elderly – need to be closely monitored for several hours after the procedure.

The intravenous anaesthetic agents, propofol and ketamine, may be used to provide sedation.[21,22] They should be administered only by a doctor who is experienced in their use, as overdose may cause anaesthesia and respiratory arrest.

ANAESTHESIA IN THE EMERGENCY DEPARTMENT

The following problems complicate anaesthesia in the trauma patient:

- Patients with major trauma are at risk of pulmonary aspiration. The stomach may contain food, alcohol or swallowed blood. Gastric stasis may also result from acute pain and opioids.
- Airway management may be difficult due to airway foreign bodies, haematoma or oedema.
- Cervical spine injury also complicates airway management, and can be exacerbated by movement during intubation.
- Chest injury may cause severe problems with artificial ventilation and oxygenation.
- Most anaesthetic agents are cardiovascular depressants, thus compounding hypotension in hypovolaemic patients.
- Trauma victims may have taken drugs or alcohol, which complicates their anaesthetic management.

General anaesthesia should ideally be undertaken in a properly equipped and staffed operating theatre. An in-depth description of trauma anaesthesia may be found elsewhere.[23] Standards for the safe provision of anaesthesia have been published by the Association of Anaesthetists of Great Britain and Ireland.[24,25] Monitoring that should be available whenever and wherever anaesthesia is induced is outlined in Table 21.6.

Table 21.6 Monitoring required for administration of general anaesthesia

Standard monitoring (all patients)	Additional monitoring (depending on clinical condition)
Oxygen analyser	Invasive blood pressure
Pulse oximeter	Neuromuscular blockade monitoring
Electrocardiography	Temperature
Non-invasive blood pressure	Central venous pressure
Capnography	
Ventilator disconnection alarm	

However, anaesthesia is required for trauma patients in the emergency department in the following situations:

- head injury with reduced consciousness level to prevent hypoxia, hypercarbia, airway obstruction and aspiration;
- actual or impending airway obstruction (such as from airway burns);
- inadequate ventilation or oxygenation, for example following chest injury;
- severe shock from any cause, with the risk of reduced level of consciousness and airway compromise.

Anaesthesia should be administered only by a doctor with suitable training and experience, either an anaesthetist or an emergency physician who has undergone anaesthetic training.[26]

> Trauma anaesthesia is a specialized field requiring appropriate training and experience.

Rapid-sequence induction of anaesthesia

All trauma patients are assumed to have a full stomach. Rapid-sequence induction of anaesthesia (RSI) allows the patient to be anaesthetized and the airway secured while reducing the risk of regurgitation and aspiration. Short-acting anaesthetic drugs are used, so that the patient can be reawakened rapidly if intubation is unsuccessful.

When performing RSI, resuscitation equipment, difficult intubation equipment and suction must be available, and the patient should be on a tilting trolley. Appropriate monitoring equipment is used, and expert assistance must be to hand.

PROCEDURE FOR RAPID-SEQUENCE INDUCTION

1. The patient is preoxygenated with high-flow oxygen via a correctly fitting facemask for 3 minutes. This 'washes out' nitrogen from the lungs, and limits hypoxaemia if intubation is unsuccessful.
2. If cervical spine injury is suspected, an assistant should maintain manual in-line cervical spine immobilization. Rigid cervical collars limit mouth opening and impede intubation: the front part of the collar should be removed before intubation is attempted.[27]
3. Intubation equipment and suction is prepared and checked; ECG, pulse oximetry and blood pressure monitoring is applied and (if needed and if time allows) anaesthetic or sedative infusions are prepared for use immediately after intubation.
4. Anaesthesia is induced with an intravenous induction agent (usually propofol, thiopentone or etomidate), followed immediately by the depolarizing muscle relaxant suxamethonium.

5. To prevent regurgitation, cricoid pressure (Sellick's manoeuvre) is applied as the patient loses consciousness, and is maintained until the airway is definitively protected: the assistant must *not* release this pressure until instructed by the intubator.

6. Suxamethonium provides adequate intubating conditions in approximately 45 seconds, and muscle fasciculations will occur as it takes effect: when these subside, the patient is intubated using a cuffed endotracheal tube. Once the position of the tube in the trachea is confirmed, the cuff is inflated and the tube secured, cricoid pressure can be released.

7. Once the patient is intubated, the lungs may be ventilated manually or using a ventilator; further sedation and muscle relaxation will be required to maintain anaesthesia.

COMPLICATIONS OF RAPID-SEQUENCE INDUCTION

Drug reactions

All induction agents cause vasodilatation and hypotension, which can be severe in the hypovolaemic patient. Of the drugs listed above, this is most likely to occur with propofol and least so with etomidate. Ketamine is an alternative for the severely shocked patient.[28] Suxamethonium has its own unique side-effects (Table 21.7). Although suxamethonium can raise intracranial pressure, it is still used in head injury as it gives the best intubating conditions. Raised intraocular pressure is a concern with penetrating eye injuries, and could theoretically lead to extrusion of intraocular contents. Potentially fatal hyperkalaemia can occur after suxamethonium in patients with a high spinal cord injury, extensive burns or upper motor neurone lesions, but this is not a problem in the acute stages immediately following injury. Anaphylactic or anaphylactoid reactions may occur with anaesthetic drugs, but are rare.

Table 21.7 The side-effects of suxamethonium

Raised intracranial pressure
Raised intraocular pressure
Bradycardia (especially in children, or following a second dose)
Hyperkalaemia
Histamine release and anaphylaxis
Prolonged apnoea, in patients who have plasma cholinesterase abnormalities
Trigger agent for malignant hyperpyrexia

Difficult/failed intubation

Intubation may be difficult in trauma patients for several reasons, including:

- facial trauma;
- in-line cervical spine stabilization which prevents neck extension;
- incorrectly applied cricoid pressure.

It is therefore essential to assess fully the patient's airway before inducing anaesthesia and paralysis. Failure to intubate a patient who was previously maintaining a partial airway and breathing may be fatal.

If difficult intubation is predicted in advance, the following options may be considered:

- Awake intubation, using local anaesthesia to the airway and either conventional or fibreoptic intubation. Fibreoptic intubation requires a skilled operator, takes time, and may be difficult if there is blood in the airway.
- Inhalational induction of anaesthesia, to preserve spontaneous breathing. Laryngoscopy can then be performed while the patient is still breathing, and before the administration of muscle relaxants. However, this technique still may lead to loss of the airway after administration of muscle relaxant, and the patient will be at risk of regurgitation and aspiration.
- Tracheostomy under local anaesthesia.

If a difficult intubation is anticipated, it is essential that the equipment and expertise for the formation of a surgical airway is immediately available.

Sympathetic stimulation

Tracheal intubation is very stimulating, and large amounts of catecholamines are released, which may cause a hypertensive surge. This may be detrimental for patients with head injuries, raised intracranial pressure or cardiovascular disease. In these patients the RSI may be modified to include agents that obtund the pressor response, such as fentanyl,[29] lidocaine,[30] labetolol or esmolol. These drugs should be administered at least 3 minutes before laryngoscopy if they are to be effective. All such agents may cause hypotension, and therefore the patient must be haemodynamically stable before they are administered.

Cardiac arrhythmias

As well as tachyarrhythmias due to sympathetic stimulation, severe vagally mediated bradycardia can also occur. This is due either to hypoxia during attempted intubation or to direct autonomic stimulation induced by laryngoscopy.

Case scenario 1

A 36-year-old man is involved in a road accident, as the driver of a car in collision with another vehicle. He is trapped in the car for 30 minutes before extrication. His injuries include a flail chest and pneumothorax, fractured pelvis and right shaft of femur, and other fractures of both lower limbs. There is no head injury. After initial resuscitation, he undergoes surgical fixation of the femoral fracture, and remains ventilated on the intensive care unit for several days.

What analgesic techniques would be suitable during the pre-hospital phase?

During pre-hospital care, carefully titrated doses of intravenous opiates are most suitable. Entonox could be given, particularly during extrication and patient movement, but would be contraindicated in this case because of the suspected pneumothorax. Intravenous ketamine could be used during extrication.

What analgesic techniques would be suitable in the emergency department?

In the emergency department, the above methods could also be used. Entonox could be given provided the pneumothorax is drained. A femoral nerve block would give analgesia for the femoral fracture. Intravenous paracetamol could be used in addition to other agents. NSAIDs should be avoided at this stage due to the risks of increased bleeding and renal failure due to hypovolaemia.

What analgesic techniques would be suitable during his subsequent care in hospital?

After the period of ventilation, he is likely to have persistent severe pain from the rib fractures, and possibly from his pelvic and lower limb injuries. Failure to provide good analgesia for his rib fractures may lead to sputum retention and pneumonia. Regular opiates can be continued, either orally or by infusion or PCA. Regular paracetamol and NSAIDs, in the absence of contraindications, will also help. Intercostal nerve blocks would relieve the pain from his rib fractures, but would have to be repeated at regular intervals. Epidural analgesia may be very effective at relieving pain from his chest or lower limb injuries, and could be continued by infusion for several days.

Case scenario 2

A 74-year-old woman is struck by a car while on a pedestrian crossing. She sustains a head injury and a suspected pelvic fracture. Although alert at the scene, her Glasgow Coma Scale score is 9 on admission to hospital.

Why are general anaesthesia and intubation needed for this patient?

Intubation and ventilation are needed to maintain and protect the airway due to her deteriorating level of consciousness, and to prevent hypoxia and hypercarbia, which would be dangerous because of her head injury (Chapter 9).

How should this be performed?

A rapid sequence induction of anaesthesia is used, to minimize the risk of pulmonary aspiration. After preoxygenation, an anaesthetic induction agent and suxamethonium are given, and cricoid pressure is applied to prevent regurgitation. Manual in-line stabilization of the head and neck is used, and the front part of any cervical collar is removed, to minimize difficulty in intubation.

What risks are involved?

Anaesthetic induction agents may cause cardiovascular collapse in hypovolaemic patients, and a relatively cardiovascularly stable agent such as etomidate should be used. The anaesthetic drugs used will precipitate airway obstruction as well as apnoea, and catastrophic hypoxia may result if the practitioner fails to intubate and cannot maintain the airway in any other way. Hypoxia also occurs with prolonged intubation attempts, and oesophageal intubation. Neck movement, arrhythmias and raised intracranial pressure may also occur.

SUMMARY

Methods for relieving pain in trauma include physical and psychological methods, oral and intravenous drugs, inhaled analgesia (Entonox) and local anaesthetic techniques. Every doctor who deals with trauma victims must be competent to provide adequate analgesia, and must understand the benefits and risks of these methods. A rapid sequence induction of general anaesthesia may be needed in trauma patients at risk of airway or ventilatory compromise. General anaesthesia in the trauma patient is challenging, and should be performed only by those with adequate training and experience.

GLOBAL PERSPECTIVES

Analgesic and anaesthetic techniques are generally similar throughout developed countries, with relatively minor differences in the availability and use of drugs. For example, diamorphine, although used widely in the UK, is not available for medical use in the USA.

In many developing countries, analgesia and anaesthesia are limited by the availability of drugs, equipment and monitoring. Medically qualified anaesthetists are in short supply, and much anaesthetic care is given by nurses or technicians. Ketamine is used widely, and is a relatively safe drug for the non-medical anaesthetist. Local anaesthetic blocks are often used, particularly spinal anaesthesia, and this is helpful when the supply of general anaesthetic drugs is limited. Thiopentone and suxamethonium are used widely, and ether and halothane which are obsolete in the UK, but safe and effective nonetheless, are still used in many countries.

Note that the drug doses given in this chapter may be excessive in some populations, due to differences in racial characteristics and body mass.

REFERENCES

1.   Subcommittee on Taxonomy. Pain terms: a list with definitions and notes on usage. *Pain* 1979;**6**:249–52.

2.   Beecher HK. *Resuscitation and Anesthesia for Wounded Men: The Management of Traumatic Shock*. Springfield, IL: Charles C. Thomas, 1949.

3.   Duggan J, Drummond GB. Activity of lower intercostals and abdominal muscle after surgery in humans. *Anesth Analg* 1987;**66**:852–5.

4.   Pate JW. Chest wall injuries. *Surg Clin N Am* 1989;**69**:59–70.

5.   Austin KL, Stapleton JV, Mather LE. Multiple intramuscular injections: a major source of variability in analgesic response to meperidine. *Pain* 1969;**8**:47–62.

6.   Sawyer RW, Bodai BI, Blaisdell FW, McCourt MM. The current state of intraosseous infusion. *J Am Coll Surg* 1994;**179**:353–8.

7.   Gutstein HB, Akil H. Opioid analgesics. In: Hardman JG, Limbird LE, eds. *Goodman and Gilman's The Pharmacological Basis of Therapeutics*, 10th edn. New York: McGraw-Hill, 2001, pp. 569–619.

8.   Budd K, Langford R. Tramadol revisited. *Br J Anaesth* 1999;**82**:493–5.

9.   Dahl JB, Kehlet H. Non-steroidal anti-inflammatory drugs: rationale for use in severe postoperative pain. *Br J Anaesth* 1991;**66**:703–12.

10.   Power I. Recent advances in postoperative pain therapy. *Br J Anaesth* 2005;**95**:43–51.

11.   Chapman WP, Arrowwood JG, Beecher HK. The analgesic effect of nitrous oxide compared in man with morphine sulphate. *J Clin Invest* 1943;**22**:871–5.

12.   Baskett PJF, Withnell A. Use of entonox in the Ambulance Service. *BMJ* 1970;**284**:41–3.

13.   Moss E, McDowall DG. ICP increases with 50% nitrous oxide in severe head injuries during controlled ventilation. *Br J Anaesth* 1979;**51**:757–60.

14.   White PF, Way WL, Trevor AJ. Ketamine – its pharmacology and therapeutic uses. *Anesthesiology* 1982;**56**:119.

15.   Shapiro HM, Wyte SR, Harris AB. Ketamine anaesthesia in patients with intracranial pathology. *Br J Anaesth* 1972;**144**:1200–4.

16.   Porter K. Ketamine in prehospital care. *Emerg Med J* 2004; **21**:351–4.

17.   Elliot JM. Regional anaesthesia in trauma. *Trauma* 2001;**3**:161–74.

18.   Lou L, Sabar R, Kaye AD. Local anaesthetics. In: Raj PP, ed. *Textbook of Regional Anaesthesia*. New York: Churchill Livingstone, 2002, pp. 177–213.

19.   Resuscitation Council (UK). *Advanced Life Support Manual*, 5th edn. London: Resuscitation Council, 2006.

20.   Heath M. Deaths after intravenous regional anaesthesia. *BMJ* 1982;**285**:913–14.

21.   Duncan RA, Symington L, Thakore S. Sedation practice in a Scottish teaching hospital emergency department. *Emerg Med J* 2006;**23**:684–6.

22.   Symington L, Thakore S. A review of the use of propofol for procedural sedation in the emergency department. *Emerg Med* 2006;**23**:89–93.

23.   Grande CM. *Textbook of Trauma Anaesthesia and Critical Care*. London: Mosby, 1993.

24.   The Association of Anaesthetists of Great Britain and Ireland. *The Anaesthesia Team*. London: AAGBI 2005.

25.   The Association of Anaesthetists of Great Britain and Ireland. *Checking Anaesthetic Equipment*. London: AAGBI, 2004.

26.   Walker A, Brenchley J. Survey of the use of rapid sequence induction in the accident and emergency department. *J Accid Emerg Med* 2000;**2**:95–7.

27.   Heath KJ. The effect on laryngoscopy of different cervical spine immobilization techniques. *Anaesthesia* 1994;**49**:843–5.

28.   Sivilotti ML, Ducharme J. Randomised, double blind study on sedatives and hemodynamics during rapid-sequence intubation in the emergency department: the SHRED study. *Ann Emerg Med* 1998;**31**:313–24.

29.   Cork RC, Weiss JC, Hameroff SR, Bentley J. Fentanyl preloading for rapid sequence induction of anesthesia. *Anesth Analg* 1984;**63**:60–4.

30.   Donegan MF, Bedford RF. Intravenous administration of lidocaine prevents intracranial hypertension during endotracheal suctioning. Anesthesiology 1980; **52**: 516–18.

22

Intensive care management of major trauma

OBJECTIVES

After completing this chapter the reader will:
- understand the relationship between trauma and multiorgan failure
- understand the implications of damage control surgery to intensive care
- understand the interplay of haemorrhage and coagulopathy after trauma
- understand the basic principles of organ support.

INTRODUCTION

Trauma is one the leading causes of mortality and morbidity worldwide across all age groups. In the UK, 35% of deaths following trauma occur within the first hour after injury and before the patient reaches hospital.[1] Pre-hospital care and protocols such as Advanced Trauma Life Support (ATLS) have had some impact on the rate of early deaths, but a bimodal distribution of mortality after trauma still exists, with the later peak occurring days or weeks after the initial injury due to multiple organ failure (MOF) and sepsis.[2] Timely and proper interventions in an intensive care unit (ICU) or high-dependency unit can reduce the size of this peak and potentially offset some of the enormous costs generated by trauma.[3]

TRAUMA AND MULTIPLE ORGAN FAILURE

After significant trauma, victims who survive the initial insult and resuscitation are commonly admitted to intensive care. Unfortunately, once on the ICU they may succumb to later septic complications and multiple organ failure.

In one study of critically ill trauma patients, approximately 21% of patients developed single organ failure (SOF) and approximately 5% developed MOF. Mortality was related to the number of organ systems which had failed, increasing from a 4% mortality for SOF to 32% for two-system failure, 67% for three-system failure and approximately 90% mortality rates for MOF.[4] The emphasis is now on the prevention of MOF.

Risk factors for developing MOF include an APACHE (Acute Physiology and Chronic Health Evaluation) III score >50 on admission to ICU, persistently elevated blood lactate levels at 24 hours and a need for more than six units of blood products in the first 24 hours.[4] A systolic blood pressure <100 mmHg and multiple transfusions[5] are both independent risk factors for the development of acute lung injury (ALI) and MOF. The Trauma and Lung Injury Group from San Francisco found that those patients who developed ALI had significantly higher Injury Severity Scores (ISS) (32 ± 11 vs. 26 ± 8) and a more severe initial metabolic acidosis (base deficit >6 mmol/L).[6] Transfusion requirements were similar between the two groups, but the incidence of lung injury was greater in the group who had received larger amounts of crystalloids within the first 24 hours. Although the incidence of hepatic, renal or gastrointestinal dysfunction was low, a raised initial prothrombin time (PT) was associated with the development of ALI. The degree of thoracic injury, particularly bilateral chest trauma, was also related to the development of ALI.

An ISS >16 is associated with acute neutrophil activation[7] and an increased risk of developing complications, depending on the host response to injury. Severe injury is associated with a systemic inflammatory response syndrome (SIRS), even in the absence of infection. This may be followed by a secondary insult due to bacterial translocation or ischaemia–reperfusion phenomenon.

> Organ failure after trauma is common and related to the degree of injury.

The role of neutrophils

Trauma results in the activation of both pro- and anti-inflammatory cascades, with over 1 million neutrophils released from the bone marrow per second. Within an hour of injury these neutrophils are primed and sequestration begins to occur.[8] Primed neutrophils release reactive oxygen species (ROS) and further express an adhesion molecule (CD11b) on their surfaces. Within the circulation they bind to the endothelial cell surfaces via expression of corresponding adhesion molecules on cell membranes, facilitating migration into the tissues, where the ROS cause further tissue damage.[9–11]

Reperfusion results in the release of previously quiescent but primed neutrophils from the gastrointestinal tract; hence, restoration of circulating volume during resuscitation can result in the delivery and sequestration of these 'sticky' neutrophils in organs distant from the site of original injury, such as the lungs and liver. This represents a potential mechanism for the development of remote tissue damage such as ALI after non-thoracic blunt trauma. This response is usually tolerated, but a greater degree of sequestration, indicated by a greater decline in circulating neutrophils at 12 hours after injury, is associated with an increased risk of developing MOF.[8]

The importance of the base deficit

Base deficit is a useful clinical marker of the degree of injury,[11] reflecting tissue hypoperfusion from 'shock' and altered cell metabolism secondary to anaerobic glycolysis. Impaired tissue perfusion also increases lactate production due to the decreased availability of oxygen at the end of the electron transport chain, and decreased uptake of lactate by the liver as a result of hepatic hypoperfusion. Base deficit measurement is readily available in the emergency department, unlike lactate measurement, and has been successfully used as a marker to guide fluid resuscitation in the trauma patient. However, the use of lactate as a measure to guide resuscitation is increasing.

Immunosuppression

Severe trauma results in an increased susceptibility to infection, but it is difficult to elucidate how much is due to direct tissue injury and how much is due to the effects of haemorrhage and massive transfusion, or a combination of the two.[12] Animal studies confirm that haemorrhage induces marked immunosuppression and that a 'second hit', such as an infective insult, significantly increases mortality.[13]

Human host defence responses vary from hyperactive through adequate to hyporeactive depending on individual circumstances and probably a genetic

disposition.[12] Those with an adequate response do well, whilst those with an exaggerated response appear to be susceptible to multiple 'hits'. In the hyporeactive group 'immune paralysis' is reflected by decreased expression of histocompatibility antigens and impaired antigen presentation by monocytes and macrophages.

A unifying theory suggests that after major trauma patients develop an early and appropriate SIRS upon resuscitation. This mild to moderate SIRS resolves with supportive care as the patient improves. However, if another 'hit' occurs, severe SIRS may then develop. After massive trauma a severe SIRS can evolve directly into MOF. With time there is a compensatory anti-inflammatory response syndrome (CARS) which limits the initial SIRS, and thus the destructive effects of inflammation.[14]

The requirement for massive transfusions of whole blood appears to be an independent risk factor for the development of MOF and not simply a reflection of the severity of injury and shock. This may be due to the immunosuppressive effect of blood transfusion. Table 22.1 summarizes the risk factors for the development of MOF.

DAMAGE CONTROL SURGERY

Historically it was thought that initial definitive repair of all injuries was associated with improved outcomes and functional results. This was true for simple isolated injuries, but multiply injured patients often died due to the 'severity of their injuries' whilst surgeons attempted to achieve a perfect surgical result. It is now appreciated that patients die not necessarily from their injuries but from the physiological derangements that occur during prolonged operative attempts at definitive anatomical repair. Thus the concept of 'damage control surgery' (DCS) has evolved: *Doing just enough to save life and limb whilst reserving definitive repair for a time when the patient is more physiologically stable and able to withstand the procedure.*[15]

The 'trauma triad of death', consisting of acidosis, coagulopathy and hypothermia, makes prolonged definitive surgery dangerous, leading Rotondo *et al.*[15] to

Table 22.1 Risk factors for developing multiple organ failure

Host factors	Age >55 years
	Male sex
	Comorbidities
Tissue injury	Mechanism of injury (blunt > penetrating)
	Glasgow Coma Scale <8
	Injury Severity Score >25
Clinical indicators of shock	Systolic blood pressure on admission <90 mmHg
	Red cell transfusion >6 units/12 h
	Arterial base deficit >8 mEq/L: worst in 24 h
	Arterial blood lactate >2.5 mmol/L

describe a multiphase approach, in which reoperation occurs when patients are more physiologically stable.[16–20] Although initially developed for abdominal injuries, the concept has now evolved to include all trauma contexts.

> Prolonged surgery for definitive repair of injuries in the physiologically compromised worsens outcome.

Hypothermia

Severe haemorrhage results in hypothermia due to cold fluid resuscitation, evaporative losses, exposure, loss of thermoregulation and reduced heat generation. Significant hypothermia further exacerbates tissue hypoperfusion due to cardiac dysrhythmias, reduced cardiac output, increased systemic vascular resistance and a left-shift of the oxygen–haemoglobin dissociation curve.

Coagulopathy

Altered coagulation occurs as a result of hypothermic inhibition of clotting cascades as well as clotting factor and platelet consumption and dilution. Platelet dysfunction occurs as a result of an imbalance between thromboxane and prostacyclin in hypothermic states.

Acidosis

Hypoperfusion results in anaerobic metabolism and lactate production. Acidosis impairs cardiovascular function, imparts an increased ventilatory burden as well as impairing coagulation and other vital functions. This can be further exacerbated by resuscitation with substantial quantities of fluids, most of which contain high concentrations of chloride. As a result, hyperchloraemic metabolic acidosis develops because of a combination of factors. For example, normal saline contains 154 mEq/L sodium and chloride, has a pH of 5–6 and possesses little buffering capacity but is used to replace blood which has a pH of 7.4 and an extensive buffering capacity. Additionally, volume expansion causes plasma bicarbonate dilution, and renal bicarbonate wasting. Other factors to consider are the effect of unmeasured strong ions[21] and the fact that proportionately more chloride ions are infused.

The triad of hypothermia, acidosis and coagulopathy results in a vicious, self-perpetuating cycle which, unless interrupted, is fatal.

The type of surgery performed affects patients' care in the ICU; thus, it is imperative to appreciate what the surgical team have achieved and have yet to do. The initial aims are rapid control of exsanguinating haemorrhage and control of gastrointestinal contamination. Haemorrhage

control may mandate temporary aortic cross-clamping, invoking a further ischaemia–reperfusion insult to the patient. Control may also be achieved by packing the cavity in question, requiring it to be left 'open'. The parameters for embarking on a DCS approach are outlined in Table 22.2, and the decision should ideally be made before the onset of clinically evident coagulopathy (Table 22.3).

> The decision to undertake damage control surgery should be made as early as possible.

The second stage of DCS occurs on the ICU, where rapid controlled correction of hypothermia takes place to facilitate attempts to correct the coagulopathy and acidosis. This requires both active and passive measures, including warming blankets, warmed humidified gases and warmed infused fluids. The aim is to raise the patient's temperature to 35°C, at which point physiological clotting begins to occur. This stage can last 48–72 hours, during which time the patient requires continued monitoring and reassessment for missed injuries and developing pathologies. An early return to theatre is indicated if there is ongoing surgical haemorrhage, limb or bowel ischaemia or an abdominal compartment syndrome.

Continued fluid resuscitation, with blood products as necessary, is guided by laboratory results, aiming for a platelet count >100 000 and an international normalized ratio (INR) <1.4 if there is persistent bleeding; remember that laboratory values for hypothermic patients are erroneous as the measurements assume a body temperature of 37°C. Cryoprecipitate is required if the fibrinogen level is less than 1 g/L. Vitamin K and calcium gluconate may also be administered. If bleeding continues despite correction of clotting factors and surgical control

Table 22.2 Indicators for the need to consider damage control

Injury pattern
Inability to achieve haemostasis (? due to coagulopathy)
Time-consuming procedure (>90 minutes)
Inaccessible major venous injury
Associated life-threatening injury in another location (e.g. head injury)
Planned re-exploration
Inability to close abdomen (gut oedema/intra-abdominal hypertension)

Table 22.3 Indicators for the development of coagulopathy[22]

Injury Severity Score	>26
Systolic blood pressure	<70 mmHg
pH	<7.10
Temperature	<34°C

Table 22.4 Goals of resuscitation

Lactate	<2.5 mmol/L
Base excess	>–4 mmol/L
Temperature	>35°C
INR	<1.25× normal
Urine output	>1mL/kg

INR, international normalized ratio.

Table 22.5 Indications for platelet transfusions

Platelet count	
<10 × 10^9/L	Transfusion definitely indicated
30–50 × 10^9/L	Transfuse if ongoing bleeding or high risk of bleeding
<100 × 10^9/L	Transfuse in acute severe trauma

of bleeding points, then recombinant activated factor VII may be considered according to local protocols. The goals of ongoing resuscitation are listed in Table 22.4.

Damage control orthopaedics

The reaming of long bones results in an increase in neutrophils, interleukin 6 (IL-6) levels and intramedullary pressures as well as blood loss. This can be associated with adverse outcome, especially in patients with concomitant severe head injury, pulmonary contusions or an ISS >18. Thus, external fixation is an appropriate temporizing measure with definitive nailing delayed for 10–14 days.[23]

HAEMORRHAGE AND COAGULOPATHY

Coagulopathy is evident on admission in a quarter of patients with an ISS >15 and in two-thirds of patients with an ISS >45. For a similar degree of trauma, patients who are coagulopathic on arrival at hospital have almost double the risk of mortality, despite a restricted fluid

administration policy.[24] A prolonged PT or activated partial thromboplastin time (aPTT) is also common in trauma patients. A ratio >1.5 has been found to predict excessive bleeding and is a strong, independent predictor of mortality.[24]

The incidence of thrombocytopenia (platelets <100 × 10^9/L) is 35–41% in trauma and surgical patients compared with 20–25% in other critically ill patient populations. This results in an increased risk of bleeding and may also indicate ongoing coagulation activity, resulting in microvascular changes and contributing to organ failure. Thrombocytopenia is also an independent predictor of ICU mortality and is inversely related to survival – a persistent thrombocytopenia for more than 4 days after admission or a drop >50% during ICU stay correlates with a sixfold increase in mortality.[25]

Any major haemorrhage results in a decrease in clotting factors and platelets due to consumption, decreased synthesis, vascular injury and ongoing loss and dilution. Furthermore, after resuscitation, a reduced haematocrit and an increased perfusion pressure may result in disruption of any clots formed, further exacerbating blood loss.

Coagulopathy can also occur independently of haemorrhage, as a result other pathologies such as fat

Table 22.6 Blood product use in coagulopathy

Product	Indication	Mechanism
Fresh-frozen plasma	Massive red blood cell transfusion International normalized ratio >1.5 + ongoing bleeding	All clotting factors
Fractionated plasma	As for fresh-frozen plasma + need to avoid large volumes	
Purified factor concentrate	As for fresh-frozen plasma + need to avoid large volumes	
Prothrombin complex concentrates	Reversal of warfarin	Factors II, VII, IX, X
Desmopressin (DDAVP)	Coagulopathy on intensive care unit; uraemic platelet dysfunction	Potentiation of primary haemostasis by unknown mechanism; releases endothelial clotting factors and von Willebrand factor
Aprotinin	Major high-risk surgery; exact role in trauma unclear	Protease inhibitor; attenuates fibrinolysis, thrombin generation, inflammatory responses
Tranexamic acid/ε-aminocaproic acid	Major high-risk surgery; exact role in trauma unclear	Anti-fibrinolytics; lysine analogues
Factor VIIa	Controversial: pH >7.1, temperature >34°C, platelets >50 × 10^9/L	Unclear in trauma

embolism, sepsis and head injury, in which neuronal injury results in the release of tissue thromboplastins; it may also pre-exist as a result of drug therapy or pre-morbid conditions such as haemophilia.[26,27] Tables 22.5 and 22.6 detail the indications for platelet therapy and other blood product use in traumatic coagulopathy.

Recombinant activated factor VII (FVIIa) is a novel agent licensed for use in haemophilia, but used off-licence as an adjunct to source control and conventional coagulation support in major haemorrhage. In blunt trauma there is a significantly reduced red cell transfusion requirement with an associated trend towards reduced organ failure and morbidity.[28]

Dutton et al.[29] compared patients who received FVIIa for traumatic haemorrhage with matched control subjects, and found an improved outcome in those patients who had a significant response to the dose administered. Thromboelastograms for a few of the patients revealed that FVIIa resulted in a faster onset and rate of clot formation. Other studies have suggested that pH at the time of administration, temperature and platelet count are important determinants of successful use of FVIIa, necessitating a pH >7.1, platelet count $>50 \times 10^9$/L and a temperature >34°C.[26]

Controversies still exist regarding the exact indications for the use of FVIIa in trauma, especially in the context of head injury, although there is increasing evidence for its use in patients with spontaneous cerebral and subarachnoid haemorrhage. The exact dose and timing of therapy have also yet to be elucidated, and phase II and III trials are awaited.

CHEST AND ACUTE LUNG INJURY

Pulmonary complications account for a significant proportion of mortality and morbidity after trauma. Apart from direct thoracic injury and pulmonary contusions, trauma can result in ALI, acute respiratory distress syndrome (ARDS), pneumonia, atelectasis and pulmonary embolism. Factors associated with the development of ARDS include higher APACHE score, more severe injury to the chest and ISS >25.[30] The mechanism of injury and timing of surgery are also important. The development of ALI/ARDS can double the mortality risk irrespective of the degree of injury.[30]

Prolonged ventilation (>4 days) is required in about 25% of patients after major trauma,[31] but intubation and ventilation are themselves associated with the development of pneumonia and aggravation of alveolar injury. Large tidal volumes result in greater alveolar stretch, which incites an exaggerated alveolar inflammatory response, increasing levels of inflammatory mediators in the systemic circulation. Guidelines exist for optimizing ventilation in trauma patients, in an attempt to prevent further ventilation-induced alveolar damage and minimize the duration of mechanical ventilation (Table

Table 22.7 Ventilation strategies in acute lung injury/acute respiratory distress syndrome

In general, appropriate initial ventilator settings in a patient with acute lung injury would be:

Tidal volume	6–8 mL/kg predicted ideal body weight
Respiratory rate	12–35 breaths/min
Positive end-expiratory pressure	+10 to +15 cmH$_2$0
Inspiratory/expiratory ratio	1:2
Plateau pressure	<35 cmH$_2$O

Adjustments should be made after review of arterial blood gases, to ensure:

Po$_2$ >8 kPa or SpO$_2$ >88%	Titrate FiO$_2$, positive end-expiratory pressure
pH >7.25	Adjust rate

(if pH <7.25 despite optimal ventilation then bicarbonate infusion may be considered)

22.7).[32,33] Hypercapnia should be tolerated unless contraindicated by concomitant pathology such as raised intracranial pressure.

> Ventilatory volutrauma may worsen acute lung injury.

In severe ARDS, when oxygenation is the predominant problem, the patient may need to be fully sedated and paralysed and transient periods of hypoxia tolerated, especially if associated with a 'de-recruiting' procedure such as endobronchial suction. In extreme cases, prone ventilation, nebulized prostacyclin or ventilation using a high-frequency oscillator may be beneficial, but trials of these novel techniques have been equivocal when long-term outcome and death are the end-points, despite clinical improvements in oxygenation at the bedside.

Fat embolism can occur when fat leaks into the systemic circulation. It results in embolic symptoms and most commonly occurs after long-bone or pelvic trauma but has been described in other situations. Fat embolism occurs after all major long bone fractures but usually goes unnoticed. Some patients will develop fat embolism syndrome (FES), which is a more serious condition affecting multiple organ systems, usually developing 24–72 hours after long-bone or pelvic trauma. A classical triad of hypoxaemia, neurological abnormalities and petechial rash is described, although not all features may occur and the symptoms may not occur simultaneously.[34,35] Fat can be detected in the lungs after even minor trauma and may pass into the systemic circulation via pulmonary capillaries or shunts or a patent foramen ovale. Fat embolus can be found in 90% of patients with long-bone fractures and invariably in all patients after reaming for intramedullary nail fixation, but FES occurs in only 1–5%. Symptoms occur as a result of direct vascular occlusion, the breakdown of free fatty

Table 22.8 Features of fat embolism

Petechial rash	Head and neck , anterior thorax, subconjunctivae, axillae
Respiratory	Tachypnoea, dyspnoea, haemoptysis, bilateral crepitations, bilateral infiltrates on chest radiograph, acute lung injury/acute respiratory distress syndrome
Neurological	Confusion, drowsiness, coma
Cardiovascular	Tachycardia, hypotension
Haematological	Thrombocytopenia (>50% decrease), anaemia (>20% decrease), erythrocyte sedimentation rate >71 mm/h, fat macroglobulaemia
Other	Fever, jaundice, renal dysfunction, retinal changes (fat or petechiae), Purscher's retinopathy

acids (FFAs) to toxic metabolites or the activation of the coagulation and fibrinolytic pathways by activated platelets (Table 22.8).

Acute respiratory distress syndrome and FES overlap in both clinical features and aetiologies, and it is possible that FES may be missed when a patient is labelled as having ARDS. The incidence of both can be reduced with prompt fixation of bony injuries.

GENERAL ORGAN SUPPORT

Even in the presence of isolated trauma, other organ dysfunction can develop. Complications common to all critically ill patients include the development of sepsis, ventilator-associated lung injury with pneumonia and renal dysfunction. In 2003 The Surviving Sepsis Campaign guidelines[36] were developed as an international collaboration to increase awareness and improve outcomes in sepsis and septic shock. The recommendations have amalgamated the recent literature, providing an evidence-based framework for the general management of a critically ill patient with sepsis. The updated guidelines were published in 2008.[37]

These measures are being implemented as locally developed bundles of care. A 'care bundles' approach is one whereby clinical processes are systematically appraised, by measuring actual provision of therapeutic interventions according to national standards and local protocols. These bundles often incorporate what are considered general, routine, inexpensive care measures as well as more specific, specialized, possibly more expensive, therapeutic options.

Adherence to the bundle involves compliance with all aspects. Overall care can be measured and literature is emerging which suggests that the bundle approach is modifying behaviour and resulting in decreased in-hospital mortality.[38] Commonly used bundles include ventilator bundles and sepsis bundles. The case scenario and Tables 22.9 and 22.10 summarize general management of the critically ill patient.

> The surviving sepsis guidelines improve outcome.

A degree of renal dysfunction is common and prevention of renal failure is a priority; thus, it is imperative to ensure adequate fluid resuscitation and mean arterial pressure to maintain renal perfusion.

Causes of renal dysfunction include:

- hypoperfusion;
- rhabdomyolysis;
- abdominal compartment syndrome;
- direct renal injury.

Renal replacement therapy (RRT) is indicated in established renal failure but is often instituted earlier if the patient is unstable due to persistent acidaemia or hyperlactaemia (Table 22.11). High-volume RRT is also instituted in many units in the presence of severe sepsis.[45] Rhabdomyolysis is an important cause of renal dysfunction in trauma. This should be anticipated and treated with a high fluid input–output strategy.

Table 22.9 Initial resuscitation/goal-directed therapy[39]

Intervention	Target
Immediate fluid resuscitation	CVP 8–12 mmHg (breathing spontaneously); CVP 12–15 mmHg (mechanically ventilated)
Vasopressors (noradrenaline/adrenaline)	MAP >65 mmHg
	MAP >80 mmHg (known hypertensive)
End-organ perfusion	Urine output >0.5 mL/kg/h
Central venous or mixed venous oxygen saturation measurement	Saturation >70%

CVP, central venous pressure; MAP, mean arterial pressure.

Table 22.10 General supportive measures

Intervention	Indications	Target/dose
Source control – cultures	Pyrexia; increasing white cell count or C-reactive protein; increasing vasodilatation	Blood (peripheral and lines); urine (catheter specimen of urine, midstream urine specimen); sputum (endotracheal); aspirates/bronchoalveolar lavage; wounds (pus/fluids); drains; stool
Source control – imaging		Cerebrospinal fluid; ultrasound; computed tomography; surgery
Broad-spectrum antibiotics	Unknown infective source	Until culture results known, then rationalize antibiotics
Steroids[40]	Septic shock; adrenal insufficiency	Hydrocortisone 200–300 mg/24 h; fludrocortisone 50 mg/24 h
Recombinant human activated protein C[41]	Septic shock and high risk of death; APACHE >25; multiple organ failure	As per local protocols
Conservative transfusion strategies[42]	Anaemia	Hb 7–8 g/dL
	Ischaemic heart disease	Hb 9–10 g/dL
	Bleeding/coagulopathy	Hb >9–10 g/dL
Glycaemic control[43]	Tight control associated with improved outcomes; adverse outcome if missed hypoglycaemia; avoid hypo- or hyperglycaemia	4–6.6 >mmol/L (tight); 4–8 >mmol/L (conservative)
Sedation, analgesia and neuromuscular blockade[44]	Accumulation in critical illness, renal failure, hepatic dysfunction results in prolonged ventilation	Daily sedation holds if stable; titrate to sedation score
Thromboprophylaxis	Prevention of deep vein thrombosis/ pulmonary embolism; critically ill are prothrombotic owing to immobility	Subcutaneous heparin or low-molecular-weight heparin if no risk of bleeding; heparin infusions if multiple surgical interventions; intermittent compression boots; graduated compression stockings; temporary inferior vena cava filter
Nutrition		Enteral; parenteral if enteral not established
Stress ulcer prophylaxis		Proton pump inhibitors; H_2 antagonists; sucralfate

APACHE, Acute Physiology and Chronic Health Evaluation.

Table 22.11 Indications for renal replacement therapy

Acutely unstable patient	Stable intensive care unit patient
Persistent acidaemia: pH >7.1	Hyperkalaemia
Hyperlactataemia	Oliguria/anuria
Pulmonary oedema	Fluid balance/overload
Hyperkalaemia and anuria	New renal impairment + creatinine 400 mmol/L, urea >40 mmol/L

Case scenario

A 27-year-old man was admitted having been stabbed several times in the upper abdomen. He walked into the emergency department from the pub next door, vomited and then collapsed. During his initial resuscitation a FAST scan demonstrated free fluid in the abdomen. As he was making only a transient and unsustained response to intravenous fluid resuscitation, he was taken immediately to the operating theatre, where he underwent an emergency laparotomy. He needed 8 units of packed red cells, clotting factors (fresh-frozen plasma and platelets) and ongoing fluid boluses. He was found to have sustained several liver lacerations and small bowel lacerations. His core temperature was now 32°C and he had a pH of 7.15.

What surgical approach is indicated?

The patient has two triggers for a damage control laparotomy – low temperature and acidosis. Active warming measures and maintenance of adequate perfusion pressure must be instituted if not already done so and an abbreviated laparotomy is required, including packing of his liver lacerations, arrest of obvious bleeding points, isolation of full-thickness small bowel injuries by stapling off injured segments and, if possible, temporary abdominal closure.

How should his management proceed from this point?

The patient should be transferred to the ICU and kept sedated and ventilated and strategies used to optimize all his systems. For example, as he had diminished lung compliance and increasing oxygen requirements, he was ventilated using lung-protective strategies – tidal volumes of 6–8 mL/kg, positive end-expiratory pressure of ~10 cmH$_2$O, accepting PaO$_2$ >8 kPa – and, as he had no original head trauma, permissive hypercarbia was tolerated. Blood pressure was maintained using fluid boluses until his central venous pressure measured 8–12 cmH$_2$O and, as there was a high risk of ongoing haemorrhage, blood was transfused to keep the haemoglobin ~10 g/dL. A low-dose noradrenaline infusion was commenced titrated to keep mean arterial pressure (MAP) >60 mmHg. End-organ perfusion was monitored initially using urine output, aiming for 0.5 mL/kg/h. Overnight the patient was actively warmed and returned to theatre the following morning for re-laparotomy and pack removal.

Over the next 48 hours he developed a pyrexia of 39°C, his blood pressure became labile and he became oliguric. His white cell count was 24 × 10^9/L and C-reactive protein 150 mg/L. Outline the intensive care response.

The patient was clearly in septic shock and was started on the 'sepsis bundle' as per the unit protocol. Intravascular filling was assessed using clinical assessment and central venous SvO$_2$ measurement. This was 56% and so he received a transfusion of packed red cells and a dobutamine infusion was commenced. Noradrenaline requirements continued to increase; thus, invasive cardiac output monitoring was instituted, which showed a cardiac index of 3.8 L/min/m^2 and systemic vascular resistance 800 dynes × s/cm^5. Noradrenaline was thus titrated to achieve MAP >70 mmHg and he was started on steroids.

What are the likely potential sources of his sepsis?

As recommended in the 'Surviving Sepsis' guidelines, this patient was started on broad-spectrum antibiotics after appropriate cultures. The most likely sources of sepsis were considered to be either pulmonary or intra-abdominal, although as his central and arterial lines had been sited in the emergency department, cultures were drawn through them and new lines sited.

Despite adequate volume loading and perfusion his urine output remained poor and his abdomen tensely distended. What abdominal condition should be ruled out as a cause of his oliguria and difficult ventilation?

The patient's clinical picture could be provoked by an abdominal compartment syndrome and steps should be taken to exclude other causes and ascertain his intra-abdominal pressure. Using an intravesical pressure transducer his abdominal pressures were found to be 30 cmH$_2$O and his airway pressures continued to increase. Chest radiography demonstrated no focal changes and his endotracheal aspirates were minimal. Bedside ultrasound of his abdomen was unhelpful and he was too unstable to be transferred for a computed tomography scan as his ventilation was precarious. Thus, it was decided to perform another laparotomy and leave his abdomen open to relieve his abdominal compartment syndrome and to facilitate ventilation and recovery of renal function, which duly happened with an eventual successful outcome.

SUMMARY

The ICU plays an integral part in the management of many trauma victims as they are at risk of organ failure distant to those areas of primary injury. Physiological restitution is the vital second phase of damage control surgery, without which the patients will not be fit to return to the operating theatre for definitive repair of their injuries. Implementation of the various 'sepsis bundles' derived by the 'Surviving Sepsis' campaign can improve outcome.

GLOBAL PERSPECTIVES

Trauma is a worldwide phenomenon and does not discriminate by age, race or prosperity.

In the elderly, it is often due to falls, whereas in the under 40s trauma due to road traffic accidents or violence is the major cause of morbidity and mortality, which has a huge economic impact. In 2004, road traffic accidents in Spain cost over 6 billion Euros, which is 1.35% of the GNP, 55% as direct costs and 45% as indirect costs owing to loss of productivity and the ongoing costs of long-term disability.[3]

REFERENCES

1. Airey CM, Franks AJ. Major trauma workload within an English Health Region. *Injury* 1995;**26**: 25–31.
2. Sauaia A, Moore FA, Moore EE, *et al.* Epidemiology of trauma deaths: a reassessment. *J Trauma* 1995;**38**:185–93.
3. Bastida JL, Aguilar PS, Gonzalez BD. The economic costs of traffic accidents in Spain. *J Trauma* 2004;**56**:883–8.
4. Durham RM, Moran JJ, Mazuski JE, *et al.* Multiple organ failure in trauma patients. *J. Trauma* 2003;**55**:608–16.
5. Moore FA, Moore EE, Sauaia A. Blood transfusion. An independent risk factor for postinjury multiple organ failure. *Arch Surg* 1997;**132**:620–5.
6. Eberhard LW, Morabito DJ, Matthay MA, *et al.* Initial severity of metabolic acidosis predicts the development of acute lung injury in severely traumatised patients. *Crit Care Med* 2000;**28**:125–31.
7. Maekawa K, Futami S, Nashida M, *et al.* Effects of trauma and sepsis on soluble L-selectin and cell surface expression of L-selectin and CD11b. *J Trauma* 1998;**44**:460–6.
8. Botha AJ, Moore FA, Moore EE, *et al.* Early neutrophil sequestration after injury: a pathogenic mechanism for multiple organ failure. *J Trauma* 1995;**39**:411–17.
9. Sauaia A, Moore FA, Moore EE, *et al.* Multiple organ failure can be predicted as early as 12 hours after injury. *J Trauma* 1998;**45**:291–301.
10. Brown GE, Silver GM, Reiff J, *et al.* Polymorphonuclear neutrophil chemiluminescence in whole blood from blunt trauma patients with multiple injuries. *J Trauma* 1999;**46**:297–305.
11. Botha AJ, Moore FA, Moore EE, *et al.* Base deficit after major trauma directly relates to neutrophil CD11b expression: a proposed mechanism for shock induced organ injury. *Intensive Care Med* 1997;**23**:504–9.
12. Martin C. Immune responses after trauma and haemorrhagic shock. In: Galley HF, ed. *Critical Care Focus: 11. Trauma.* Oxford: Blackwell Publishing, 2005.
13. Stephan RN, Kupper TS, Geha AS, *et al.* Haemorrhage without tissue trauma produces immunosuppression and enhances susceptibility to sepsis. *Arch Surg* 1987;**122**:62–8.
14. Moore FA, Sauaia A, Moore EE, *et al.* Post injury multi organ failure: a bimodal phenomenon. *J Trauma* 1996;**40**:501–12.
15. Rotondo KL, Schwab CW, McGonigal MD, *et al.* 'Damage control': an approach for improved survival in exsanguinating penetrating abdominal injury. *J Trauma* 1993;**5**:375–83.
16. Johnson JW, Gracias VH, Schwab CW, *et al.* Evolution of damage control for exsanguinating penetrating abdominal injury. *J Trauma* 2001;**51**:261–71.
17. Mohr AM, Asensio JA, Garcia-Nunez LM, *et al.* Guidelines for the institution of damage control in trauma patients. *International Trauma Care (ITAACS)* 2005;fall:185–9.
18. Moeng MS, Loveland JA, Boffard KD. Damage control: beyond the limits of the abdominal cavity. A review. *International Trauma Care (ITAACS)* 2005;fall:189–96.
19. Dutton RP. Damage control anaesthesia. *International Trauma Care (ITAACS)* 2005;fall:197–201.
20. Lee JC, Peitzman AB. Damage control laparotomy. *Curr Opin Crit Care* 2006;**12**:346–50.
21. Kellum JA. Disorders of acid–base balance. *Crit Care Med* 2007;**35**:2630–6.
22. Cosgriff, N, Moore EE, Sauaia A, *et al.* Predicting life-threatening coagulopathy in the massively transfused trauma patient: hypothermia and acidosis revisited. *J Trauma* 1997;**42**:857–61; discussion 861–2.
23. Roberts CS, Pape H, Jones AL, *et al.* Damage control orthopaedics. Evolving concepts in the treatment of patients who have sustained orthopaedic trauma. *J Bone Joint Surg* 2005;**87A**:434–49.
24. Brohi K, Singh J, Heron M, Coats T. Acute traumatic coagulopathy. *J Trauma* 2003;**54**:1127–30.
25. Levi M, Opal SM. Coagulation abnormalities in critically ill patients. *Crit Care* 2006;**10**:222.
26. Schreiber MA. Coagulopathy in the trauma patient. *Curr Opin Crit Care* 2005;**11**:590–7.
27. Hess JR, Hiippala S. Optimizing the use of blood products in trauma care. *Crit Care* 2005(Suppl. 5):S10–S14.
28. Boffard KB, Riou B, Warren B, *et al.* Recombinant factor VIIa as an adjunctive therapy in bleeding control in severely injured trauma patients. *J Trauma* 2005;**1**:8–15.
29. Dutton RP, McCunn M, Hyder M, *et al.* Factor VIIa for correction of traumatic coagulopathy. *J Trauma* 2004,**57**:709–18.

30.   Treggiari MM, Hudson LD, Martin DP, *et al.* Effect of acute lung injury and acute respiratory distress syndrome on outcome in critically ill trauma patients. *Crit Care Med* 2004;**32**:327–31.

31.   American College of Surgeons. National Trauma Data Bank™, 2003.

32.   Nathens AB, Johnson JL, Minei JP, *et al.* Guidelines for the mechanical ventilation of the trauma patient. *J Trauma* 2005;**59**:764–9.

33.   The Acute Respiratory Distress Syndrome Network. Ventilation with lower tidal volumes as compared with traditional tidal volumes for acute lung injury and acute respiratory distress syndrome. *N Engl J Med* 2000;**342**:1301–8.

34.   Georgopoulos D, Bouros D. Fat embolism syndrome. Clinical diagnosis is still the preferable diagnostic method. *Chest* 2003;**123**:982–3.

35.   Glover P, Worthley LIG. Fat embolism. *Crit Care Resusc* 1999;**1**:276–84.

36.   Dellinger RP, Carlet JM, Masur H, *et al.* Surviving Sepsis Campaign guidelines for management of severe sepsis and septic shock. *Intensive Care Med* 2004;**30**:536–55.

37.   Dellinger RP, Levy MM, Carlet JM, *et al.* Surviving Sepsis Campaign: international guidelines for management of severe sepsis and septic shock. *Intensive Care Med* 2008;**34**:17–60.

38.   Nguyen HB, Corbett SW, Steele R, *et al.* Implementation of a bundle of quality indicators for the early management of severe sepsis and septic shock is associated with decreased mortality. *Crit Care Med* 2007;**35**:1105–12.

39.   Rivers E, Nguyen B, Havstad S, *et al.* Early goal directed therapy in the treatment of severe sepsis and septic shock. *N Engl J Med* 2001;**345**:1368–77.

40.   Annane D, Sebille V, Charpentier C, *et al.* Effect of treatment with low doses of hydrocortisone and fludrocortisone on mortality in patients with septic shock. *JAMA* 2002;**288**:862–71.

41.   Bernard GR, Vincent JL, Laterre PF, *et al.* Recombinant human Protein C Worldwide Evaluation in Severe Sepsis (PROWRESS). Efficacy and safety. *N Engl J Med* 2001;**344**:699–709.

42.   Herbert PC, Wells G, Blajchman MA, *et al.* A multicenter randomised controlled trial of transfusion in critical care. *N Engl J Med* 1999;**340**:409–17.

43.   Berghe G, Wouters P, Weekers F, *et al.* Intensive insulin therapy in critically ill patients. *N Engl J Med* 2001;**345**:1359–67.

44.   Kress JP, Pohlman AS, O'Connor MF, Hall JB. Daily interruption of sedative infusions in critically ill patients undergoing mechanical ventilation. *N Engl J Med* 2000;**342**:1471–7.

45.   Ronco C, Ricci Z, Bellomo R. Importance of increased ultrafiltration volume and impact on mortality: sepsis and cytokine story and the role of continuous veno-venous haemofiltration. *Curr Opin Nephrol Hypertens* 2001;**10**:755–61.

Patient transfer

OBJECTIVES

After completing this chapter the reader will:
- understand the indications for inter- and intra-hospital transfer of the trauma patient
- be able to recognize the dangers involved in patient transfer
- appreciate how to perform safe transfer, with particular regard to communication and planning, optimal timing and mode of transport, stabilization before transfer, drugs, equipment and monitoring en route and arranging escorts.

The good work done in the resuscitation room is then undone during the journey.[1]

INTRODUCTION

Transfer is inherently undesirable. It becomes necessary when the care the patient can receive elsewhere is better than that which can be provided locally, taking due consideration of the risks of transferring the patient between the two locations.

> The ability to deliver better care elsewhere is the basis of all secondary transfers.

There is an inescapable logic for the continuing need to transfer trauma patients: there is too little work for supraregional specialties such as neurosurgery to justify setting up a specialist service in each acute hospital and patients are still generally taken from the scene to the nearest acute hospital rather than triaging them all directly to a regional trauma centre. A typical district general hospital with a catchment population of 250 000 will need to transfer about one or two major trauma patients per month.

Inter-hospital transfer is a potentially dangerous time for the critically injured patient.[2] The main problems arise from:

- deterioration in the patient's underlying condition, including his or her injuries, concurrent medical problems and complications;
- physical disturbance from vibration, acceleration and deceleration, including the risk of an ambulance crash;
- loss of temperature control (usually, but not invariably, cooling);
- specific problems associated with altitude in transfers by air;
- limited access to the patient;
- difficulty in making clinical assessments and interventions while moving;
- inexperienced escorts;
- lack of access to specialized help or facilities en route;
- limited drugs and equipment;
- equipment failure;
- unexpected delays during the journey;
- errors in planning and communication.

Many of these factors also apply to transfer within a hospital,[3] and it is important not to become complacent because of the short distance involved. An endotracheal tube can become dislodged just as easily in a hospital corridor as in an ambulance.

> Similar care is needed for *intra*-hospital as for *inter*-hospital transfers.

Many patients are transferred by inexperienced doctors and nurses with little formal training in patient transfer and with varying standards of equipment and monitoring. While guidelines and training courses have been developed to help address this, poor compliance with the guidelines, limited course uptake and inadequate audit data leave the problems unresolved.

THE RISKS OF TRANSFER

The patient is already at risk because of the injuries sustained, so in order to benefit from care at the destination, the risks of transfer must be acknowledged and minimized. It is not only the patient who is exposed to risk; escorts are also vulnerable. Damage to valuable equipment may also occur, escalating the cost and the risks to the patient.

The risks for patients

Dangers to the patient include the following.

AIRWAY

- Airway compromise due to:
  - a deteriorating conscious level
  - increasing airway swelling from oedema or haematoma, especially after burns and injuries to the face and neck
  - obstruction of an endotracheal tube or displacement out of the larynx or into a main stem bronchus
  - endotracheal cuff pressure injury or cuff rupture at high altitude.
- Further spinal injury from failure to immobilize the neck adequately in a neutral position.

OXYGENATION AND VENTILATION

- Hypoxia due to:
  - worsening pulmonary contusion
  - failure of the oxygen supply
  - low partial pressure of oxygen at altitude.
- Hypoventilation due to:
  - a deteriorating consciousness level
  - a high spinal cord injury interfering with intercostal or diaphragmatic function
  - a flail chest with pain-related splinting
  - tension pneumothorax (especially during air travel) or an increasing haemothorax
  - ventilator disconnection or failure.
- Chest drain blockage, disconnection or displacement.

Hypoventilation, hypoxia and hypercarbia are difficult to detect clinically during transfer, the pulse oximeter may be ineffective in the face of poor peripheral perfusion and the capnograph may yield an end-tidal CO_2 level that is not representative of the arterial level.

CIRCULATION

- Bleeding either internally or externally, often exacerbated by movement or by hypothermia.

- Displacement of intravascular lines (peripheral venous, central venous or arterial) or their connections, leading to:
  - loss of drug or fluid effect
  - loss of monitoring information
  - further bleeding from the site (a particular risk when an arterial line becomes disconnected)
  - air embolism when a central line is disconnected in an underfilled patient
  - delay or difficulty in attempting to recannulate en route.

NERVOUS SYSTEM

- Worsening cerebral perfusion from:
  - hypotension from bleeding, other causes of shock or oversedation
  - raised intracranial pressure associated with hypoxia, hypercarbia, inadequate sedation, exacerbated by coughing or gagging, or an increase in the size of the underlying intracranial lesion
  - hypoglycaemia (see below)
  - acceleration or deceleration of the vehicle
  - a head-down position in an airborne helicopter.
- Discomfort and distress in an undersedated patient.
- Pain from inadequate splinting of fractures.

METABOLISM

- Oliguria and uraemia from uncorrected hypovolaemia.
- Loss of glucose control:
  - hyperglycaemia, as a stress response or in known diabetics
  - hypoglycaemia, especially in small children, intoxicated adolescents or insulin-treated diabetics.

HOST DEFENCE

- Hypothermia, leading to:
  - vasoconstriction with reduced tissue perfusion
  - shivering with increased oxygen demand
  - coagulopathy
  - susceptibility to infection.
- Contamination of inadequately dressed or re-exposed wounds.
- Further injury from excessive movement, poorly secured equipment or a further crash, especially if the transfer vehicle has been travelling at high speed.

Specific risks of air transfer

In air transfers, there are particular risks that relate to altitude:[4]

- Exposure to low atmospheric pressure, leading to:
  - a fall in the partial pressure of atmospheric oxygen, increasing the risk of hypoxia and the need for oxygen supplementation
  - expansion of closed gas-containing structures within the patient such as pneumothoraces, pneumoperitoneum, bowel and pneumocephalus (a consequence of Boyle's law, which states that pressure is inversely proportional to volume)
  - expansion of closed gas-containing structures within equipment that may lead to harm, e.g. of endotracheal tube cuffs, risking cuff pressure damage or cuff rupture; of air splints and air trapped under encircling casts, risking compartment syndrome; and of vacuum mattresses, risking ineffective immobilization.
- Reduced humidity at altitude, affecting airway humidification.

The risk to escorts

Transfer may be hazardous not only for the patient, but also for the escorting staff and members of the public, especially when the vehicle is travelling at high speed. Adequate insurance provision is required, such as that provided to members of the Association of Anaesthetists of Great Britain and Ireland (AAGBI). There are also other risks to escorts, such as falls when moving around in a moving vehicle, impact from dislodged equipment, needlestick and ampoule injuries from drawing up drugs en route and back injuries from poor lifting technique.

TYPES OF TRANSFER

Outside hospital

There are three main types of transfer outside hospital, reflecting different phases of care:

- *Primary transfer to hospital.* The transfer of the injured patient from the scene of the incident to the primary receiving hospital by:
  - land ambulance staffed by paramedics with or without immediate-care doctors
  - specialist immediate-care helicopter services
  - hospital-based flying squads responding to the scene, usually in mass casualty incidents, in situations that require extraordinary clinical interventions at the scene or when the ambulance service is unable to provide advanced life support skills to a trapped patient.
- *Secondary transfer between hospitals for clinical reasons.* The movement of the patient from the primary receiving hospital to a secondary admitting hospital for care that is not available locally because:
  - the specialist care required for a particular injury, such as a major head injury requiring a neurosurgical unit, or for a particular patient, such as a critically injured child needing paediatric intensive care, is not normally available at the primary hospital
  - resources that are normally available are exhausted or temporarily unavailable – typically a lack of intensive care beds.
- *Tertiary transfer between hospitals for non-clinical reasons.* These transfers should not to be confused with secondary transfer to a 'tertiary' supraregional centre. These include:
  - repatriation for social reasons, such as being closer to family after a period of acute care in the primary or secondary hospital
  - transfer for financial reasons where insurance cover is not available or the cost of continuing care elsewhere is prohibitive, usually abroad.

PRIMARY TRANSFER

Primary transfer can be to the closest hospital or, where the predicted needs of the patient exceed the resources available in the local hospital, to a trauma centre or other major acute hospital with a full range of specialist services. Bypassing the nearest hospital increases the time to reach hospital but reduces the time to definitive care when regional specialist intervention is needed. Helicopter transport reduces the time difference for journeys between different hospitals, provided time is not wasted by road ambulance transfers between the helipad and the hospital receiving area. In primary transfers there is generally little opportunity to stabilize a patient at the scene, especially if the patient is bleeding; nevertheless, the general principles are similar to those of secondary transfers.[5]

INTER-HOSPITAL TRANSFER

In the UK, head injury is the commonest reason for inter-hospital transfer, partly because of the high incidence of head injury in road traffic collisions (RTCs) but also because most severely injured patients are taken to the nearest district general hospital whilst neurosurgical expertise is limited to regional centres typically serving six or more district hospitals. Patients with head injuries fare much better in neurosurgical units, even when surgical intervention is not required.[6] Mediastinal injuries represent another indication for centralized care, although the increased availability of high-quality computed tomography (CT) scanners in district hospitals has reduced the need to transfer simply to exclude injuries when the mediastinum is widened on the plain chest radiograph. Unstable pelvic injuries that require reconstructive surgery are also best treated in a specialist centre.

Children have specialized needs. It is not appropriate to nurse a child on an adult ward. Critically injured children need to be transferred to a paediatric intensive care unit.

Tertiary transfers are undertaken for non-clinical reasons and the patient should therefore be stable or the transfer be deferred.

Within the hospital

Intra-hospital transfer may be needed for investigation or treatment and the source or destination may be the emergency department, imaging suite, operating theatre, critical care unit or other acute ward. Imaging is a frequent indication for intra-hospital transfer, especially from the emergency department, to define injuries during the secondary survey, or from the intensive care unit to repeat the head CT scan at a time of concern. These are generally return journeys, to and from the imaging suite, although in some emergency situations the final destination will be different, for example when the imaging indicates a need for immediate operative intervention. Such uncertainty must be incorporated into the planning process.

The same standards of equipment, monitoring and escort staff training should apply to transfers within the hospital as apply to those between hospitals. The temptation to 'cut and run', even for short distances must be avoided, unless the intervention for which transfer is being made is critically time dependent for survival and temporary under-resuscitation is accepted as part of best management. Some aspects of care cannot be overlooked even in severely time-limited stabilization; for example, patients with a decompensating head injury and a dilating pupil must have their $PaCO_2$ checked on the transport ventilator prior to transfer to avoid inadvertent hypercarbia.

The journey time is shorter within the hospital and, although drugs, equipment and oxygen supplies can be 'scaled down' accordingly, unexpected delays such as getting stuck in a lift can still occur. The bed or trolley still needs a 'driver' as escorts should not have to push it, and it is also useful to have the equivalent of a 'police escort' with designated personnel holding open doors and lifts and clearing the corridor to prevent delays.

THE NEED TO TRANSFER

Inter-hospital transfer should be undertaken only if it is likely to lead to an improvement in the patient's overall condition. It is vital to consider the risks and benefits carefully and to demand senior involvement in the decision-making. The decision to transfer requires agreement between the sending and receiving hospitals, and this hinges on effective communication.

> Decisions regarding patient transfer must be taken at consultant level.

There are important resource implications for any transfer as losing a member of staff and an emergency vehicle for several hours may put undue pressure on the transferring hospital and its local ambulance service. Some transfers may be avoided by the specialist providing advice and support from what would be the receiving hospital, or even bringing the specialist to the patient; however, this places the specialist in unfamiliar surroundings, may necessitate the transfer of specialist surgical equipment as well and may have implications for the staffing of the specialist unit.

When transfer is necessary as a result of 'overflow', such as lack of intensive care beds, rather than lack of expertise, an ethical issue arises. If the trauma patient is unstable it may be safer to transfer out a more stable intensive care patient. This may not be in the latter's best interests but represents the safest option overall. A common alternative is to keep a patient in an operating theatre recovery ward instead of transferring out, providing surrogate but suboptimal intensive care. This will also deplete the on-call service as a doctor will usually have to stay with the patient for an even longer period than a transfer would have taken.

A national intensive care bed information service has been established in the UK, contactable on 0207 407 7181, to help identify the next closest appropriate hospital.

THE NEEDS OF TRANSFER

After agreeing transfer with an appropriate receiving unit, the needs of the patient during transfer should be considered. The urgency of transfer and the level of care provided en route are prime concerns. A suitable mode of transport must be chosen to support these needs. Escorts may be provided by the sending hospital, by the receiving unit or by a dedicated transfer agency.

Mode of transport

Inter-hospital transfer may be by land or air depending on the urgency and distance, the time to arrange transfer, weather and traffic conditions, the training of escorts and cost.

LAND AMBULANCE

This remains the commonest mode of transfer and is generally the quickest to arrange and carry out for transfers up to 50 miles. Ambulances are relatively low cost, quickly mobilized and operate over 24 hours in most weather conditions. In addition, they generally allow better access to the patient. They are more familiar to hospital staff and, crucially, are able to *stop* if necessary for critical procedures to be performed.

HELICOPTERS

Helicopters are generally faster over distances greater than 50 miles and are particularly useful if road access is difficult. This is of particular value in primary transfers in remote regions. Not all hospitals have helipads, and a separate land ambulance leg to the journey may be needed. Over shorter distances, helicopters may *not* be faster if they take longer to arrange or if the patient has to be loaded on and off a land ambulance at each end of the journey. Their disadvantages include expense, limited availability and possible restrictions at night or in poor weather conditions. They are also very noisy, unpressurized and prone to vibration. Although they typically fly at about 3000 feet, this is still high enough to cause hypobaric problems such as the expansion of gas-filled spaces. They cannot stop to allow patient interventions. Monitoring equipment and defibrillators must not interfere with the helicopter's navigation systems.

FIXED-WING AIRCRAFT

These are particularly suitable for distances over 200 miles. Like helicopters, they are expensive and of limited availability. However, they are often more spacious and less affected by movement, noise and vibration. They may or may not be pressurized and, if they are, the cabin pressure will be equivalent to the pressure 5000–8000 feet above sea level, rather than to that at sea level. Fixed-wing aircraft generally require an airport landing strip, so that relay land vehicles will be needed at both ends of the journey.

Urgency and speed

When a transfer is to allow immediate life-saving surgery there must be no unnecessary delays. Attempts to stabilize the patient must be under way even before transfer has been agreed. The choice of transport should reflect the need for speed. A list of transport agency contacts and an agreed categorization of urgency and vehicle requirements should be available in advance to minimize delay in making practical arrangements. Transfers that are less urgent can be undertaken during working hours to allow escorts to be spared more easily from the referring hospital. This may also be more convenient for the ambulance service.

Weather and daylight conditions are important when considering air transfers. The pilot has ultimate responsibility for mission safety and can overrule any decision to transfer a patient by air, however urgent, on the basis of worsening atmospheric conditions. A slower transfer by land may be necessary.

In general, emergency transfers can be accomplished at speed. An ambulance is not an adequate substitute for a hospital, and time en route should be kept to a minimum. A police escort facilitates a smooth passage through a busy urban environment. Transfer of patients with spinal injuries was previously undertaken at a 'snail's pace', but this is not necessary if the patient is carefully packaged, the route is well chosen and the police keep the road clear. The driver may proceed quickly but smoothly on the straights, slowing down appropriately for bends and roundabouts.

Escorts

The make-up of the transferring team will vary according to the needs of the patient. A simple categorization (Table 23.1) of the severity of the patient's condition serves as a guide to the choice of escorts, as well as indicating the urgency with which the transport vehicle needs to respond to the request for transfer.[7]

Patients who are considered to be 'ill-unstable' or 'time-critical' require an advanced life support practitioner in the team. 'Intensive' patients with brain injuries should be accompanied by a doctor with specific training, skills, competencies and experience of brain injury transfer. Patients who need intensive care require a minimum of two escorts in addition to the vehicle's crew.[8] One should be a medical practitioner with appropriate training in intensive care medicine, anaesthesia or other acute specialty. The other should generally be a nurse with a post-registration qualification in critical care, which should include educational elements on the transfer of critically ill patients. Alternatively, the second escort may be a paramedic or operating department practitioner with suitable specific training.

> All escorting staff must have minimum standards of training and experience.

Ideally, the team should have had the opportunity to train together and have repeated exposures to transfers to prevent skill decay. They should be familiar with the layout of their local ambulance service vehicles, particularly the oxygen supply and connections, suction and electrical supply and outlets.

The medical escorts must have suitable indemnity insurance, and all escorts require life and personal injury insurance. Staff should take suitable outdoor clothing, money, credit cards and a telephone. Advance arrangements for their safe and timely return should be made so they do not become stranded when the transfer vehicle is summoned to another mission.

Table 23.1 A guide to the level of escort and equipment for transfers (Modified from Safe Transport and Retrieval)

Degree of illness	Vehicle	Escorts			Extra equipment	Urgency of vehicle response
		Ambulance	Nursing	Medical		
Intensive	Capable of high speed Siren Single-cot Stretcher Suction Oxygen Basic life support kit Defibrillator	Driver and technician or paramedic	Trained intensive care unit or emergency department nurse with critical care experience from sending or receiving unit	Appropriately trained critical care doctor	Advanced life support kit and drugs Ventilator Monitor Syringe pumps Extra intensive care unit kit and drugs	20 minutes
Time-critical		Driver and paramedic	Trained emergency department nurse	Appropriately skilled emergency care doctor	Advanced life support kit	8 minutes
Ill – unstable		Driver and paramedic	Trained emergency department nurse	Appropriately competent doctor for inter-hospital transfer and according to perceived risk for transfer across site	Monitor Sometimes syringe pumps	30 minutes
Ill – stable		Driver and technician	Trained emergency department nurse for inter-hospital transfer and according to perceived risk for transfer across site	Not generally required for transfer across site but appropriately competent doctor according to perceived risk for inter-hospital transfer	Monitor Occasional syringe pump	60 minutes

Transferring out versus retrieval

For inter-hospital transfers, the transferring team is usually from the sending rather than the receiving hospital, because of the inherent delay in getting a retrieval team to the patient. However, a well-drilled retrieval team may still prove to be as quick as an ad hoc team assembled at the primary hospital, provided that the team can respond immediately and be transported rapidly to the primary hospital.

Paediatric retrieval, mainly for medical conditions, is well established in the UK and reduces complications en route.[9,10] Few dedicated, regional retrieval services for adults exist in the UK, and those that do principally serve the more remote regions such as the Scottish Highlands.[11,12]

For patients who do not need urgent surgical intervention at the receiving hospital, a specialist retrieval team is ideal, particularly when dealing with conditions or types of patients that are unfamiliar to the sending hospital staff such as paediatric intensive care retrievals. However, if urgent surgical intervention is needed after transfer, waiting for just an extra 30 minutes for the retrieval team to arrive is undesirable.

The escorts in a dedicated retrieval service should have no other clinical responsibilities, so that they can respond immediately without having to make cover arrangements. The service may run into problems when the demands on it exceed staff and vehicle availability as a single team cannot do two transfers at once. If the clinicians in the primary receiving hospitals have come to depend on this service, they may be ill-prepared to undertake the transfer themselves. Increasing the service area and the number of escorts available makes a retrieval service less vulnerable to competing demands but increases costs and the time to reach the more distant hospitals. It will also lead to prolonged periods of inactivity during quiet spells.

Communication

Good communication underpins every successful transfer and impinges on all aspects:

- initial contact with the receiving hospital including consultation, referral and implementing any advice given;
- arranging transport;
- briefing and coordinating the transport team;
- alerting the receiving area on leaving and providing an estimated time of arrival;
- informing relatives (and the patient if awake) and giving them instructions on how to get to the receiving hospital;
- repeated contact with the receiving hospital to deal with further problems;
- handover at the receiving hospital;
- debriefing the transfer team to review performance and learn lessons.

PREPARATION FOR TRANSFER

Patient preparation

In general, the patient should be fully resuscitated and stabilized before departure, although in some conditions full resuscitation is possible only after transfer, such as in the case of a ruptured aorta. Stabilization, however, remains a central concept in safe transfer. It must be achieved swiftly if the patient's condition is liable to deteriorate acutely, bearing in mind that definitive management is possible only at the receiving unit. In these circumstances, there is an inevitable conflict between stabilization and delay.

Some assessments may be delayed in order to achieve timely definitive care of life-threatening conditions at the receiving centre. In urgent transfers, a full set of radiographs of peripheral limb injuries or full spinal clearance may be pending, so it is important to record and communicate what has *not* been done, as well as what has, so that these tasks can be completed at the receiving unit.

Key considerations in patient preparation are described below.

AIRWAY CONTROL

The airway must be secure. It is best to intubate electively before transfer if there is any doubt (Table 23.2). It is very much harder to achieve if needed in a critical situation en route.

> Intubate before transfer if the airway is at risk.

Table 23.2 Indications for intubation and ventilation for transfer after brain injury (adapted from the Association of Anaesthetists of Great Britain and Ireland guidelines[13])

Glasgow Coma Scale score ≤ 8
Significantly deteriorating consciousness level, i.e. fall in motor score of two points or more
Loss of protective laryngeal reflexes
Hypoxaemia – PaO_2 <13 kPa on oxygen
Hypercarbia – $PaCO_2$ >6 kPa
Spontaneous hyperventilation causing $PaCO_2$ <4 kPa
Bilateral fractured mandible
Copious bleeding into the mouth such as a skull base fracture
Seizures
Burns with risk of airway obstruction

A gastric tube should be passed in any ventilated patient to reduce the risk of regurgitation/aspiration and decompress gastric dilatation. If basal skull fracture is suspected, the oral route should be used. It should be aspirated and then left on free drainage.

OXYGENATION AND VENTILATION

Oxygenation and ventilation must be adequate. Continual clinical assessment is paramount but needs to be backed up by monitoring. Pulse oximetry is an essential guide to oxygenation but gives no indication of ventilation. Capnography is now mandatory in ventilated patients undergoing transfer, but end-tidal readings may differ considerably from arterial $PaCO_2$, particularly in the face of hypotension, low cardiac output states and other causes of ventilation–perfusion mismatch in the lungs. A blood gas measurement before departure is essential to ensure optimal control en route. In ventilated, brain-injured patients, hypoxia and hypercarbia must be avoided. The targets for oxygenation and ventilation are:[14]

- PaO_2 >13 kPa;
- $PaCO_2$ 4.5–5 kPa if there is no evidence of raised intracranial pressure;
- $PaCO_2$ 4–4.5 kPa if there is clinical or radiological evidence of raised intracranial pressure.

The patient should be kept on the same ventilator en route as employed for stabilization in the emergency department. Changing over in the vehicle is likely to alter the blood gas control and risk inadvertent hypo- or hyperventilation.

> The patient should be stabilized on transport equipment as soon as possible.

Not all ventilated patients with rib fractures need chest drains, but in aeromedical transfers the consequences of an overlooked pneumothorax are higher; consequently, the index of suspicion should be higher and the threshold for inserting a chest drain lower.

CIRCULATION

Major trauma patients need reliable large-bore venous access. Central venous lines are often helpful, but insertion should not be the cause of delays in an urgent transfer. All lines must be firmly secured.

Haemodynamic stability is important, although different conditions require different targets. Maintaining a *mean* arterial pressure of over 80 mmHg is recommended in patients with severe head injuries, while keeping the *systolic* pressure below 100 mmHg is the aim in patients with suspected aortic rupture. Tissue perfusion depends on the mean pressure whereas the risk of displacing a clot relates more to the peak pressure. An arterial line allows beat-to-beat blood pressure readings and is essential in such cases.

Uncontrolled internal bleeding must be recognized and treated to avoid hypotension en route. External bleeding is usually obvious and will need surgical control if it does not stop with applied pressure. Persistent scalp bleeding is usually easily controlled with temporary deep sutures.[15]

Central venous lines may be needed if inotropes or vasopressors are being administered, but are rarely indicated in immediate trauma care, except to achieve an adequate mean arterial pressure in patients with severe head injury after correcting hypovolaemia. Monitoring central venous and pulmonary artery pressure has become less popular for judging volume status and is not necessary specifically for transfer. Pulmonary artery catheters may wedge inadvertently in a small branch of a pulmonary artery, leading to pulmonary infarcts. If used, the trace must be displayed continuously to aid the recognition of wedging, or the catheter should be pulled back to avoid wedging.

Blood that has been cross-matched should be transferred from the blood fridge to a cool box for taking on the transfer.

NERVOUS SYSTEM

All intubated patients should receive appropriate sedation and analgesia. Muscle relaxation is generally recommended for transfer. The eyes are often covered for protection during transfer, but in a severely head-injured patient the pupils must be checked frequently to recognize deterioration.

If the patient has had a fit, loading with an anticonvulsant such as phenytoin should be considered, remembering that hypotension can readily occur during the infusion.

Neurological deterioration, especially with lateralizing signs, merits the consideration of either mannitol or hypertonic saline after discussion with the neurosurgical team or following agreed guidelines.

METABOLISM

A urinary catheter is an important monitor of organ perfusion and mannitol will generate a large diuresis; the bag will need to be emptied before leaving.

Poor glucose control is associated with a worse outcome in critically ill patients. Head-injured patients are vulnerable to both hypoglycaemia (especially adolescents after alcohol binges) and hyperglycaemia, as a stress response. The glucose level should be controlled before setting off.

HOST DEFENCE

Wounds and burns should be dressed with non-constrictive dressings and fractures stabilized. Patients with open fractures should receive antibiotics. Tetanus cover should be considered.

If the spine has not been cleared, immobilization should continue en route, but a spinal board should be avoided for long periods or for secondary transfers. A vacuum mattress is more suitable for land ambulance journeys but is prone to lose rigidity in air transfers.

The transfer team

Ideally, the escorts should have been part of the resuscitation team. Otherwise, they must be given time to familiarize themselves with the mechanism of injury, the injuries identified, the results of investigations and the treatment administered. They should assess the patient's condition independently. Although no time can be wasted if the transfer is urgent, there is often a tendency for preparations to be rushed, especially when the ambulance crew arrives. If the patient has deteriorated, the team should not be afraid to delay departure, even if the transport has to be re-booked when the problem has been treated.

VEHICLE

The design of intensive care ambulances has been considered by the Intensive Care Society[16] and relates to the vehicle, the services and equipment.

The vehicle should :

- be driven by suitably trained personnel;
- be able to carry up to four members of hospital staff in addition to ambulance crew;
- have seats for staff, which should ideally be rear or forward facing;
- have seats fitted with head restraints and three-point inertia reel seat belts;
- have a hydraulic ramp, winch or trolley system designed to enable single-operator loading;
- have a centrally mounted patient trolley allowing all-round patient access;

- provide a stable comfortable ride with minimal noise and vibration levels;
- be subject to regular servicing and maintenance contracts.

SERVICES

Services should include:

- A standard 12-volt DC supply plus 240-volt 50-Hz AC power supply from an inverter or generator. The recommended minimum output is 750 watts, which is generally sufficient to power a portable ventilator, monitor or infusion pumps.
- At least two standard three-pin 13-amp outlet sockets in the patient cabin.
- A minimum of two F-size oxygen cylinders in secure housings (Table 23.3). Oxygen concentrators may be an alternative. The duration of oxygen supply depends on the rate of use, but sufficient oxygen must be available for the duration of the journey.
- A manifold system with automatic cylinder changeover, and audible oxygen supply failure alarm.
- A minimum of two wall-mounted outlet valves for oxygen.
- A medical air supply is also desirable but the space required by additional cylinders or compressors may be a limiting factor.
- Adequate lighting, heating, air conditioning and humidity control.

EQUIPMENT

Equipment should include:

- mobile telephone facilities to enable communication with the referring and receiving hospitals (compatibility with medical equipment must be assured);
- a defibrillator and suction equipment;
- adequate storage and stowage for ancillary equipment.

Equipment

Equipment should be comprehensive enough to permit critical care management to be continued at the same level during transfer as during stabilization, but chosen so as not to be cumbersome and unusable within the confines of the transfer vehicle. The following should be readily available:[17]

- airway equipment including suction devices;
- an adequate supply of oxygen;
- a portable ventilator;
- chest decompression equipment;
- a portable multifunction monitor;
- defibrillator;
- battery-powered syringe and volumetric pumps;
- warming blanket.

AIRWAY EQUIPMENT

Whether or not the patient has been intubated beforehand, a full set of equipment for manual mask ventilation and intubation should be carried with back-up equipment for failed intubation. This includes:

- a self-inflating bag, valve and mask;
- laryngoscopes with spare batteries and bulbs;
- endotracheal tubes with a bougie and stylet;
- oropharyngeal and nasopharyngeal tubes;
- laryngeal masks;
- suction devices including a manual device as back-up;
- surgical airway equipment.

OXYGEN SUPPLY

Enough oxygen should be taken to last for twice the expected journey time or at least one hour for very short journeys and calculations should be based on maximum flow rates. The oxygen consumption equates to the minute volume multiplied by the inspired oxygen fraction plus any oxygen required to drive the ventilator. Table 23.3 outlines the capacity of the various oxygen cylinder sizes and the time to empty from full at 10 L/min.

> Calculate oxygen cylinder supplies against patient requirements ... and then double it.

TRANSPORT VENTILATOR

The portable ventilator should have airway pressure alarms for high peak pressure and low pressure indicating

Table 23.3 The capacities of oxygen cylinders

	Cylinder size					
	C	D	E	F	G	J
Height (inches)	14	18	31	34	49	57
Capacity (litres)	17	340	680	1360	3400	6800
Time to empty from full when using 10 L/min	¼ hour	½ hour	1 hour	2¼ hours	5½ hours	11¼ hours

disconnection. A positive end-expiratory pressure (PEEP) valve should be available if not built into the ventilator, especially in cases of pulmonary contusion that can worsen en route.

Transport ventilators should be checked daily with further checks immediately before connecting them to a patient.

TRANSPORT MONITOR

The level of monitoring should be similar to that used during anaesthesia and intensive care. It should match the patient's condition rather than be stepped down for convenience during a journey.

The ideal transport monitor should be:

- robust, compact, lightweight and trolley mountable;
- powered by a long-life battery with a charge indicator and mains back-up;
- easy to see in differing light conditions and from different angles;
- fitted with visible as well as audible alarms;
- simple and intuitive to operate.

The following features should be available:

- capnography;
- pulse oximetry;
- ECG;
- non-invasive blood pressure;
- at least two channels for invasive pressure monitoring of arterial, central venous or pulmonary artery pressure;
- temperature.

The monitor must have a reliable battery. It should be plugged in when not in use and when in use up to the time of departure to ensure a full battery when setting off.

Oxygen saturation, ECG and non-invasive blood pressure should be monitored in all patients. If the patient is ventilated, capnography and invasive arterial monitoring are necessary. An arterial line is also invaluable in any trauma patient with potential haemodynamic instability, allowing beat-to-beat blood pressure readings with a visible waveform to support their validity. Non-invasive devices provide intermittent readings that take about 1 minute to perform. Unobtainable readings may be due to movement artefact or cardiovascular collapse, creating confusion and further delay. However, the arterial line may fail too and leaving a cuff in place is a valuable back-up.

Drugs and fluids

The choice of drugs should cover ongoing treatment, predictable problems and resuscitation, but should be rationalized to keep their use as simple as possible in the confines of the ambulance:

- sedative agents such as propofol and midazolam;
- analgesics;
- muscle relaxants;
- anticonvulsants;
- mannitol (and frusemide if the combination is advocated in the local neurosurgical guidelines);
- inotropes, vasopressors and other resuscitation drugs;
- intravenous fluids;
- cross-matched blood and fresh-frozen plasma if major haemorrhage is present.

For an ongoing infusion, such as propofol for sedation, an extra syringe should be prepared before departure. If there is a reasonable likelihood of needing specific drugs en route, it is wise to draw them up and label them in advance. The seemingly simple task of preparing them can prove to be troublesome when distracted by the problem in hand in a moving, imperfectly lit ambulance.

MANAGEMENT DURING TRANSFER

If stabilization has been effective, the journey itself is generally smooth and uneventful. However, it is important to prevent dislodgement of tubes and lines by careful positioning and taping. They should be laid out carefully to prevent entanglements.

Monitoring

The same ventilator and monitoring equipment used for stabilization prior to transfer should remain attached to the patient for the transfer itself. An inadvertent change in the minute ventilation resulting from changing the ventilator can lead to rises in intracranial pressure from hypoventilation or risk cerebral ischaemia from hyperventilation. If PEEP has been needed during stabilization, it should not be discarded for transfer. The end-tidal capnograph may yield values that are significantly different from the arterial PCO_2. However, a high end-tidal reading does indicate that the arterial value will be high, as the arterial value is always greater than the end-tidal. A low reading has alternative explanations, ranging from hyperventilation to low cardiac output and hypotension.

Transport trolley

A well-designed transport trolley facilitates the journey to, from and within the ambulance. It must comply with CEN (European Committee for Standardization) regulations,[18] which require all equipment to be secured so as to withstand 10G deceleration in five directions. The trolley should:

- be lightweight and robust;
- have a facility to attach the ventilator, infusion pumps, suction and monitoring devices;
- have a low centre of gravity when loaded with the patient and equipment;
- have a firm base to allow its use as a suitable surface for patients with actual or potential spinal injuries and to permit cardiopulmonary resuscitation if needed;
- be provided with cot sides;
- have the ability to tip head down to help dealing with vomiting in a non-intubated patient.

Some ambulance vehicles have a central trolley attachment that uses a collapsing trolley. This requires less lifting to load the trolley into the vehicle, but precludes the use of the space beneath the patient for the relatively heavy monitoring equipment, infusion pumps and the ventilator, resulting in a more unstable, top-heavy trolley.

Troubleshooting en route

The same system control approach should be maintained during transfer as during stabilization beforehand. While the environment is more confined and the drugs and equipment are more restricted, the same standard of care should be administered.

REASSESSMENT

A 'physiological system check' should be performed at key stages during the transfer: just prior to setting off from the hospital, after securing the patient in the ambulance, just before arriving at the destination, on reaching the receiving clinical area, and at any stage if a problem is suspected en route.

> When in doubt, do a physiological system check.

- Catastrophic haemorrhage (<C>). This must be definitively controlled before transfer.
- Airway (A):
  - patency
  - security.
- Breathing (B):
  - oxygenation
  - ventilation.
- Circulation (C = 3 'H's):
  - haemodynamics
  - haemoglobin
  - haemostasis.
- Nervous system (D = disability):
  - consciousness (including sedation)
  - pain
  - raised intracranial pressure.

- Metabolism (EFGH):
  - electrolytes, fluids, gut, hormones
  - don't ever forget glucose!
- Host defence (all the 'I's):
  - injuries missed or new ones caused by poor positioning
  - infection – unlikely in early trauma care but gut perforations can be missed
  - intoxication from overlooked patient overdose or iatrogenic drug effect
  - immune reaction or allergy to drugs given.

INTERVENTIONS

Interventions are difficult in a moving vehicle. Life-saving measures may require the vehicle to be stopped or the aeroplane to land, but there is a trade-off between immediate benefit if successful and delay in arriving in hospital if unsuccessful. The best insurance policy is thorough stabilization before setting off and gentle handling so as not to disturb the patient or dislodge tubes and lines on loading.

ADVICE

Advice can be sought en route by using the ambulance radio or a mobile phone. In the case of a transfer out, the referring hospital is still responsible for the patient, so a senior colleague can be contacted back at base. Alternatively, the problems can be discussed with the receiving specialist team. In the case of a retrieval, the escorts are either from the receiving hospital or from a regional or stand-alone specialist retrieval team and may refer to their base for help.

RECORDS

Despite the challenges of the transport environment and the distraction of caring for a critically injured patient, it is important to maintain a record of events and observations during the transfer. Standardized documentation may be supplemented by a print-out from the electronic memory in the monitor and by extra notes written after handing over the patient.

ARRIVAL AND HANDOVER

This is an important time. Handing over verbally to a new team while ensuring that there is no disruption in the care delivered as the monitoring and ventilator are changed requires considerable concentration and attention to detail.

The transferring team

Unloading the patient from the vehicle is just as dangerous as loading. Sedation must be continued and a top-up dose of muscle relaxant considered if the patient is not on a continuous infusion, in order to prevent coughing or gagging on unloading and transferring to the bed in the receiving area. Standards of monitoring and vigilance must be maintained until handover has been completed and responsibility has shifted to the receiving team. It is generally best to liaise with the team to set up the new ventilator before concentrating on the formal handover.

The handover process is facilitated by the use of a template[19] (Table 23.4). The patient's condition on arrival should be recorded and the following documents handed over:

- the patient's clinical notes;
- the transfer records;
- investigation results;
- radiographs;
- contact details of partner, relatives or close friends, as appropriate.

The receiving team

Members of the receiving team need to ensure that key details are not overlooked. They must

- reassess the patient (ABCD);
- receive a handover from the transferring team;
- change over the ventilator and monitors;
- liaise with the transferring team to optimize the settings;
- set aside the transfer equipment for the transfer team to retrieve.

Courtesy is an important part of the process. The transfer team should be offered facilities for rest and refreshment.

Table 23.4 Handover template

Immediate information
1. Personnel: introduce yourselves
2. Patient: introduce your patient
3. Priority: indicate and deal with any major problem that needs immediate attention

Case presentation
1. Presentation: mechanism and time of injury
2. Problems: list of injuries and other problems (medical conditions, drugs, allergies)
3. Procedures: list of major investigations and interventions (including those awaited or still to be done)
4. Progress: system review
   - Airway – intubation details
   - Breathing – oxygenation and ventilator settings
   - Circulation – haemodynamic status and blood transfused
   - Nervous system – conscious level and sedation/paralysis
   - Metabolism – urine output and glucose level
   - Host defence – temperature, antibiotics, wound care

It is important to thank the escorts for their endeavours. If there are aspects of care that are perceived to have been carried out poorly, this should be pointed out politely. High-handed criticism should be avoided as the fault may lie elsewhere. It is not appropriate to voice concerns, especially in front of other personnel, when the patient needs full attention. Serious concerns should be raised later at senior level.

SYSTEM PLANNING AND AUDIT

Transfers are infrequent and unpredictable. A proactive approach is essential for an efficient response when needed. The AAGBI recommends that there should be designated consultants in all referring hospitals and neuroscience units to take overall responsibility for the transfer of patients with brain injuries. The key issues to consider are setting up a training programme, developing regional guidelines and auditing practice against agreed standards.

Training

Every clinician who is likely to act as an escort should be trained formally in advance. Instruction should cover:

- the principles of trauma management;
- the pathophysiology of transport;
- manual handling of the patient;
- ambulance and aircraft safety and communication;
- drugs and equipment for transfer.

National courses such as the Safe Transfer and Retrieval (STaR) course have been developed. These emphasize the need for cooperation and communication. In some regions, local variants have been devised with a particular emphasis on practical skills.

Guidelines

Transfer guidelines have been published and updated by the AAGBI,[13] the Intensive Care Society[8] and the Paediatric Intensive Care Society,[20] as well as by many international organizations. The Brain Trauma Foundation has produced and updated a set of evidence-based guidelines[21,22] on the stabilization of head-injured patients that is relevant to preparation for transfer.

Each hospital should develop its own set of guidelines that are compatible with those recommended nationally. Local guidance also needs to address how escorts are identified when the need arises and how the hospital's emergency cover is reconfigured to cope with their absence.

Audit

Details of every transfer undertaken should be kept, together with a copy of the transfer record. This allows errors to be identified and corrections made to the system of care. Specific standards should be agreed[23] and corresponding audit cycles completed as part of a formal quality assurance programme.

SUMMARY

The aim of transferring trauma patients between hospitals is to provide better care elsewhere. The likelihood of benefit must outweigh the risks of transfer. Good communication and attention to detail in achieving system control are vital. Careful physiological stabilization without undue delay before setting off reduces the risk of deterioration en route. Proactive organization in the form of training, guideline development and standard setting is essential.

REFERENCES

1. Gentleman D, Dearden M, Midgley S, Maclean D. Guidelines for resuscitation and transfer of patients with serious head injury. *BMJ* 1993;**307**:547–52.
2. Andrews PJD, Piper IR, Dearden NM, Miller JD. Secondary insults during intrahospital transport of head-injured patients. *Lancet* 1990;**335**:327–30.
3. Venkataraman ST. Intrahospital transport of critically ill children – should we pay attention? *Crit Care Med* 1999;**27**:694–5 .
4. Davies G. Aeromedical evacuation. In: Greaves I, Porter K, eds. *Pre-hospital Medicine*. London: Arnold, 1999, pp. 651–9.
5. Martin T. Aviation medicine. In: Greaves I, Porter K, eds. *Pre-hospital Medicine*. London: Arnold, 1999, pp. 661–74.
6. Patel HC, Woodford M, King AT, Yates DW, Lecky FE. Trends in head injury outcome from 1989 to 2003 and the effect of neurosurgical care: an observational study. *Lancet* 2005;**366**:1538–44.
7. Advanced Life Support Group. *Safe Transfer and Retrieval: the Practical Approach*. London: BMJ Books, 2006.
8. Intensive Care Society. *Guidelines for the Transport of the Critically Ill Adult*. London: Intensive Care Society, 2002.
9. Britto J, Nadel S, Maconochie I, Levin M, Habibi P. Morbidity and severity of illness during interhospital transfer: impact of a specialised paediatric retrieval team. *BMJ* 1995;**311**:836–9.
10. Mok Q, Tasker R, Macrae D, James I. Impact of specialised paediatric retrieval teams. *BMJ* 1996;**312**:119.
11. Corfield AR, Thomas L, Inglis A, Hearns S. A rural emergency medical retrieval service: the first year. *Emerg Med* 2006;**23**:679–83.
12. Caldow SJ, Parke TRJ, Graham CA, Munro PT. Aeromedical retrieval to a university hospital emergency department in Scotland. *Emerg Med* 2005;**22**:53–5.
13. Association of Anaesthetists of Great Britain and Ireland. *Recommendations for the Safe Transfer of Patients with Brain Injury*. London: AAGBI, 2006 (www.aagbi.org).
14. Association of Anaesthetists of Great Britain and Ireland. *Recommendations for the Safe Transfer of Patients with Brain Injury*. London: AAGBI, 2006, p 9 (www.aagbi.org).
15. Fitzpatrick MO, Seex K. Scalp lacerations demand careful attention before interhospital transfer of head injured patients. *J Accid Emerg Med* 1996;**13**:207–8.
16. Intensive Care Society. *Guidelines for the Transport of the Critically Ill Adult*. London: Intensive Care Society, 2002, p. 7.
17. Association of Anaesthetists of Great Britain and Ireland. *Recommendations for the Safe Transfer of Patients with Brain Injury*. London: AAGBI, 2006, pp. 13–14 (www.aagbi.org).
18. European Committee for Standardization. *Medical Vehicles and their Equipment – Road Ambulances*, EN 1789, 1999 (www.cenorm.be).
19. Oakley PA. Interhospital transfer of the trauma patient. *Injury* 1999;**1**:61–70.
20. Paediatric Intensive Care Society. Standards document 2001: section 12 (www.ukpics.org).
21. Brain Trauma Foundation. Guidelines for the management of severe head injury. *J Neurotrauma* 1996;**13**:641–734.
22. Brain Trauma Foundation. *Management and Prognosis of Severe Traumatic Brain Injury 1995 and 2003 update* (www.braintrauma.org).
23. Oakley PA. Setting and living up to national standards for the care of the injured. *Injury* 1994;**25**:595–604.

24

Psychological reactions to trauma

OBJECTIVES

After completing this chapter the reader will:
- understand normal reactions to trauma
- be able to identify acute psychiatric reactions to trauma
- recognize the general principles of 'breaking bad news'
- be familiar with basic methods of managing acute reactions to trauma
- appreciate the impact of trauma care on staff.

INTRODUCTION

Most psychological reactions after trauma are normal and should be dealt with as such. Premature psychiatric interventions run the risk of impeding the normal healing practices of individuals and their families, or even of communities.[1]

Only occasionally is expert psychiatric help required in the earliest phases of care, for example in the case of psychotic illness, serious pre-existent mental illness, serious suicidal risk and the psychiatric complications of head injury.

There are, however, several, generally less serious, psychiatric symptoms and conditions which can emerge in the early stages of trauma management, and these may need to be dealt with lest they compromise ongoing medical and surgical care.

> It is essential to be able to recognize normal reactions.

NORMAL REACTIONS TO TRAUMA

Some of the normal post-traumatic reactions are described below.

Numbness, shock and denial

This shields victims from potentially overwhelming stress. However, in this state, patients may find it difficult to absorb information. This should be given in small 'doses', and possibly repeated and/or written down.

Fear

Fear is an essential trigger to the 'fight/flight' mechanism, and therefore it is biologically adaptive. Every effort must be made to reassure patients that fear is a normal reaction and not a sign of weakness.

Depression, apathy and hopelessness

Trauma nearly always involves loss, and loss commonly leads to low mood and apathy. Such reactions are also likely to be seen when the individual has suffered the loss of a loved one (see 'Bereavement reactions', p. 278). Because of low mood, loss of drive and sense of hopelessness, survivors may find it difficult to cooperate with rescuers and medical personnel.

Elation

This is similar to what the military describe as 'combat rush'. It may be associated with the relief of having survived, or it may represent the influence of major neuroendocrine changes including the release of endorphins, representing the body's biological response to major trauma. Elated patients may fail to realize how serious their injuries are, particularly as the pain threshold is raised: compliance with medical instructions may be compromised. Sedation is unlikely to be useful and may hinder diagnosis.

Irritation and anger

Trauma victims are often angry, particularly if the trauma had been due to human negligence or malice; but a legitimate target for these feelings may not present itself. Rescuers and medical personnel may become the target, as patients criticize what they (mis)perceive to be delayed or inadequate care or efforts to help.[2] Confrontation and defensive justifications ('I'm only doing my best') do not help. The patients' grievances should not be taken personally. A more empathic approach ('I can understand why you feel so upset about what's happened to you ...') will help.

Guilt

Some survivors, particularly when there have been fatalities and when children have been involved, may feel guilty. They may even describe guilt at having survived when others have died ('survivor guilt'). Others may believe that they did not do enough to avert the tragedy ('performance guilt'). Where legitimate, reassurance that they were not responsible should be given, but it is important to avoid pre-judging circumstances on inadequate information and giving false reassurance. If in doubt, it is best to listen empathically and not to make judgements or 'take sides', as in some cases guilt may be justified.

Flashbacks

These are involuntary, dramatic replays of the trauma or elements thereof, accompanied by intense emotional and autonomic changes. Flashbacks are commonly visual, but they may involve any or all sensory modalities. They are often triggered by obvious reminders of the trauma. They tend to subside over time.

Cognitive and perceptual disturbances

Survivors of trauma commonly report that events occurred as though in slow motion. Commonly, there will be gaps in their recall as a result of, for example, temporary unconsciousness and 'tunnel vision'. The latter occurs when the individual focuses on one particular feature of the environment – usually the main source of threat – to the exclusion of peripheral details. Survivors commonly report the passage of events in the wrong order.

Where possible, corroboration of the patient's account should be obtained, particularly if it is relevant to medical care. If the facts are known with certainty, it can be helpful to fill in some gaps – particularly with regard to what has happened. Many victims arrive at emergency departments without knowing what has taken place. Alternatively, they may have overheard or misheard what rescuers and others said at the scene of the trauma or on the way to hospital.

> Normal reactions to trauma are varied and patients should be reassured about this. There is no 'right' way to respond.

Autonomic hyperarousal and hypervigilance

Trauma overstimulates the autonomic nervous system, resulting in an exaggerated acoustic startle response and hyperacusis. Patients may also be overly sensitive to what they perceive as further threat, and this may include efforts to rescue or to help them. The routine use of medication is not indicated, although it may be required in extreme cases.

> Psychiatric help is unlikely to be required or be helpful for reactions within the first 4 weeks.[1]

Bereavement reactions

Many victims of trauma have not only been traumatized but also bereaved. In addition to the features above, they may also display features of an acute grief reaction.

> Grief reactions may be precipitated by losses other than bereavement such as loss of function or looks or limb amputation.

Typical acute grief reactions include:

- denial and disbelief ('I can't believe he's dead');
- apathy ('I don't care whether I live or die');
- pining and searching in despairing efforts to find evidence that the tragedy has not occurred;
- acute distress – often in waves with episodes of irresistible tearfulness and paroxysmal sobbing.

Bereavement can affect almost all physiological systems and functions, including how we think, feel and react socially. It may also lead to the reporting of physical symptoms, sometimes echoing the symptoms reported by the deceased. Headaches are common.

> Dealing with a death and mourning varies between cultures and religion – sensitivity is needed.

Table 24.1 Prognostic factors for an abnormal grief reaction

Type of death	Type of relationship	Type of person
Sudden, unexpected	'Love/hate'	Insecure, anxious
Mutilating	Highly dependent	Psychiatric history
No body available	Concurrent problems of living	Lack of support

Whilst it is correct to regard most reactions to a death, or other significant loss, as 'normal', certain factors can lead to an 'abnormal' grief reaction which may require professional help.[3] An abnormal grief reaction may be identified when its intensity is overwhelming, when its onset is delayed, when it is disproportionately prolonged or when it is a 'masked' one. The last occurs when the bereaved do not acknowledge their grief but present to doctors with physical symptoms. This can often be seen in children and adolescents. Factors leading to an abnormal grief reaction are listed in Table 24.1.

Management of acute grief reactions

The management of the grieving patient inevitably overlaps with that of the traumatized patient. However, the following points should be noted.

- *Listening* is likely to be more effective and less intrusive than *talking*; unnecessary talking is due to anxiety at the silences created by the bereaved.
- Clichés and platitudes can be hurtful such as this comment to a mother who lost a son in an RTC *You're lucky – you might have lost both sons.*
- Reassurance that the reactions are normal, the patients are not being silly or 'neurotic', and they are not losing their minds are helpful.
- Tolerance of the patient's irritability and apparent lack of appreciation and gratitude should be remembered.

> In a normal bereavement, the intensity of grief reactions reduces by about 6 months, although normal adjustment commonly takes another 18 months.

> Traumatic bereavement may lead to adjustment periods of several years. Patients and relatives should be forewarned of an acute re-emergence of grief at around a year after the death – the 'anniversary reaction'.

ACUTE PSYCHIATRIC REACTIONS

This section considers acute stress reactions, post-traumatic stress disorder, panic attack, and dissociation, and violent behaviour using the taxonomy of *International Classification of Mental and Behavioural Disorders* (ICD-10).[4]

Acute stress reaction

This condition is a ... *transient disorder of significant severity which develops in an individual without any other apparent mental disorder in response to exceptional physical and/or mental stress and which usually subsides within hours or days ... The risk of this disorder developing is increased if physical exhaustion or organic factors (for example , in the elderly) are also present.*

Patients will characteristically display an initial state of shock, a constricted field of consciousness and concentration, and disorientation, followed by a fluctuating picture which may include depression, agitation, anxiety, social withdrawal and autonomic over-reactivity.

This condition may interfere with medical care, and it may represent a very distressing experience for patients and their relatives.

Post-traumatic stress disorder

Unless the patient remains in hospital for over a month, most trauma staff will not see cases of post-traumatic stress disorder (PTSD) because its core symptoms are deemed 'normal' unless they continue beyond this time. These core symptoms are also seen in the acute stress reaction, namely intrusive phenomena (flashbacks, memories and nightmares), avoidant behaviour (of reminders of the trauma) and hyperarousal, usually with hypervigilance.

Post-traumatic stress disorder is most likely to occur *not* as a simple diagnosis but in conjunction with anxiety, depression or substance misuse. Although children over about 8 years of age may manifest the same core PTSD symptoms, younger children may display their post-traumatic distress in other ways, including through antisocial behaviour and repetitive play relating to their trauma.

Panic attack

Panic attacks are of unpredictable onset and are associated with sudden and severe anxiety, palpitations, profuse sweating, an inexplicable sense of impending doom, tremor, dyspnoea, an almost irresistible urge to flee, chest pain, paraesthesiae, choking or smothering sensations and feelings of unreality.

These attacks usually peak within 10 minutes and are usually short-lived, but they may last for several hours. They are often aborted when the patient feels safe and secure. They may also be associated with hyperventilation, although it is not clear whether hyperventilation causes the panic attack or vice versa. Hyperventilation may also lead to the 'hyperventilation syndrome', characterized by palpitations, dizziness, faintness, tinnitus, peripheral tingling and chest pain. Physical causes should also be excluded, including pulmonary embolism, acute or chronic pulmonary disease, asthma and the excessive ingestion of aspirin.[5]

Dissociation

This psychogenic condition involves a partial or incomplete integration of cognitive processes such that the patient may display amnesia, loss of identity, stupor and disturbances of physical function, such as a paralysis or loss of sensation in the absence of any physical aetiology. There is usually a sudden and complete recovery shortly after the source of stress has been removed or reduced. This term has replaced 'hysterical symptoms' because of the latter's pejorative associations.

MANAGEMENT OF ACUTE REACTIONS

Patients should be reassured that their condition is benign, and it should be explained that the symptoms are usually short-lived and self-limiting. Benzodiazepines may be used for short-term relief if the symptoms are overwhelming and are likely to jeopardize medical care. Usually lorazepam (2–4 mg) given intramuscularly is sufficient to bring these symptoms under control. A beta-blocker (propranolol 40–60 mg daily) may reduce autonomic over-reactivity, but it has little effect on anxious thoughts or on panic symptoms. Neuroleptics have no role unless there is also markedly aggressive or self-destructive behaviour. Hyperventilation may be aborted by rebreathing into a paper bag for a few minutes, but cardiorespiratory causes of anxiety should be excluded first. Patients should also be instructed to take slow, measured breaths. Symptoms recede as the CO_2 levels return to normal.

For PTSD, the National Institute for Health and Clinical Excellence (NICE) Guidelines[1] advocate trauma-focused cognitive–behavioural therapy (CBT) or eye movement desensitization and reprocessing therapy as the first line of therapy, provided by specialists. In terms of psychotropic medication, paroxetine and mirtazapine (for use by non-specialists) and amitriptyline and phenelzine (for use by mental health specialists) are recommended.

> Benzodiazepine therapy should be short term, and used with caution in patients with a head injury and patients with a history of benzodiazepine dependence.

Violent behaviour

Medical and emergency personnel are increasingly likely to encounter violent or potentially violent situations. Violent or threatening behaviour can be distressing and alarming and may jeopardize patient care. It is important to be able to anticipate and to abort potentially violent situations, by conducting rapid assessment, containment and resolution.[6]

It is best to anticipate a potentially violent scenario. It is often not possible in a clinical emergency to assess a situation thoroughly or to obtain historical data which would help to identify the likelihood of a violent outbreak. Caution should be exercised if the patient:

- has a history of violence;
- displays threatening, challenging or abusive behaviour;
- reports an irreconcilable grievance against authority including medical, nursing and emergency personnel; or
- has an identifiable psychiatric condition (especially schizophrenia, depression, alcohol/substance abuse, paranoia, antisocial or explosive personality disorder, or an organic cerebral disorder, including epilepsy and frontal lobe damage).

MANAGEMENT OF VIOLENT EPISODES

Dealing with a violent situation often depends on its cause, but the following are useful general pointers remembering that violence is often precipitated by fear and misunderstanding.

- Try not to deal with the situation alone.
- Always try to explain throughout what *is* happening and *is going to* happen, particularly when it is necessary to approach closely and to touch the patient. The patient may be very defensive of his or her 'psychological space'. Try not to approach the patient unexpectedly from behind.
- It may be helpful to leave a door or screen open to avoid a patient feeling trapped.
- It is vital to maintain a calm, reassuring and confident manner. Being challenging, threatening and confrontational will not help; indeed, it is likely to inflame the situation. Courtesy is more likely to calm a potentially violent situation than is an abrasive or authoritarian attitude.
- Slow movements, and regular forewarning of what is going to happen, are less likely to precipitate a violent reaction than are sudden, dramatic and unexpected actions.
- Excessive eye contact should be avoided, as this can be regarded as confrontational and challenging.
- Physical restraints should be avoided unless absolutely necessary. It is vital not to attempt to restrain someone unless there are sufficient staff to ensure that the exercise can be conducted safely and successfully. (It is

helpful to identify staff who are trained in appropriate restraint techniques.) A 'free for all' in which staff and patient could be injured must be avoided. Before beginning to restrain the patient, a carefully prepared plan, in which everybody knows what they are supposed to do and when, must be in place.

Occasionally, sedation may be required, but injections should be avoided unless the patient is securely immobilized and restrained. Restraints should be removed slowly only when you are certain that the risk of violent behaviour has been sufficiently reduced. A psychiatric opinion should be sought before using psychotropic medication and prolonged or high doses should be avoided.[7]

PSYCHOLOGICAL FIRST AID

How we react to victims of trauma in the early stages after their traumatic experience may influence to a considerable extent how they adjust subsequently to it. 'Psychological first aid' is a widely respected early intervention[8] after major incidents, and a modified version is described below. It enshrines an important principle of psychological intervention to deal with vital physical, biological needs (for example, food, water, warmth, and safety) before addressing higher order emotional or psychological needs.

Comfort and protect

In their bewildered and shocked state, survivors of trauma need to be comforted and protected from further, unintended, risks to their own safety such as wandering across busy roads. Comfort can be conveyed by words, but sometimes a compassionate touch may be more eloquent than a carefully prepared script.

Counteract helplessness

In the case of the 'walking wounded' or uninjured, they can be invited to help temporarily at the scene of the accident. This may counter the sense of helplessness and subsequent guilt commonly reported by victims. They may be able to comfort the injured, warn others of the accident or relay important messages.

Reunion with friends or relations

Attempts should be made to help victims to establish contact with other relevant persons such as family members, friends and other survivors.

Re-establish order

Characteristically, trauma victims feel out of control and vulnerable as their world has been turned upside-down. They welcome signs that order and control have been re-established. Information about what is going to happen, the availability of contact with family and friends, and even a cup of tea help to convey the impression that chaos and uncertainty have ended.

Expression of feelings

Particularly in the early stages of trauma, it is unlikely to be helpful to do more than to allow victims of trauma to spontaneously express how they feel. 'Emotional mining' – forcing individuals to describe their feelings – is not helpful, and may even do harm. It is important to avoid 'taking sides' regarding culpability as it is possible that such opinions may be cited by others at a later stage with potential legal and financial implications.

Provision of *accurate* information

This is related to inducing a sense of order and control. However, concessions must be made. In the earliest phase after trauma victims will find it difficult to absorb information, and they may hear only what they want to hear. Slow delivery and the repetition of information are likely to be necessary (see 'Breaking bad news', below).

Psychological triage

The majority of individuals will eventually adjust to even the most horrific events, but a number will go on to develop chronic and/or severe problems of post-traumatic adjustment. It is helpful to be alert to 'at-risk' factors[9] which can be related to the trauma or the individual (Table 24.2). Previous trauma may have a complex relationship with adjustment to a subsequent one and there may be an additive effect if the person has not adjusted to the earlier one. Alternatively, there may be an 'inoculating' effect; having dealt with a previous trauma makes it easier to cope with a subsequent one. The key factor may be to what extent the person *believes* he or she has coped successfully with an earlier trauma and it is good practice to enquire about coping after previous trauma.

BREAKING BAD NEWS

Giving bad news to patients and their relatives is never an easy task, and there is no standard script. What is said, to whom, when and where must always be tailored to suit

Table 24.2 Factors that suggest 'at risk' of chronic/severe post-traumatic adjustment

Related to the trauma	Related to the individual
Extended exposure to trauma (e.g. being trapped)	'Serious' physical injury. This may be serious to the patient but medically minor
Severity of trauma	
(Perceived) threat to life (even if there were no objective risk)	Younger age
Multiple deaths/and mutilation	Previous psychiatric history
Sudden and unexpected events	Childhood abuse
Man-made events (rather than 'acts of nature')	Severe acute stress reaction (following the trauma)
	Particularly anxious personality
	Female gender
	Lack of support
	Concurrent life stresses (there may be major problems in the patient's life which compromise his/her ability to cope with the most recent trauma)
	Low economic status

individual circumstances,[10–12] and the following guidelines provide a helpful framework.

Preparation

Preparation before speaking is essential:

* ensuring that we know to whom we are going to speak;
* establishing as much information as possible about the circumstances, the socioeconomic status and the occupation of those involved to gauge at what level the discussion is pitched;
* finding out what they may have already been told, accepting that they may have been previously misinformed or may have heard wrongly or selectively;
* anticipating what they may wish to know;
* covering up or removing any of our clothing which is stained with blood or other body fluids;
* finding a suitable site which offers privacy and minimizes the risk of interruption (pagers and telephones should be turned off if possible).

Delivery of information

This should be made in stepwise fashion from basic to more complex information. An introduction is important (name, status and involvement in the proceedings). The identities of those present should be confirmed and a suitable non-threatening posture adopted. There is an initial assessment stage in which it is important to find out what the relatives already know; what they want to know (as unsolicited truths can be as hurtful and distressing as a veil of secrecy) and to listen as this helps in establishing what others want to hear, gives them a chance to digest unpalatable news, to compose themselves and to identify further questions. It is important to use clear, simple English with a slowish delivery with pauses. Diagrams and

notes can facilitate communication and understanding. Clichés and platitudes must be avoided as we are unlikely to know 'just how you feel'. The dose of information should be titrated to what patients and relatives seem able to absorb and avoid overwhelming them with too many facts, especially medical details, as shocked and distressed individuals cannot think as quickly or as clearly as normal. It is important to be honest. There is no shame in admitting that one does not know the answer to a question – the requested information can usually be found and the questioner should be reassured that it will be sought. It is necessary to be cautious about being 'squeezed' by patients and relatives into offering unrealistically optimistic prognostications.

Follow-up

The delivery of bad news is the first step towards adjustment for patients and relatives and clinical staff can facilitate it. They should be allowed privacy while they come to terms with the news and to compose themselves; it is useful to ask if they wish someone to accompany them, such as a nurse or a chaplain. It is essential to ensure that they know what will happen next in relation to medical care and the return of any possessions and clothing and to explain the reasons for any damage or if the police need to retain items. Relatives should be forewarned if there are likely to be legal proceedings involving the coroner or procurator fiscal or if a post-mortem examination will be required, bearing in mind personal, religious or cultural sensitivities to such an event.[13] The possibility of organ donation should be discussed as sensitively as possible. It is helpful to provide information about sources of help in the community and the details of those organizations that deal with the survivors of trauma and the bereaved are usually available from a local library or via the internet. Relatives should be told how to obtain further information if required.

VIEWING THE BODY

This is an emotive and contentious issue, particularly if it has been badly mutilated or burned. To increase the likelihood of relatives finding this to be a positive experience it is necessary to:

- prepare them for what they will see, smell and feel;
- describe and explain any damage to the body, including resuscitation marks and other signs of medical intervention;
- offer them time to be alone with the body, although some may wish to have a member of staff with them;
- have a member of staff to meet them after they have viewed the body, to ensure that they are all right, and to answer any questions which this experience may have generated.

IMPACT OF TRAUMA CARE ON STAFF

The training and careful selection of staff are powerful antidotes to the potentially disturbing effects of dealing regularly with severely injured or dying patients and their relatives. Extended experience of such work may also contribute to trauma care personnel developing their own successful methods of coping with these rigours.

Despite these protective mechanisms not even senior staff are impervious to the emotional impact of their work.[14] 'Compassion fatigue' has also been identified among those who provide dedicated care to the victims of trauma.[15] Those who are involved in such work should be aware that, however rewarding their work, it is capable of exacting a substantial emotional toll which has the potential to have a deleterious cumulative effect.[16]

Most staff will cope with unpleasant incidents. However, there are some warning signs which suggest that certain staff may be struggling and require some extra help:

- excessive use of substances – alcohol, tobacco and food;
- unusual poor time-keeping and work record;
- unexpected overwork or underwork;
- excessive irritability and moodiness;
- unusual carelessness and/or proneness to accidents;
- inability to attain a realistic view of an incident; unable to stop talking about it and reliving it;
- excessive denial that such events 'trouble' them.

Minimizing the emotional impact of work on staff

PEER SUPPORT

Good, supportive relationships with colleagues are probably the most potent antidote to the adverse effects of trauma work, outside the network of support provided by family and friends. Unfortunately, peer support is sometimes unavailable because there are concerns about confidentiality and about being seen to be 'weak' in the eyes of one's colleagues, a circumstance which could easily compromise promotion opportunities.[16] Also, colleagues are sometimes reluctant to approach their peers who have had a 'hard' time for fear of saying the wrong thing or of being seen as being interfering.

Managers must aim to establish a 'climate of care' in order that employees feel free to acknowledge when they feel under pressure and that their colleagues feel free to provide support.

ORGANIZATIONAL AND MANAGERIAL PRACTICES

The way an organization reacts to its employees has a major bearing on their ability to adapt to unpleasant tasks, such as body handling after major catastrophe.[17]

Valuable features include:

- having opportunities to openly discuss their feelings and reactions;
- mutual support among all colleagues, senior as well as junior;
- a clear definition of purposeful duties;
- 'black' or 'gallows' humour, although this may be inappropriate when children are the casualties;
- attention by management to the physical needs of trauma care staff;
- good leadership.

PSYCHOLOGICAL DEBRIEFING

Psychological debriefing after unpleasant events is not a new concept; it has been used for many years by the military and other organizations, such as the emergency services.[18,19] It has an intuitive appeal, and is generally viewed favourably by participants. It has many committed advocates in Western countries, although most emphasize that it should be one element of a package of welfare provisions, often referred to as Critical Incident Stress Management. Research has not supported its role as a preventative measure against PTSD,[1] and some studies suggest that one-off debriefing sessions may make participants worse.

One conclusion on which there is a wide agreement is that mandatory debriefing is not recommended as that assumes all participants are equally ready to talk through an incident and that all individuals would benefit from talking about their feelings.

Case scenario

A 42-year-old married man with two sons was hit in his car by an oncoming lorry on the wrong side of the road; he was wearing a seat belt and had not been drinking. He sustained complex and multiple fractures of both lower limbs, and amputation of his more badly damaged right leg remained a threat for several months. He struggled to sleep beyond 2–3 hours per night because of pain and disturbing nightmares.

Would night sedation be a useful intervention for him?

Ward staff were initially opposed to night sedation because of worries about dependence. After being convinced that this was unlikely, especially when made clear to the patient that it was a short-term measure to improve the sleep architecture and initiate a more normal sleep pattern, sedation was used in the form of 10 mg of temazepam prescribed for 10 days. This achieved its aims and the patient's mood subsequently improved; he became less critical of the ward staff, and his state of hyperarousal was reduced.

How might his trauma impact on his family relationships ....

The patient's general irritability and anger at what had happened to him caused friction between him and his spouse. Three meetings between a psychologist and the patient and his spouse helped them to better understand why he reacted as he did, and how each could reduce the likelihood of 'flare-ups' between them, and how they could communicate more successfully with each other.

... and employment?

Initially, the patient's employer was impatient at his colleague's 'lack of progress', and pressurized him to set a target date for his return to work. With the patient's written permission, his psychologist met with the employer's representative on a regular basis over several weeks to discuss the patient's progress.

What should happen after discharge?

To combat the symptoms of post-traumatic stress disorder and an associated fear of driving, the patient received 10 sessions of CBT, to which he responded very successfully. Cognitive–behavioural therapy employs a number of well-established methods to achieve stress management and a more realistic set of thoughts, attitudes and personal expectations. It is a formal psychiatric treatment which has to be delivered by a professional with specialist training. The patient never lost all anxiety about driving but was, nonetheless, able to resume gainful employment.

SUMMARY

Historically, the psychological care of trauma victims has been neglected to the detriment of their overall care. Even in well-adjusted individuals, trauma can trigger powerful emotional reactions, most of which are normal reactions to abnormal events. However, for a significant number of individuals such events can give rise to frank psychopathology. Although personal resilience of patients and staff is the most common reaction to trauma, this circumstance does not justify complacency. We must all be alert to 'at-risk' factors, and know how to help those persons who suffer badly after trauma. In particular, staff should know of local and other agencies and websites which might be of help to their patients and their relatives.

There are basic methods of easing the psychological suffering of victims of trauma without expert psychiatric help, which represent 'good practice'. Breaking bad news and viewing human remains are emotive and challenging issues, even for experienced clinicians, but there are guidelines which allow staff to help patients and relatives in these situations. Trauma care is challenging and rewarding for most staff, but it is also emotionally demanding, and it can take its toll of even senior and experienced staff. Identifying staff who are under pressure and responding to their emotional needs is a neglected but important aspect of trauma care.

GLOBAL PERSPECTIVES

The ICD-10 *Classification of Mental and Behavioural Disorders* from the World Health Organization and the *Diagnostic and Statistical Manual of Mental Disorders* of the American Psychiatric Association[20] have variable diagnostic criteria and epidemiological and clinical findings must be interpreted in relation to which classification scheme has been used. For example, ICD-10 will more often classify a patient as having PTSD than will the American taxonomy.

We also must recognize that an individual's chance of encountering a traumatic event varies considerably[21] across the globe with variation even within countries such as the USA and South Africa.

It must also be acknowledged that diagnostic terms widely prevalent and understood in Western industrialized countries may be unknown or inappropriate in other cultures. For example, it is only relatively recently that Sri Lankans became familiar with the word 'depression'.

Researchers and clinicians must be familiar with intercultural differences with regard to psychiatric terminology and to how psychological distress and ill-health is expressed. Some cultures express these through physical symptoms; in other words, they 'somatize' their feelings.[22]

All of these observations serve as important caveats for those who seek to help trauma victims from other cultures. We must be very careful, particularly when working overseas after major catastrophes, that we do not impose inappropriately and unhelpfully Western concepts of psychopathology and treatment.[23]

REFERENCES

1. National Institute for Health and Clinical Excellence. *Post-traumatic Stress Disorder. The Management of PTSD in Adults and Children in Primary and Secondary Care.* London and Leicester: Gaskell and the British Psychological Society, 2005.
2. Alexander DA. Burn victims after a major disaster: reactions of patients and their caregivers. *Burns* 1993;19:105–9.
3. Parkes CM. Bereavement. *Br J Psychiatr* 1985;146:11–17.
4. World Health Organization. *ICD-10 Classification of Mental Health and Behavioural Disorders. Clinical Depression and Diagnostic Guidelines.* Geneva: WHO, 1992.
5. Smith C, Sell L, Sudbury P. *Key Topics in Psychiatry.* Oxford: Bios Scientific Publishers, 1996, pp. 159–61.
6. Gill D. Violent patients. In: Smith C, Sell L, Sudbury P, eds. *Key Topics in Psychiatry.* Oxford: Bios Scientific Publishers, 1996, pp. 353–7.
7. Royal College of Psychiatrists. *High-dose Antipsychotic Medication: New Consensus Statement from the Royal College of Psychiatrists.* London: Royal College of Psychiatrists, 2006.
8. Raphael B. *When Disaster Strikes: How Individuals and Communities Cope with Catastrophe.* New York: Basic Books, 1986.
9. Bowman ML, Yehuda R. Risk factors and the adversity-stress model. In: Rosen GM, ed. *Post Traumatic Stress Disorder. Issues and Controversies.* Chichester: John Wiley and Sons, 2004, pp. 15–38.
10. Alexander DA, Klein S. Bad news is bad news; let's not make it worse. *Trauma* 2000;2:11–18.
11. McLaughlan CAJ. Handling distressed relatives and breaking bad news. In: Skinner D, Driscoll P, Earlam R, eds. *ABC of Trauma,* 2nd edn. London: BMJ Publishing Group, 1996, pp. 103–8.
12. Hind CRK. *Communication Skills in Medicine.* London: BMJ Publishing Group, 1997.
13. Gibson M. *Order from Chaos,* 3rd edn. Bristol: The Policy Press, 2006, pp. 166–70.
14. Alexander DA, Atcheson SF. Psychiatric aspects of trauma care: a survey of nurses and doctors. *Psychiat Bull* 1998;22:132–6.
15. Figley CR. *Compassion Fatigue. Coping with Secondary Traumatic Stress Disorder in Those who Treat the Traumatized.* New York: Brunner/Mazel, 1995.
16. Alexander DA, Klein S. Ambulance personnel and critical incidents. *Br J Psychiatr* 2001;178:76–81.
17. Alexander DA. Stress among police body handlers. *Br J Psychiatr* 1993;163:806–8.
18. Mitchell JT, Everly GS. *Critical Incident Stress Debriefing: CISD.* Ellicot City: Chevron Publishing, 1995.
19. Dyregrov A. The process of psychological debriefings. *J Traumat Stress* 1997;10:589–605.
20. American Psychiatric Association. *Diagnostic and Statistical Manual of Mental Disorders,* 4th edn. Washington, DC: American Psychiatric Association, 1994.
21. Klein S, Alexander DA. Epidemiology and presentation of post-traumatic disorders. *Psychiatry* 2006;5:225–7.
22. Patel V, Sumathipala A. Psychological approaches to somatization in developing countries. *Ad Psychiatr Treat* 2006;12:54–62.
23. Summerfield D. Cross-cultural perspectives on the medicalisation of human suffering. In: Rosen GM, ed. *Post-traumatic Stress Disorder: Issues and Controversies.* Chichester: John Wiley and Sons Ltd, 2004, pp. 233–45.

FURTHER READING

Alexander DA. Early mental health intervention after disasters. *Advanc Psychiatr Treat* 2005;11:12–18.
Stroebe MS, Stroebe W, Haussan R. *Handbook of Bereavement, Theory, Research and Intervention.* Cambridge: Cambridge University Press, 1993.
Brewin CR, Rose S, Andrews B, *et al.* Brief screening instrument for post-traumatic stress disorder. *Br J Psychiatr* 2002;181:158–62.
Greenberg N, Cawkill P, Sharpley J. How to TRiM away at post traumatic stress reactions: trauma risk management – now and the future. *J R Naval Med Ser* 2005;91:26–31.
http://www.stish.org – The Sudden Trauma Information Service Helpline website. Useful information on trauma-related issues pertaining to health, children, employment, finance, and the law.
http://www.rcpsych.ac.uk – The Royal College of Psychiatrists' website. Useful information and links on bereavement, post-traumatic stress disorder and stress at work.

25

Rehabilitation after trauma

OBJECTIVES

After completing this chapter the reader will:
- understand the principles of rehabilitation for amputees and patients with brain and spinal cord injuries
- appreciate how outcome is dependent on the decisions made during the acute phase of care
- understand why the multidisciplinary team and the use of goal setting are so important in rehabilitation.

INTRODUCTION

The priority for the surgical team following trauma is to save life and reduce morbidity. Many of the decisions made during resuscitation and initial surgery will have significant bearing on long-term outcome and rehabilitation potential; for example, the eventual mobility of an amputee is critically dependent on the length of the residual limb and the fashioning of a healthy stump. Rehabilitation starts in the acute phase of treatment, and it is usual for patients to be begin rehabilitation while on acute wards. Input from the surgical team is greatly valued by the patient and other members of staff because of their medical knowledge and insight into the nature of the injuries. However, the process of rehabilitation can often appear slow, complicated and even frustrating, and can cause the acute doctor to be unsure of the best way of becoming involved. The aim of this chapter is to clarify the role of the acute doctor by explaining the general principles of rehabilitation and then discussing the specific concerns for patients following amputation, spinal cord injury and traumatic brain injury.

GENERAL PRINCIPLES OF REHABILITATION

To understand why rehabilitation is different from many other clinical specialties, it is helpful to consider the problems that can beset any patient with long-term ill-health aside from the original problem. A previously fit and healthy young man who is recovering following operative fixation of a traumatic pelvic fracture is susceptible to the consequences of immobility – deep vein thrombosis, loss of muscle mass, flexibility and balance, malnourishment or even excess weight gain. He may become anxious or depressed as a consequence of the shock of the incident and other injuries may be unmasked, such as a ruptured anterior cruciate ligament or a traumatic brain injury. Relationships with family and friends may be profoundly affected. He will need to move around even if he cannot walk, and later he will need to return to work. Irrespective of the direct treatment of the fracture, this patient's condition will be immeasurably better if all of these issues can be predicted, identified and addressed.

Rehabilitation aims to minimize complications and restore physical, emotional, social and intellectual *function*, even if the patient cannot return to full health. A patient with such serious injuries as in the example above may have a wide range of needs, which may be physical, psychological, functional, social or financial. Some of these are best dealt with by a doctor, but many other health care professionals are needed, and this has led to the development of the multidisciplinary team (MDT). The make-up of a rehabilitation team is determined by the type and severity of the patient's injuries. It will usually consist of medical and nursing staff, psychologists, occupational therapists, physiotherapists, speech and language therapists and social workers. The team must have the facilities to seek assistance from other professions, such as the acute medical specialties, particularly in the early stages of rehabilitation, and in the case of patients with multiple injuries, in whom recurring problems associated with the original injuries may require attention. Later on the help of orthotists and prosthetic limb fitters may be required.

The strengths of the MDT are that it can provide holistic care and can be very good at problem-solving because of the wide range of skills available; its weakness is a tendency to a loss of focus because of the complexity of the case and the number of people involved. For this reason, the team needs to be well led, to meet regularly to discuss the patient's progress and to set clear goals so that all of the members of the team and the patient know where to concentrate their efforts.

Goal setting is an MDT process of identifying the problems that are important, developing concrete strategies for dealing with them and reviewing progress at a realistic time. A useful acronym for this is SMART: **S**pecific; **M**easurable; **A**ttainable; **R**ealistic; **T**imely. Both short- and long-term goals are appropriate, e.g. in a patient with acute anterior cruciate ligament rupture the short-term goal of reducing swelling contributes to the long-term goal of a return to sport. Accurate and detailed notes must be kept to facilitate good communication among the team members and reduce misinterpretation by the patient and family. It will also make referring back to the documentation easier in the years ahead as many patients will have legal and compensation cases ongoing.

> Realistic goal setting is an integral part of the rehabilitation process.

Successful rehabilitation relies on the active participation of the patient. It requires good communication with the team so that the correct goals can be set. Most patients do not fully appreciate the significance of their injuries in the acute stages. One of the most important jobs for the team is to provide support and education so that the patient is aided to an acceptance of the situation.

The role of the acute doctor

The following questions provide a structure for acute medical practitioners when assessing patients with regard to rehabilitation. The members of the MDT are particularly dependent on the medical team for the answers to the first three, whilst the last two questions are less 'medical' but of intense interest to the patient and are the principal focus for the rest of the team.

IS THE DIAGNOSIS CORRECT?

Although the primary diagnosis may be clear-cut, other conditions may remain undiagnosed. Mild traumatic brain injury after any major trauma is a common example.

ARE THERE ANY SECONDARY MEDICAL COMPLICATIONS?

This includes pressure sores, urinary tract infection, poor nutrition, anaemia and electrolyte disturbance. Neurological complications of spinal cord injury include spasticity and contracture. Immobility leads to loss of muscle bulk, flexibility and balance.

WHAT IS THE PROGNOSIS?

This is very helpful to the patient and the team. In many instances it is not immediately clear, but an honest assessment helps in setting goals.

WHAT ARE THE DISABILITIES RESULTING FROM THE INJURY?

In other words, what function has the patient lost? Examples include walking, climbing stairs or loss of short-term memory. Once identified, these problems may be overcome if not cured.

WHAT ARE THE HANDICAPS?

In the longer term, what does the patient want to do with his or her life? Will it be possible to return to the original home? Will it be possible to resume employment? What will be the long-term effects on finances and relationships?

AMPUTATION

Amputee care is a rapidly changing and improving field, stimulated by new technologies in prosthetic components and in stump and socket care. The eventual function that an amputee can now expect is far better than it was a generation ago. However, during the acute phase, the principle of an experienced surgeon working closely with the rehabilitation team remains as important as ever. This section discusses some of the most important factors that a surgeon should be aware of during the acute phase of treatment that can transform the eventual outcome. These factors include stump fashioning, choice of level and length of amputation, preoperative preparation by the rehabilitation team, avoidance of chronic pain and early mobilization.

Within Western culture, poor arterial circulation and diabetes mellitus-associated vascular disease are the main causes of amputation (Table 25.1). Traumatic amputees tend to be young adults, particularly men, involved in road traffic and industrial accidents.[1] Worldwide, lower limb amputation as a result of residual ordnance (land mines) is increasingly common, with over 10 000 lost limbs a year.

> Trauma is the indication for amputation in only 5% of cases but usually involves previously fit, motivated, young people.

Most traumatic amputations involve the lower limb and usually have acute vascular and/or neural damage with

Table 25.1 Aetiology of amputation in the Western society[2]

Aetiology	Percentage
Vascular problems (peripheral vascular disease vs. diabetes)	90 (60 vs. 30)
Trauma	5
Neoplasm	1
Other causes including renal failure and infection following implant surgery	4

associated bone and soft-tissue injury. If damage is irreparable, primary amputation may be the best course of action, although it may be best to delay consideration of amputation until an accurate demarcation between viable and non-viable tissues can be delineated. It is now clear that in the injured extremity amputation does not necessarily have to be at the level of bone injury, as internal fixation of the fracture at a level of otherwise healthy soft tissue can allow amputation with a longer residual limb[3] (Figure 25.1). Amputation surgery is especially prone to complications, particularly infection, haematomas and wound breakdown, and is best carried out by experienced surgeons. Special care is required to optimize the condition of the skin and muscle flap in the residual limb as these will be the weight-bearing structures.

> Amputation need not necessarily be at the level of bony injury.

Amputations are described by the level at which they are performed, but there is often confusion between the *level* and the *length* of amputation. The level in traumatic amputees is defined by international descriptions (Table 25.2) and there are advantages and disadvantages for each level. In general, more distal amputations require less energy for walking (Table 25.3) and are more successful. The transtibial amputation preserves the anatomical knee joint and allows a comfortable functional and cosmetically acceptable prosthetic limb replacement. The through-knee amputation provides a potentially strong

Table 25.2 The level and proportion of lower limb amputations[2]

Amputation level (British Standard 1993)	Proportion (%)
Transtibial (below knee)	50.6
Transfemoral (above knee)	38.3
Knee disarticulation	2.8
Toes	2.3
Partial foot	0.7
Ankle disarticulation	0.6
Hip disarticulation	0.6
Hemipelvectomy (hindquarter amputation)	0.2

(3.9% reported as double lower limb amputation)

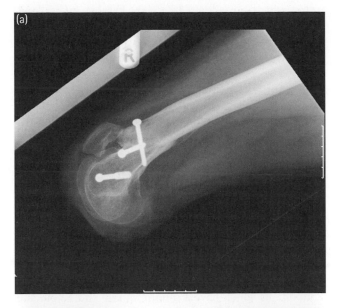
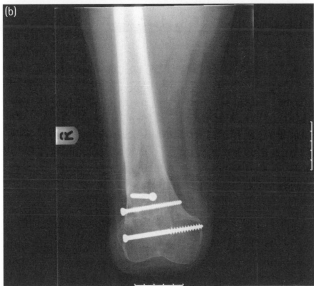

Figure 25.1 (a and b) Healed Y distal intercondylar fracture of the femur in a through-knee amputee following limited internal fixation. Had the limb been amputated at the fracture site, a transfemoral amputation would have resulted in significantly reduced function (courtesy of the Editor, *Journal of the Royal Army Medical Corps*,[3] and the Defence Medical Rehabilitation Centre, Headley Court).

Table 25.3 Energy expenditure for different levels of lower limb amputation[4]

Level of amputation	Mean oxygen consumption above normal at rest (%)
Transtibial	9
Transfemoral	49
Hip disarticulation	125
Bilateral transfemoral	280
Crutch walking	45

stump which can allow end weight-bearing for walking, but, as the knee joint is at the end of the socket, it creates a leg length discrepancy that is most noticeable with the patient seated as one thigh appears longer than the other; this effect is reduced with modern prosthetic knee units. Ideally, the knee joint should be preserved, but 'through-knee' disarticulation patients often walk earlier than patients who have undergone transtibial amputations and are usually very satisfied with their outcome.

The length refers to the most distal segment of the residual limb. This has a significant bearing on outcome, functionality and cosmetic appearance. The residual limb acts as the interface between the body and the prosthesis and allows the transmission of force and sensory input. The length is a compromise between a long lever arm and clearance for prosthetic components. A longer lever arms reduces the physiological energy demands for ambulation, but there is less room available for the prosthetic components which have a minimum size and length and must be fitted on to the socket.

> Good surgical technique and decision-making at amputation can directly improve functional outcome in rehabilitation.

If there is time, the patient should ideally be seen by the rehabilitation team before surgery. From the physical point of view, amputation predisposes the patient to hip flexor contractures and weakness around the hip joint, which can be prevented by prescribing a simple exercise programme for the pre- and postoperative period. From the psychological point of view, it is very helpful for the patient to meet the team who will be tasked with helping him or her to regain function after surgery.

Good control of pain in the pre- and perioperative periods probably reduces the incidence of chronic pain in the residual limb and there is growing evidence that local anaesthetic nerve infusions reduce the severity of phantom pain. Neuromas are unavoidable, but gentle traction on the nerve at surgery prior to transaction to allow the neuroma to form in the muscle reduces pain. Adequate analgesia and the use of neuromodulators such as gabapentin, pregabalin and low-dose tricyclic antidepressants are also effective measures for neuroma and phantom pain, although, when considering which analgesic modalities to prescribe, careful direct questioning is usually needed to differentiate between phantom pain, phantom sensations and phantom limb.

An amputee should be mobilized as soon after surgery as the wounds and other injuries allow. There are a number of early walking aids (EWAs) which can be used as early as 5–7 days after surgery, and the evidence suggests that early mobilization encourages wound healing. EWAs should be used only under the guidance of an appropriately trained specialist and may be useful in assessing an amputee's suitability for later provision of a prosthesis.

A prosthesis consists of a socket, an interface between the socket and stump, such as a silicone sleeve, a suspension system to keep the socket and stump together, and the other components such as a knee joint. The type of prosthesis prescribed by the limb-fitting team should be compatible with the function of the amputee; a young traumatic amputee will have very different functional expectations and requirements from an elderly patient who has undergone an amputation for the complications of peripheral vascular disease. Whilst many factors determine the success of limb fitting, the single most important is the interface between the residual limb and the prosthesis, highlighting the absolute importance of fashioning an adequate stump at acute surgery – if the fit and comfort of the socket are not satisfactory the prosthesis will fail. Table 25.4 highlights some of the other factors that may affect outcome after amputation.

The level of function can be recorded using the SIGAM (Special Interest Group of Amputee Medicine) scale (Table 25.5). Unfortunately for young traumatic amputees, it is an insensitive scale for measuring progress, as most will get to level E or F very rapidly.

SPINAL CORD INJURY

Following surgical stabilization, the greatest risks to a patient with a spinal cord injury (SCI) are the complications that the immobility and loss of neurological function promote. Following surgery, the patient will probably spend several months in a rehabilitation unit. During this time, spinal shock will resolve and the degree of recovery of neurological function will become evident. It is the first priority of a rehabilitation programme during this time to assess the risk of each of the complications discussed below and put measures in place to prevent or treat them. The process of helping the patient to regain function can be successful only if this 'groundwork' has been properly done.

The American Spinal Injuries Association (ASIA) scoring system provides a format for describing the level and degree of injury (Figure 25.2). It is useful in providing a format for describing the degree of neurological deficit and helps in predicting complications and the degree of disability that is likely to result from the injury.

Deep vein thrombosis (DVT) is common in the early stages of the injury because the muscles are flaccid while the cord is in shock. Most rehabilitation units have a formal policy of DVT prevention including the use of anticoagulants. Spinal shock is described in detail in Chapter 12.

Spasticity

Once the spinal cord has recovered from spinal shock, spasticity is almost universal. Spasticity is an exaggeration of

Table 25.4 Factors affecting outcome after amputation

Factor	Rationale
Age and level of fitness	These may preclude the use of a prosthesis or limit the functional outcome
Gender	Young women often find it harder to socialize following amputation
Cause of amputation	Diabetic patients may well have reduced proprioception. This will make the use of a prosthetic limb very difficult
Pre-existing medical condition	Chronic medical conditions such as chronic obstructive pulmonary disease or ischaemic heart disease will limit the patient's ability to be fully mobile post amputation
Type of limb	Most amputees will use a lower limb prosthesis even if it is only for assisted transfers. Less use is made of an upper limb prosthesis as the technology is less advanced and there are more ways to replace hand function
Contralateral limb function	If the contralateral limb is injured, this will delay prosthetic rehabilitation and will also reduce the long-term potential outcome
Provision of rehabilitation services	Limb fitting and rehabilitation tend to be regionalized. Some regions have a larger budget and are thus able to offer more intensive rehabilitation and training and more expensive prostheses
Social circumstances	If a patient lives in nursing or residential accommodation, the requirements to be mobile are less than those of a young person living alone and in employment
Mental state	It is very difficult to teach someone with dementia the techniques necessary to use a prosthesis
Family support	People living alone will often be forced to use their prosthetic limbs or become socially and economically isolated

the normal stretch reflexes and occurs when a muscle is stretched leading to an inappropriately strong contraction of that muscle. In an able-bodied person, the stretching of the muscle will stimulate the reflex arc, but inhibitory control from the brain via the spinal cord modifies the response of the muscle. In SCI, this inhibitory influence is cut off. Consequently, minor stimuli such as a slight movement of the limb, or even touching the skin, can stimulate the reflex arc and lead to powerful muscle contractions, joint stiffness, loss of movement, muscle spasms and contractures. The spasms are very painful and can be powerful enough to throw someone out of their wheelchair. Measures to control spasticity include stretching, postural management and drugs such as baclofen and tizanadine.

Contractures

Muscle contractures can be prevented with regular stretching programmes, splinting and intramuscular botulinum toxin injections as required. These measures reduce the requirements for surgical tendon-lengthening procedures.

Pressure sores

Pressure sores cause chronic infection and are a cause of premature death. They occur in skin over bony prominences and it is important to inspect the skin regularly as it is insensate. Each patient's risk should be assessed and a care plan implemented that includes the correct programme of moving and turning the patient, and cushions and mattresses that spread the pressure away from the vulnerable points.

Autonomic dysreflexia

Autonomic dysreflexia is a poorly appreciated problem that is a medical emergency. It can occur in any patient

Table 25.5 The SIGAM scale[5]

Grade	Disability	Definition
A	Non-limb user	Those who have abandoned the use of an artificial limb or use only non-functioning prostheses
B	Therapeutic	Wear prostheses *only* in the following circumstances: for transfer, to assist nursing, walking with the physical aid of another *or* during therapy
C	Limited/restricted	Walks up to 50 m on even ground with or without walking aids: a = frame, b = two crutches/sticks, c = one crutch/stick, d = no walking aids
D	Impaired	Walks 50 m or more on level ground in good weather with walking aids: a = two sticks/crutches, b = one stick/crutch
E	Independent	Walks 50 m or more without walking aids. Expects to improve confidence in adverse terrain or weather
F	Normal	Normal or near-normal walking SIGAM

Special Interest Group of Amputee Medicine.

(a)

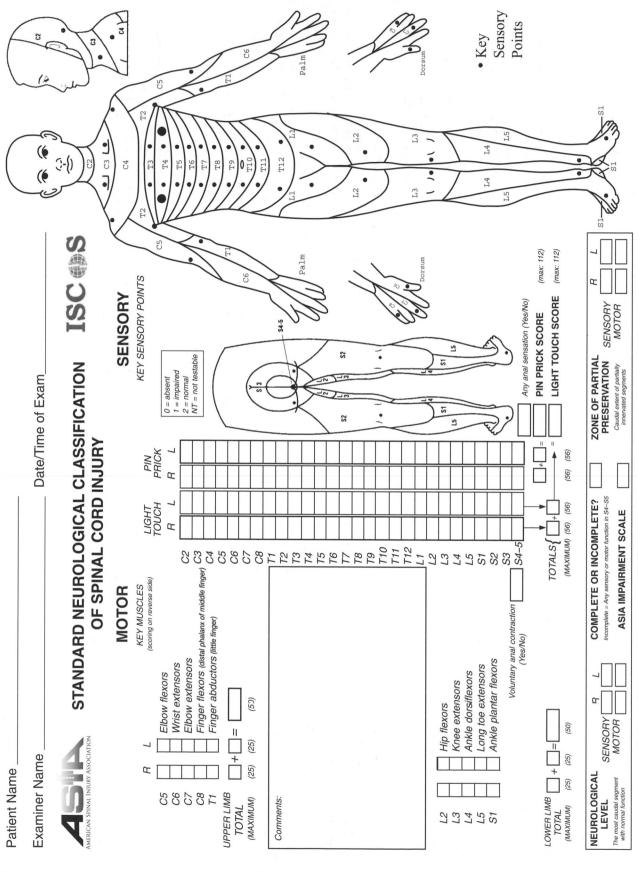

(b)

MUSCLE GRADING

0 total paralysis

1. palpable or visible contraction

2. active movement, full range of motion, gravity eliminated

3. active movement, full range of motion, against gravity

4. active movement, full range of motion, against gravity and provides some resistance

5. active movement, full range of motion, against gravity and provides normal resistance

5* muscle able to exert, in examiner's judgement, sufficient resistance to be considered normal if identifiable inhibiting factors were not present

NT not testable. Patient unable to reliably exert effort or muscle unavailable for testing due to factors such as immobilization, pain on effort or contracture.

ASIA IMPAIRMENT SCALE

☐ **A = Complete:** No motor or sensory function is preserved in the sacral segments S4–S5.

☐ **B = Incomplete:** Sensory but not motor function is preserved below the neurological level and includes the sacral segments S4–S5.

☐ **C = Incomplete:** Motor function is preserved below the neurological level, and more than half of key muscles below the neurological level have a muscle grade less than 3.

☐ **D = Incomplete:** Motor function is preserved below the neurological level, and at least half of key muscles below the neurological level have a muscle grade of 3 or more.

☐ **E = Normal:** Motor and sensory function are normal.

CLINICAL SYNDROMES (OPTIONAL)

☐ Central cord
☐ Brown-Séquard
☐ Anterior cord
☐ Conus medullaris
☐ Cauda equina

STEPS IN CLASSIFICATION

The following order is recommended in determining the classification of individuals with SCI.

1. Determine sensory levels for right and left sides.

2. Determine motor levels for right and left sides.
    Note: in regions where there is no myotome to test, the motor level is presumed to be the same as the sensory level.

3. Determine the single neurological level.
    This is the lowest segment where motor and sensory function is normal on both sides, and is the most cephalad of the sensory and motor levels determined in steps 1 and 2.

4. Determine whether the injury is Complete or Incomplete (sacral sparing).
    *If voluntary anal contraction = **No** AND all S4–S5 sensory scores = **0** AND any anal sensation = **No,** then injury is COMPLETE. Otherwise injury is incomplete.*

5. Determine ASIA Impairment Scale (AIS) Grade:

Is injury **Complete?**   If **YES,** AIS=A   Record ZPP
                            (For ZPP record lowest dermatome or myotome on
                            each side with some (non-zero score) preservation)

        NO
         ↓

Is injury
motor **underlined** incomplete?   If **NO,** AIS=B
                            (Yes=voluntary anal contraction OR motor
                            function more than three levels below the motor
        YES   level on a given side.)
         ↓

Are at least half of the key muscles below the (single) neurological level graded 3 or better?

        NO   YES
         ↓   ↓
       AIS=C   AIS=D

If sensation and motor function is normal in all segments, AIS=E
Note: AIS E is used in follow-up testing when an individual with a documented SCI has recovered normal function. If at initial testing no deficits are found, the individual is neurologically intact; the ASIA Impairment Scale does not apply.

Figure 25.2 The American Spinal Injuries Association scoring system for level and degree of spinal cord injury.

with a SCI above the level of T5 and occurs because of the disruption of the sympathetic nervous system; the symptoms are directly attributable to this loss of sympathetic control. Common symptoms are hypertension, often with a blood pressure greater than 200/100mmHg accompanied by pounding headache; a flushed face; red blotches on the skin; sweating above the level of spinal injury but a cold, clammy skin below; nasal stuffiness; nausea secondary to vagal parasympathetic stimulation and bradycardia (pulse <60 beats/min). It can be triggered by any noxious stimuli that would ordinarily act as a painful stimulus to areas of the body below the level of spinal injury. The management is to identify and remove the offending stimulus, which may be all that is required. The patient should be sat up with frequent blood pressure checks until the episode has resolved. The medication recommended in the UK is sublingual nifedipine 10 mg to reduce the blood pressure.

Evacuatory disturbance

Denervation of the bladder can lead to incontinence, urinary retention and reflux with risk of permanent renal impairment. Urodynamic studies and ultrasound scanning are used in all patients to assess bladder function. Bladder management may be intermittent self-catheterization or insertion of a suprapubic catheter, both of which reduce the risk of infection and renal failure. Drugs such as oxybutinin and tolterodine may be required to reduce bladder pressures.

Loss of innervation to the lower bowel can lead to constipation and overflow incontinence. An effective bowel care regime may include regular toileting, stimulation of the bowel using the gastrocolic reflex, manual evacuation and the use of bulking agents and aperients. Advice should be given on diet to maintain good nutrition and to avoid obesity.

Most patients go through a very difficult time as the degree of the injury and the lack of recovery becomes clear to them. Early psychological support of the patient, family and carers cannot be overemphasized.

> Recognition of the potential complications of spinal cord injury is paramount.

TRAUMATIC BRAIN INJURY

Traumatic brain injury (TBI) can be devastating. Even apparently trivial head injury may have long-term cognitive and functional sequelae. As outlined in Chapter 9, the initial emergency management of TBI is prevention of secondary injury by maintenance of an airway and oxygenation, maintaining cerebral circulation, perfusion

and pressure and prompt diagnosis and management of intracerebral pathology.

Brain injuries can be defined by their severity (Chapter 9), which gives prognostic information both in the acute stages and for longer-term outcome.

As soon as patients are medically stable and transferred from the intensive care unit (ICU), they should be assessed by the MDT and considered for transfer to a rehabilitation unit. Long- and short-term goals should be set with regular reviews. A treatment planning meeting involving all the members of the team follows the initial assessment period. This will determine management and treatment duration. Patients with brain injury often respond better in structured environments free of distractions. Daily structured programmes with regular rest periods should be allotted to each patient (Figure 25.3).

Early and regular communication with the patient and his or her family is important. Honesty, although difficult and often painful, is best when discussing long-term prognosis, as it is better to be wrong when a patient makes a significantly better recovery than predicted than the converse.

There is often a variable period after TBI before functional memory and the ability to store new memories returns, known as post-traumatic amnesia (PTA). It has previously been used as a measure of brain injury severity, although it is not used currently by most neurosurgical services. Loss of memory immediately prior to the injury is common and is called retrograde amnesia; in contrast to PTA, retrograde amnesia can resolve to some degree. Incomplete recovery from TBI has significant long-term cognitive, emotional, behavioural, social and economic effects.

The post-concussional syndrome refers to a syndrome of headaches, dizziness, poor concentration, memory impairment and personality change which usually resolve after about a year but can persist.

There are many ways of assessing outcome after TBI, of which the Glasgow Outcome Score (Table 25.6) is simple, validated and probably the most well known. It can be used to compare outcomes between individual studies of treatment.

Table 25.6 The Glasgow Outcome Score

Good recovery	Able to resume pre-injury lifestyle
Moderate disability	Independent, but unable to resume full pre-injury activities
Severe disability	Dependent on the care of others for the activities of daily living
Vegetative	No sign of psychologically mediated responses
Dead	

Time	Monday	Tuesday	Wednesday	Thursday	Friday
0800–0830	Nursing ADL	Nursing ADL		Nursing ADL	Nursing ADL
0830–0900	Nursing ADL	Nursing ADL	OT washing and dressing	Nursing ADL	Nursing ADL
0900–0930	Nursing ADL	Nursing ADL	OT washing and dressing	Nursing ADL	Nursing ADL
0930–1000	Nursing ADL	Nursing ADL	OT washing and dressing	Nursing ADL	Nursing ADL
1000–1030	OT treatment	Nursing ADL	Psychology	OT treatment	Rehabilitation workshop or computers
1030–1100	Break	Break	Break	Break	Break
1100–1130		Ward round			PT
1130–1200		OT treatment		Rehabilitation workshop or computers	PT
1200–1230	Lunch	Lunch	Lunch	Lunch	SLT
1230–1300	Lunch	Lunch	Lunch	Lunch	OT treatment
1300–1330	Lunch	Lunch	Lunch	Lunch	Lunch
1330–1400	PT	PT	PT	PT	Lunch
1400–1430	PT	PT	PT	PT	
1430–1500				SLT	
1500–1530	Break	Break	Break	Break	
1530–1600		SLT	SLT		
1600–1630					
Evening activities					
Evening activities					

Figure 25.3 A typical structured timetable for the rehabilitation of traumatic brain injury. ADL, activities of daily living; OT, occupational therapy; PT, physiotherapy; SLT, speech and language therapy.

SUMMARY

This chapter provides a general framework for considering how to provide rehabilitation following trauma with emphasis on three conditions, each of which highlights differing aspects of the rehabilitation process. In amputee care, the emphasis is on recognizing the importance of the decision-making in the acute phase and its consequences for eventual function. In spinal cord injury, the avoidance of complications is paramount and requires meticulous attention to detail, whereas the challenge of rehabilitation of patients with traumatic brain injury is the recognition of the impairment and the need to find strategies to allow the patient to adapt to the limitations that it imposes.

REFERENCES

1. *Amputation Statistics for England, Wales and Northern Ireland.* London: HMSO, 1987.

2. *A Series of 4584 Lower Limb Amputees Referred to Limb Fitting Centres in England and Wales*: NASDAB Steering Group, 1997/8.

3. Clasper J. Lower Limb Trauma Working Group. Amputations of the lower limb: a multidisciplinary consensus. *J R Army Med Corps* 2007;**153**:172–4.

4. Huang CT, Jackson JR, Moore NB, *et al.* Amputation: energy cost of ambulation. *Arch Phys Med Rehabil* 1979;**60**:18–24.

5. Ryall NH, Eyres SB, Neumann VC, Bhakta BB, Tennant A. The SIGAM mobility grades: a new population-specific measure for lower limb amputees. *Disabil Rehabil* 2003;**25**:833–44.

26

Trauma scoring

After completing this chapter the reader will:
* understand the principles of trauma scoring

* understand the importance of trauma scoring in auditing and developing best practice.

INTRODUCTION

No two trauma patients are identical, but there are definite patterns of injury associated with particular mechanisms. These allow a high index of suspicion to be maintained and occult injuries to be detected. However, even when the mechanisms of injury are almost identical, casualties may suffer wildly differing injury patterns. Across the spectrum of trauma, there is an almost infinite variety of separate and combined injuries. Other variables, such as the age and pre-injury health of the patient, will also affect the outcome. In this context, comparing outcomes is problematical and showing new interventions and changes to the structure of trauma care to be clinically beneficial and cost-effective is difficult. Trauma scoring systems are tools to allow analysis and comparison of individual patients and groups. Table 26.1 outlines the uses to which these scoring tools can be put.

Trauma scoring was first developed in the USA during the 1960s, and has become increasingly sophisticated. The overall usefulness and validity of trauma scoring is dependent on personnel within trauma teams ensuring adequate and accurate data collection. Any scoring system must be accurate, valid, reproducible and free from observer bias. Scoring systems are based on anatomical or physiological data, or a combination of both. Anatomical systems have the advantage in that the amount of tissue damage is amenable to clinical examination and radiological, operative or post-mortem findings. In addition, the findings usually remain constant after the initial injury, as opposed to physiological systems, which rely on data that will change during resuscitation. The initial set of observations in the resuscitation room is currently used for calculations, but may not reflect the true nature of the situation. The physiological data used in the calculation of a trauma score may be collected before the compensatory mechanisms of a pregnant or young casualty are exhausted, causing an overestimation of the probability of survival. Despite this, physiological systems can give a more accurate reading of the overall condition of the patient. This is particularly seen in patients with closed head injuries. Combined systems that use both sets of data are the most accurate, but are the most complicated to use.

Table 26.1 Uses of trauma scoring

Epidemiology
Research
Triage
Outcome prediction
Anatomical and physiological evaluations of injury severity
Intra- and inter-hospital evaluation of trauma care
Trauma registers
Planning of and resource allocation within trauma systems

Case scenario

This scenario is used to calculate all the following trauma scores.

A 45-year-old female cyclist is hit by a car. She has suffered a depressed skull fracture and a small subdural haematoma. There are facial abrasions and three fractured ribs but no flail segment. There is no abdominal or pelvic content injury. There are open radius and ulna fractures on the right side and no external injuries. Initial observations in the resuscitation room are a respiratory rate of 28, a systolic blood pressure of 140 mmHg and a Glasgow Coma Scale (GCS) score of E1, M4, V2 = 7.

ANATOMICAL SYSTEMS

Abbreviated Injury Scale

The Abbreviated Injury Scale (AIS)[1] was developed by the Association for the Advancement of Automotive Medicine and was first introduced in 1971. It assigns a six-figure code and a severity score to individual penetrating and blunt injuries. The most recent revision in 1990 (AIS 90) lists over 1200 injuries. The code allows easier computer entry and retrieval of data. The severity score ranges from 1 to 6 (Table 26.2) and is non-linear, as the differentials between each point are not the same (an injury with a score of 4 is not necessarily twice as severe as an injury with a score of 2). The Maximum AIS (MAIS) – the highest single AIS of a multiply injured patient – was initially used as a predictor of outcome and is a good discriminator for survival.[2] It is also used for research into the design of safer vehicles. Staff with training and experience should collect data and perform scoring, and a quality control system be in place. This ensures consistency, and involving the trauma surgeons in this process improves accuracy.[3]

Organ injury scaling

Scaling systems for injuries to individual organs have been developed by the American Association for the Surgery of Trauma. The scales, like the AIS, run from 1 to 6, with 6 equating to a largely unsurvivable injury. The Mangled Extremity Severity Score is used to identify patients for primary amputation with irretrievably injured limbs.[4]

Injury Severity Score

In the Injury Severity Score (ISS)[5,6] the patient's injuries are coded with AIS 90 and divided into six body regions: head and neck, face, chest, abdomen and pelvic contents, extremities and bony pelvis, and external (skin). The highest severity score from each of the three most seriously injured regions is taken and squared. The sum of the three squares is the ISS, which has a range of 1–75. A score of 75

is incompatible with life, and therefore any patient with an AIS 6 injury in any one region is awarded a total score of 75.

Since the ISS is based on the AIS it is also a non-linear measure. In addition, certain scores are common and others impossible. The non-linearity is a disadvantage as a patient with an isolated AIS 5 injury is more likely to die than a patient with both an AIS 4 injury and an AIS 3 injury. However, both patients will have an ISS of 25. An ISS >15 signifies major trauma – as a score of 16 is associated with a mortality rate of 10%.

New Injury Severity Score

The New Injury Severity Score (NISS)[7] takes the three highest AIS severity scores, regardless of body area. The scores are squared and added. Again, a range of 1–75 is produced, and any single AIS of 6 gives a total score of 75. This system is simpler to calculate and is a better predictor of outcome than ISS[8-11] as multiple injuries to one body area are given their full weight. For example, a patient with bilateral closed femoral shaft fractures can exsanguinate into the thighs and is obviously more seriously injured than a patient with a single fracture, but both would have an ISS of 9. With both injuries counting in NISS the score is 18. Similarly, severe closed head injuries are underscored by ISS. At present, NISS is unlikely to replace ISS completely because of the key role of the latter in Trauma and Injury Severity Score (TRISS) methodology (see below). Calculation of a representative ISS and NISS are detailed in Table 26.3.

Anatomic Profile

The Anatomic Profile (AP)[12] scoring system takes injuries with AIS scores of >2 and groups them into three components: A – head, brain and spinal cord; B – thorax and the front of the neck; C – all remaining injuries. The AP provides the anatomical part of ASCOT, which is illustrated later. Although the AP discriminates survivors from non-survivors better and is more sensitive[11,12] the ISS remains the most widely used system.

Table 26.2 Examples of severity scores in the Abbreviated Injury Scale

1	Mild	450212.1	Single rib fracture
2	Moderate	450220.2	Two or three rib fractures, stable chest
3	Serious (non-life-threatening)	450230.3	More than three rib fractures on one side, three rib fractures on other side, stable chest
4	Severe (life-threatening)	450260.4	Unilateral flail chest
5	Critical	450266.5	Bilateral flail chest
6	Fatal	413000.6	Bilateral obliteration of large portion of chest cavity

The presence of a haemothorax and/or pneumothorax adds a point to the injuries scoring 1–4.

Table 26.3 An example of Injury Severity Score and New Injury Severity Score calculation

Head and neck				
Depressed parietal skull fracture	150404	3	squared	9
Small subdural haematoma	140652	4	squared	16
Face				
Abrasions	210202	1		
Chest				
Three rib fractures of right chest, stable chest	450220	2	squared	4
Abdomen and pelvic contents	nil			
Pelvis and extremities				
Open fracture of radius	752804	3	squared	9
Open fracture of ulna	753204	3		
External (skin)	nil			

ISS = 16 + 4 + 9 = 29

NISS = 16 + 9 + 9 = 34

International Classification of Disease Injury Severity Score (ICISS)[13–15]

This system has developed since the early 1990s. Although it is based on the *International Classification of Diseases*, 9th edition (ICD-9), it has also been validated for ICD-10 codes.[16] The calculation of survival risk ratios (SRRs) for all possible injuries is central to this method (Table 26.4), and operative procedures have also been coded. The SRRs were determined from large trauma registries in the USA. The ICISS is the product of the SRRs for each of the patient's 10 worst injuries. It is claimed that the ICISS has greater predictive accuracy than ISS and TRISS (see below), especially when combined with factors allowing for physiological state and age, but the system has yet to be adopted on a widespread basis. Since patients are already coded for the ICD, it is also considered that this reduces the effort required in assigning AIS values.

Wesson's criteria[17]

This is a crude calculation for assessing the effectiveness of a trauma system. It provides a simple expression of performance based on ISS and calculates the percentage of all potentially salvageable patients who did actually survive, where a salvageable patient is defined as:

15 >ISS <60 where there is no head injury with an AIS >5.

PHYSIOLOGICAL SYSTEMS

Glasgow Coma Scale score[18]

This was first introduced in 1974 as a research tool for studying head injuries. Its full details and paediatric modifications are dealt with in Chapters 9 and 15.

Trauma Score

The Trauma Score (TS)[19] assesses five parameters, awarding weighted points, to give a score of 1–16, but has been generally superseded by the Revised Trauma Score (RTS) and is not discussed further here.

The Revised Trauma Score and Triage Revised Trauma Score

The Revised Trauma Score (RTS)[20] records only three parameters – respiratory rate, systolic blood pressure and GCS score. Each parameter scores 0–4 points, and this figure is then multiplied by a weighting factor. The resulting values are added to give a score of 0–7.8408. The percentage probability of survival (P_s) for the nearest whole number is then read from the chart. The weighting factor allows the RTS to take account of severe head injuries without systemic injury, making it a more reliable indicator of outcome. The first recorded value for each parameter after arrival at hospital is used to ensure consistency in recording, though it has been shown that field values for GCS are predictive of arrival ones and make little difference to the accuracy of scoring.[21]

The triage modification of the RTS, the Triage Revised Trauma Score (TRTS), allows rapid physiological triage of multiple patients. It uses the unweighted sum of the RTS values to allocate priorities. This system is currently used as a triage system by many ambulance services. It has been suggested that the TRTS is as good a discriminator of outcome as the RTS.[22]

Table 26.5 calculates the RTS and TRTS for the patient from the case scenario.

Table 26.4 International Classification of Diseases Injury Severity Score (ICISS)

$$\text{Survival risk ratio (SRR) for injury ICD code} = \frac{\text{Number of survivors with injury ICD code}}{\text{Number of patients with injury ICD code}}$$

ICISS = SRR (injury 1) × ... × SRR (injury 2) × ... × SRR (injury 10)

Where injury 1 is the injury with the lowest SRR in that patient

Table 26.5 The Revised Trauma Score (RTS) and Triage Revised Trauma Score (TRTS)

Respiratory rate (RR; per min)	0	1–5	6–9	30+	10–29
Score	0	1	2	3	4
RTS	α = score × 0.2908				
TRTS	A = score				
Systolic blood pressure (SBP; mmHg)	0	1–49	50–75	76–89	90
Score	0	1	2	3	4
RTS	β = score × 0.7326				
TRTS	B = score				
Glasgow Coma Scale score (total)	3	4–5	6–8	9–12	13–15
Score	0	1	2	3	4
RTS	χ = score × 0.9368				
TRTS	C = score				

RTS = (4 × 0.2908) + (4 × 0.7326) + (2 × 0.9368) = 1.1632 + 2.9304 + 1.8736 = 5.9672.

TRTS = A + B + C = 4 + 4 + 2 = 10.

Probability of survival against RTS

Nearest whole number	8	7	6	5	4	3	2	1	0
P_s (%)	99	97	92	81	61	36	17	7	3

Triage priorities using TRTS

TRTS	12	10–11	1–9	0
Priority	3	2	1	
	Delayed	Urgent	Immediate	Dead

P_s, probability of survival.

The Paediatric Trauma Score

The RTS has been shown to underestimate injury severity in children. The Paediatric Trauma Score (PTS)[23,24] (Table 26.6) combines observations with simple interventions and a rough estimation of tissue damage. The PTS tends to overestimate injury severity, but it is used as a paediatric pre-hospital triage tool in the USA.

COMBINED SYSTEMS

Trauma Score–Injury Severity Score

The *Trauma Score–Injury Severity Score* (TRISS)[25] uses the RTS and ISS as well as the age of the patient. Different weighting factors are used for blunt and penetrating

trauma. The equation for P_s is shown in Table 26.7. Different study groups can use their own coefficients to take account of the characteristics of the trauma seen in their populations. By convention, patients with a P_s of <50% who survive are 'unexpected survivors', and those with a P_s >50% who die are 'unexpected deaths'. TRISS is not validated for children under the age of 12 years.

It must be stressed that the P_s is a mathematical expression of the probability of survival, and not an absolute statement of the patient's chances. One in four patients with a P_s of 75% will still be expected to die. While these cases may be highlighted for audit to see whether there are any lessons to be learned, conclusions about performance should not be drawn from single patients. Other calculations can be made from TRISS values that better reflect a unit's results against the regional or national standards.

Table 26.6 The Paediatric Trauma Score

	+2	+1	−1
Weight (kg)	>20	10–20	<10
Airway	Normal	Simple adjunct	Endotracheal tube/surgical
Systolic blood pressure (mmHg)	>90	50–90	<50
Consciousness level	Alert	Decreased/history of loss of consciousness	Coma
Open wounds	None	Minor	Major/penetrating
Fractures	None	Minor	Open/multiple
	Total range – 6 to 12		

Table 26.7 TRISS equation

$$P_s = 1/1 + e^{-b}$$

where $b = b_0 + b_1 \text{(RTS)} + b_2 \text{(ISS)} + b_3 \text{(age coefficient)}$ and $b_0 - b_3$ = coefficients for blunt and penetrating trauma (will vary with the trauma system being studied)

Original coefficients	b_0	b_1	b_2	b_3
Blunt trauma	−1.2470	0.9544	−0.0768	−1.9052
Penetrating trauma	−0.6029	1.1430	−0.1516	−2.6676

e = 2.718282 (base of Naperian logarithm).
RTS and ISS = calculated scores for RTS and ISS.
Age coefficient = 0 if ≤54, 1 if ≥55.

Example: Patient S.W., 45-year-old female cyclist hit by car; injuries and observations as before
RTS = 5.9672, ISS = 29
$b = b_0 + b_1 \text{(RTS)} + b_2 \text{(ISS)} + b_3 \text{(age factor)}$
$b = -1.2470 + (0.9544 \times 5.9672) + (-0.0768 \times 29) + (-1.9052 \times 0)$

$b \geq 2.2209$

$P_s = 1/1 + e^{-b} = 1/1.1085 = 0.9021$ or 90.21%

ISS, Injury Severity Score; RTS, Revised Trauma Score.

A Severity Characterization of Trauma (ASCOT)

A Severity Characterization of Trauma (ASCOT)[26] is a more recent system, first described in 1990. It has proved more reliable than TRISS in predicting outcome in both blunt and penetrating trauma and provides a more accurate assessment of a patient's anatomical and physiological injury status,[27] but is a more complicated calculation (Table 26.8). ASCOT uses the AP to take account of all injuries classified as serious by AIS (scores 3–5). TRISS is flawed because of its reliance on using ISS, which counts only the worst injury within a single body

Table 26.8 The ASCOT (A Severity Characterization Of Trauma) calculation

$$P_s = 1/1 + e^{-k}$$

where $k = k_0 + k_1 \text{(GCS)} + k_2 \text{(SBP)} + k_3 \text{(RR)} + k_4 \text{(A)} + k_5 \text{(B)} + k_6 \text{(C)} + k_7 \text{(age)}$ and $k_0 - k_7$ are fixed coefficients for blunt or penetrating trauma

Original coefficients	k_0	k_1	k_2	k_3	k_4	k_5	k_6	k_7
Blunt trauma	−1.1570	0.7705	0.6583	0.2810	−0.3002	−0.1961	−0.2086	−0.6355
Penetrating trauma	−1.1350	1.0626	0.3638	0.3320	−0.3702	−0.2053	−0.3188	−0.8365

e = 2.718282 (base of Naperian logarithm).
GCS (Glasgow Coma Scale score), SBP (systolic blood pressure) and RR (respiratory rate) are coded values (0–4) as per RTS.
A = √(sum of the squares of all Abbreviated Injury Scale (AIS) codes 3, 4 or 5 in the head and rear of neck).
B = √(sum of the squares of all AIS codes 3, 4 or 5 in the chest and front of neck).
C = √(sum of the squares of all AIS codes 3, 4 or 5 in all other body areas).
Age = coded value for defined age ranges: 0 = 0–54 years, 1 = 55–64, 2 = 65–74, 3 = 75–84, 4 = 85+.

Example: Patient S.W., 45-year-old female cyclist hit by car; injuries and observations as before
A = √(9 + 16) = 5, depressed parietal skull fracture AIS 3, small subdural haematoma AIS 4.
B = √(0).
C = √(9 + 9) = 4.2426, open fracture radius AIS 3, open fracture ulna AIS 3.
$k = k_0 + k_1 \text{(GCS)} + k_2 \text{(SBP)} + k_3 \text{(RR)} + k_4 \text{(A)} + k_5 \text{(B)} + k_6 \text{(C)} + k_7 \text{(age)}$
$k = -1.1570 + (0.7705 \times 2) + (0.6583 \times 4) + (0.2810 \times 4) + (-0.3002 \times 5) + (-0.1961 \times 0) + (-0.2086 \times 4.2426) + (-0.6355 \times 0)$

$k = 1.7552$

$P_s = 1/1 + e^{-k} = 1/1.1729 = 0.8526$ or 85.26%

region and ignores other serious ones. ASCOT also has a more detailed age classification. ASCOT has not replaced TRISS because the improvement in performance is small and is outweighed by the increased difficulty in calculation.

MULTICENTRE STUDIES

The Major Trauma Outcome Study (MTOS) started in the USA during the early 1980s,[28] and is now established internationally. This study expanded into the UK in 1988 following the report of the Royal College of Surgeons criticizing trauma care. Now called the Trauma Audit Research Network (TARN), it is based at the North West Injury Research Centre. Around 90 UK hospitals that receive trauma cases contribute data to TARN. The initial aim of MTOS was to develop and test coefficients and P_s values to increase the predictive accuracy of scoring systems, and to give feedback to contributing trauma units. The data collected have become more detailed. Pre-existing morbidity, mechanism of injury, operations, complications and the seniority of staff are all included as the patient is followed from the scene of injury through the emergency department and hospital to discharge. The feedback allows audit and comparison of performance over time and between units. The approach to the injured patient has changed as a result, with the introduction of trauma teams and, increasingly, senior staff leading them. Entry criteria for the MTOS are shown in Table 26.9. Other studies are also in progress in the UK, for example the Scottish Trauma Audit Group (STAG). Each study group may develop different coefficients for TRISS and ASCOT to reflect their own trauma populations.

FUTURE DEVELOPMENTS

None of the systems developed so far is perfect,[29,30] but succeeding systems are continually improving reliability and predictive performance. New systems are under development to take the process further[31] or simplify calculation.[32]

Measuring mortality rates and calculating survival probabilities looks at only one outcome for the trauma patient. For every patient killed, another two suffer

residual problems. Measuring the degree of these problems is difficult, especially in relation to musculoskeletal injuries. An Injury Impairment Scale is currently undergoing evaluation, and the UK TARN study assesses morbidity at 3 months. The ICISS can generate expected results for the cost and length of hospital stay.

The pre-morbid condition of the patient is not currently taken into account. In the previously hypertensive patient a normal systolic blood pressure may indicate substantial blood loss. A previously fit and independent patient is likely to cope with injury better than one of the same age with chronic disease processes. Studies into this issue have been published, and are continuing.[33,34]

Pre-hospital care is a developing field with increasing medical input alongside the paramedics. Currently physiological and combined scoring systems, by convention, use the first set of observations after arrival in the resuscitation room as this is a relatively 'fixed point'. Evidence is required as to the value of pre-hospital medical care, and different strategies such as 'stay and play' versus 'scoop and run' could be evaluated by extending scoring to cover the pre-hospital environment.

SUMMARY

Trauma care teams must be able to show that they are providing as good a service as possible. The optimal organization of trauma care in the UK is still a matter of debate, and any new systems must be based on evidence and assessed in practice. The time, effort and skill that teams bring to patient care may be wasted without proper analysis of their results. In this way good practice can be recognized and spread, and lessons learned from poor outcomes. Trauma scoring systems provide the data to allow this analysis to be made. Trauma teams must appreciate the importance of scoring, and ensure adequate and accurate data collection.

Table 26.9 Entry criteria for trauma patients into the Major Trauma Outcome Study

Admitted to hospital for 3+ days
Died in hospital
Intensive care required
Inter-hospital transfer required for specialist care
Patients with fractures of the distal radius and single pubic ramus
    excluded

REFERENCES

1.   Association for the Advancement of Automotive Medicine. *The Abbreviated Injury Scale*, 2005 Revision. Des Plaines, IL: Association for the Advancement of Automotive Medicine, 2005.
2.   Kilgo PD, Osler TM, Meredith W. The worst injury predicts mortality outcome the best: rethinking the role of multiple injuries in trauma outcome scoring. *J Trauma* 2004;**55**:599–606.
3.   Mikhail JN, Harris YD, Sorensen VJ. Injury Severity Scoring; influence of trauma surgeon involvement on accuracy. *J Trauma Nurs* 2003;**10**:43–7.
4.   Johansen K, Daines M, Howey T, Helfet D, Hansen ST Jr. Objective criteria accurately predict amputation following lower extremity trauma. *J Trauma* 1990;**30**:568–72.

5.   Baker SP, O'Neill B, Haddon W, Long WB. The Injury Severity Score: a method for describing patients with multiple injuries and evaluating emergency care. *J Trauma* 1974;**14**:187–96.

6.   Baker SP, O'Neill B. The Injury Severity Score: an update. *J Trauma* 1976;**16**:882–5.

7.   Osler T, Baker S, Long W. A modification of the Injury Severity Score that both improves accuracy and simplifies scoring. *J Trauma* 1997;**43**:922–6.

8.   Balogh ZJ, Varga E, Tomka J, Süveges G, Tóth L, Simonaka JA. The new injury severity score is a better predictor of extended hospitalisation and intensive care unit admission than the injury severity score in patients with multiple ortopaedic injuries. *J Orthop Trauma* 2003;**17**:508–12.

9.   Frankema SP, Steyerberg EW, Edwards MJ, van Vugt AB. Comparison of current injury scales for survival chance estimation: an evaluation comparing the predictive performance of the ISS, NISS and AP scores in a Dutch local trauma registration. *J Trauma* 2005;**58**:596–604.

10.   Harwood PJ, Giannoudis PV, Probst C, Van Griensven M, Krettek C, Pape HC; The Polytrauma Study Group of the German Trauma Society. Which AIS based scoring system is the best predictor of outcome in orthopaedic blunt trauma patients? *J Trauma* 2006;**60**:334–40.

11.   Frankema SP, Steyerberg EW, Edwards MJ, van Vugt AB. Comparision of current injury scales for survival chance estimation: an evaluation comparing the predictive performance of the ISS, NISS and AP scores in a Dutch local trauma registration. *J Trauma* 2005;**58**:596–604.

12.   Copes WS, Champion HR, Sacco WJ, *et al.* Progress in charecterising anatomic injury. *J Trauma* 1990;**30**:1200–7.

13.   Rutledge R, Fakhry S, Baker C, Oller D. Injury severity grading in trauma patients: a simplified technique based upon ICD-9 coding. *J Trauma* 1993;**35**:497–507.

14.   Rutledge R. Injury severity and probability of survival assessment in trauma patients using a predictive hierarchical network model derived from ICD-9 codes. *J Trauma* 1995;**38**:590–601.

15.   Rutledge R, Osler T, Emery S, Kromhout-Schiro S. The end of the Injury Severity Score (ISS) and the Trauma and Injury Severity Score (TRISS): ICISS, an International Classification of Diseases, ninth revision-based prediction tool, outperforms both ISS and TRISS as predictors of trauma patient survival, hospital charges and hospital length of stay. *J Trauma* 1998;**44**:41–9.

16.   Kim Y, Jung KY, Kim CY, Kim YI, Shin Y. Validation of the International Classification of Diseases 10th Edition-based Injury Severity Score (ICISS). *J Trauma* 2000;**48**:280–5.

17.   Wesson DE, Williams JI, Salmi LR, Spence LJ, Armstrong PF, Filler RM. Evaluating a pediatric trauma program: effectiveness versus preventable death rate. *J Trauma* 1988;**28**:1226–31.

18.   Teasdale G, Jennett B. Assessment of coma and impaired consciousness: a practical scale. *Lancet* 1974;**1**:81–4.

19.   Champion HR, Sacco WJ, Carnazzo AJ, *et al.* The Trauma Score. *Crit Care Med* 1981;**9**:672–6.

20.   Champion HR, Sacco WJ, Copes WS, *et al.* A revision of the Trauma Score. *J Trauma* 1989;**20**:623.

21.   Davis DP, Serrano JA, Vilke GM, *et al.* The predictive value of field versus arrival Glasgow Coma Scale score and TRISS calculations in moderate-to-severe taumatic brain injury. *J Trauma* 2006;**60**:985–90.

22.   Moore L, Lavoie A, Abdous B, *et al.* Unification of the revised trauma score. *J Trauma* 2006;**61**:718–22.

23.   Tepas JJ, Mollitt DL, Bryant M. The Paediatric Trauma Score as a predictor of injury severity in the injured child. *J Paediatr Surg* 1987;**22**:14–18.

24.   Kaufmann CR, Maier RV, Rivara P, Carrico CJ. Evaluation of the Paediatric Trauma Score. *JAMA* 1990;**263**:69–72.

25.   Boyd CR, Tolson MA, Copes WS. Evaluating trauma care: the TRISS method. *J Trauma* 1987;**27**:370–8.

26.   Champion HR, Copes WS, Sacco WJ, *et al.* A new characterisation of injury severity. *J Trauma* 1990;**30**:539–46.

27.   Champion HR, Copes WS, Sacco WJ, *et al.* Improved predictions of severity characterisation of trauma (ASCOT) over Trauma and Injury Severity Score (TRISS): results of an independent evaluation. *J Trauma* 1996;**40**:42–8.

28.   Champion HR, Copes WS, Sacco WJ, *et al.* The major trauma outcome study: establishing national norms for trauma care. *J Trauma* 1990;**30**:1356–65.

29.   Gabbe BJ, Cameron PA, Wolfe R. TRISS: does it get better than this? *Acad Emerg Med* 2004;**11**:181–6.

30.   Chawda MN, Hildebrand F, Pape HC, Giannoudis PV. Predicting outcome after multiple trauma: which scoring system? *Injury* 2004;**35**:347–58.

31.   Gabbe BJ, Cameron PA, Wolfe R, Simpson P, Smith KL, McNeil JJ. Predictors of mortality length of stay and discharge destination in blunt trauma. *Aust N Z J Surg* 2005;**75**:650–6.

32.   Kilgo PD, Meredith JW, Osler TM. Incorporating recent advances to make the TRISS approach universally available. *J Trauma* 2006;**60**:1002–8.

33.   Hannan EL, Mendeloff J, Farrell LS, Cayten CG, Murphy JG. Multivariate models for predicting survival of patients with trauma from low falls: the impact of gender and pre-existing conditions. *J Trauma* 1995;**38**:697.

34.   Gabbe BJ, Magtengaard K, Hannaford AP, Cameron PA. Is the Charlson Comorbidity Index useful for predicting trauma outcomes. *Acad Emer Med* 2005;**12**:318–21.

27

Organ donation

OBJECTIVES

After completing this chapter the reader will:
- recognize the ongoing severe shortage of organs (and tissues) for donation
- understand that the diagnosis of brainstem death is good intensive care practice and should occur irrespective of any possibility of organ donation
- recognize the option of non-heart-beating organ donation in patients in whom treatment is being withdrawn
- know that the organ donor register should always be checked if a patient is a possible donor
- understand how optimal medical management of the organ donor increases the number and outcome of potential solid organs suitable for transplantation.

INTRODUCTION

It was not until the 1940s that the role of the immune system in rejection of transplanted organs was recognized and two decades of work began on the immunosuppressive therapy which would make transplantation possible. All donated organs were originally from asystolic donors; however, the advent of artificial ventilation and intensive care in the 1950s resulted in the first brainstem-dead, heart-beating patients. The first such patient was documented in the medical literature in Paris in 1959 as 'coma depassé'.[1] Diagnostic criteria for brainstem death were subsequently developed, and in 1968, following a complex ethical and philosophical debate, brainstem death was accepted as being equivalent to somatic death by the World Medical Association, as it represented a state when 'the body as an integrated whole has ceased to function'. In the UK this position was accepted in a 1976 memorandum from the Conference of the Medical Royal Colleges and their Faculties.[2,3] This allowed discontinuation of ventilation in patients whose brains had irreversibly ceased to function; the diagnosis and implications of brainstem death have changed little since then. The development of the concept of brainstem death also made possible organ transplantation from brainstem-dead, heart-beating donors.

Organ donation by living donors, who may be relatives of the intended recipient or merely altruistic, is not discussed further here. Deceased donors may be heart beating (brainstem dead) or non-heart-beating organ donors (NHBODs). Recent advances in the management of the brainstem-dead, heart-beating donor have led to increased numbers and superior function of organs for donation. In addition, better understanding of organ ischaemia and pre-transplant assessment of organ function, particularly renal, and the realization that other organs such as lungs may be successfully transplanted from these donors has led to resurgence in interest in non-heart-beating organ donation.

THE ORGAN DONOR SHORTAGE

The number of patients on the waiting list for an organ transplant continues to grow whilst the numbers of organs donated remains static (Figure 27.1). Approximately 6500 patients in the UK are on the waiting list for a transplant, three-quarters of whom are awaiting kidneys, of whom about 10% will die each year without a transplant. In the year to March 2005, 1783 kidney transplants were performed in the UK, of which 475 came from living donors, 143 from NHBODs and 1565 from donors certified by brainstem testing.

Reasons for the increase in demand for donor organs include improved surgical techniques, leading to improved outcomes, the ability to successfully treat older and sicker patients with organ donation and the addition to the waiting list of patients who have previously

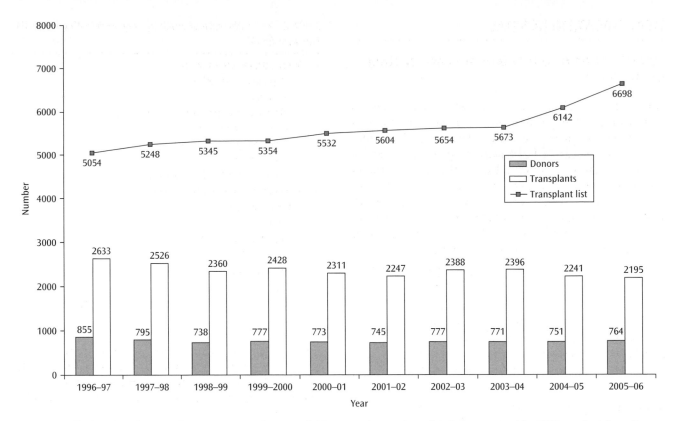

Figure 27.1 Each cadaveric organ donor represents the potential for several transplants (statistics prepared by UK Transplant from the National Transplant Database maintained on behalf of transplant services in the UK and Republic of Ireland).

undergone organ transplantation that has resulted in chronic rejection. The reasons for the decline in donor numbers include fewer road deaths following the introduction of seat belt legislation and improved outcomes in neurotrauma critical care. However, the situation is complex, and potential organs for donation are also lost due to resource issues in critical care, suboptimal donor management and, most significantly, the refusal of relatives to permit donation. The desire to increase the number of donated organs has led to consideration of several options, including restructuring of donation services, introduction of 'presumed consent' legislation,[4] the use of more marginal donors,[5] including NHBODs, and even the possibility of paid donation[6,7] which is being actively discussed in certain countries, most notably Israel.

There is a limit to the potential for transplantation from heart-beating donors (those certified dead by brainstem testing) that is less than the previous estimates of approximately 3000 brainstem-dead potential donors in the UK.[8] A recent analysis of over 50 000 intensive care deaths in the UK over two and a half years revealed that fewer than 1400 potential heart-beating organ donors are available annually.[9] The issue of donation is raised in about 95% of cases; however, in about 10% of cases there is a contraindication to transplantation or the coroner refuses donation, and 41% of families refuse to allow donation to proceed, leaving approximately 750 cadaveric donors annually.

The true potential for non-heart-beating organ donation is unknown, but of the 1300 potential NHBODs from intensive therapy units in the UK each year, donation is discussed in only a quarter of cases. Family refusal rates are as high as for brainstem-dead potential donors, and so only 6% of the total potential NHBODs lead to successful donation.[10] This may be an overestimate as the criteria for non-heart-beating organ donation are less well documented and subsequent data collection is more difficult, but certainly significant potential exists in both intensive care units and emergency departments.

COST

A successful transplant not only increases individual life expectancy and transforms quality of life but results in cost benefits to the NHS. Each of the 20 000 UK patients on haemodialysis costs the National Health Service (NHS) £22 000 per year, with the result that 3% of the total annual NHS budget is spent on kidney failure services. The cost of a kidney transplant (£17 000) and immunosuppression (£5 000 per patient per year) over the average 12-year lifespan of a patient following kidney transplant saves the NHS approximately £200 000 per renal transplant. In 2003–04 the 18 000 people living in the UK with a functioning renal transplant saved the NHS £290 million in dialysis costs.[11]

HEART-BEATING DONORS

Identification of the potential heart-beating organ donor

Although the diagnosis of brainstem death allows consideration of organ donation, it is vital that the two subjects are considered separately. Diagnosing brainstem death is simply good intensive care practice; it refutes other potential confounding diagnoses, allows discontinuation of intensive care treatment in a patient with no chance of recovery and allows the family to understand that the patient has died before treatment was withdrawn. The timing of death in the UK occurs at completion of the first set of brainstem death tests, before which no treatment in respect of organ donation should be administered since it is not of direct benefit to the patient.

> Brainstem death is documented after the first set of brainstem tests, before which no 'donation-centred' treatment may be given.

Most contraindications to transplantation are relative and depend on recipient characteristics – for example an organ from a hepatitis C-positive donor may be suitable for transplant if the proposed recipient is also hepatitis C positive. The only absolute contraindications to transplantation are human immunodeficiency virus (HIV) infection, Creutzfelt–Jakob disease (CJD) and disseminated malignancy. It is therefore good practice to discuss all potential organ donors with the transplant team.

Brainstem death

The UK criteria for the diagnosis of brainstem death are well known (Table 27.1). They are a sequence of clinical tests of brainstem function and can be performed only if the cause of brainstem death is known and confounding factors such as hypothermia, sedative drugs, muscle relaxants and hormonal and biochemical derangement have been excluded as contributing to coma. Ancillary testing such as electroencephalography, transcranial Doppler studies or cerebral angiography is not required, but rarely may be useful to support the diagnosis if all the tests cannot be performed, for example following massive facial trauma. No further supportive tests are usually required if a computed tomography (CT) scan is compatible with the diagnosis such as massive cerebral injury with herniation of the brainstem, and one would proceed to clinical testing. The time of the first set of tests is legally regarded as the time of death, and it is usually after this that the relatives are approached to discuss organ donation. It is only after brainstem death has been diagnosed that the emphasis of care must shift to the

Table 27.1 Certification of death by brainstem testing in the UK (www.ics.ac.uk)

- Absent brainstem functions
  - Pupillary light reflex
  - Corneal reflex
  - No facial movement to painful stimulus
  - Oculovestibular reflex
  - Orophayngeal reflex ('gag')
  - Cough reflex
  - Apnoea with $PaCO_2$ >6.65 kPa
- Irreversible – due to known cause
- In the absence of
  - Drug intoxication
  - Metabolic derangement
  - Abnormal biochemistry
  - Hypothermia
  - Shock

preservation and optimization of organ function. The general standards of intensive care treatment provided for the patient before brainstem death must continue after this diagnosis is made to allow the organs to be removed in optimum condition.

Approach to the donor's family

As for any intensive care patient the family should be fully informed of the patient's progress at every stage. Family members will usually be facing a sudden, catastrophic loss and a thoughtful and compassionate manner is essential. It is important to discuss the meaning of brainstem death and its implications in appropriate detail. The concept of brainstem death may be difficult for many families to understand and may require time and careful explanation; the use of diagrams or CT scans may occasionally be helpful. Families themselves may raise the subject of organ donation, otherwise the timing and manner of such a request is a matter for the individual clinician. Families who donate appear to benefit from this experience, but some who do not may regret this lost opportunity.[12]

> Always consult the donor register, the transplant coordinator and the coroner's office before raising the issue of donation with the family.

Before approaching the family to discuss organ donation, the organ donor register should be checked (tel. 01179 75 75 75), the local transplant coordinator should be contacted in case donation is not appropriate and the coroner (or procurator fiscal in Scotland) should be contacted to determine that donation is allowed, e.g. following trauma or surgery. Some centres have found that a joint request from the intensivist and transplant coordinator is associated with lower family refusal rates, and studies from the USA have shown that more time spent with families also reduces the refusal rate, presumably because it allows questions and concerns to be answered.[13] Occasionally relatives may wish to be present during brainstem testing, and this may be beneficial provided appropriate support and explanation is available.

Physiological changes associated with brainstem death

The pathophysiological effects of brainstem death are well recognized (Table 27.2). Characteristic Cushing's responses (hypertension and bradycardia) are usually seen initially in these patients as intracranial pressure rises and the brainstem is rendered ischaemic. Later, as brainstem infarction causes death of the vasomotor centres, endogenous sympathetic activity is lost and the patient develops a relative vasodilatory hypovolaemia, which if left untreated will inevitably progress to asystole, usually within 72 hours. The sympathetic catecholamine storm leads not only to end-organ damage but also to a systemic inflammatory response syndrome (SIRS)-type response, resulting in increased tissue permeability and oedema formation, as well as increased immune activation. It is increasingly clear that hormonal derangement following failure of the hypothalamic–pituitary axis and immune changes consequent on brainstem death adversely affect outcome in donated organs.[14] Not all the features described are seen in every case, often depending on the aetiology and time course of brainstem death.

CARDIORESPIRATORY SYSTEM

The sympathetic storm produces areas of myocardial necrosis as the myocardium outstrips its own blood supply, leading to arrhythmias and biventricular dysfunction. Neurogenic pulmonary oedema is common and is related to a combination of elevated pulmonary capillary hydrostatic pressure from acute left ventricular dysfunction and increased capillary permeability, seen as part of a more generalized inflammatory response. This patient population may also have concomitant pulmonary aspiration, contusion, pneumonia and atelectasis and

Table 27.2 Incidence of physiological changes following death of the brainstem

Hypotension	81%
Diabetes insipidus	65%
Disseminated intravascular coagulation	28%
Cardiac arrhythmias	27%
Pulmonary oedema	18%
Metabolic acidosis	11%

hypovolaemia as part of the underlying illness and treatment.

ENDOCRINE SYSTEM

Progressive failure of the hypothalamic–pituitary axis leads to a gradual but inexorable decline in hormone levels, in particular antidiuretic hormone (ADH), thyroid hormones, cortisol and, indirectly, insulin. Lack of ADH produces diabetes insipidus, leading to the production of large volumes of dilute urine. If left untreated, this results in dehydration and metabolic derangements including hypernatraemia, increased serum osmolality, hypomagnesaemia and hypocalcaemia, and a state of relative hypovolaemia, contributing to cardiovascular collapse. Thyroid hormone levels, particularly free triiodothyronine (T_3), invariably fall as a result of both impaired thyroid-stimulating hormone (TSH) secretion and impaired peripheral conversion of thyroxine (T_4), with an increase in inactive reverse T_3. Loss of free T_3 has been implicated in the progressive loss of cardiac contractility associated with depletion of high-energy phosphates, increased anaerobic metabolism and accumulation of lactate and contributes to metabolic acidosis, together with poor peripheral perfusion. Serum cortisol falls, resulting in hypoadrenalism and impaired donor stress response, which, together with the sick euthyroid state, contributes to cardiovascular collapse. Finally, insulin secretion is usually impaired, secondary to a decreased stress response, and hyperglycaemia is common, contributing to metabolic acidosis.

TEMPERATURE REGULATION

Hypothalamic temperature regulation is lost and hypothermia is common unless temperature is actively corrected. It is essential that normothermia is maintained in this group of patients not only for brainstem death testing, but also to optimize organ function. This is achieved by using fluid warmers, forced air warming blankets and active inspired gas humidification.

HAEMATOLOGY

Coagulopathy occurs as a result of the release of thromboplastin and other mediators from ischaemic brain tissue. This may need to be corrected by the administration of clotting factors, particularly before organ retrieval.

IMMUNOLOGICAL EFFECTS

The process of brain death itself appears to increase the immunogenicity of solid organs by a variety of mechanisms that are still being investigated but appear to include upregulation of major histocompatability class II antigens and an increased rate of acute rejection.[15] Steroids may help to modulate this process, and theoretically these effects may be reduced in organs transplanted from NHBODs.

Approach to managing the potential organ donor

Management priorities on the intensive care unit (ICU) change after certification of death to become care of a potential organ donor. Much of the management strategy is not specific to the organ donor and should reflect optimum ICU care, which should be continued beyond brainstem death testing. Strict asepsis, particularly regarding insertion of central lines, treatment of arrhythmias and infection and chest physiotherapy, for example, should all be continued. It is reasonable to assume that interventions recently associated with improved outcome in the general intensive care population, such as maintenance of normoglycaemia, might be equally applicable to the donor population.

However, in several areas of management that are specific to the potential organ donor, high-quality donor management increases the number of transplantable organs by up to 60%.[16] In particular, there is a renewal of interest in more aggressive hormone 'resuscitation' of brainstem-dead organ donors, which may result not only in more organs successfully transplanted, but also in better allograft function post transplantation.[17] Organ donor management remains a compromise as optimal support of one system may be detrimental to another; for example, fluid loading and inotropic support may maximize abdominal organ perfusion but may generate pulmonary oedema or render the heart unsuitable for transplantation. Each case is judged individually according to which organs are being considered for transplant.

VENTILATION

The donor lung is particularly vulnerable and must be able to achieve a PaO_2 of around 50 kPa on an FiO_2 of 1.0 and a positive end-expiratory pressure (PEEP) of 5 cmH_2O to be suitable for transplantation. Ventilatory strategies aim to protect the lung whilst optimizing oxygenation and include tidal volumes of 6–8 mL/kg and the use of PEEP of 5–10 cmH_2O to treat pulmonary oedema and prevent alveolar collapse. Higher PEEP and tidal volumes (12–15 mL/kg) are associated with volutrauma, increased alveolar cytokine release, alveolar damage and decreased cardiac output. The donor lung is particularly prone to developing pulmonary oedema, since the left ventricle is often significantly impaired in comparison with the right and the central venous pressure (CVP) may not accurately reflect left ventricular filling.

Fluid loading to a CVP greater than 6–10 mmHg may worsen alveolar arterial oxygen gradient in brainstem-dead donors.[18] If the lungs are considered for transplantation, fluid should be given cautiously and measurement of left-sided filling pressures considered. The role of pulmonary artery occlusion pressure (PAOP) monitoring in cardiovascular manipulation in the critically ill remains controversial; it has not been shown to be helpful in the general ICU population[19] but is still occasionally used to stabilize heart–lung donors, in whom targets include PAOP of 10–14 mmHg and cardiac index of >2.1 L/min/m^2.

CIRCULATION

The aims of treatment are to protect the heart itself from ischaemic or other damage while maximizing its ability to perfuse other organs. Absolute or relative hypovolaemia is commonly present in these patients due either to increased losses from mannitol and diuretic therapy or to diabetes insipidus and profound vasodilatation. Fluid resuscitation of several litres is usually necessary whilst avoiding fluid overload; invasive haemodynamic monitoring (including CVP) is essential; cardiac output measurement may be required:

- CVP 6–10 mmHg or PAOP 10–15 mmHg;
- cardiac index 2.2–2.5 L/m^2;
- mean arterial pressure 60–80 mmHg.

If the heart is being considered for transplantation, a mean arterial pressure of 60–70 mmHg in the absence of hypovolaemia is a reasonable compromise, providing good organ perfusion in a vasodilated circulation, with an offloaded left ventricle. Aiming for higher systemic blood pressures may require higher inotropic requirements, making the heart less suitable for transplantation by utilizing adenosine triphosphate (ATP). Transoesophageal echocardiography or PAOP measurement may be requested by the cardiac transplant team to further assess the organ's suitability and, in combination with 'hormone resuscitation', increases the number of organs retrieved. If the heart is not considered, systemic pressures may be driven higher, particularly in older donors, in whom the abdominal organs may require higher perfusion pressures.

If hypotension remains a problem despite correction of hypovolaemia, low-dose vasopressin replacement is increasingly used as first-line inotropic therapy. Both sepsis and brainstem death are associated with low vasopressin levels, and replacement is seen as restoring 'physiological' vasomotor tone. The dose should be limited to 2.5 international units (IU) per hour as higher doses in septic patients may induce cardiac arrest.

If hypotension still persists, further inotropes are required and the choice is less clear-cut, but high-dose adrenaline should be avoided because of its deleterious vasoconstrictor effects on organ perfusion and depletion of myocardial ATP. Dopamine is usually needed in high doses and may necessitate the addition of low-dose noradrenaline to deliver an adequate perfusion pressure.

ENDOCRINE REPLACEMENT

The deterioration in endocrine function following brainstem death has led to renewed interest in the replacement of those hormones essential for maintenance of homeostasis and organ function (Table 27.3).

If polyuria occurs despite vasopressin, urine and serum osmolalities should be used to confirm diabetes insipidus and treatment with intermittent desmopressin (DDAVP) may then also be required.

Intravenous T_3 *potentially* improves cardiovascular stability in the donor, but does improve function of the donor heart in the recipient. Intravenous T_4, which is significantly cheaper, does not undergo peripheral conversion to T_3 in the brainstem-dead patient and may therefore be of less benefit. High-dose methylprednisolone can attenuate the effects of proinflammatory cytokines, improve oxygenation and increase lung donor recovery and may be indicated if lung transplantation is planned or 'hormone resuscitation' considered. Hyperglycaemia is common and should be treated with insulin.

Three-drug 'hormone resuscitation' is included in the standardized management protocol of the United Network for Organ Sharing (UNOS), which demonstrated a 22% increase in numbers of organs recovered.[20] Currently in the UK each regional transplant team has its own donor management protocol.

NON–HEART-BEATING ORGAN DONATION

It is increasingly recognized that organs donated from NHBODs may be successfully transplanted due to advances in the understanding of ischaemia and the evaluation of organs before transplantation. Many authorities no longer consider controlled NHBODs as marginal donors.[21,22] Organ retrieval occurs after asystole and subsequent certification of death. This usually follows withdrawal of active treatment in the ICU, but may occasionally occur in less controlled settings, such as in the emergency department and occasionally on a medical ward, usually following a fatal and untreatable head injury or stroke or a failed attempt at cardiopulmonary resuscitation. NHBODs have been classified into five categories (Table 27.4).

Table 27.3 Standard hormone 'resuscitation' (adapted from United Network for Organ Sharing)

Vasopressin	1-unit bolus, infusion at 0.5–2.5 units/h, titrated to systemic vascluar resistance 800–1200 dynes × s/cm^5
Triiodothyronine (T_3)	4-μg bolus, infusion at 3 μg/h
Methylprednisolone	15 mg/kg bolus
Insulin	1 unit/h minimum, titrated against glucose level

Table 27.4 The modified Maastricht classification of non-heart beating donors[23]

Category I	Dead on arrival
Category II	Unsuccessful resuscitation
Category III	Awaiting cardiac arrest
Category IV	Cardiac arrest in a brainstem-dead donor
Category V	Unexpected cardiac arrest in a critically ill patient

The Maastricht III group comprises patients in whom cardiac arrest is expected, i.e. from whom treatment has been withdrawn and who will not be resuscitated after cardiac arrest. Patients in whom treatment is being withdrawn in the ICU and who may be considered as potential organ donors include patients with severe cerebral injury, irretrievable trauma or burns and patients with cardiorespiratory failure.[24] In the emergency department setting, where patients usually fall into categories I, II or V, this would necessitate the rapid establishment of lack of objection from a family member or that the patient was registered on the Organ Donor Register, which should be quickly checked.

In addition to usual contraindications to organ donation, most units also have an upper age limit for NHBODs of around 65 years, though this depends more on biological age, and any *potential* donor should be discussed with transplant teams. Treatment withdrawal or limitation precedes death in 80–90% of deaths in the ICU, and the medical staff making the decision to withdraw treatment must be independent of the transplant team. Decisions to withdraw treatment are based purely on what is in the best interests of the patient irrespective of any possibility of organ donation. In addition, no treatment may be administered to the patient before death has been certified, and treatment withdrawal should be in accordance with the usual practice and protocols of the ICU and hospital. Treatment for organ donation may be instituted only after the certification of death, which should be performed at least 5 minutes after cessation of cardiorespiratory function.[25] After certification of death, the relatives may value a brief respectful period, usually around 5–10 minutes, to sit with the deceased, after which steps are taken to minimize the warm ischaemic time.

Organs from NHBODs are at risk of significant damage from ischaemia, most damage occurring rapidly during warm ischaemia whilst cells are still physiologically active. Anaerobic metabolism produces high levels of lactic acid, which causes cellular dysfunction and the normal membrane pumps stop working. If the environment is corrected, the cells recover, but if the insult is sustained cell death ensues. In addition, after cardiac standstill, intravascular coagulation occurs and the resulting organs may never work. Successful transplant programmes utilizing NHBODs generally have very robust quality control procedures, so that non-viable kidneys are identified and not transplanted. At their simplest these viability tests are based on the knowledge of the circumstances of the death and the duration of warm ischaemia as well as the appearance of the organ. More complex criteria depend upon flow characteristics determined by machine perfusion (Figure 27.2) as well as enzyme levels from the perfusion fluid.

Steps must be taken rapidly to preserve organs in NHBODs (usually kidneys, liver and, rarely, lungs), usually within 20 minutes following asystole. This necessitates either rapid transfer to the operating theatre, where the abdomen is packed with ice, or the insertion of femoral artery catheters and instillation of cold preservation fluid, which may be done in the emergency department or ICU with subsequent organ retrieval in theatre.

Long-term donor renal function following non-heart-beating organ donation is similar to that following transplantation of kidneys donated from brainstem-dead, heart-beating donors[26] (Figure 27.3), and the number of kidneys donated from this source has steadily risen in the UK in the past few years (Figure 27.4).

UK guidelines for organ donation, including the addition of non-heart-beating organ donation, were published in October 2004 by the Intensive Care Society (www.ics.ac.uk).[27] Any potential patients suitable for donation should be discussed with the transplant coordinator, ideally before this possibility is offered to the family, to confirm suitability as a potential NHBOD.

HUMAN TISSUE ACT

The Human Tissue Act came into force in the UK in September 2006. This new legislation emphasizes that the wishes of the individual are paramount and an expressed wish during life to donate after death will carry more authority to allow organ donation. It also emphasizes the

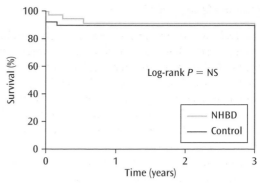

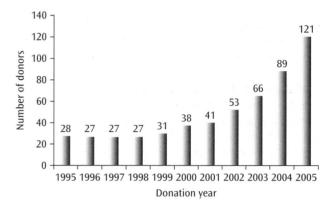

Figure 27.3 Long-term renal function appears identical between heart-beating and controlled non-heart-beating organ donors (adapted from Gok *et al*.[26]).

Figure 27.4 Number of non-heart-beating organ donors in the UK to 2005 (statistics prepared by UK Transplant from the National Transplant Database maintained on behalf of transplant services in the UK and Republic of Ireland).

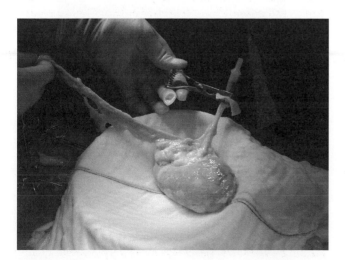

Figure 27.2 Pale kidney removed after washout with cold preservation fluid being cannulated in order to be assessed by machine perfusion (courtesy of D Talbot).

position of a designated person able to make decisions on the patient's behalf with regard to organ donation if he or she had not expressed an opinion during life. In order to allow the option of donation for relatives, it also allows the minimum necessary treatment to be commenced without consent to preserve organ function. For example, the insertion of perfusion catheters after death in the emergency department without consent from the family would appear to be supported by the Act if this then allows the family to have the option of donation when they arrive at the hospital. The Act cannot be used to condone treatment before death to facilitate donation, such as 'elective ventilation'. This was performed in the UK in some centres in the 1980s, when patients with severe stroke whose families wished organ donation to take place were intubated and ventilated and transferred to the intensive care unit with the sole expectation that brainstem death would ensue, allowing them to become organ donors. Ventilation under these circumstances was not in the best interests of the patients as it did not benefit them; indeed, it could increase their chances of surviving in a brain-damaged state and could constitute an assault.

TISSUE DONATION

It is important to remember that, even if organ donation cannot be performed, tissue donation is usually possible from many people who die in the emergency setting; this includes traumatic deaths where the pathologist may even remove these tissues during the autopsy if suitable consent is organized in time. Tissues suitable for transplantation include:

- eyes for corneal and sclera
- heart valves
- bone
- tendon
- menisci
- skin.

Corneas may be taken up to 24 hours and heart valves, bone, skin and tendon up to 48–72 hours after death. Contraindications include HIV, CJD, hepatitis viruses, systemic malignancy, immunosuppressive drugs and chronic neurological disease. Any possible tissue donors should be discussed for suitability with the transplant team. The number of patients suitable for tissue donation is huge, but, unfortunately, few families are offered this option. To know, for example, that corneal donation has restored someone's sight may give families much comfort following a death.

> Tissue donation may be possible where organ donation is not.

Case scenario

A 19-year-old man crashed his car, sustaining a severe traumatic brain injury. He was found to be apnoeic at the scene and was intubated without drugs by the paramedics. In the emergency department he had a GCS score of 3, with a fixed and dilated right pupil. Clinically, he had a base of skull fracture with brain visible in the nares and cerebrospinal fluid rhinorrhoea. A plain cervical spine film showed a craniocervical transection (Figure 27.5) and a CT scan showed multiple intracerebral haemorrhages, bleeding in the brainstem, extensive base of skull fractures and craniocervical transection. He was seen by the neurosurgical team, who confirmed that this was a fatal injury. They discussed this situation with his family, who agreed that treatment should be withdrawn as any further treatment was not in his best interests, and they offered the possibility of organ donation.

The transplant coordinators were contacted and they organized the retrieval team to attend and discussed donation with his family. The patient was moved to a side room on a ward where the family spent time with him before treatment withdrawal. Permission for donation was sought from the coroner and the police, who were initially wary about proceeding with donation as his death followed a road traffic accident; however, the Home Office pathologist agreed to attend the retrieval operation to document injuries sustained, and this allowed the retrieval operation to go ahead.

Treatment was withdrawn at a time convenient to the family, once they had spent time with him. He was certified dead 20 minutes later, and after 10 minutes with his family he was transferred to the operating theatre, where his lungs, liver and kidneys and tissues were harvested the following day. His family were grateful that six transplants (including corneas) were successfully performed following his tragic death.

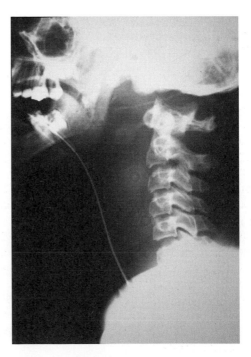

Figure 27.5 Lateral cervical spine radiograph showing craniocervical transection.

SUMMARY

Organ transplantation saves lives, transforms the quality of patients' lives and saves the NHS millions of pounds annually. The number of potential heart-beating donors in the UK is low and may fall further with the increased popularity of neurosurgical techniques such as decompressive craniectomy following severe head injury. Future developments such as xenotransplantation remain years away. Optimum management of the heart-beating, brainstem-dead organ donor not only has the potential to improve the number of organs available for successful transplantation, but may also contribute to improved survival of each transplanted organ. As organ function after controlled non-heart-beating organ donation is equivalent to that after heart-beating donation, and the number of non-heart-beating organ donors is likely to increase, organ donation should be considered in all patients in whom treatment is withdrawn. This has the potential to significantly increase the number of organs donated in the UK, including making use of a largely untapped potential source in emergency departments. Most patients are suitable tissue donors, and this request should always be considered; families appreciate the offer of allowing donation and get comfort if it is carried out. Continual support, understanding, communication and explanation with the donor family is essential throughout.

REFERENCES

1. Mollaret P, Goulon M. Le coma depasse. *Rev Neurol* 1959;**101**:3–15.

2. Diagnosis of brain death. Statement issued by the honorary secretary of the Conference of Medical Royal Colleges and their Faculties in the United Kingdom on 11 October 1976. *BMJ* 1976;**2**:1187–8.

3. Conference of Medical Royal Colleges and their Faculties in the United Kingdom: diagnosis of death. *BMJ* 1979;**1**:322.

4. Kennedy I, Sells R, Daar A, *et al.* The case for 'presumed consent' in organ donation. *Lancet* 1998;**351**:1650–2.

5. Bhorade SM, Vigneswaran W, McCabe MA, Garrity ER. Liberalization of donor criteria may expand the donor pool without adverse consequence in lung transplantation. *J Heart Lung Transplant* 2000;**19**:1199–204.

6. Roff R. Thinking the unthinkable; selling kidneys. *BMJ* 2006;**333**:51 .

7. Harris J, Erin C. An ethically defensible market in organs. *BMJ* 2002;**325**:114–15.

8. Gore SM, Cable DJ, Holland AJ. Organ donation from intensive care units in England and Wales: two year confidential audit of deaths in intensive care. *Br Med J* 1992;**304**:349–55.

The majority of countries in the world accept certification of death using brain or brainstem death criteria with different requirements for ancillary testing. However, organ donation rates differ dramatically between countries[28] (Figure 27.6). The reasons include cultural factors, such as the prevailing religious or societal beliefs, the existence or otherwise of specialized organ procurement teams, which increase the rate of transplantation in many countries, and the prevailing legal framework, e.g. 'presumed consent' legislation. Presumed consent has long been advocated in the UK but it has never been proven to be of benefit. The issues involved are more complex than they first appear. For example, for many years the highest organ donation rate in the world has been in Spain, a Catholic country where life is revered and donation seen as preserving life. In a highly pro-donation system, every hospital has in-house coordinators, often physicians, who approach families to discuss donation. However, the number of *potential* donors in UK hospitals (23.2 per million population) is lower even than the *actual* donor rate in Spain (33.6 per million), suggesting that other factors, such as the fact that Spain has one of the highest mortality rates from road traffic collisions in Europe, may be relevant. It is also possible that the number of organ donors may be higher in countries where conditions such as stroke are treated more intensively, i.e. where older patients with stroke may be admitted to an intensive therapy unit. Perhaps more illuminating is a comparison of the rates of refusal to donate by relatives: this is approximately 20% in Spain but approximately 41% in both the USA and the UK, countries where society may place more emphasis on individual choice than on the sanctity of life. The UK is currently developing some of the ideas taken from the Spanish model, such as advocating collaborative requesting and developing in-house coordinators in those hospitals with potential for donation.

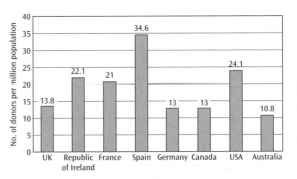

Figure 27.6 Cadaveric donors 2004. Some international comparisons (adapted from Council of Europe[28]).

9. Barber K, Falvey S, Hamilton C, Collett D, Rudge C. Potential for organ donation in the United Kingdom: audit of intensive care records. *BMJ* 2006;**332**:1124–16.

10. www.uktransplant.org.uk/ukt/statistics/potential_donor_audit.

11. www.uktransplant.org.uk/ukt/newsroom/fact_sheets/cost_effectiveness_of_transplantation.jsp.

12. Ormrod J, Ryder T, Chadwick R, Bonner SM. Experiences of families when a relative is diagnosed brainstem dead. Understanding of death, observation of brainstem death testing and attitudes to organ donation. *Anaesthesia* 2005;**60**:1002–8.

13. Siminoff LA, Gordon N, Hewlett J, Arnold RM. Factors influencing families' consent for donation of solid organs for transplantation *JAMA* 2001;**286**:71–7.

14. Pratschke J , Wilhelm MJ, Kusaka M, *et al.* Brain death and its influence on donor organ quality and outcome after transplantation *Transplantation* 1999;**67**:343–8.

15. Wilheim MJ, Pratchke J, Beato F, *et al.* Activation of the heart by donor brain death accelerates acute rejection after transplantation. *Circulation* 2000;**102**:2426–33.

16. Wheeldon DR, Potter CDO, Oduro A, Wallwork J, Large SR. Transforming the unacceptable donor: outcomes from the adoption of a standardised donor management technique. *J Heart Lung Transplant* 1995;**14**:734–42.

17. Rosendale JD, Kauffman HM, McBride MA, *et al.* Hormonal resuscitation yields more transplanted hearts, with improved early function. *Transplantation* 2003;**27**:1336–41.

18. Pennefather SH, Bullock RE, Dark JH. The effect of fluid therapy on alveolar arterial oxygen gradient in brain dead organ donors. *Transplantation* 1993;**56**:1418–22.

19. Harvey S, Harrison DA, Singer M, *et al.* Assessment of the clinical effectiveness of pulmonary artery catheters in management of patients in intensive care (PAC-Man): a randomised controlled trial. *Lancet* 2005;**366**:472–7.

20. Rosendale JD, Kauffman MH, McBride MA, *et al.* Aggressive pharmacologic donor management results in more transplanted organs. *Transplantation* 2003;**75**:482–7.

21. Weber M, Dindo D, Demartines N, Ambuhl P, Clavien P. Kidney transplantation from donors without a heartbeat. *N Engl J Med* 2002;**347**:248–55.

22. Nicholson M, Metcalfe M, White S, *et al.* A comparison of the results of renal transplantation from non-heart-beating, conventional cadaveric and living donors. *Kidney Int* 2000;**58**:2585–91.

23. Kootstra G, Daemen JH, Osmen AP. Categories of non-heart beating donors. *Transplant Proc* 1995;**27**:2893–4.

24. Manara AR, Pittman JAL, Braddon FEM. Reasons for withdrawing treatment in patients receiving intensive care. *Anaesthesia* 1998;**53**:523–8.

25. Institute of Medicine. *Non-Heart-beating Organ Transplantation. Practice and Protocols.* Washington, DC: National Academy Press, 2000.

26. Gok M, Buckley P, Shenton B, *et al.* Long-term renal function in kidneys from non-heart-beating donors: a single-center experience. *Transplantation* 2002;**74**:664–9.

27. Ridley S, Bonner S, Bray K, Falvey, S, Mackay J, Manara A; ICS Working Party on Organ Donation. UK Guidance for Non-Heart Beating Donation. *Br J Anaesth* 2005;**95**:592–5.

28. Council of Europe. *International Figures on Organ Donation and Transplantation Activity 2004.* Madrid: Council of Europe, 2005.

Index

THE
BOXER

THE
BOXER

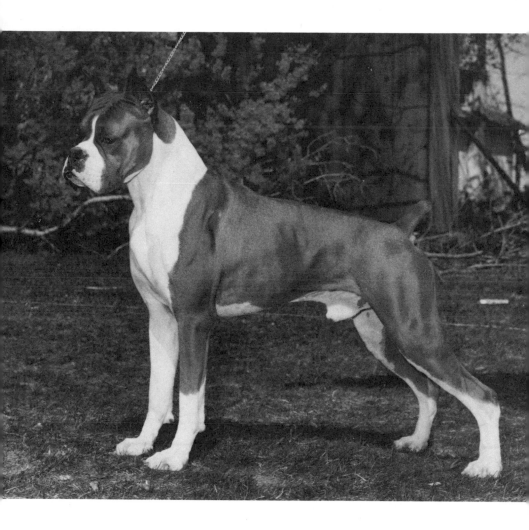

ANNA KATHERINE NICHOLAS

Front cover photo: Ch. Turo's Cachet, owned by Leonard Magowits of New York City.

Back cover photo: Ch. Spring Willow's Suzy Q is the foundation bitch of Evergreen Kennels, owned by Jane Nolt Flowers, Buffalo, Minnesota.

Title page photo: Ch. Sunset Image of Five T's, known to his friends as "Bosco," has done much good winning for his owners, Bruce and Jeannie Korsan, Laurel Hill Kennels, Oyster Bay, N.Y.

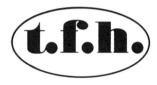

Distributed in the UNITED STATES by T.F.H. Publications, Inc., 211 West Sylvania Avenue, Neptune City, NJ 07753; in CANADA by H & L Pet Supplies Inc., 27 Kingston Crescent, Kitchener, Ontario N2B 2T6; Rolf C. Hagen Ltd., 3225 Sartelon Street, Montreal 382 Quebec; in ENGLAND by T.F.H. Publications Limited, 4 Kier Park, Ascot, Berkshire SL5 7DS; in AUSTRALIA AND THE SOUTH PACIFIC by T.F.H. (Australia) Pty. Ltd., Box 149, Brookvale 2100 N.S.W., Australia; in NEW ZEALAND by Ross Haines & Son, Ltd., 18 Monmouth Street, Grey Lynn, Auckland 2 New Zealand; in SINGAPORE AND MALAYSIA by MPH Distributors (S) Pte., Ltd., 601 Sims Drive, # 03/07/21, Singapore 1438; in the PHILIPPINES by Bio-Research, 5 Lippay Street, San Lorenzo Village, Makati Rizal; in SOUTH AFRICA by Multipet Pty. Ltd., 30 Turners Avenue, Durban 4001. Published by T.F.H. Publications Inc., Ltd. the British Crown Colony of Hong Kong.

Contents

About the Author

Since early childhood, Anna Katherine Nicholas has been involved with dogs. Her first pets were a Boston Terrier, an Airedale, and a German Shepherd. Then, in 1925, came the first of the Pekingese—a gift from a friend who raised them. Now her home is shared with a Miniature Poodle and a dozen or so Beagles, including her noted Best in Show dog and National Specialty winner, Champion Rockaplenty's Wild Oats, a Gold Certificate sire (one of the breed's truly great stud dogs), who as a show dog was Top Beagle in the Nation in 1973. She also owns Champion Foyscroft True Blue Lou, Foyscroft Aces Are Wild, and in co-ownership with Marcia Foy, who lives with her, Champion Foyscroft Triple Mitey Migit.

Miss Nicholas is best known throughout the Dog Fancy as a writer and as a judge. Her first magazine article, published in *Dog News* magazine around 1930, was about Pekingese; and this was followed by a widely acclaimed breed column, "Peeking at the Pekingese" which appeared for at least two decades, originally in *Dogdom*, then, following the demise of that publication, in *Popular Dogs*. During the 1940's she was Boxer columnist for *Pure-Bred Dogs/American Kennel Gazette* and for *Boxer Briefs*. More recently many of her articles, geared to interest fanciers of every breed, have appeared in *Popular Dogs, Pure-Bred Dogs/American Kennel Gazette, Show Dogs, Dog Fancy*, and *The World of the Working Dog*. Currently she is a featured regular columnist in *Kennel Review, Dog World*, and *Canine Chronicle*. Her *Dog World* column, "Here, There and Everywhere," was the Dog Writers Association of America winner of the Best Series in a Dog Magazine Award for 1979.

It was during the late 1930's that Miss Nicholas's first book, *The Pekingese*, appeared, published by and written at the request of the Judy Publishing Company. This book completely sold out and is now a collector's item, as is her *The Skye Terrier Book*, which was published by the Skye Terrier Club of America during the early 1960's.

In 1970 Miss Nicholas won the Dog Writers Association of America award for the Best Technical Book of the Year with her *Nicholas Guide to Dog Judging.* Then in 1979 the revision of this book again won the Dog Writers Association of America Best Technical Book Award, the first time ever that a revision has been so honored by this association.

In the early 1970's, Miss Nicholas co-authored, with Joan Brearley, five breed books which were published by T.F.H. Publications, Inc. These were *This is the Bichon Frise, The Wonderful World of Beagles and Beagling* (winner of a Dog Writers Association of America Honorable Mention Award), *The Book of the Pekingese, The Book of the Boxer,* and *This is the Skye Terrier.*

During recent years, Miss Nicholas has been writing books consistently for T.F.H. These include *Successful Dog Show Exhibiting, The Book of the Rottweiler, The Book of the Poodle, The Book of the Labrador Retriever, The Book of the English Springer Spaniel, The Book of the Golden Retriever,* and *The Book of the German Shepherd Dog.* Currently she is working on *The Book of the Shetland Sheepdog,* which will be another breed spectacular, and in the same series with the one you are now reading, *The Chow Chow, The Keeshond, The Cocker Spaniel, The Maltese,* and several additional titles. In the T.F.H. "KW" series, she has done *Rottweilers, Weimaraners,* and *Norwegian Elkhounds.* She has also supplied the American chapters for two English publications, imported by T.F.H., *The Staffordshire Bull Terrier* and *The Jack Russell Terrier.*

Miss Nicholas, in addition to her four Dog Writers Association of America awards, has on two occasions been honored with the *Kennel Review* "Winkie" as Dog Writer of the Year; and in both 1977 and 1982 she was recipient of the Gaines "Fido" award as Journalist of the Year in Dogs.

Her judging career began in 1934 at the First Company Governors' Foot Guard in Hartford, Connecticut, drawing the largest Pekingese entry ever assembled to date at this event. Presently she is approved to judge all Hounds, Terriers, Toys and Non-Sporting Dogs; all Pointers, English and Gordon Setters, Vizslas, Weimaraners, and Wire-haired Pointing Griffons in Sporting breeds and, in Working Group, Boxers and Doberman Pinschers. In 1970 she became the third woman in history to judge Best in Show at the prestigious Westminster Kennel Club Dog Show, where she has officiated on some sixteen other occasions through the years. In addition to her numerous Westminster assignments, Miss Nicholas has judged at such other outstandingly important events as Santa Barbara, Trenton, Chicago International, the Sportsmans in Canada, the Metropolitan in

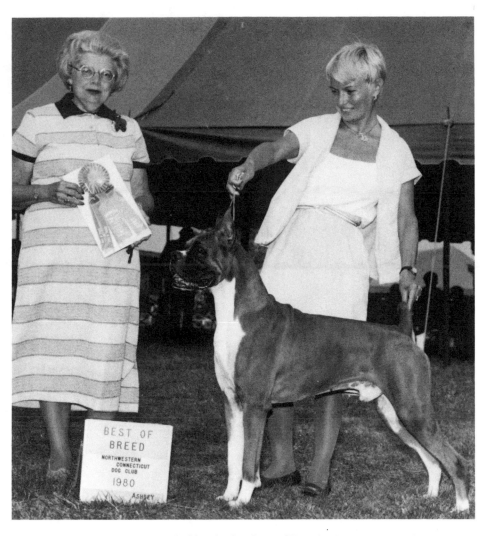

Ch. Moreleen Meralota v Imladris winning Best of Breed at Northwestern Connecticut in 1980, with Carmen N. Skinner handling for Suzie Campbell and G. Hughes and Anna Katherine Nicholas judging.

Canada, and Specialty Shows in several dozen breeds both in the United States and in Canada. She has judged in almost every one of the mainland United States and in four Canadian provinces, and her services are constantly sought in other countries.

Through the years, Miss Nicholas has held important offices in a great many all-breed and Specialty clubs. She still remains an honorary member of several of them.

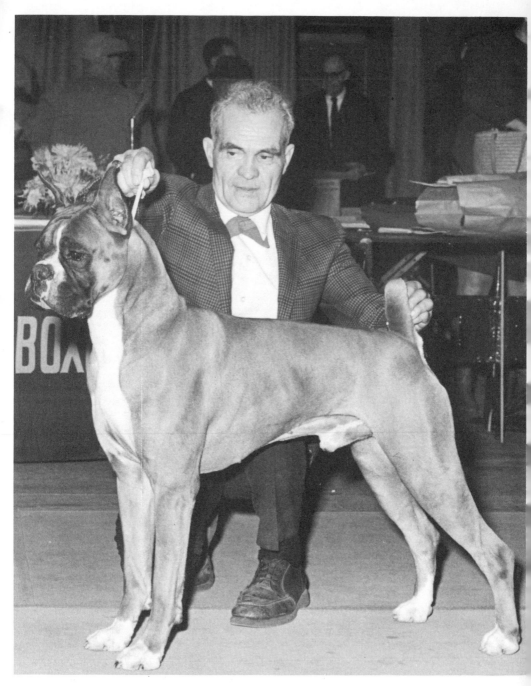

Ch. Rocky of Shawnee Trail, a winner from the late 1960's, owned by Doris Ketchow, handled by Chic Ceccarini.

Chapter 1

History of the Boxer

Origin of the Boxer

One of the oldest divisions of the canine world is the Mastiff family, its members known by various names but all massive in appearance. All are said to have originated in Asia, their common denominator being size and substance, breadth of heads with blunt, wide and deep muzzles, and a unique formation of the jaws. These dogs are noted for tremendous courage, having been used as guard dogs, fighting dogs, and in hunting lions and wild boar. They are referred to in the earliest history not only of the modern Mastiff and Bullmastiff, but also in that of the Great Dane, Bulldogs, and our Boxers.

Recognizable drawings of these dogs have been found on Egyptian monuments from as long ago as 3000 B.C. They are said to have participated in Assyrian Wars between 2300 and 600 B.C. They are referred to in Chinese literature dated to 1121 B.C. And Caesar is said to have expressed admiration for them in 51 B.C.

Canine members of the Mastiff family were seen in Greece during those early times, too, especially in the Grecian city known as Molossis, for which reason they were given that name.

During the second century A.D. some of the British branch of the Mastiff family were imported by the Romans. Closely resembling the Molossis, they were known as English Mastiffs or English Bullenbeissers, but they are said to have been of greater strength, size, agility and power. These English Bullenbeissers were highly prized by the Teutonic and Celtic tribes. It would seem quite logical that these Bullenbeissers were combined with the Molossis to create the German Bullenbeisser and that from the latter the Brabanter, the direct ancestor of our modern Boxer, was evolved.

We are told that early Bullenbeissers were seen throughout Europe. During the Middle Ages, this was Germany's only hunting dog, re-

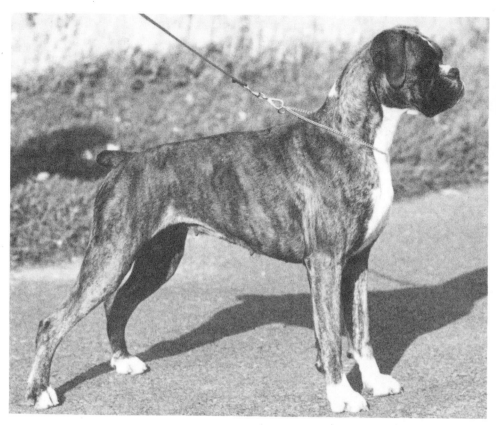

Eng. Ch. Moljon Dream Again of Marbelton, by Dandy V Starenschloss of Marbelton, Sch.H. 1, is a German import. Mrs. M. Hambleton, Ormskirk, Lancashire, England, has handled this great Boxer for Mrs. M. Davies, Moljon Boxers, Tenby, Pembrokeshire, England.

taining all of its original characteristics. Bullenbeisser owners in Great Britain, on the other hand, undoubtedly experimented with crossing various of their hounds with the Bullenbeissers, creating a faster, more agile dog of lighter build, more elegant but still large and powerful. These were called the English Dogge, and in due course they appeared in Germany.

The Germans bred Bullenbeisers to their English Dogges, it is believed, creating the early ancestors of the Great Dane, to become known as the National Dog of the Fatherland. Undoubtedly Danes and Bullenbeissers were interbred upon occasion, since both were very numerous in Germany at that period.

The Bullenbeisser's popularity was strong and steady, the dog being outstanding in his field, which included animal baiting and fighting. In those days these were entirely acceptable forms of entertainment and sport. A rather small dog of courage and power was essential for this purpose, which finally divided the breeding of Bullenbeissers into two sizes, the smaller one becoming the Brabanter. This was accomplished not by outcrossing but rather by selecting smaller specimens to be bred together to reduce the size of the progeny. The larger dogs became known as Danzigers. There was little difference between the two beyond that of size; both retained the original features of the Bullenbeisser.

It is from the Brabanter that the Boxer is believed to have been bred. He is almost entirely of German descent, although admittedly an occasional Bulldog outcross was introduced in these early days.

It was in southern Germany during the latter part of the nineteenth century that the transition from Bullenbeisser to Boxer actually took place. Twice in registered pedigrees are Bullenbeisser breedings to Bulldogs noted—once with a Bulldog named Trutzel which was said to had little impact and once with a Bulldog named Tom which led to lasting and beneficial results. It was this litter which produced a very famous white bitch, Champion Blanka von Andertor, dam of the highly influential Meta von der Passage, generally credited with having been the grand matriarch of Boxers.

Differences of opinion were strong on this point, one side feeling that head type could be greatly and quickly improved by an infusion of Bulldog blood; the other objecting for fear of roached back, shortness of leg, clumsiness of body structure, and an overabundance of white coloring. So bitter was this controversy that the Deutscher Boxer Club, founded in Munich in 1895, consisting of members who were opposed to the Bulldog influence, was soon opposed by numerous other Specialty Clubs at odds with this feeling. Eventually all was at peace, however; the Deutscher Boxer Club viewpoints and Standard were adopted, and the other Specialty Clubs combined with it as one true organization for the benefit of Boxers. The present Deutscher Boxer Club is descended from this one which at first been briefly known as the Munich Boxer Club.

It took less than ten years for the Boxer to rise to popularity, and by the early twentieth century a mutual goal had been settled upon—that of producing powerful Boxers of sound conformation and good musculation without loss of elegance and nobility.

Development of the Boxer in Germany

It was in 1887 that George Alt brought to Munich from France a bitch named Alt's Flora No. 49 whom he bred there to a Boxer dog. Unfortunately no record exists of the names of either the dog or his owner. Among the puppies was one registered in the stud book as Lechner's Box No. 48, owned by George Lechner, who also was from Munich. Eventually a mother-son breeding took place between these two dogs. The resulting litter produced two bitches who were bred to two very different dogs, each producing progenitors of our current leading Boxer strains.

One sister, Alt's Schecken No. 50, was bred to the Bulldog Tom, producing the white Champion Blanka von Angertor No. 4, the dam of the great Meta von der Passage No. 30. The other sister, Alt's Flora No. 11, was further inbred to her sire and half-brother Lechner's Box. She produced the breed's first truly influential sire, Maier's Lord No. 13.

Other early contributers to setting breed type for Boxers were three stud dogs: Flock St. Salvator No. 14, Wotan No. 46, and Bosco Immergrun No. 24, also the bitch Mirzl No. 44. All of these played their part in standardizing the Boxer.

Meta von der Passage was a fantastic producer. She herself somewhat favored the Bulldog part of her ancestry in general conformation, was "lippy" and weak in underjaw. But she produced type far superior to her own. She was by Piccolo von Angertor No. 19 (a brother to Mirzl No. 44) from Champion Blanka von Angertor as mentioned above.

Bred to Flock von Salvator, Meta produced three sons, Hugo von Pfalzgau No. 85, Schlag Bitru No. 111, and Schani von der Passage No. 128, who, in color were fawn, brindle, and light fawn respectively. Bred to Wotan for another litter, these puppies included Champion Gigerl No. 113 and Prinz Mark von Graudenz No. 118, both brindles.

Champion Gigerl is credited with having almost completely eliminated white and parti-color from Boxer coloring, overcoming the earlier tendency toward white and partis. His brindle color carried on to later generations of his offspring. He did much to overcome other Bulldog tendencies, too, his topline and hindquarters having been excellent and in keeping with those considered desirable for Boxers.

A half-brother to Gigerl (sired by Wotan), Moritz von Pfalzgau No. 14, was sire of the first German Club Champion Bitch, Champion Nora von Lauterbach No. 543. He and Hugo von Pfalzgau No. 85, by

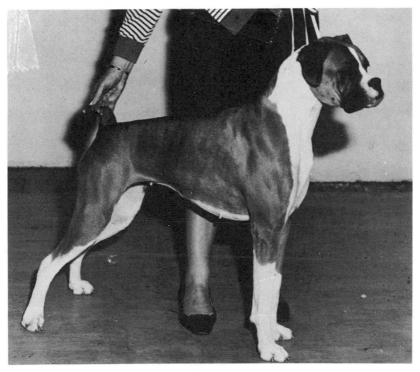

English Ch. Wardrobes Wilsiclea Autumn Serenade, owned by Mrs. C. Wilson Wiley. Photo by C. M. Cooke and Son.

Flock from Meta, became the property of Herr Otto Roth in Mannheim, where they helped to found the noted Mannheim strain.

Still another son of Flock ex Meta, Champion Shani von der Passage, was owned by Joseph Frey. Shani's son, Champion Rigo von Angertor, became a widely acclaimed winner for whom his breeder, Joseph Widman (Angertor Kennels) is said to have been paid the record price of 1,000 marks when persuaded to sell the dog. Rigo confirmed his excellence when he sired thirteen champions.

Hugo von Pfalzgau was losing no time in making his mark on the breed for Mannheim Kennels and Herr Roth. Four of his sons made prestigious names for themselves in the ring and as sires. The most notable, where future history is concerned, was Kurt von Pfalzgau No. 481, who in his turn became the sire of the magnificent Champion Rolf von Vogelsberg No. 1183.

15

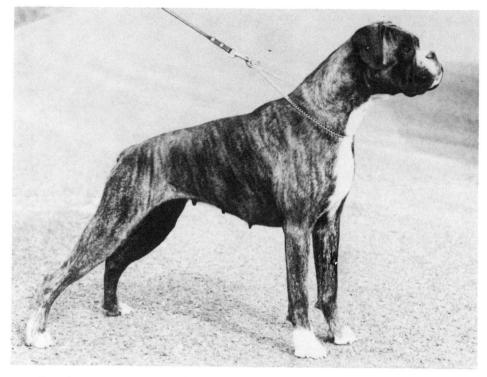

Eng. Ch. Wanderobo Hurley Burly of Marbelton, was sired by Dandy V Staren-schloss of Marbelton, Sch.H. 1, a German import. Owned by Marbelton Boxers, Mrs. Mary Hambleton, Ormskirk, Lancashire, England.

Everything we have ever read about Rolf substantiates his greatness. He was a brindle dog of tremendous quality (his color has been credited with turning the tide of popularity from the fawns back to the brindles); he seemed to have inherited all of the best Boxer features of the great dogs who preceded him. Rolf was strongly linebred to his paternal grandsire, Hugo von Pfalzgau, his dam, Venus von Vogelsberg, having been Hugo's grandaughter. Undefeated in the show ring, Rolf I'm sure must stand alone in history as being the only dog whose show career was temporarily interrupted while he served his country as a war dog in World War I, then in celebration of his safe homecoming, returned to the show scene, winning the open class and his fifth Sieger title at Munich. Rolf lived to be twelve years of age, and his descendants live on to this day since he was used at stud by the Philip Stockmanns (who purchased him from Dr. J. Schulein) in the establishment of the von Dom strain.

16

Rolf was the sire of Sieger Siegfried von Hirschpark No. 1774, Champion Rolf Walhall No. 3091, Sieger Dampf von Dom No. 2469, Schelm von Angertor No. 1500, Wotan von Dom No. 2176, Siegerin Rassel von Dom No. 4045, and Morna von Dom No. 3895.

His son, Rolf Walhall, sired close to a dozen truly important Boxers. The most notable of which were Champion Egon von Gumburtusbrunnen and Champion Moritz von Goldrain. Both of these dogs made important contributions, probably the greatest of which must be credited to Moritz who became the grandsire of the magnificent and justly famed Champion Caesar Deutenhofen, the next link in the chain of excellent producers.

It was Caesar who sired the Boxer who did so much for the breed in the United States, Champion and Sieger Check von Hunnerstein. This dog who was brought to America by Cirrol Kennels and became the first Boxer to win a Best in Show at an all-breed event here. Check left only a couple of litters behind him in Germany when he came to the States around 1930, but among them was a daughter, Saxonia's Andl, who became the dam of Champion Dorian von Marienhof of Mazelaine. Check was also the foundation sire at Mazelaine, having sired the first Boxer litter bred by Mazie and Jack Wagner.

It was a son of Caesar, Sieger Buko von Biederstein, who sired, along with several other memorable Boxers, a dog named Iwein von Dom, whose claim to fame is having produced the dog often referred to as "father of the breed in the United States," International Champion Sigurd von Dom of Barmere.

These dogs are the progenitors of many of our modern Boxers.

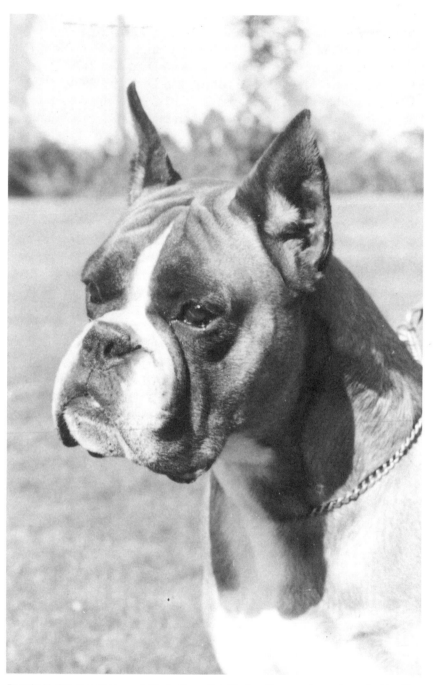

Dandy V Starenschloss of Marbelton, Sch.H. 1, a German import, owned by Mrs. M. Hambleton, Aughton, Ormskirk, Lancashire, England.

18

Chapter 2

Boxers in Great Britain

Only one Boxer gained championship in Great Britain prior to World War II. This was Horsa of Leithhill who did so in 1939. He was a brindle son of Sieger Hansl von Biederstein ex Gretl von Boxerstadt, owned by Mrs. H. M. Caro and bred by Mrs. Sprigge. He was also the first of his breed to win a British Challenge Certificate, which he did under Mrs. Cyril Pacey on this first occasion, at the Ladies Kennel Association.

Mr. Allon Dawson was the outstanding British breeder of Boxers during the 1930's. His Stainburndorf Boxers produced three especially notable homebreds. Stainburndorf Asdor and Stainburndorf Vanda each accounted for a Challenge Certificate, while Stainburndorf Wendy gained two, all during the year 1939. These three were sired by the German Sieger who was to become International Champion Lustig von Dom of Tulgey Wood (and to be owned by Tulgey Wood Kennels in the United States) from a German dam, Burga von Twiel. Mr. Dawson remained active in Boxers over the next twenty years or longer, finishing some handsome dogs. It is notable that a Stainburndorf dog was sire of Mrs. Wilson Wiley's Champion Wardrobes Cherryburton Wild Honey, winner of four Challenge Certificates.

Only 74 Boxers were registered with the Kennel Club in 1939 which number had risen to 707 when the first of the postwar shows took place. Only one set of Challenge Certificates was offered that year, at the British Boxer Club Specialty judged by Mr. John P. Wagner from the United States. Panfield Serenade won her first Challenge Certificate that day, starting her on the road to becoming Britain's first postwar Boxer Champion and the first for Mrs. Elizabeth Somerfield who became so famed and successful a breeder.

Mrs. Somerfield's Panfield Boxers are noted throughout the Boxer world, with descendants of her dogs to be found almost everywhere that

19

the breed is known. Her second to win the title was a fawn dog, Panfield Tango, who gained title towards the close of the forties. He was a half-brother to Serenade, being from the same dam, Alma von der Frankenwarte, but while Serenade had been sired by Juniper of Bramblins, Tango was a son of Panfield Flak (a son of Stainburndorf Zulu).

Champion Panfield Serenade excelled in the whelping box as well as in the show ring, and was England's Top Producing Boxer Bitch on more than one occasion. Tango proved equally successful as a stud dog. These two combined to produce Mrs. Somerfield's third champion, the fawn dog Champion Panfield Ringleader; and, in a repeat of that breeding, the fawn bitch, Champion Panfield Rhythm, one of three Panfields to gain title during 1950.

Panfield Boxers owned the leading Boxer Challenge Certificate winner of the forties in Champion Panfield Ringleader with eight. This dog sired seven champions during his lifetime who accounted for a total of forty Challenge Certificates.

As the forties were drawing to a close, Gremlin Moonsong owned by Mrs. Marion Fairbrother scored the first big win for a Boxer in all-breed competition by taking Reserve Best in Show under Leo G. Wilson at the Brighton Championship Show. Mrs. Fairbrother made notable contributions to Boxer progress through her famous Gremlins, another important British kennel that had its start during the forties.

The first Gremlin champion, which finished in the forties, was owned by Mrs. Pugh. The first of Mrs. Fairbrother's own Boxers to gain the title was the fawn homebred Champion Gremlin Inxpot, by Mrs. Somerfield's Axel von Bad Oeyn ex Gremlin Inxpot, by Mrs. Somerfield's Axel von Bad Oeyn ex Gremlin Moonbeam, who collected a neat total of seven Challenge Certificates. Among some very notable progeny of this dog was the magnificent Champion Gremlin Inkling, from Mandy Lou of Wrymark and bred by Mr. A. J. Wright, whose imposing total of twenty-four Challenge Certificates made Gremlin Top Kennel and Mr. Wright Top Breeder for a two-year period in the mid-fifties.

In the early 1960's Mrs. Fairbrother joined forces with Martin Summers of Summerdale Boxers. Previous to this time they had co-owned an American importation, Champion Rainey Lane's Sirocco and fawn littermates by him, Champions Summerdale Shamus and Snazy, from Summerdale Selmus Debutante. Sirocco very definitely turned out to have been money well spent, as he sired twelve or so champions whose combined Challenge Certificates totalled 65 or more.

In 1967, Mrs. Fairbrother finished title on Champion Summerdale Stormkist, almost twenty years after finishing her first.

Major D. F. Bostock was a very prominent English breeder in the 1950's, President of the British Boxer Club, and owner of some very outstanding champions which carried the kennel prefix Burstall. Major Bostock was one of those who imported Boxers from the United States to blend successfully into his own stock. These included one from Keith Merrill's Southdown Kennel in Virginia; two from Beaulaine, a New Jersey establishment belonging to Mr. and Mrs. R. C. Harris; and Rob Roy of Tomira, from the Ray Stoyles of Long Island. The latter dog sired some quality champions for him.

Probably one of the most exciting success stories in our dog show world is that of Wardrobes owned by Mr. and Mrs. Wilson Wiley at Princes Risborough, in Buckinghamshire. It was at the close of the forties that the Wileys attended their first dog show, taking with them Max, a puppy dog who had been a gift for Mrs. Wiley's birthday, and Queenie, who had been purchased as a companion for him.

Queenie delighted her owners by placing third in the maiden bitch class, (from that moment on they thought dog shows were the greatest); and the following week she was bred to an importation from the United States, Finemere's Flip of Berolina, who had been brought over by Captain and Mrs. Jellicoe.

This very first litter had a dog puppy, Top Hat of Wardrobes, and a bitch named Mitzi who died, but then was replaced with another young bitch from Klesby Kennels, a daughter of Champion Panfield Ringleader. She was the first of Mrs. Wilson Wiley's champions, Wardrobes Alma of Greenovia, who finished in 1951.

Wardrobes' foundation stock included Wardrobes Gay Taffeta, a Champion Panfield Ringleader daughter; and Wardrobes Starlight of Belfoynem, a Champion Winkinglight Viking son. A litter of three bitches from these two was the true beginning of the Wardrobes Saga. Two of these three became champions: Wardrobes Sari, Wardrobes Hunting Pink, and Wardrobes Silver Spurs.

Silver Spurs has gone down in history as the supreme dam in the British Boxer World, a title she was still holding in 1973 and quite possibly right up until the present time. She produced five champions whose aggregate number of certificates reached a formidable total. Most famous of them was Champion Wardrobes Miss Mink, acknowledged by many authorities to be one of the world's greatest Boxers, a fact which could hardly be questioned when one considers that she has won 27 Challenge Certificates. This stood as a breed record for sixteen years, to be broken only by her direct descendant Champion Wardrobes Claire de Lune on the day during the 1970's when she gained her 28th!

Champion Wardrobes Miss Mink won Best in Show four times at all-breed British Championship Dog Shows, making a record for the breed. She was voted Best Bitch of All Breeds in 1956 in Great Britain. Entered in 73 dog shows, Miss Mink was defeated in the breed only once—conquered by her sister, Champion Wardrobes Miss Sable, at Crufts in 1957.

Miss Mink was retired in 1957 after winning, for the second time, Best of Breed at the British Boxer Club Specialty and, also for the second time, the Champion of Champions award. Bred to her full brother, Champion Wardrobes Swinging Kilt, she produced three champions, one of which was Champion Wardrobes Wild Mink. He by the close of 1967, had become one of England's most important Boxer sires, with eleven champions having earned 76 challenge certificates. His two littermates were Champion Wardrobes Saphire Mink and Wardrobes Ranch Mink who went to Australia and became a champion there.

The breeding which had produced Miss Mink was repeated and was again excitingly successful. It was from this breeding that Champion Wardrobes Swinging Kilt was born, (the sire of Wild Mink) along with some others of superior quality.

Wild Mink's progeny left considerable impact on the breed, which has carried down through the generations. To tell the complete story of Wardrobes would be a volume in itself, and for that reason we had to limit these notes to highlights.

On the following pages are stories of some of the currently active British Boxer kennels to keep you current on what is taking place there up to the present time. We have tremendous admiration for the Boxers in Great Britain and feel that reading of them will be shared with interest by all fanciers of the breed.

Marbelton

The Marbelton Boxers, owned by Mrs. M. Hambleton of Aughton, Ormskirk, England, have earned respect and prestige throughout the world of purebred dogs.

Much credit here goes to a stud dog from the 1960's, English Champion Marbelton Top Mark, sire of six champions including Champion

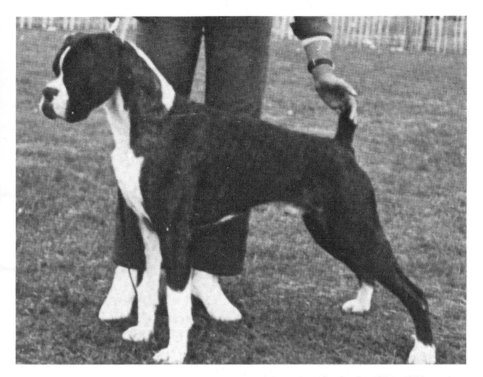

Eng. Ch. Marbelton Desperate Dan, Best of Breed at Crufts in 1971, 1973, and 1975. A winner of 29 Challenge Certificates and record holder for many years, this champion is owned by Mrs. M. Hambleton, Ormskirk, Lancashire, England.

Marbelton Double O Seven, Best of Breed at Crufts in 1970 and himself the sire of champions.

One of the most famous of Mrs. Hambleton's dogs is English Champion Marbelton Desperate Dan, who was Best of Breed at Crufts in 1971, 1973 and 1975. The winner of 29 Challenge Certificates, Dan was a record holder for many years. Additionally, Desperate Dan sired Champion Marbelton Super Trouper who won the bitch Challenge Certificate at Crufts in 1974.

Mrs. Hambleton imported a most useful Boxer from Germany, Dandy V Starenschloss of Marbelton, Sch. H.1, who seemed to blend in perfectly with the bitches in her breeding program. Among the splendid Boxers sired by him are English Champion Wardrobes Hurly Burly, and English Champion MolJon Dream Again of Marbelton, the latter the winner of six Challenge Certificates and five Bests of Breed, including Crufts in 1984. Dream Again is handled by Mrs. Hambleton for Mrs. M. Davies.

23

Moljon

Moljon Boxers are at Tenby in Pembrokeshire, England. Their owner, Mrs. Mollie Davies, and her husband have been Boxer owners since 1954, but have been showing their dogs only since the mid-1970's. In partnership with Mary Hambleton, Mr. and Mrs. Davies own the gorgeous bitch, English Champion Moljon Dream Again, who is linebred to that great Boxer, International Champion Witherford Hot Chestnut. Her dam, Moljon Sporting Favor, is by a Witherford dog and carries the best of the Witherford bloodlines. She is out of a daughter of Gremlin Satin Shorts, a litter sister to the noted Challenge Certificate record holder, Champion Gremlin Summer Storm. Dream Again was not shown until she was fourteen months of age, having been rather a slow starter. But once she started her show career, she really made her presence felt.

At her first championship show, Dream Again qualified for Crufts by winning the Junior Bitch Class with 32 entries. Then she won, at Windsor Championship Show, first in Junior, first in Novice, the bitch Challenge Certificate and Best of Breed. At the Welsh Kennel Association Championship Show she took first in Junior. At the Scottish Kennel Club Championship Show she won first in Junior, Challenge Certificate, and Best of Breed, repeating these honors at Belfast and Midland Counties, took first in Junior and the Challenge Certificate at the Irish Boxer Club Championship Specialty, then at Crufts 1984, she went from first in Open B to the Challenge Certificate and Best of Breed. These are the only shows she has attended with the exception of being placed third in Open at a Championship Show when she unfortunately went lame due to treatment on a cut foot.

Solely due to the fact that the distance from West Wales to the Championship Shows is too great, Mary Hambleton handles Dream Again in the ring.

Mrs. Davies has a lovely dog in Moljon Sporting Chance, a litter brother of Moljon Sporting Favour, who is the winner of sixteen Bests of Breed, and a Best in Show at an Open All-Breeds event where 560 dogs were entered.

Opposite page: Eng. Ch. Moljon Dream Again of Marbelton, winner of six Challenge Certificates and five Bests of Breed, including Best of Breed at Crufts in 1984. Sired by Dandy V Starenschloss of Marbelton, Sch.H. 1. Owner, Mrs. M. Hambleton, Ormskirk, Lancashire, England.

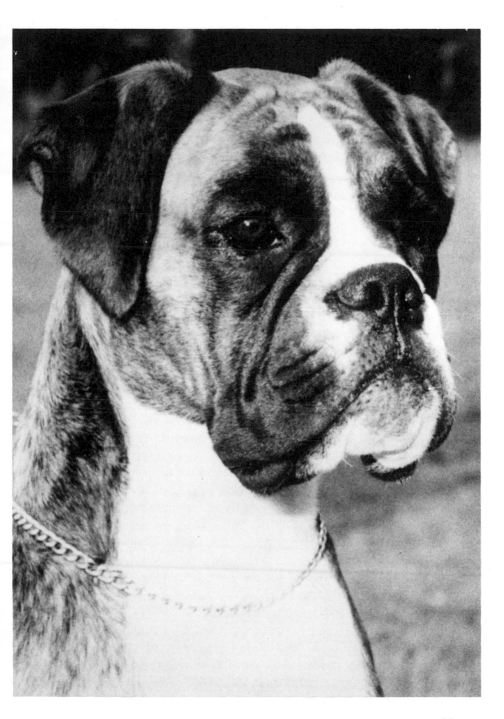

Seefeld

Seefeld Boxers were founded by Pat Heath, Axbridge, Somerset, England, in the 1960's, and have gained renown worldwide for quality and excellence.

The First two champions owned by Pat Heath were a dog, Champion Seefeld Holbein, C. D. X., and a bitch, Champion Seefeld Musk Rose. Holbein was by Seefeld Radden Rembrandt (the sire of three British Champions) who was by 1968's Top Sire, Falcign Faro (American Champion Rainey Lane Raffles ex Champion Toplocks Walladay of Sheafdon) ex Champion Wardrobes Miss Sable. The dam of Holbein was Mixonne Mitzi Moonbeam (Second Top Dam of 1964), who was a double granddaughter of Gremlin Sirocco of Felden.

Champion Seefeld Musk Rose was by the American import Champion Wardrobes Delharts Mack The Knife (sire of four British Champions) who was by American Champion Jered's Spellbinder from a daughter of American Champion Barrage of Quality Hill (by Bang Away).

Pat Heath bred her two early champions to each other, producing a very smart and stylish puppy in the litter whelped on November 12th 1968, which she named Seefeld's Picasso. Right from the beginning this puppy had an air of quality about him, leading to excitement on the part of his breeder who felt that she had, indeed, produced something unusually outstanding.

Picasso made his debut with instant success. At seven months he won his first puppy award; at eleven months his first Reserve Best in Show; at nineteen months his first Challenge Certificate. His total show record upon retirement consisted of 24 Challenge Certificates, seventeen Reserve Challenge Certificates, Dog of the Year all breeds in Ireland in 1971, sixteen times Best in Show (with three Bests in Show, twice Reserve Best in Show, and eight Working Groups at *all-breed Championship shows* in England and Ireland), plus second in the Working Group at Crufts in 1972. Adding particular glory to his wins is the fact that many of them were made under the most highly respected judges of England, Ireland, the United States (Alva Rosenberg and Percy Roberts), Canada, New Zealand, and Scandinavia.

As a sire, Picasso distinguished himself in a notable manner. In Great Britain he sired 25 different Challenge Certificate winners (eighteen of them champions), winning among them the impressive total of 105 Challenge Certificates and five Working Groups at Championship shows. In addition to these, Picasso had champion offspring

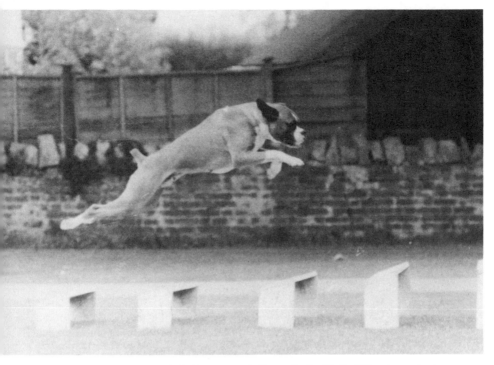

Eng. Ch. Seefeld Holbein, C.D.(Ex), the only Boxer in the United Kingdom who is a show champion and qualified for working trials. A first-prize Obedience winner, here he Is clearing a nine-foot jump. This dog is the sire of champions, including the famous Int. Ch. Seefeld Picasso. Owned by Mrs. Pat Heath.

in many other countries of the world, and when his son, Seefeld Rolfadan Reign Beau, became a champion in Singapore, this brought Picasso's overall total of champion offspring to fifty.

There are, and have been, numerous other extraordinary Boxers at Seefeld in addition to Picasso. To name one, his sire, Champion Seefeld Holbein C.D.X. had the distinction of being the only show champion Boxer in the United Kingdom to qualify at Working Trials, and he was also a first prize Obedience winner.

Champion Seefeld Sunbeam, by Picasso from Caefennie Abby and bred by Mrs. Barnett, has won Best in Show and is the sire of champions.

Champion Seefeld Mustard Seed, bred and owned by Pat Heath, is the dam of three champions and herself a daughter of Norwegian Champion Cavajes Herakles of Seefeld from Seefeld Rose Marie. Also by Herakles but from Seefeld Beau Folly, the homebred Champion

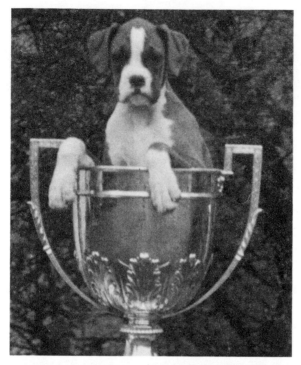

Future Int. Ch. Seefeld Wynbok Dominic, son of Int. Ch. Seefeld Picasso, at four months of age sitting in the Crufts Cup won by his sire for second place in the Working Group. Bred by Mrs. Marley. Owned by Mr. and Mrs. Wilberg.

English Ch. Seefeld Shadowfax, one of the famed Boxers belonging to Mrs. Pat Heath, Seefeld Kennels, England.

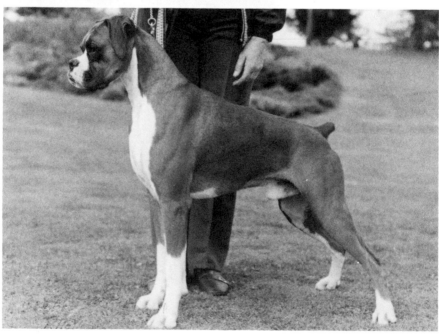

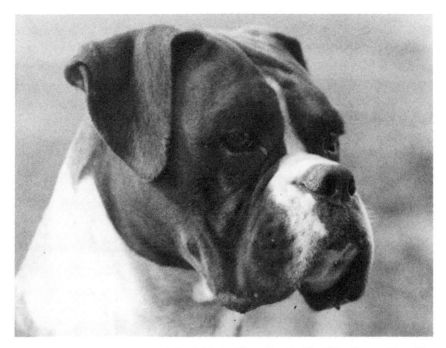

Nor. Ch. Cavajes Herakles of Seefeld, by Nor. Ch. My-R's Side Car ex Nor. Ch. Cavajes Fleur, bred by Mr. K. Anderson and owned by Mrs. Pat Heath. Imported to England in 1974, this sire of eight champions is 90% American breeding through Salgray and Boxella.

Seefeld Shadow is a Best in Show all-breed winner and the sire of seven champions. This dog started on the road to his title with a Best of Breed and a Challenge Certificate from the Novice Class at Black pool under no less an authority than Mr. Dawson, then quickly followed with the Challenge Certificate and Best in Show at both the Irish Boxer Club and the South Western Boxer Club. He also won Best in Show all-breeds, and reserve Best in Show at all-breed events prior to reaching twenty months of age.

The Best in Show winner, Champion Seefeld Smarty Pants, was sired by Shadowfax from Seefeld Fancy Pants, owned and bred by Mrs. Heath with Mrs L. Gunns.

Another Picasso son of particular note, International Champion Wynbox Dominie, was bred by Mrs. Marley from Wynbok Wilhelmina and owned by Mr. and Mrs. Wilberg. This dog started out by becoming Top Boxer Puppy in England; then became Top Boxer in Norway, Sweden, and Finland. He won the International Title under F.C.I. rules qualifying in the show ring in three different countries, and qualifying in Obedience, Temperament and Working Trial tests. Now, as a Veteran, he is still winning Groups and Reserve Best in Show.

The Norwegian Champion Cavajes Herakles of Seefeld was imported to England in 1974. The sire of eight champions, this dog is 90% American breeding, primarily Salgray and Boxella. He is by Norwegian Champion My-R's Side Car (American) ex Norwegian Champion Cavajes Fleur, was bred by Mr. Anderson and belongs to Mrs. Heath.

The famous American Champion Salgray's Minute Man, by American Champion Salgray's Ambush ex Am. Ch. Salgray's Jitterbug, bred by Phyllis and Daniel Hamilburg, spent one year in England, under Pat Heath's ownership, en route to his new home in Australia where he went to Mr. T. Carter. In England he sired thirteen litters which included twenty first-prize winners, one Irish Champion, an English Challenge Certificate and Reserve Challenge Certificate.

Minute Man's grandson, Braemerwood Proclamation, has now been imported into England and is owned by Mrs. Heath. It is hoped that he will be as successful at stud as all the many previous famous Seefeld sires.

Pat Heath is widely sought after in all parts of the world as a judge. The author recalls the pleasure of meeting her on one of her judging trips to the United States, when we dined together with mutual friends including Jane and Bob Forsyth and Eleanor Linderholm. Her knowledge of Boxers is impressive, as is the quality of her dogs.

Skelder

The Skelder Boxers belong to Mrs. Joy Malcolm at Blandford Forum, Dorset, England.

It was in 1943 that Mrs. Malcolm started breeding Boxers, and she has quite consistently remained with her original bitch line since then, judiciously selecting top winning dogs which she has admired from other bloodlines for breeding with them from time to time in order to guard against her kennel becoming too closely inbred.

English Champion Skelder Burny Almond has the honor of having gained twenty Challenge Certificates during his show career, the twentieth in September 1983 at seven and a half years of age.

Other current champions at Skelder include Champion Skelder Scorching, Champion Skelder Sky High, Champion Snarestone Sky Rocket of Skelder, to name a few.

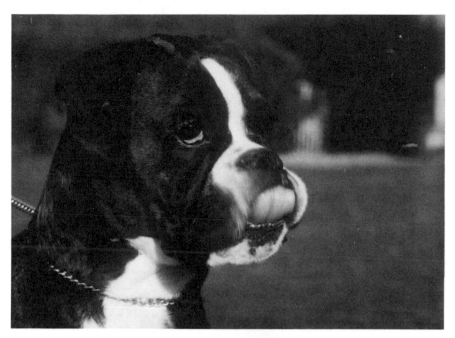

Ch. Skelder Burnt Almond, by Ch. Skelder Sweet Talking Guy ex Burning Bright of Skelder. Owned by Mrs. Joy Malcolm, Blandford Forum, Dorset, England.

Right to left: Eng. Ch. Skelder Scorching, by Ch. Starmark Sweet Talking Guy ex Burning Bright of Skelder, winner of ten Challenges, leading Boxer in the United Kingdom, pictured with his son, Ch. Snarestone Sky Rocket of Skelder. Owned by Mrs. Joy Malcolm. Blandford Forum, Dorset, England.

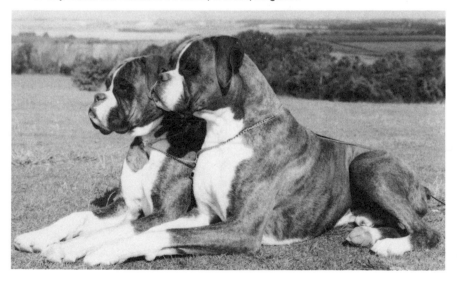

Winuwuk

Winuwuk Boxers are owned by Ivor and Marion Ward-Davies of Schoolhouse, United Kingdom. During a visit to the United States, these folks became acquainted with Mrs. Margaret Krey of the Kreyon Boxers who showed them a brindle dog whom they immediately admired. They finally succeeded in persuading Mrs. Krey to allow this gorgeous Boxer to return to Great Britain with them. This was Kreyon's Back In Town, by Champion Schor Khoun's Shadrack from Champion Kreyon's Firebrand. The first litter sired by him for his new owners produced three litter sisters who placed first,

Ch. Kinbra Uncle Sam of Winuwuk, by the American import Kreyons Back in Town, was bred by Mr. and Mrs. Coombs and is owned by I. and M. Ward-Davies.

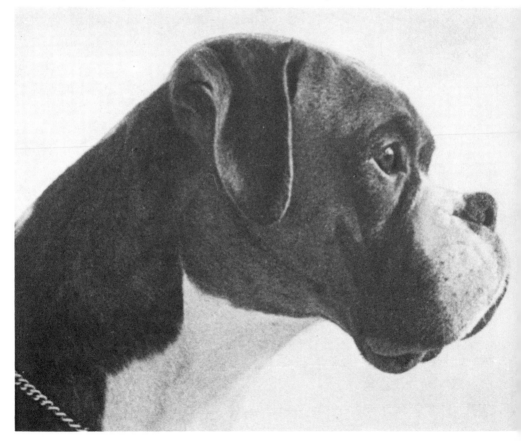

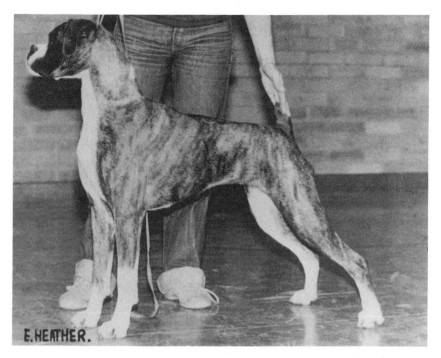

E.HEATHER.

English Ch. Winuwuk Good Golly is the Top Winning Bitch of all time in the United Kingdom and the British Boxer Club Champion of Champions in 1983. Bred and owned by M. and I. Ward-Davies, Winuwuk Kennels.

second and third in the Special Puppy Class at the British Boxer Club Championship Show.

Back In Town sired four English Champions, including Champion Kinsra Uncle Sam of Winuwuk who was 1977's Top Boxer Male in the United Kingdom. Sam was retired early, but came out of retirement at six years of age when he went Best in Show at a Boxer Championship Specialty under an Australian judge.

Back In Town was a highly influential sire. Another very successful son of his was Rainey Lane's Grand Slam who sired no less than thirteen Australian champions. Mr. and Mrs. Ward-Davies have lost count of Back in Town's winning children and grandchildren both at home and overseas.

Later Mr. and Mrs. Ward-Davies paid another visit to the United States, and again brought home a dog. This time it was Milray's Red Baron of Valvay, by Champion Schor Khoun's Abednego from Milray's Flame of Candlewood. She seemed ideal for the Back In

Town offspring, which proved to be correct. Mating Baron to the Back In Town daughter Winuwuk Goodness Gracious produced the lovely bitch Champion Winuwuk Good Golly, who finished her championship title at Crufts in 1980 and went on to win two Challenge Certificates up to now. In England the competition for Challenge Certificates is open, so you must beat all the champions in order to win. Good Golly is the top winning brindle bitch of all time in the United Kingdom, and presently holds the coveted British Boxer Club Champion of Champions Award, this for 1983.

The American import, Milray's Red Baron of Valvay, taken in a quarantine kennel on arrival in the United Kingdom, en route to his new home at Winuwuk Boxers in England.

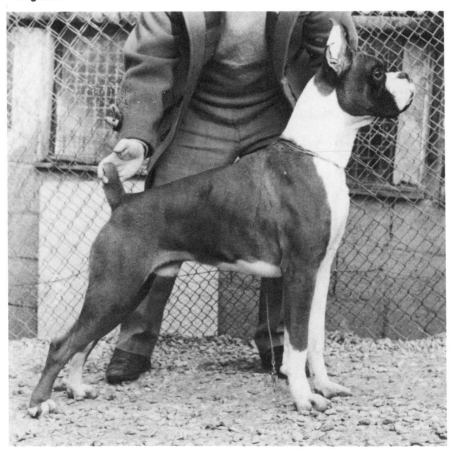

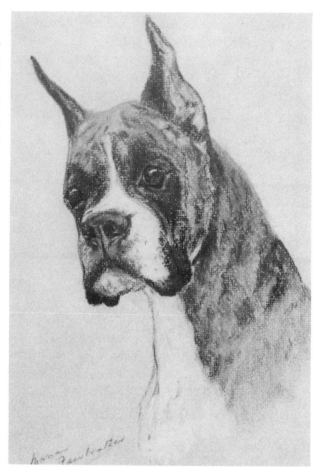

Am. Ch. Kreyon's Back in Town, by Int. Ch. Schor Khoun's Shadrack ex Am. Ch. Kreyon's Fire Brand, was bred by M. Krey in the United States and is owned by M. and I. Ward-Davies.

Red Baron has sired two other champions, and has champion off-spring overseas. Both of these dogs have passed on their many virtues and are behind most of the top winners in the United Kingdom.

Back In Town died in 1983, but rests under a magnolia on the river bank at Winuluk. He will be remembered not only as a great stud dog, but also as a most gentle dog with a superb temperament that he handed on to the breed. Red Baron is still alive and well and happy.

35

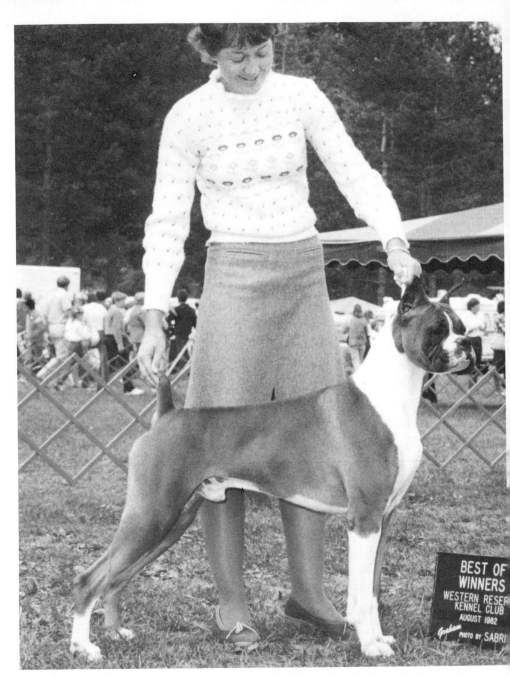

Am. and Japanese Ch. Jacquet's Urko, by Ch. Happy Ours Fortune de Jacquard ex Ch. Jacquet's Candy Dancer, here is going Best of Winners under judge Charlotte McGowan. Finished in three weekends of showing with three Bests of Breed and Group placement. Went on to Japan to become Top Winning Dog in Japan. Owned by Dr. Hideaki Nakazawa, Tokyo, Japan. Breeder, Richard Tomiko, Jacquet Boxers, Paramus, New Jersey.

Chapter 3

Boxers in the United States

In the early part of the present century, probably about 1905, Valentine Martin of the Stuttgarter Kennels began breeding Boxers here from the excellent dogs he had brought with him from Germany. A picture of Mr. Martin was once shown to us, taken at Stuttgart, Germany, in 1908, with two dogs, Febo and Leo. In the caption under it the gentleman is referred to as being "one of America's leading fanciers," as indeed he was! Stuttgarter Kennels are believed to have been in operation here in the States for several years at that time.

The attention of the American public was called to Boxers as a breed of dog when, a few years later, future Governor of New York and Mrs. Herbert H. Lehman imported the 1912 Sieger, Dampf von Dom who was sired by the highly influential German winner and sire Sieger Rolf von Vogelsburg. Dampf became the first Boxer to attain championship honors in the United States, which he did in 1915.

Some ten years after the above event, around 1925, two Boxers appeared among the dogs entered at Westminster. They were a bitch, Dina von Thuringer, and a dog, Ali von Haldenburg, both owned by Dr. J. G. William Greeff.

By 1926 the Lehmans were showing a dog and a bitch, Artus von Hornfeld and Betty, and during that year the second American Champion Boxer gained title, Blutcher von Rosengarten. It was not until the 1930's that the first American-bred Boxer gained title, this honor going to Banner of Barmere owned by Mrs. William Z. Breed who was a highly influential early Boxer breeder. The first champion born in the United States from a breeding which had taken place in Germany was Dodi von der Stoeckensberg.

Mr. and Mrs. Alexander Nitt, breeders from Long Island, are other fanciers of the 1920's who remained active in the breed. The first of their dogs were Lenz von Dom, Zerna von Muchlen, and Germania von Haag, imported and representing finest German bloodlines.

It was during the early part of the 1930's that Mr. and Mrs. John P. (Mazie and Jack) Wagner started their involvement with Boxers which led to the establishment of Mazelaine Kennels. The first of their Boxers was purchased from the Birkbaum Kennels, owned by Dr. Birk and Mr. Greenbaum, located where they, too, lived at Milwaukee, Wisconsin. She grew up to become Champion Landa of Mazelaine, the first of Mazelaine's long roster of champions.

Landa was bred to Champion Check von Hunnerstein, whelping Mazelaine's first Boxer litter on November 11th 1933. It was a bitch from this litter, Anitra of Mazelaine, who became the Wagners' special house pet. It was she who, in due time, founded one of the leading Mazelaine lines with her litter by International Champion Dorian von Marienhof of Mazelaine, which gave the Wagners their first homebred champion, Kavanaugh of Mazelaine, along with Champions Kobald, Kohath and Keturah. A repeat Dorian-Anitra breeding produced Champion Warrior of Mazelaine. Then Anitra was bred to Champion Argus of Konigsee of Mazelaine, producing Dagmar of Mazelaine who, bred to Dorian, produced Champions Nocturne and Nemesis of Mazelaine and Champion Tweedle Dum of Tulgy Wood. Champion Renown of Barmere also was from this combination in a later litter.

Champion Nemesis of Mazelaine founded the Bladan Kennels of Dr. and Mrs. Dan. M. Gordon. By Champion Brokaw von Germanstolz she produced Champion Sir Galahad of Bladan and Champion Sir Royal of Bladan. With International Champion Lustig von Dom of Tulgey Wood several more Nemesis champions were produced, among them Champion Bladan's U-Chetnik.

Champion Nocturne of Mazelaine, sister to Nemesis, when bred to Champion Utz von Dom of Mazelaine created the famous V litter. Dirndl von Stolzenhof, a bitch of whom he had heard interesting reports, was imported by Jack Wagner in the early 1930's and became Mazelaine's first Boxer champion, followed by three other importations that same year and by the first bitch, Lande, the following year.

Between 1934 and 1951 alone, Mazelaine finished a minimum of two champions annually, usually five or six each year, and several times in the region of a dozen.

The Wagners imported a number of outstanding Boxers from Germany, using them successfully in the creation of outstanding homebreds. Champion Dorian von Dom of Mazelaine was one of the greatest of those to come over, a true "pillar of the breed" who in his short lifetime (he lived to be only eight years old) left an indelible impact on the breed. Dorian was never defeated by any other Boxer in the United States or in Germany, and at the time of his retirement had won the amazing total of 22 Bests in Show in the United States.

International Champion Utz von Dom of Mazelaine was the next memorable importation to come to the Wagners from Germany. He was a younger brother to Champion Lustig von Dom of Tulgey Wood, and had aroused the admiration of the Wagners when they had seen him while in Germany.

Throughout the forties and the fifties, Mazelaine turned out magnificent dogs who made great names for themselves at an amazing rate. Among them were such notable Boxers as Champion Mazelaine's Zazarac Brandy, Westminster Best in Show winner and one of the Top Best in Show winners of any breed in the United States; Champion Warlord of Mazelaine, a Best in Show and Best American-bred in Show winner at Westminster on separate occasions, and literally dozens more. They said in those days "The winning strain is Mazelaine"—and believe me, they said it only because, for at least a couple of decades, it was true, and the descendants of these dogs are still in the limelight up until the present.

The American Boxer Club was founded in 1935 by a group of fanciers who felt that at the rate breed interest was growing, such an organization was needed for the breed's future protection. The Club's first President was Harold Palmedo, Alexander Nitt the Treasurer, and Mrs. Palmedo's mother, Mrs. Rudolph Gaertner, the Secretary. Membership to the American Kennel Club was approved the following May.

The Club's first Specialty Show took place in 1936, in conjunction with the Greenwich Kennel Club. The first independent separate Specialty Show of the American Boxer Club took place at the Hotel McAlpin in New York City on January 5th 1944, with 104 Boxers in competition for the opinion of the famous and highly respected judge Alva Rosenberg.

The American Boxer Club was incorporated in 1939. Delegate to the American Kennel Club was Richard C. Kettles, Jr. The first two affiliated Boxer Clubs, which started at about this time, were the Mid-West and Eastern Boxer Clubs.

Many devoted and talented Boxer fanciers played a part in the breed's development and rapid rise to popularity here. As the 1930's started to unfold Cirrol Kennels, in New York City, imported one of the "greats" from Germany, who became the first of his breed to win a

Best in Show in the United States. This was under judge T.E.L. Kemp, and was followed shortly thereafter by a second Best in Show for the dog, at North Westchester in 1932. Check's owners here were Joseph and Marcia Fennessey of New York City. Check, prior to coming over, sired two excellent producing bitches left behind to carry on his line. These were Siegerin Yva von Marienhof and Saxonia's Andl, the latter eventually becoming the dam of International Champion Dorian von Marienhof of Mazelaine. Here in the States, among others, Check sired the first litter bred at Mazelaine Kennels.

Barmere Kennels is another to have started in the early 1930s. This was owned by Mrs. Miriam Hostetter Breed, or, as she was at the time, Mrs. Hostetter Young, and became the home of the dog generally referred to as "father of American Boxers," International Champion Sigurd von Dom of Barmere. Five years old when imported, he was already established as a quality sire in Germany, where his progeny included Sieger Fachinger von Neu Drosedow, Sieger Zero von

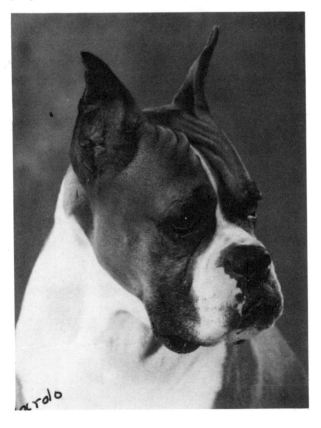

Ch. Holly Lane's Delovely Replay owned by Donald M. Edwards, M.D., Fullerton, California.

40

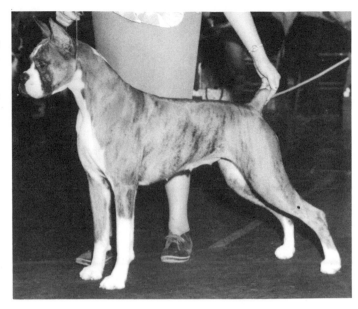

Brig's Daisy Mae, the foundation bitch at Vihabra Boxers, Dr. H.L. and Mrs. V.J. Bradley, Los Altos Hills, California.

Dom, International Champion Xerxes von Dom, American Champion Just von Dom and the highly successful sire Zorn von Dom along with such bitches as Siegerin Yva von Marienhof and Siegerin Zeila von Dom. It is indeed impressive to consider that Sigurd's son, Xerxes, was the sire of International Champion Dorian von Marienhof of Mazelaine plus other famed champions; and that another son, Zorn, sired International Champion Lustig von Dom of Tulgey Wood and International Champion Utz von Dom of Mazelaine. Just trying to contemplate the number of champions sired by and descended from Dorian, Lustig, and Utz is downright mindboggling. The impact of these dogs on the development of the modern Boxer can never be overestimated. As already noted, Dorian and Utz were owned in the United States by Mr. and Mrs. John P. Wagner. Lustig was brought here by Mr. and Mrs. Erwin Freund for their Tulgey Wood Kennels, which also imported International Champion Lisl von der Blutenau of Tulgey Wood and Champion Pitt von der Wurm of Tulgey Wood. Like Dorian, Lustig was undefeated by any Boxer in Germany or in the United States.

Sumbala Kennels, owned by Mrs. Lillian Palmedo, was an esteemed Boxer stronghold in the thirties, probably its best known representative having been the excellent bitch Champion Biene von Elbe-Bogen se Sumbala, who was an imported daughter of Dorian.

Mr. and Mrs. Charles Ludwig, Sr., were active importers and breeders of Boxers at that time. Their daughter, Lena Ludwig, who passed away early in the 1980's, was a breeder-exhibitor and highly respected judge.

Other names to be remembered from the years of Boxer development here include:

Dr. and Mrs. S. Potter Bartley, Shinnecock Kennels, founded in the early 1930's, whose dogs included Champion Dora von Uracher-Wasserfall. The Bartleys were breeders, exhibitors, and great enthusiasts. Dr. Bartley was a judge, and the second President of the American Boxer Club.

Francis A. Bigler, Bravenhartz Kennels, started with a Sigurd daughter. Frank was a widely read and interesting columnist on Boxer activities in his day.

Walter F. Foster, Fostoria Kennels, breeder and professional handler, was the owner of the first American-bred Group winning Boxer, Champion Baldur of Fostoria. He handled many great Boxers including Champions Warlord and Serenade of Mazelaine and Champion Kurass v.d. Blutenau of Dorick for the Richard C. Kettles and Champion Merry Monarch for Mr. and Mrs. Edward V. Quinn.

Frederick I. Hamm was a widely liked and hard-working member of the American Boxer Club from the thirties to the fifties, serving terms as Treasurer and as President. His Mahderf Kennels gained fame as the home of Champion Mahderf's Miss Eva, who became the dam of the famous Champion Mahderf's El Chico.

Charles O. Spannaus was another who started during this period. His Charos Kennels owned Champion Edra of Barmere. Mr. Spannaus was a long-time Secretary of the American Boxer Club and also served as its President.

Throughout the forties Boxers continued to prosper, gaining in popularity at an amazing rate of speed. By 1950, enthusiasm, number of entries, number of important wins, and number of breeders becoming involved had reached almost astronomical heights. As I have written in the past, these years can only be thought of as having been "The Golden Era" in the Boxer world, so numerous and so outstanding were the breed's accomplishments.

In 1947, 1949 and 1951 three separate Boxers, all of them American-bred, won Best in Show at Westminster Kennel Club's prestigious annual dog show at Madison Square Garden in New York. These were, in that order, Champion Warlord of Mazelaine, owned by Mr. and

Mrs. Richard C. Kettles, Jr., and handled by Nate Levine (1944, Warlord, handled by Walter C. Foster, had won Best American-bred in Show here); in 1949, Champion Mazelaine's Zazarac Brady, owned by Mr. and Mrs. John Phelps Wagner, handled by Phil Marsh; and in 1951 Champion Bang Away of Sirrah Crest, owned by Dr. and Mrs. Rafael C. Harris, handled by J. Nate Levine. In 1970 another Boxer joined this list: for the first time, a bitch Champion Arriba's Prima Donna, owned by Dr. and Mrs. P.J. Pagano and Dr. Theodore S. Fickes handled by Jane K. Forsyth. These four are the only Boxers to date who have gained the supreme award of Best in Show here. All of these Boxers had notable ring careers to their credit. Brandy and Bang Away each had, for a time, the record of most all breed Bests in Show of any dog of any breed in the United States, and Warlord had the honor of about a dozen such victories, many Specialties and Working Groups, and the previously gained Westminster Special Award for Best American-bred in Show. All of these dogs were highly successful sires, leaving literally hundreds of excellent descendants. The bitch, Prima Donna, was a multiple Best in Show dog and had been Top Show Dog in the Country the previous year. Boxers over which to thrill with pride, each and every one of them!

There are so many dogs and so many people to whom we would dearly love to pay tribute on these pages. This book however is not designed to be a huge one, and thus it is impossible to do more than to skim the surface of the past. These people, dogs, and accomplishments will never be forgotten!

Box M

Box M Kennels are the result of Lois Matthews having attended a dog show, in the early 1950's, to "root for" a friend's Collie. While there she saw a Boxer, which prompted her to make the most obvious of all novice "boo boos" in speaking of the breed—"look at the cute Bulldog." Lois's friend with the Collie soon lost interest in dogs and dropped out. Lois became more enthusiastic by the moment and still, more than thirty years later, is as in love with dogs and dog shows as anyone I know.

Several years after her first sight of a Boxer, Lois actually met an individual member of the breed (in the past it had been more a matter of seeing them than of becoming truly acquainted). He was Banner Blues Casanova, known as "Butch" to his friends, who was sired by Champion Dauber of Tulgey Wood, a son of the great Champion Lustig von

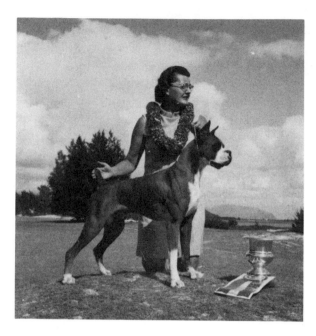

Ch. Jondem's Makiki, by Ch. Treceder Selection ex Jondem's Pikake (a Sequel daughter), winning Best in Show at the Hawaiian Kennel Club in 1969. Lois M. Matthews, owner, Kailua, Hawaii.

Dom of Tulgey Wood, one of the truly *important* dogs in the early history of the breed here in the United States. A year or two following this introduction, Lois purchased a son of "Butch," a fawn and white, from Rhythm of Sirrah Crest, a Champion Utz v.d. of Mazelaine daughter (another pioneer sire in the breed). Lois named the puppy Joachim v Sturm, and her hopes were high, based on the breeding behind him, that he would become a champion. He did not, although to quote Lois "If he could have had a Reserve Championship for Reserve Winners wins he would have." He did, however, earn a C.D. title, to his owner's pleasure.

Joachim lived to be almost fifteen years old, and he made a lifetime Boxer fan of Lois Matthews even before he had become a grown dog.

For about 25 years now Lois Matthews has been a resident of Hawaii. A Californian when Boxer interest first struck, she moved from there to Washington, D.C., then back to Southern California prior to settling in Hawaii.

Lois has had a very successful period as a Boxer breeder. Among those champions who bear her Box M prefix are Pinafore, Broker's Tip, Betzel, Royal Hawaiian, Punchline Precedent, Kamehameha, Bandana (Canadian Champion), Royal Illusion, Tropic Storm, Mona Lisa, Hawaiian Commander, and Sonny's Souvenir.

Other champions which Lois has owned or co-owned include Champion Stapleton's Special Model, Champion Laur-Faun's Touchdown, Champion Jondem's Jason, American and Canadian Champion Jondem's Makiki, Champion Maileaka's Miss Meta, Champion Merrilane's Love Song of Jofra, Champion Merrilane's Holiday Fashion, Champion Princess Mauna Kea, Champion Mauna Kea Misty of Box M, and Champion Beau Monde Boquet of Box M. Three of these Boxers are Best in Show winners.

Lois Matthews is a very popular judge, and her travels in connection with her dog show interests have taken her to Australia, Canada, England and Japan as well as to all parts of the United States. She is also an excellent writer and columnist for the Hawaiian dog magazine, *Ilio*.

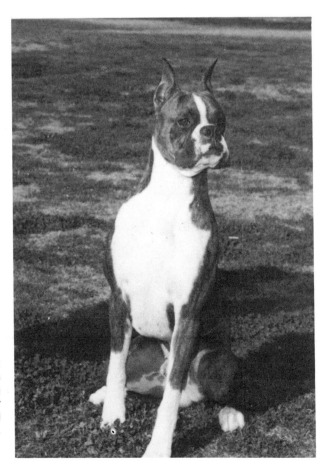

An informal portrait of Ch. Merrilane's Holiday Fashion owned by Eleanor Linderholm Wood and Lois Matthews.

Evergreen

The Evergreen Boxers, located at Buffalo, Minnesota, are owned by Jane Nolt Flowers and widely admired for their excellence and quality.

Foundation bitch here was the lovely Champion Spring Willow's Suzy Q, who made a nice record in the show ring and as a producer. She is the dam of three champions: Champion Evergreen's Delight (by Champion Vel-Kel's Big Ben); Champion Evergreen's Cassiopeia (by International Champion Mephisto's Soldier of Fortune); and the outstanding dog, Champion Evergreen's Orion (also by Soldier of Fortune).

The young Orion dog is rapidly making a name for himself as a sire, with three champions already to his credit. These are Champion Evergreen's Indian Penny, Champion Megan Monten of Evergreen, and Champion Evergreen's Gold Dust.

Ch. Megan Monten of Evergreen, by Ch. Evergreen's Orion ex Ms. Ghana, is shown finishing with her third major under judge Betty Frohock at Heart of America Specialty in March 1983. Stan Flowers handling for Al and Jo Monten, Burnsville, Minnesota.

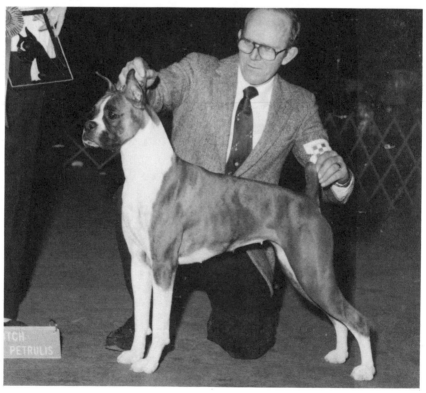

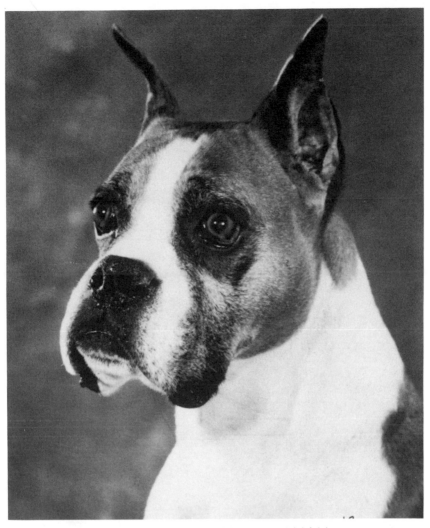

Ch. Spring Willow's Suzy Q is owned by Jane Nolt Flowers, Buffalo, Minnesota.

Indian Penny completed her title under judge Alice Downey in July 1981, doing so with three majors at a mere ten months of age.

Magen took her third major in March 1983 under judge Betty Frohock at the Heart of America Boxer Specialty, completing her title that day.

Gold Dust won her third major from the Bred-by Exhibitor Class under judge Glen Sommers at Tampa Bay in January 1984.

Evergreen Boxers are handled by Jane's husband, Stan Flowers.

Galanjud

Galanjud Boxers were established by Mr. and Mrs. Judson L. Streicher of Scarsdale, New York, back in the early 1950's, initially with obedience dogs with which they succeeded well. Almost immediately this popular couple became closely involved with the breed, and with the American Boxer Club, their interests growing to include conformation competition, too, in which they are still actively engaged.

The Streichers have owned a number of champions over the years, among them at least several very famous winners. These include the marvelous brindle dog, Champion Galanjud's Blue Chip, who was a

Ch. Mystery's Show Biz taking one of numerous Working Groups, this time under judge Bob Wills, for Mr. and Mrs. Judson Streicher of Scarsdale, N.Y.

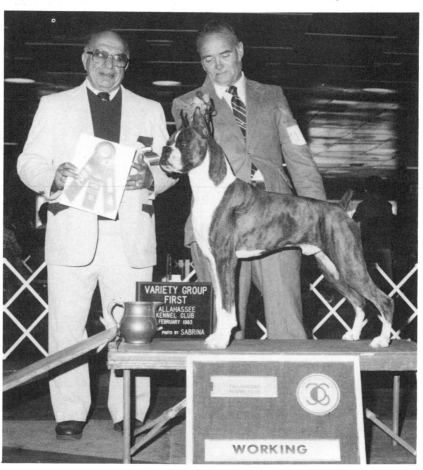

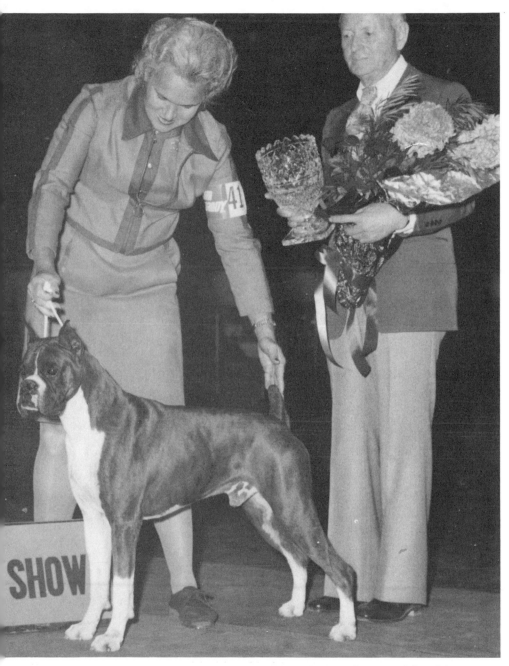

Ch. Galanjud's Blue Chip, multiple Best in Show, Working Group and Specialty Best of Breed winner, was handled by Jane Forsyth to a long list of exciting victories for Mr. and Mrs. Judson L. Streicher of Scarsdale, New York.

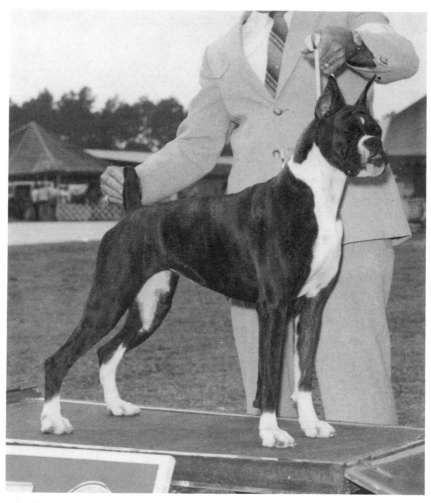

Ch. D.J.'s Hot Lips, owned by Mr. and Mrs. Judson L. Streicher, Scarsdale, New York, has been doing some very spectacular winning for these long-time fanciers.

multi-Group and Best in Show winner, plus taking Best in Show at an American Boxer Club Specialty, under Jane Forsyth's handling, a few years back. Then there was the magnificent bitch, Champion My Cyn's Winter Wheat, who piled up an imposing record, also handled by Jane Forsyth.

More recently, the Streichers have been well represented at the shows by a handsome dog and a very stunning bitch. These are Champion Mystery's Show Bix and Champion D.J.'s Hot Lips respectively, who are going strong for them, handled by Johnny Johnson.

Heldenbrand

Heldenbrand Boxers are the result of Elvinia Heldenbrand, of Manhattan, Kansas, having purchased, in 1970 from Earl and Jan Russell, a puppy named Bach's Dear as a 4-H project for daughter, Lillis. Dear proved to have been very aptly named. A "carefree, happy puppy and *so* intelligent." She attained her C.D. degree with scores in the 190's in three trials, and still, at fourteen years of age, remains Elvinia's constant companion.

In 1972, Elvinia found that she had caught the "dog training bug" when Saruman was given to her by the Russells. He was "nine months old and had been disciplined a lot," but patience and perseverance paid off with his achieving a C.D.X. and was ready to start towards his U.D. when he was stricken with kidney failure in 1980.

The first litter bred by Elvinia produced the U.D. dog, Heldenbrand's Proud Ruler. He was by Holly Lane's Bold Ruler ex Bach's Dear, C.D.—a big brindle male who was a happy, enthusiastic worker. Proud and his uncle, Saruman, were Elvinia's obedience brace.

Longing for a conformation dog, Elvinia purchased Holly Lane's

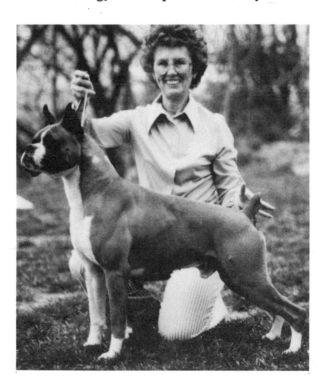

Ch. Holly Lane's Dream Peddler, C.D., with owner Elvinia Heldenbrand, Manhattan, Kansas.

51

Dream Peddler and Holly Lane's Aureate Halo in 1975. Peddler was shown to all but one major by Elvinia, attained his C.D. degree, and is trained for Open, as is Halo. But Elvinia cannot bear to jump them the required heights.

Halo has points, but hated the show ring so she was retired to whelp the litter that produced Champion Heldenbrand's Kansas Twister, Elvinia's first homebred champion. Along with Twister, this litter contained Augury (who with Twister made up Elvinia's conformation brace), Heldenbrand's Kansas Pumpkin and Heldenbrand's Happy Go Lucky. The last two were of lovely quality but shown infrequently if at all.

Ch. Heldenbrand's Jedi Knight, a son of Ch. Heldenbrand's Kansas Twister ex Misty Mountain Rhodes, finishing at the age of seventeen months. Owner-handled by Elvinia Heldenbrand, Manhattan, Kansas.

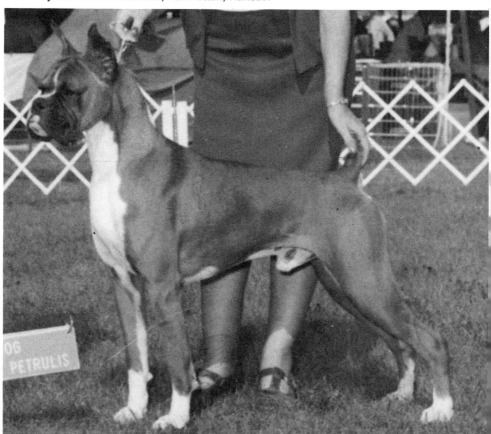

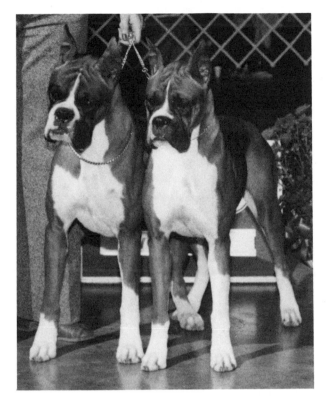

Ch. Heldenbrand Kansas Twister and his litter-sister, Heldenbrand Augury, C.D., going Best Brace of Working Dogs at Tulsa in November 1979. Owner-handled by Elvinia Heldenbrand, Manhattan, Kansas.

In January 1980, another litter by Peddler and Aureate produced Champions Heldenbrands KS Kid and Heldenbrands I'm A Peddler Too, plus Elvinia's current brood matron, Blythe Spirit, who was Reserve Winners Bitch at the 1982 American Boxer Club Regional.

Twister died of bloat in March 1984—a heartbreaking loss, as he had been a joy to own. His winning career started when he began winning Best of Breed over "specials" at eleven months of age. At one time he was rated Number Five in the *Canine Chronicle* statistics—owner-handled. Three of his kids finished in 1983, they being Champion Heldenbrands Jedi Knight, Wheatlands Intimidator, and Wheatlands Bluestar Buffie. Jedi's litter sister, Jetta, is pointed and being campaigned to finish. Their dam is Misty Mountain Rhodes and their breeders were Judy and Forrest Rhodes. Jedi finished, owner-handled, at seventeen months; his wins included a five-point major at the Wichita Boxer Club Specialty when nine months old. He will be specialed and obedience trained.

Wheatlands Gem V Heldenbrand was sired by Peddler ex Foxfire's

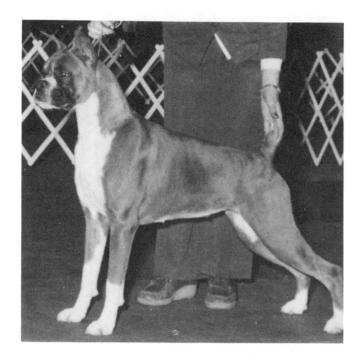

Honey In The Hay. Although Elvinia is not listed as the breeder, Gem was whelped and raised at Heldenbrand. She was a litter of one, born following eight hours of labor and minus a sac. She came down with pneumonia, and was deserted by her dam. But Elvinia spent two weeks nursing and reviving this frail puppy whom the vets said would never survive. She did, thanks to Elvinia's having cared, and now is a beautiful bundle of energy, who has acquired two Bests of Breed from the classes, both majors, and a total of ten points from the American-bred Class.

Champion Wheatlands Bluestar Buffie is owned by the Heldenbrands' daughter, Lillis Peck, for whom the original Boxer was purchased. She has a Grand Sweepstakes win to her credit, and a Best of Breed owner-handled.

Heldenbrand's Peddlers Dream is the last pup from Aureate sired by Peddler. She has a Grand Sweeps to her credit and will be shown by Elvinia.

The Peddler-Aureate cross produced so well, but due to Aureate's problems with mastitis she was bred only three times.

For the future, Elvinia is looking towards Heldenbrand's Dream Courier and Tambell's Quest V Heldenbrand. Courier was named for his grandsire, Aracrest's Courier, who was owned by Mark Steels in Johannesburg, South Africa. Courier is by Peddler ex a Twister daughter. Quest is by Peddler ex Tambells Enchantress, a Soldier of Fortune daughter. Courier was bred by Elvinia and Tim and Jane Greiser, Quest by Chuck and Jean Kennedy.

Heritage

Heritage Boxers at East Aurora, New York, tell a highly successful story of owner Jane B. Moog, whose dogs have completed eighteen championships in the past ten years.

Among the most exciting of these have been Champion Hydalis U-Betcha, with three majors during one weekend in Louisville, Kentucky, September 1973.

Ch. Cover Girl of Heritage, by Ch. Quisto's Cornerstone ex Holly Lane's Captivating Wind, finished with three majors, two of them from the puppy class. Pictured here winning the Peoria Boxer Club Sweepstakes. Cover Girl is a full sister, from a repeat breeding, which had previously produced Champions Morning Star and Evening Star. Owned by Jane B. Moog.

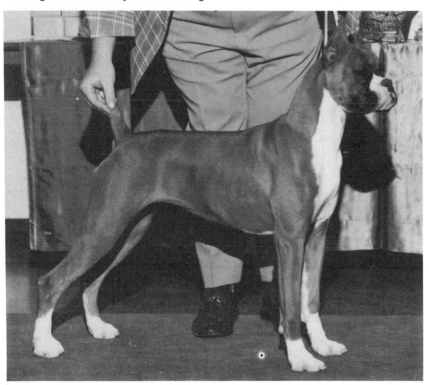

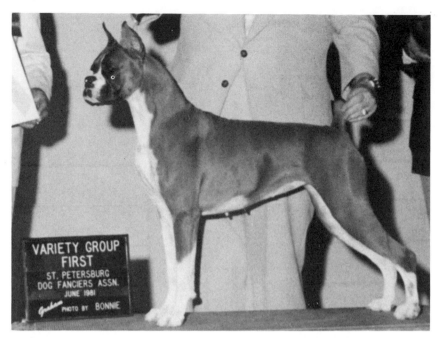

Ch. Heritage Carolina Hala, by Ch. Heritage Assault ex Ch. Wilderson's Kelly, is pictured winning the Group at St. Petersburg in June 1981, owned by Jane B. Moog.

Champion Morning Star of Heritage, whom handler Charles E. Steel tells us is the youngest Boxer *bitch* to have finished, doing so in eight months and fifteen days with three majors. She was Best of Opposite Sex at the 1976 Regional Specialty in Denver.

Champion Evening Star of Heritage, finished with points which included those won in two majors at Specialty Shows.

Champion Cover Girl of Heritage finished with three majors, two of them from the Puppy Class.

Champion Tempo's Ode to Joy finished with four majors, two of them at Specialties.

Champion Heritage Up Tempo finished with three majors.

Champion Heritage Up and Coming finished with three majors and Champion Heritage Assault with three majors from the Puppy Class.

Champion Heritage Carolina Hala, who had three majors from the Puppy Class, and as a Special was 63 times Best of Breed, has four Working Groups, six Specialty Bests in Show, and an award from the American Boxer Club for Group wins by a bitch.

Champion Paragon's Nite Rider finished with three majors.

Champion Turo's Sugar of Five T's, a multiple breed and Specialty winner with numerous Group placements; Best of Winners at the American Boxer Club Specialty 1978.

Champion Heritage Match Point finished with three majors, two at Specialties including Best of Winners at the American Boxer Club 1983.

Champion Wesan's Maggie Maggee finished with three Specialties, then became a multiple breed and Specialty winner.

Champion Crescendo's Aria finished with three majors, including Best of Winners at the American Boxer Club Regional Specialty in San Francisco in 1978.

Champion Hi Hill's Winter Classic dam of Champion Heritage Match Point had two majors in one week-end from the 9 to 12-month Puppy Class, finishing with a four-point major at Baltimore.

Champion Heritage Fancy That finished entirely from the Puppy and American-bred Classes and is a multiple Best of Breed and Group placer.

Mrs. Moog's dogs are handled by Charles E. Steele.

Ch. Turo's Sugar of Five T's owned by Jane G. Moog, East Aurora, New York.

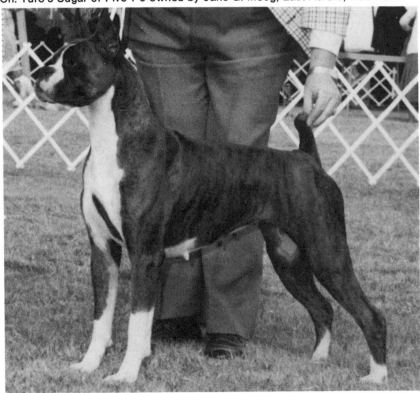

Hi-Hat

Hi-Hat Boxers, at Hamden Connecticut, are owned by Jerry and Leni Kaplan and their daughter Eileen.

The Kaplans started out in the mid-1970's with their first champion and foundation brood bitch, American and Canadian Champion Hi-Hat's Cameo of Donessle, by Champion Gray Roy's Minstrel Boy ex Canadian Champion Donessle's Miss Fancy, a Shadrack daughter. Cameo proved herself to be an excellent show bitch as well as a top producer.

Cameo was bred first to Champion Merrilane's Holiday Fashion, who was a son of Fashion Hint, from which she produced her first champion daughter, Champion Hi-Hat's Flowing Velvet. For her next litter she was again bred to a Fashion Hint son, this one Champion Becrelen's Import by whom she produced two champions, Hi-Hat's Other Side of Midnite, 1979 American Boxer Club Regional winner; and Champion Hi-Hat's Summer Prelude.

The above dogs are the ones from which the Kaplans have been breeding most of the splendid winners they've been putting in the rings.

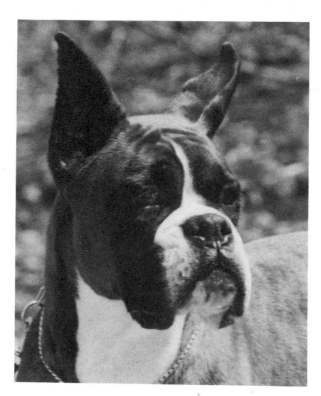

Ch. Hi-Hat's Summer's Prelude, by Ch. Becrelen's Import (Fashion Hint son) ex Am. and Can. Ch. Hi-Hat's Cameo of Donessle. Mr. and Mrs. Jerry Kaplan, owners, Hamden, Connecticut.

58

Ch. Hi-Hat's Flowing Velvet, by Ch. Merrilane's Holiday Fashion ex Am. and Can. Ch. Hi-Hat's Cameo of Donessle, winning at Hockamock in 1977 to complete her title. Eileen Kaplan handling for Mr. and Mrs. Jerry Kaplan, Hamden, Connecticut.

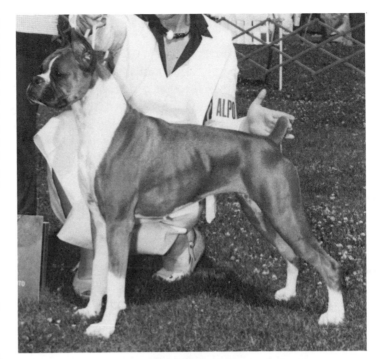

Ch. Hi-Hat's Other Side of Midnite, born June 1977, by Ch. Becrelen's Import ex Am. and Can. Ch. Hi-Hat's Cameo of Donessle, was an American Boxer Club Regional winner. Owned by Mr. and Mrs. Jerry Kaplan, Hamden, Connecticut.

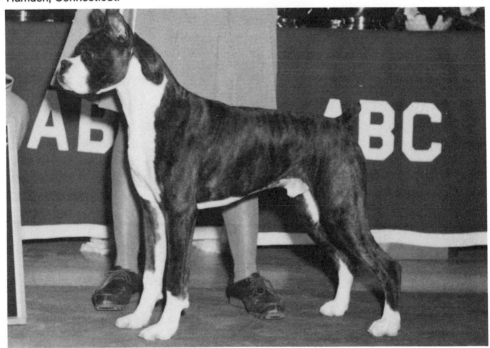

59

Hollycrest

Hollycrest Boxers are located at Riverside, Illinois, where they are owned by Cheryl Colby and Leon De Priest.

Cheryl Colby's first show dog, and first champion, was the handsome Champion C.C. Bobber of Bethel who sad to tell died of kidney failure just prior to this book going to press—a deeply felt loss as he was a dearly loved pet as well as show dog.

Bobber was by Champion Regail Bo-Jack ex Bethel's Pretty Direct, whose breeders were M. Dunner and B. Guerra. He is the dog who earned Ms. Colby's devotion to his breed, and her determination to accomplish something outstanding for it as a breeder.

There are several outstanding Boxers currently at Hollycrest. Champion Hollycrest's Southern Gent for one, "Jackson" to his friends, who finished at fourteen months with three majors, two

Ch. Brittendale's Sheer Madness, by Ch. Vel Kel's Big Ben ex Ch. Turo's Magic Spell was bred by Bob and Betty Jo Phillips. Owned by Cheryl Colby and Leon De Priest.

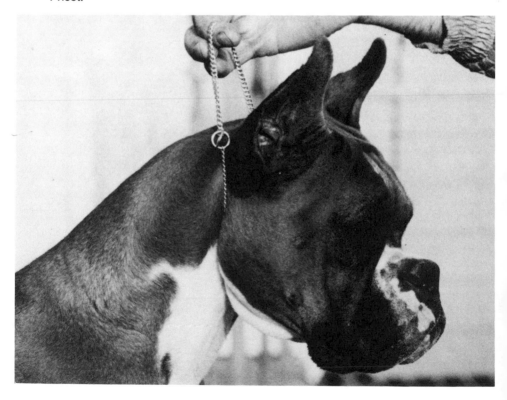

Ch. Hollycrest's Southern Gent, known for his alert and beautiful expression, is a son of Ch. Wildwood's Imagemaker ex Bullet of Prospect, was bred by M. and J. Anderson, and is owned by Cheryl Colby and Leon De Priest.

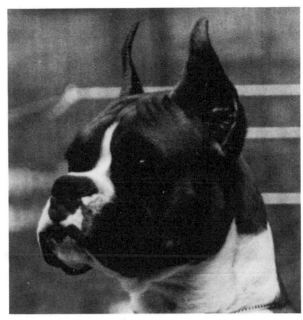

Hollycrest Born Free, by Ch. Wildwood's Imagemaker ex Mello-Oaks Lady Love. Bred by Karen Ochocki and owned by Nita Harper and Ron Reynolds.

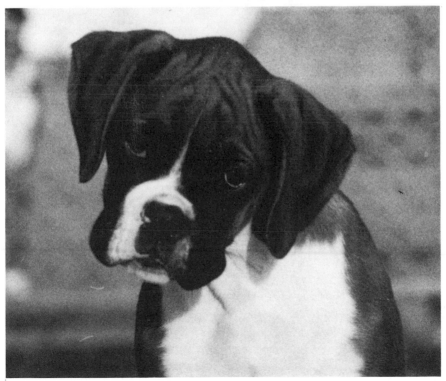

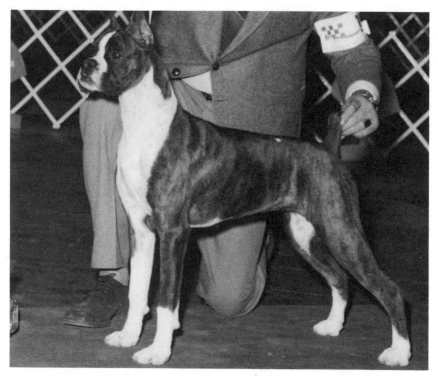

The fantastic puppy, Ch. Hi-Hill's Rave Review acquired four majors and three Sweepstakes on the way to completing her title at thirteen months. Owned by Cheryl Colby and Leon De Priest, Hollycrest Boxers, Riverside, Illinois.

Grand Sweepstakes awards, and numerous wins at the puppy matches. A son of Champion Wildwood's Imagemaker ex Bullet of Prospect, he was bred by M. and J. Anderson.

The lovely bitch, Champion Hi-Hill's Rave Review, is a daughter of Champion Heldenbrand's KS Kid by Peddler ex Hi-Hill's Summer Shadows, bred by Donna Titus. "Floozy" also was a youthful champion, gaining title when only nine months of age, acquiring four majors and three Grand Sweepstakes awards along the way. She was entered and shown on only thirteen occasions.

Champion Brettendale's Sheer Magic is another successful member of this family, by Champion Vel-Kel's Big Ben ex Champion Turo's Magic Spell, bred by Bob and Betty Jo Phillips.

And for the future, keep an eye on Hollycrest's Born Free, by Champion Wildwood's Imagemaker ex Mello-Oaks Lady Love, bred by Karen Ochoki, belonging to Nita Harper and Ron Reynolds.

Jacquet

Jacquet Boxers are owned by Richard Tomita and located at Paramus, New Jersey. The first litter there was whelped in 1971. From this litter the puppy which was to become Champion Jacquet's Ronel Ricah was kept and campaigned to the title. This dog was not only Jacquet's first homebred champion, but also went on to become *Boxer Review's* "Top Boxer In The East" for 1973. Sad to say, he was lost in a tragic automobile accident just at the time he was awarded this distinction.

Jacquet's Sirius, by Ch. Jacquet's Branston ex Zucchini of Silver Spring, taking Winners Dog at the New Jersey Boxer Club's 1983 Specialty Show judged by a famous English breeder, Mrs. Pat Heath. Owned by Lisa and Richard Button.

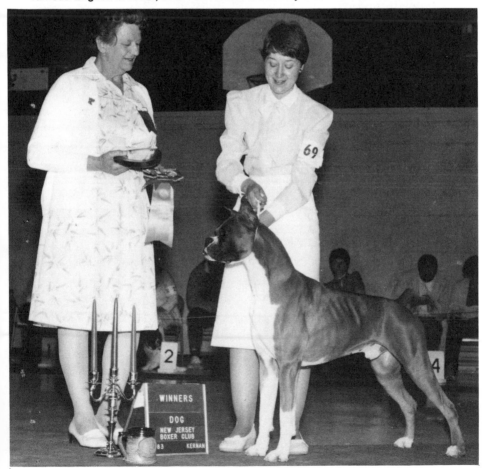

Since Ronel Ricah there have been a total of forty-four American Champions and twelve foreign champions under the Jacquet banner, with many more pointed Boxers currently being shown to their titles. Some of the most outstanding ones include: Champion Jacquet's Brass Image, now in England, who was rated Number Ten Boxer in 1981; Champion Jacquet's Urko finished here with breeds and Group placements won from the classes, then went to Japan where he became Top Winning Dog in that country; Champion Jacquet's Garnier was rated Number Five Boxer during 1983 in addition to winning the American Boxer Club Award for the Puppy Winning Most Blue Ribbons that year. At the 1979 American Boxer Club National Specialty, Winners Dog and Winners Bitch were Jacquet Boxers. There are also three Jacquet dogs with obedience degrees.

In addition, there are two Sires of Merit at the kennel, these being Champion Happy Ours Fortune de Jacquet and Champion Jacquet's Brass Idol. Also two Dams of Merit, Champion Jacquet's Jolie and Jacquet's Perigal. In 1981 and 1982 the Kennel Making Most Champions Award was received by Jacquet from the American Boxer Club, and in both 1982 and 1983 Jacquet earned the Kennel Breeding Most Champions Award.

To Richard Tomita, the most important thing in breeding top quality dogs is having good producers. Perigal is a granddaughter of Champion Salgray's Flying High, himself a Sire of Merit. She was bred to Champion Merrilane's April Fashion, another Sire of Merit, and produced Champion Jacquet's Brass Idol, also a Sire of Merit. This breeding resulted in Jacquet's 1979 American Boxer Club wins. As Rick Tomita says "It was tremendously exciting to have both Winners Dog (Brass Idol) and Winners Bitch (Shana of Talisman) from Jacquet"—a feeling with which any true dog fancier would certainly agree!

Champion Jacquet's Jolie, a Dam of Merit, bred to Brass Idol, produced four champions. Painted Lady bred to Champion Merrilane's April Fashion, a Sire of Merit, produced Champion Jacquet's Faline, the first plain black-faced bitch to finish in many years.

Rick Tomita has truly concentrated on linebreeding, established with the Eldic line by Champion Eldic's Landlord. From him Jacquet acquired wonderful temperament in their Boxers, but, of course, they are still full of fun and exuberance. Since most of the Jacquet dogs leaving there go to homes with children, temperament is considered to be of prime importance. The other trait acquired from Landlord is elegance, also something which Rick Tomita appreciates and values.

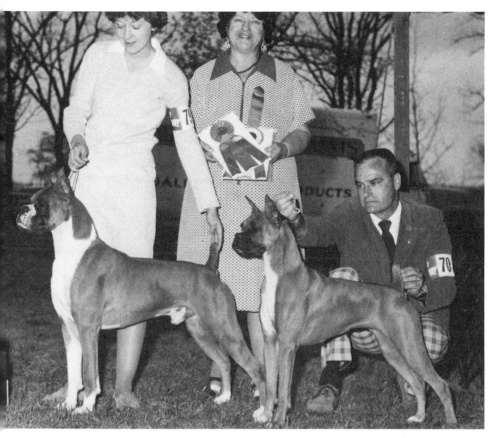

Ch. Jacquet's Brass Image, *left*, and Ch. Jacquet's Faline, Best of Breed and Best of Winners (Eastern Boxer Club 1981), judged by Mrs. William Anderson. Brass Image was Number Ten Boxer in 1981 is now in England, owned by Newlaithe Boxers (Christine Beardsall) and Lynpine Boxers (June Walker). Faline owned by Georgine Schwerdfeger and Richard Tomita. Marylou Wilderson handled Brass Image, Bob Phillips handled Faline. Both by Ch. Merrilane's April Fashion.

Jacquet started with a Landlord daughter from Ronel Kennels, a brindle bitch whom they bred to Champion Rocky of Shawnee Trail, also an Eldic Darius grandson. "Micah," her son, was Jacquet's first champion, winning handsomely for them. Following the aforementioned accident, they were so fortunate as to produce by repeat breeding, a full brother "Zephan," who has to date sired six champions.

Strong heads and excellent bites came from the bitch, Champion Barday's Chatterbox, strongly linebred from Brayshaw. She in turn was bred to a Millan's Fashion Hint son to produce Painted Lady's dam, Barday's Lady Tiara, and also Markham who is untitled yet with

65

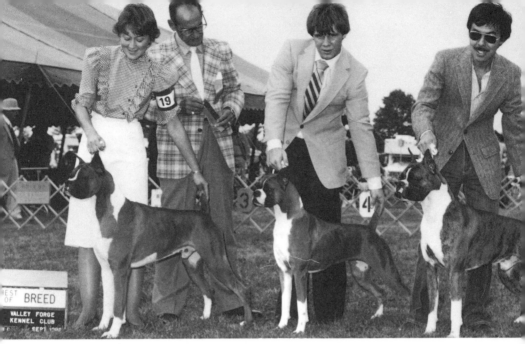

Left to right: Am. and Jap. Ch. Jacquet's Urko, Ch. Jacquet's Garnier, and Ch. Jacquet's Dark Donner winning Best of Breed, Winners Bitch and Winners Dog under Don Bradley at Valley Forge K.C. Urko owned by Dr. Hideaki Nakazawa, Tokyo, Japan. Garnier by Sandy Powell and Richard Tomita; Dark Donner by Dr. Cyrus L. and Nancy M. Mineo.

Left to right: All handled by Marylou Wilderson. Ch. Happy Ours Fortune de Jacquet, Winners Dog; Ch. Jacquet's Brass Image. Best of Breed; Ch. Jacquet's Duchene, Winners Bitch. All by Ch. Merrilane's April Fashion, bred by Richard Tomita. Happy Ours owned by Mr. Tomita; Brass Image by Newlaithe and Lynpine Kennels, Duchene by Susan Fontana. Marie Moore is judge.

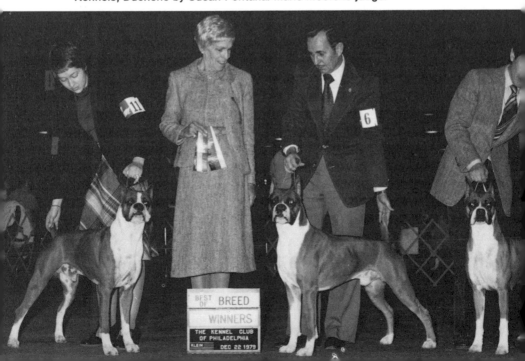

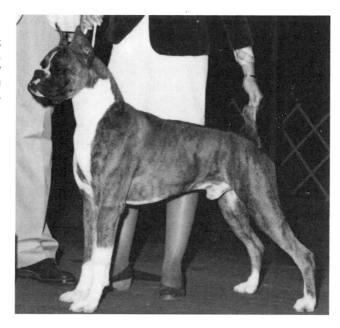

Ch. Jacquet's Dark Donner owned by Dr. Cyrus L. and Nancy Mineo. Handler, Marylou Wilderson.

five champions to date. She was bred to Zephan, a Landlord grandson and Jacquet's second champion.

Then a most exciting dog appeared in the East from the West Coast, Champion Merrilane's April Fashion, who Rick saw for the first time at the American Boxer Club Specialty in New Jersey. "Punki" brought beautiful heads, smooth bodies, and, most important, showmanship. Jacquet produced his first litter, from which came two champions. Two subsequent breedings with the Jacquet bitch Perigal produced five champions. Meanwhile Painted Lady, the Barday's Chatterbox grandaughter, moved to the West Coast and was bred to April Fashion's litter brother, Champion Merrilane's April Holiday, which produced Champion Happy Ours Fortune for Rick Tomita.

Several Zephan and Markham daughters have been bred to Brass Idol with excellent results. When Happy Ours Fortune moved East, April Fashion daughters and Brass Idol daughters were bred to him, producing champions. Urko, used only twice before going to Japan, produced seven promising youngsters. Dark Donner has excellent prospects on the ground now, as does Gaspard, a Markham grandson.

The new young hopeful at Jacquet is Agassiz, who became a champion in Bermuda.

Kameo

Kameo Boxers are owned by Robert H. and Shirley L. Hickam at Exeter, California, where they are famous for two very outstanding Boxer bitches, Champion Mac-A-Nor's Sirocco Suzi Q and her daughter, Champion Kameo's Show Girl.

Suzi was born May 24th 1977, a daughter of Champion Notelrac's Sirocco ex Diamond's Gay Mitzi of Mac-A-Nor. She was bred by C.N. and Elnora McLean, and handled by Cheryl Cates. Shown on the West Coast during 1980, 1981 and 1982, she piled up 38 Bests of Breed, including the Golden Gate Boxer Club judged by Mrs. Marion Fairbrother from England, and Working Group honors.

On October 22nc 1979, Suzi Q whelped a litter by Champion Notelrac's Major Beau. Among the puppies was one who would become Champion Kameo's Show Girl who has been very outstanding in the ring. Her current total of awards stands at 54 times Best of Breed, and ten Group placements. Among her honors was that of taking Best of Breed at the Boxer Club of Southern California Specialty under judge Rufus Burleson and best of Opposite Sex at the American Boxer Club Specialty in May 1983 judged by Mrs. Alice Downey.

Litter sisters to Show Girl, Champion Encore Kameo Debutante and Champion Creme de la Creme de Kameo, also have completed title, and another of Suzi's offspring is close to finishing.

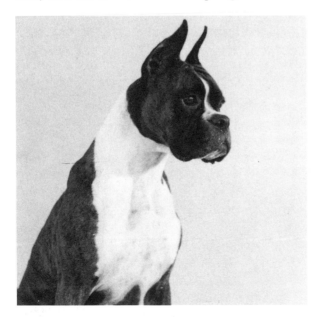

Ch. Mac-A-Nor's Sirocco Suzi Q was bred by C.N. and Elnora McLean and the owners are Robert H. and Shirley L. Hickam, Exeter, California.

Ch. Mac-A-Nor's Sirocco Suzi Q owned by Robert H. and Shirley L. Hickam, Exeter, California.

Ch. Kameo's Show Girl, by Ch. Notelrac's Major Beau ex Ch. Mac-A-Nor's Sirocco Suzi Q, bred and owned by Robert and Shirley Hickam. In July 1982 she was Best of Breed at the Boxer Club of Southern California Specialty and in 1983 Best of Opposite Sex at the American Boxer Club Specialty.

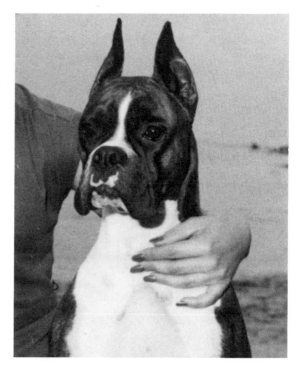

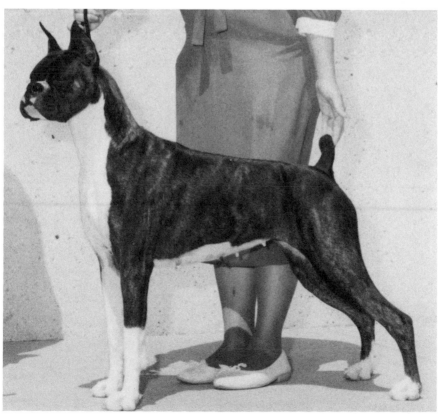

Katu

Katu Boxers are a fairly young kennel, but one which has nonetheless been extremely successful. Owned by Dick and Kathy Frohock at Westford, Massachusetts, Katu already has two excellent champions to their credit.

Their first Boxer to finish was Champion R.J.'s Token President, who went through to his title in good time, and did a bit of winning as a Special as well, under Doug Holloway's handling.

Ch. Hexastar's Ted Stamp of Ruhland, co-owned by Dick and Kathy Frohock, and Agnes Buchwald, Sao Paulo, Brazil. This handsome young dog has had a splendid career in the United States under Doug Holloway's handling, and has now returned to Mrs. Buchwald in South America.

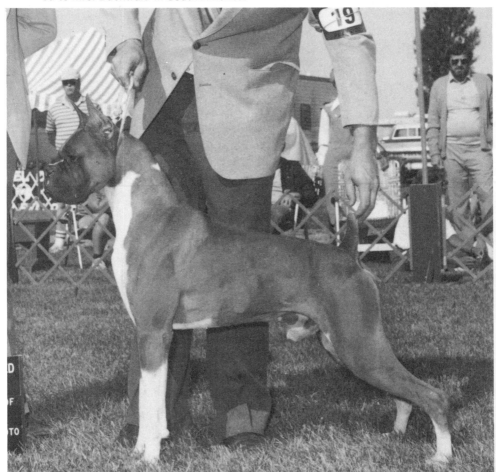

70

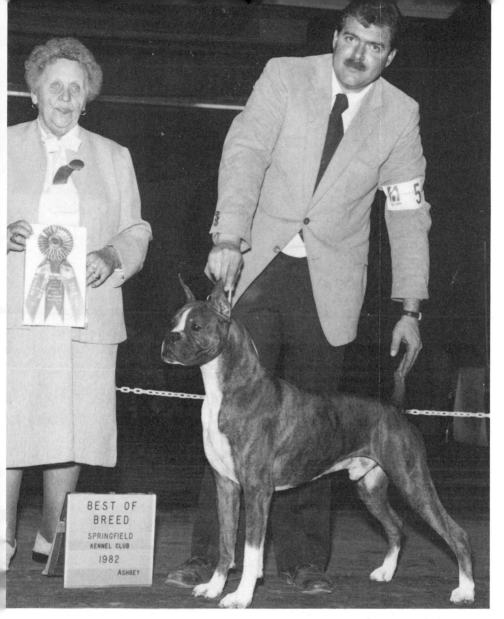

Ch. R.J.'s Token President, by Ch. Arriba's Red Spritz ex R.J.'s Twice as Nice, owned by Kathleen Frohock, Westford, Massachusetts.

Then, in co-ownership with Agnes Buchwald, Hexastar Boxers from Brazil, Katu has campaigned an excellent dog in Champion Hexastar's Ted Stamp of Ruhland, who just recently has returned to his former home after a good career in the United States.

We understand that there are some promising youngsters at the kennel, so watch for Katu as the future unfolds.

Laurel Hill

Laurel Hill Boxers, at Oyster Bay, New York, started off when, in 1974, Jeannie and Bruce Korsan purchased Dieterich's Lord Joker from Muriel Dieterich, shortly thereafter acquiring Brayshaw's Lady Brat from Charlotte Brayshaw. "Brat" was to become their foundation bitch.

In 1975, after returning from a trip to Africa, the Korsans' first errand was to travel directly from Kennedy Airport on Long Island to Carmel, New York, where their two Boxers had been boarding during their owners' absence, only to discover that, as planned, Joker had bred Brat. Sixty-three days later Laurel Hill had their first Boxer litter—of eleven puppies! From among them came Bermudian Champion Korsan's Friar Tuck.

The several years following these events were spent by the Korsans in learning all about their breed and traveling many miles to dog shows. Also, a house in the country was needed, as all those dogs were regarded with horror by the board of directors of the New York City apartment where Jeannie and Bruce had been living. During that period they purchased Brayshaw's Jam Session who became a Bermuda Champion and went on to produce Brazilian Champion Laurel Hill's Charlemagne who was to become a multiple All-Breed Best in Show winner in Brazil.

Charlemagne was sired by Champion Sunset Image of Five T's, known as "Bosco," whom the Korsans had purchased from Jo and Don Thompson in 1977. "Bosco" was Winners Dog at the American Boxer Club National Specialty in 1978. He finished his title three weeks later, won the working Group his first time out as a Special, and went on to win over 125 Bests of Breed, numerous Groups and Group placements.

In 1979 the Korsans purchased another Five T's dog from Jo and Don Thompson, Champion Sunset Spirit of Five T's. In May of 1980 "Sonny" followed "Bosco's" pawprints by taking Winners Dog at that year's National Specialty. What a thrill to have made this win twice at the National!

"Sonny" finished his championship a few months later. In the meantime, Brat had been bred to Champion Merrilane's April Fashion and produced the Korsans' first homebred champions, Laurel Hill's Autumn Leaves and Laurel Hill's Arabian Knight. Both won the American Boxer Club annual award for the dog and bitch winning the most first prizes in the puppy classes.

Laurel Hill's foundation bitch, Brayshaw's Lady Brat, is the dam of Ch. Laurel Hill's Autumn Leaves, Ch. Laurel Hill's Arabian Knight, Bermudian Ch. Korsan's Friar Tuck, and the granddam of Ch. Laurel Hill's Call Me Brat and Ch. Laurel Hill's Silver Cloud.

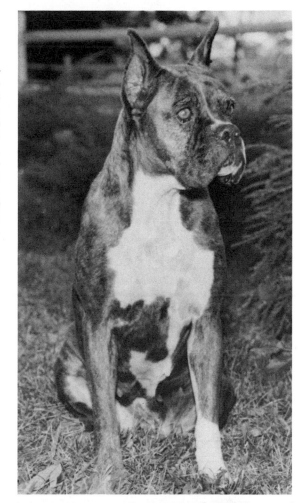

"Bosco" celebrating one of his important wins. Ch. Sunset's Image of Five T's owned by Bruce and Jeannie Korsan, Oyster Bay, N.Y.

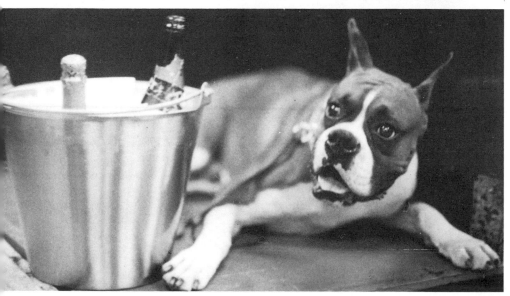

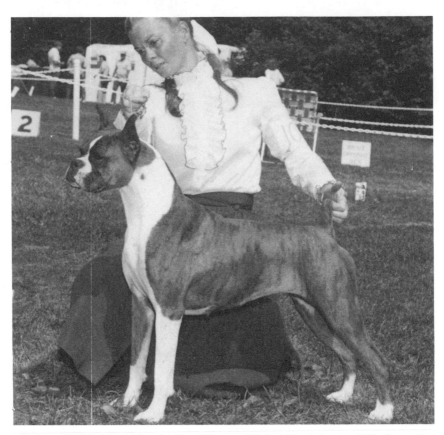

Ch. Laurel Hill's Silver Cloud taking Winners Bitch at Westchester 1982. Owned by Bruce and Jeannie Korsan, Oyster Bay, New York.

Through their years of showing, Laurel Hill has finished twelve American Champions, five of which were homebred. Champion Laurel Hill's Silver Cloud was Reserve Puppy in the Futurity at the American Boxer Club. She was sired by Champion Laurel Hill's Arabian Knight from the Korsans' Champion Ivy Lawn's Chat'r'Box, a Champion Katoman of Five T's daughter.

Champion Laurel Hill's Call Me Brat was sired by Champion Bent's Shawn of Five T's from Laurel Hill's Buttons'n'Bows, a Brat daughter.

The Korsans' newest champion as we write, in March 1984, is Champion Laurel Hill's Rudolf, who is co-owned by Ann Harr of Treceder. Rudy finished in California. He was sired by Champion Sunset Spirit of Five T's from Laurel Hill's Jingle Bells, a "Bosco" daughter. Jingle Bells' dam was the Korsans' Champion Turo's Gabriel of Five T's.

Merrilane-Woodcrest

Merrilane Boxers are owned by Eleanor Linderholm Wood, who has been a Boxer enthusiast since childhood and has become one of the Fancy's most successful Boxer breeders of the present time. This is hardly to be wondered at when one considers Ellie's experience with the breed, plus the fact that she received her "basic training" in it while working for the Henry W. Larks at Meritaire and for the John P. Wagners at Mazelaine. In fact it is in honor of these two famed kennels that her own kennel prefix, Merrilane, was coined.

Eleanor Rowe, as she was then, and her first Boxer became acquainted all the way back in 1939, when a family friend allowed her to care for his young Boxer bitch while he traveled to the Orient. This arrangement worked out so well that it was repeated during two later summers, with Eleanor's fondness for the breed growing on each occasion, until finally her parents purchased it as a birthday gift for their daughter so she could have it for her very own.

This bitch came originally from Fred Hamm's Mahderf Kennel. In 1941 her first litter was born, just one big fawn male, who was later donated to The Seeing Eye and became the first Boxer and one of the first males of any breed trained there.

The bitch, who was a Champion Ferbo von Konigstor daughter, was bred again and this time whelped a litter of six. Through these puppies Eleanor became acquainted with Mary and Al Cousins, to whom they were taken for cropping.

The Cousins became good and helpful friends to Eleanor, and when they moved to Milwaukee the following year to manage the Mazelaine Kennels, it was at their suggestion that Mazie and Jack Wagner invited her to come there to work during her summer vacation, at which she was most happy.

During the school year, Eleanor was occupied with Boxers, too, working at "loving and training" the earliest Woodcrest dogs which led to Carl and Alice Wood's kennel which became one of the most respected in the East. Eleanor showed their first Boxer for them, Robin Hood of Mazelaine, and also made them their first champion, Ysolde of Mazelaine.

It had been Eleanor's ambition to become a veterinarian. But during her second year at Cornell, where she was working on a solid background with which to enter vet school, she found that this would be impossible. Since the war had ended, returning veterans were being offered the first chance for any available openings.

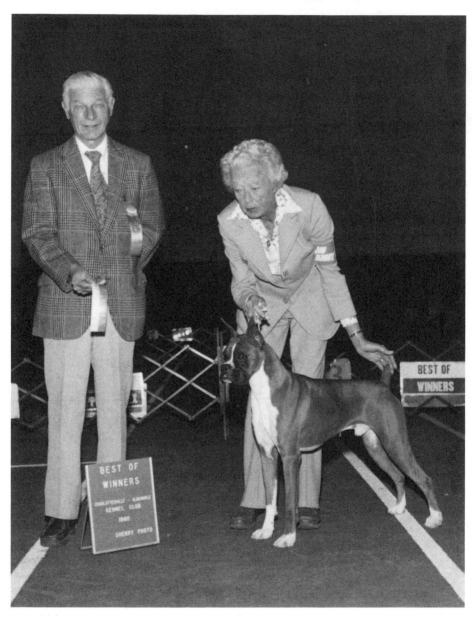

The late Peter Knoop and the late Alice Wood of Woodcrest fame photograph when both were nearing the end of their long careers. The dog is X-Cellent of Woodcrest, sired by Ch. Super Duper of Woodcrest ex Ch. Woodcrest's Alicia, from Woodcrest's 76th litter, whelped October 7th 1978. Owner Carl Wood and the Woodcrest Boxers are now at La Selva, California.

The summer between her two years at Cornell had been spent at the Meritaire Kennels of Henry and Isabel Lark in Dewart, Pennsylvania. When she left college, she returned there on a full time basis. The Larks were very seriously interested in breeding excellent Boxers, and there Eleanor was able to put into practice what she had learned at Mazelaine along with developing her experience at raising, breeding, and handling. In the latter department, she had the fun of showing Champion Yller of Mazelaine to her Best in Show awards, and also numerous other Boxers who became American Boxer Club Annual Award winners.

Eleanor was married in 1947 and divorced in 1954. During those years she dabbled a bit in Boxers and did a fair amount of handling from 1951 to 1954, after having daughters Ann (in 1948) and Gail (in 1950).

Following her divorce, Eleanor returned to Mazelaine, working for awhile at the kennel located in Texas then, and, when it returned to the Chicago area, for awhile there as well. Then she moved to Nevada, concentrating principally on raising her daughters. During this time there were, of course, Boxers with her.

A friend of Eleanor's in Carson City bred a lovely Boxer bitch to Frances Lowman's Champion Space Man of Jofra, from which litter Eleanor purchased the fawn puppy. He was to become Champion Merrilane's Silver Dollar, who completed title at seventeen months three times along the way taking Best of Breed from the classes over Specials. He won eleven Bests of Breed, including the East Bay Specialty, before Eleanor retired him from competition. She had decided to start handling again in earnest and thus could not keep him out against clients' dogs.

In 1969 Eleanor moved to California where she started the Boxer kennel of which she so long had dreamed and also a full-time highly successful career as a professional handler. During her years of handling she was enormously successful, finishing a great many champions and gaining an imposing array of top awards for her clients. Also her first two and a half years on the Coast saw eight homebred Merrilane champions complete title; Silver Dollar's daughter, Merrilane's Mad Passion, C.D., became the kennel's foundation bitch with seven or more champions in her first litter.

Between July 1971 and March 1984, forty-four homebred Merrilane champions have gained their titles. A number of these dogs have gone to new owners overseas, where they have made impressive records in their new countries. Some of these are Champion Merrilane's Happy

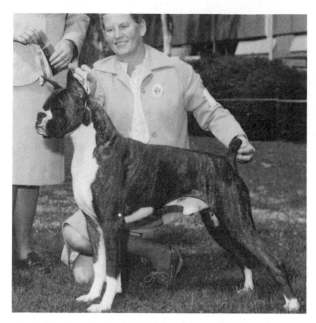

Ch. Merrilane's Ode to Vihabra, by Ch. Merrilane's Salute To April ex Ch. Vihabra's Stardust (a Ch. Merrilane's Fashion Star daughter), shown finishing with a 5-point major going Best of Breed. Bred, owned, and handled by Eleanor Linderholm Wood, La Selva Beach, California. One of Merrilane's *stars* that just finished in 1984.

Ch. Merrilane's April Holiday, an American Boxer Club Sire of Merit, subject to an award in 1985, as sire of seven champions as of March 1984. He is by Ch. Merrilane's Holiday Fashion ex Ch. Merrilane's April Love and litter brother to Ch. Merrilane's April Fashion. Owned by Valerie and Larry Duncan, San Jose, California.

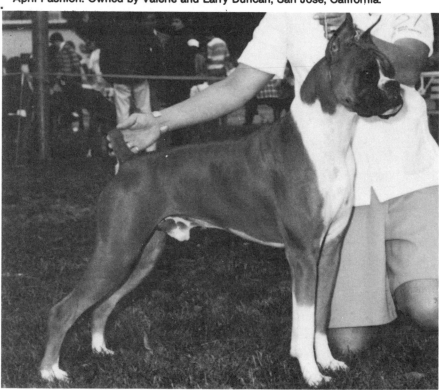

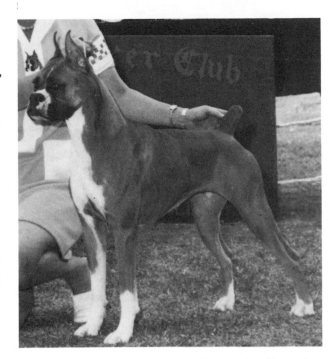

Ch. Merrilane April Love, by Ch. Merrilane's Love Life of Jofra ex Ch. Diamond Lil of Rio Vista, owned by Larry and Valerie Duncan. Bred by Eleanor Linderholm Wood. Her only litter produced three champions: Ch. Merrilane's April Fashion, Ch. April Holiday (both American Club Sires of Merit), and April Showers. Love was Reserve Winners Bitch (A.B.C. Specialty 1975) and is a Specialty Best in Show winner.

To Meet You, one of three champions from a litter by Champion Benjamin of Five T's out of the litter sister to Champion Merrilane's Holiday Fashion. This lovely bitch known as "Howdy" is currently owned by Dr. Miyagawa in Japan.

Champion Merrilane's Salute To April, Reserve Winners Dog at the American Boxer Club Specialty in May 1981, is currently owned by Paul Scott, Kennel Formula, Stabekk, Norway. And Champion Merrilane's It Must Be Him, by Champion Merrilane's April Holiday from a Silver Dollar daughter, is currently owned by Thomas and Joan Greenwood, Johannesburg, South Africa.

Eleanor Linderholm and Carl Wood were married a few years ago, Alice Wood having passed away previously. Since Carl is a popular American Kennel Club approved judge, Eleanor thereby was no longer eligible to handle dogs professionally, so she has retired to breeding and showing her own and, as all of us who respect her knowlege and dedication, hopes soon to join her husband as a judge. Ellie and Carl started married life in Virginia, where Carl and the Woodcrest dogs were established. But they then decided that the California climate suited them better, so Merrilane and Woodcrest Kennels are now located at La Selva Beach.

Both Eleanor and Carl continue their interest in Boxers, and I believe that both kennels are doing a bit of breeding.

My-R

Lorraine Meyer and her late husband, Ken, of Rockford, Illinois, became interested in Boxers in the late 1930's. Soon after their marriage in 1942, they purchased their first of the breed, who proved to be a great companion but was sadly lacking in breed quality. She did, however, become the first of the My-R obedience Boxers.

With a limited breeding program, starting in 1948, the Meyers' forty-two litters in 36 years produced a total of twenty American champions bred at My-R plus five foreign champions.

Probably the most rewarding part of a breeding program is the pleasure of watching the continuation and continuity of successful breedings. From a litter by Champion Captain Lookout of Thorhall from a bitch by his son, Champion Marjack's Golden Windjammer, one of the three resulting champions was My-R's Magic Spell, who was Best Puppy in the American Boxer Club's Futurity in 1961. Her

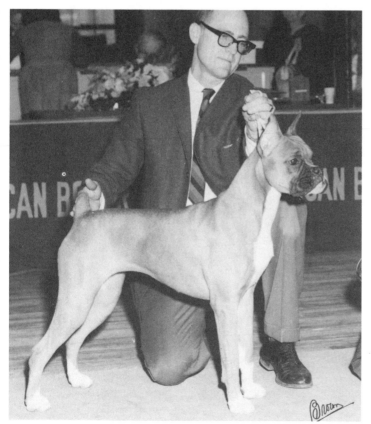

Ch. My-R's Magic Spell, owned and bred by Lorraine C. Meyer, Rockford, Ill. Handled by Larry Downey at the American Boxer Club Specialty in 1961.

Ch. My-R's Sensation, bred and owned by Lorraine C. Meyer, Rockford, Illinois.

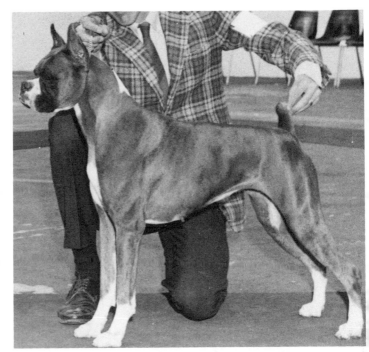

Ch. My-R's Haybinder of Holly Lane, bred by Lorraine C. Meyer, owned by Eileen McClintock, Holly Lane Boxers, Topeka, Kansas.

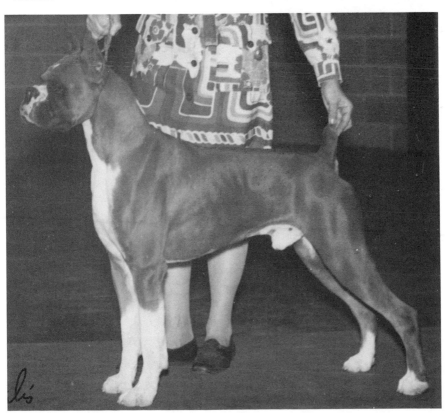

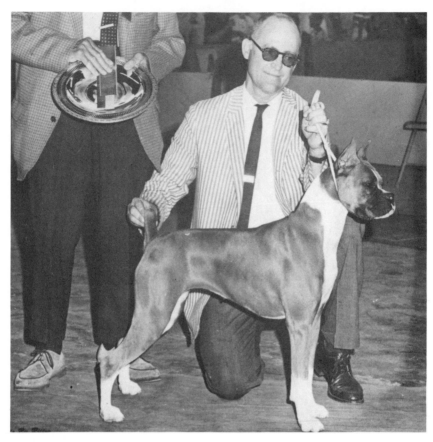

Ch. My-R's Brag About, by Ch. Salgray's Fashion Plate ex Ch. My-R's Magic Spell, bred and owned by Lorraine C. Meyer, Rockford, Illinois. Handled here by Larry Downey.

daughter by Champion Salgray's Fashion Plate was Champion My-R's Brag About, best Puppy at the 1965 American Boxer Club Specialty. Bred back to her sire—the *only* time that My-R ever has bred so closely, her daughter, My-R's Sensation, finished her championship at the 1970 American Boxer Club Specialty.

After such a close breeding, the Meyers felt it was time to go outside of the line, to a male from a breeding which had produced multiple champions. So Sensation was bred to Champion Holly Lane's Wildwind, from which came Champion My-R's Haybinder of Holly Lane, who became a Sire of Merit. Then, to My-R came the Haybinder daughter, Champion Holly Lane's Sun Flower, recipient of an Award of Excellence at the American Boxer Club's 1983 Specialty.

Richaire

Richaire Boxers are located at Tucson, Arizona, where they are owned by Dick and Claire Tolagian. Formerly from Colorado, the Tolagians while living there became friends with Sam and Carole Asseff who had been breeding Boxers for some dozen years, and they, too, developed an interest in these lovely dogs.

The Tolagians purchased a stag red bitch, granddaughter of Champion Benjamin of Five T's, whom they named Tiffany of Brookwood. As a birthday gift for Claire, a flashy brindle dog was acquired, Josh of Dublin who was sired by Sunar Dorian. These two were subsequently bred, and the Tolagians were won over to the idea of raising Boxers.

Following their move to Tucson, it was decided to breed Tiffany to a champion stud dog, and after studying pedigrees, Champion Telstar's Highflyer was selected. The litter consisted of six brindle puppies, two of which the Tolagians kept. Richaire's Domino, from this litter, went out with professional handler Dixie McCauley and by fourteen months of age he had completed his championship. He then stayed home for awhile to mature, after which he started out with

Ch. Richaire's Domino winning Best in Show, March 1983 under judge Robert Moore for Richard and Claire Tolagian, Tucson, Arizona.

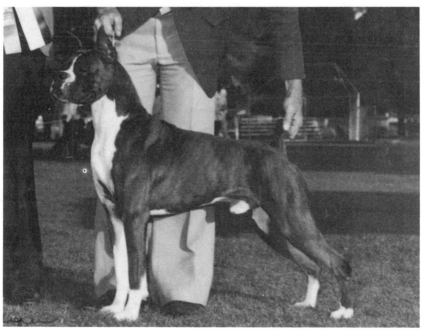

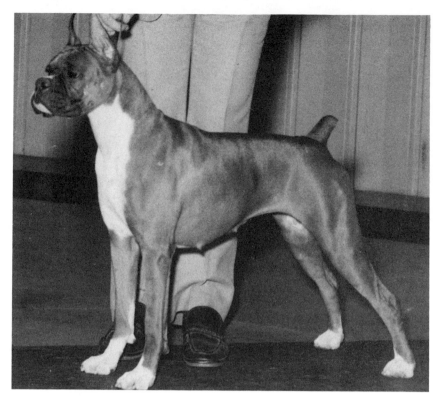

Richaire's Lady Victoria, by Candlewood's Lite My Fire ex Richaire's Christa Crat, Grand Sweepstakes Winner, Boxer Club of Colorado 1983. Owners, Richard and Claire Tolagian, Tucson, Arizona.

Richard Mysliwiec as a Special. Domino took Best in Show at Tucson six weeks prior to the American Boxer Club Specialty, went on to that prestigious event, and won Best of Breed over a star-studded galaxy of Specials under judge Mrs. Alice Downey. Now retired from the show ring, Domino is producing puppies over which the Tolagians are greatly excited.

The bitch puppy, Domino's litter sister, is a flashy brindle bitch. Following more study of pedigrees it was decided to breed this bitch, Richaire's Christa Crat, to her litter brother, Domino. Four beautiful puppies have resulted, including one plain dog, two flashy bitches and a flashy dog. The dog, Richaire's Mark of Time, will be residing with John and Audrey Peach of Calgary, Alberta, Canada, to be shown both there and in the United States.

The Tolagians have several litters due as we are writing, linebred, and their expectations are high for some truly great Boxers to join Domino in their future.

Ruhlend

Ruhlend Boxers, at Gig Harbor, Washington, were started by Ruth and Bill Leek back in the 1960's.

One of their early Boxers was Champion K-9's Swiss Yodeler, C.D., who was whelped January 15th 1966 in Denver, Colorado. His sire, Champion Von Schorer's Mountain Music, and dam, Calypso Heidi, both were sired by Champion Willow Round's Fortissimo, the latter having been Mountain Music's first champion.

Yodeler completed his championship in five majors before reaching two years of age. He got his C.D. exactly one year later, and in three straight shows. He was the sire of Champion Ruhlend's Swiss Miss, and himself a successful show dog, with several Bests of Breed to his credit and a Best of Opposite Sex at the Heart of America Boxer Specialty from the Veterans Class at eight years of age. He died in 1976.

American and Canadian Champion Peablo's Black Bishop was born August 20th 1970 and died at the age of three. He completed his American championship at twenty months of age, then went on to take a Canadian title as well. Black Bishop was of Champion Millan's Fashion Hint breeding, a most beautiful dog whose loss was strongly felt at Ruhlend.

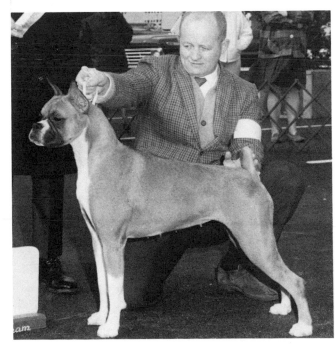

Ch. Ruhlend's Swiss Miss finishing her title at Clearwater, Jan. 1970, handled by John Connolly for owners Ruth and Bill Leek, Gig Harbor, Washington.

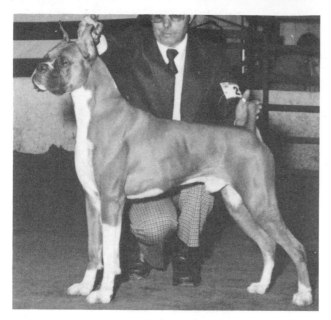

Ch. Ruhlend's Swiss Konig wins Best of Breed and second in Group at Whidbey Island Kennel Club. Handled by James E. Pasano for Ruth F. and Wm. J. Leek.

Ch. K-9's Swiss Yodeler, Best of Opposite Sex from the Veteran's Class, American Boxer Club Specialty, at eight years of age. Owned and handled by Ruth F. Leek, Gig Harbor, Washington.

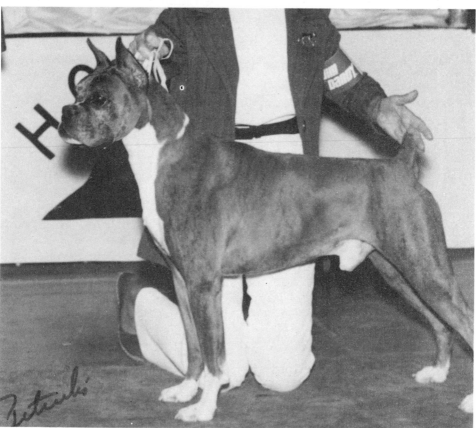

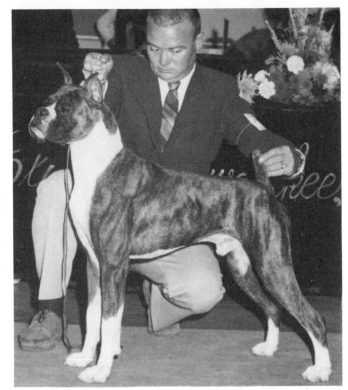

Am. and Can. Ch. Peablo's Black Bishop, by Tri-Int. Ch. Millan's Fashion Hint, finished his championship in the United States at 20 months, his Canadian title just short of three years. He lived to be only three years old, and is still greatly missed by his owner, Mrs. Ruth F. Leek, Gig Harbor, Washington.

Champion Ruhlend's Swiss Miss was born May 26th 1968, by Champion K-9's Swiss Yodeler, C.D. ex Amber's Annah. This lovely bitch had six Bests of Breed and eight times Best of Opposite Sex to her credit, shown in the mid-West and on the West Coast. Bred to Champion Peablo's Black Bishop, she became the dam of Champion Ruhlend's Swiss Konig, born in September 1972 who lived to the age of ten. Swiss Konig sired Champion Lake Bay's Pal Joey, Champion Kar-Neil's Swiss Mocha, Champion Kar-Neil's Swiss Delight, Champion Harris' Bronze Image, and Brazilian Champion Pattie. He was shown very little once he had gained his title.

Ruth Leek speaks with special pride of Ruhlend's Contessa of Abara, by Champion Salgray's V.I.P. ex Champion Braemerwood's Bishop Jitter, thus a grandaughter of Champion Peablo's Black Bishop. Contessa went to Brazil in April 1977, to join Agnes Buchwald's Hexastar Kennels. There she became the dam of three sons who came to America to complete their American championships; they did so with style. They are American and Brazilian Champion Hexastar's Legacy of Ruhlend, American and Brazilian Champion Hexastar's Native Dancer of Ruhlend, and American Champion Hexastar's Ted Stamp of Ruhlend.

Sakura

Active involvement in the Boxer breed began in 1966, for Dr. Donald W. Edwards when he purchased a two-and-a-half-year-old Boxer dog following a burglary at his home. Although they had owned him only six months prior to his being poisoned in the Edwards' own yard, he made a lasting impression on Dr. Edwards and his family.

It was resolved that the Boxer to replace this original one must have a similar pedigree, and would be a show dog as well as a guard dog. After months of search, a brindle son of Champion Rogales Roquito and Champion Brindle Beauty of Britania was purchased from Don Berlant

Ch. Sakura's Whispering Breeze winning a Working Group for Donald W. Edwards, M.D., Fullerton, California.

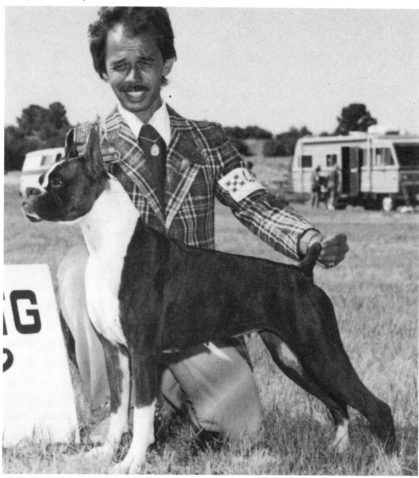

of Portland, Oregon. At the same time a fawn bitch was also purchased, sired by Champion Valatham's Barbwire. She was named Sakura of Twin Willows and was destined to be Dr. Edwards' foundation bitch and the one in whose honor the kennel was named. A lovely head study of this bitch, done by Kathleen Noel, is used as the kennel logo.

Although both of these purchases were shown, neither finished. Saki was retired at an early age, and her kennel mate was retired after three years of showing during which he had accumulated eight points with one major. Saki was bred, and after three attempts, produced a surviving plain fawn bitch with Champion Cajon's Calling Card as her sire. This bitch was in turn bred to Champion Norhaven's Kaleidoscope owned by Mr. and Mrs. James Harris, and produced Sakura's Lollipop Rhapsodie. She was bred initially to Champion Holly Lane's Diamond Replay and produced ten lovely puppies. Two of these remained in Dr. Edwards' kennel and were shown, but due to ear problems were not successful. A fawn male who showed great promise was sent to Canada to be raised and trained for the show ring by Cora Verhulst and attained his Canadian championship readily. However, Alvin Lee, Sr., who was Dr. Edwards' handler, did not feel that the dog had gained sufficient stature to compete successfully in the States.

Lollipop was then bred to Champion Holly Lane's Inherit the Wind with five puppies resulting, one of which was Champion Sakura's Whispering Breeze. She finished rapidly with Best of Winners at Golden Gate Boxer Club under Mrs. Marion Fairbrother, Best of Winners at Boxer Club of Arizona under Mrs. Beverly Sachs, Best of Breed at Scottsdale Dog Fanciers Association under Mr. Robert Moore, Best of Winners and Best of Opposite Sex at Tucson Kennel Club under Mrs. John Patterson for a total of eighteen points, thirteen of them on that fabulous weekend in Arizona. During her show career she had thirty-five Bests of Breed, and received the American Boxer Club Award in 1982 for the greatest number of Group wins by a Boxer bitch.

A repeat breeding of Lollipop to Inherit the Wind resulted in two puppies: one fawn, one brindle. These are Champion Sakura's Bubbling Brown Sugar and Champion Sakura's Cinnamon Spice, the latter a multiple Best of Breed winner and Group placement winner.

During the period in the early 1970's when Dr. Edwards had nothing of his own breeding to show, he purchased a fawn bitch from Dr. and Mrs. McClintock. This was the Edwards' beloved Champion Holly Lane's Delovely Replay who became the eleventh champion for

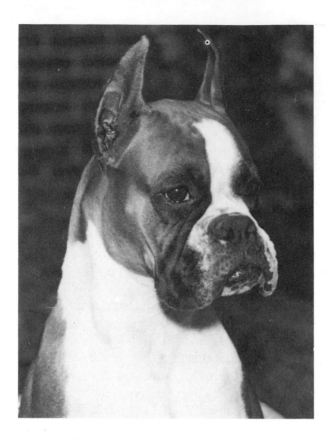

her dam, Champion Holly Lane's WindStorm, which tied her for the world record for Boxer bitch producing the most champion offspring.

Following Delovely Replay's show career, she was bred to Champion Edger of Faldr producing a fawn dog who was slow to mature. At two and a half years of age Mr. Lee felt the dog was finally ready for the Open Class. Bruno gained both majors from his first two Open Classes, and finished in successive shows, thereafter becoming Champion Sakura's Bronze Centurian.

Not having a top contender, Dr. Edwards purchased Champion Doggone Carsman from Mrs. Duana Young of Concord, California. He had been a consistent winner. In six months of showing he gained 21 Bests of Breed, had placed in the Group on nineteen of these occasions, winning it six times and going on to Best in Show twice.

Sakura Boxers hope to produce some quality puppies from their girls with which to carry on the line. There have been lots of heartaches and periods of depression, Dr. Edwards comments, as well as a sense of accomplishment and the joy of having a top winner associated with their establishment.

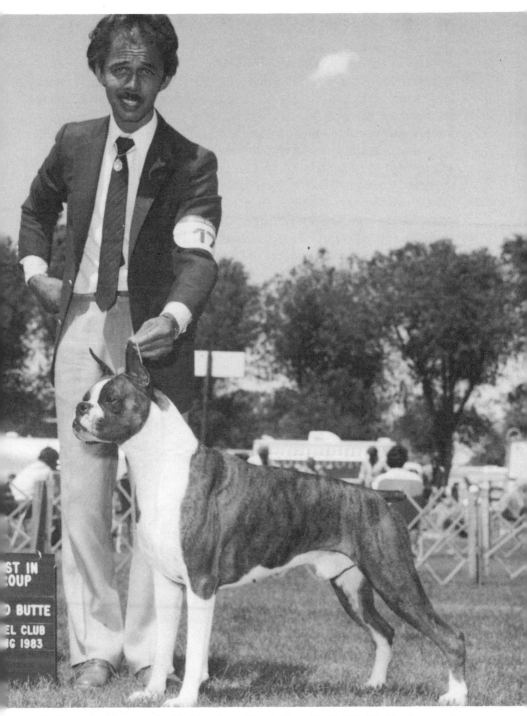

Ch. Doggone Oarsman, by Ch. Mephistos Vendetta ex Ch. Orrkids First Lady, owned by Donald M. Edwards, M.D., Fullerton, California.

Salgray

Salgray Boxers were established in 1952 by Mr. and Mrs. Daniel Hamilburg of Brookline, Massachusetts, when they purchased, as a pet for their children, a bitch named Sally of Grayarlin (for which Salgray was coined as their kennel name) from Jane Kamp Forsyth. Sally was an instant success with the entire family, to the extent that it was decided she should be shown. In very little time she was sporting the title "Champion" before her name.

Sally's final points were gained at Morris and Essex, where another young Boxer from Grayarlin, namely, Sabot, took the purple in dogs. In all the excitement of Sally's finishing, the Hamilburgs decided that they would like to have him, too, and so he was purchased from Jane.

Ch. Salgray's V.I.P., Best in Show and Group winner handled by Stan Flowers for Mr. and Mrs. Daniel Hamilburg, Plymouth, Massachusetts.

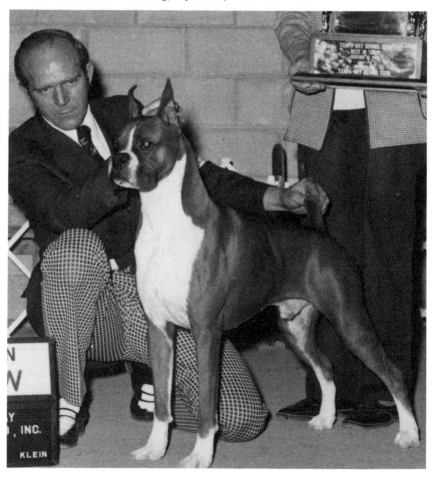

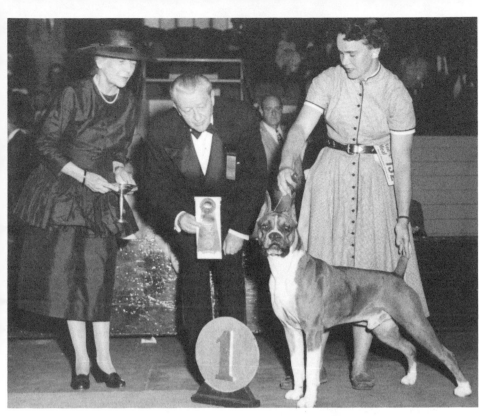

Ch. Sabot of Grayarlin, foundation stud dog and the second Boxer owned by Dan and Phyllis Hamilburg. Sabot was the Hamilburgs' first important winner, handled by his breeder, Jane Kamp Forsyth. In this photo, Mrs. Alice Roosevelt Longworth is presenting the trophy won by Sabot for Best in Show at the Potomac Boxer Club Specialty of 1955, under judge John P. Wagner of Mazelaine fame.

Along with Sabot, his litter sister was acquired, Champion Slipper of Grayarlin. These two represented the finest of the "old" Boxer breeding, being by Champion Meritaire's Fancy Free (Champion Bang Away of Sirrah Crest ex a daughter of Champion Yobang of Sirrah Crest, he by Champion Utz von Dom of Mazelaine ex a Champion Symphony of Mazelaine bitch). The dam of Sabot and Slipper was Cinder Ponds Primadonna, descended from Champion Warlord of Mazelaine, two of the great Lilac Hedge champions, Utz, and the very successful Best in Show winning bitch Champion El Wendie of Rockland. Surely all the factors present to form the background for so great and influential a kennel as Salgray became!

Slipper was bred to Bang Away's great son, Champion Barrage of Quality Hill, belonging to Mrs. Jouett Shouse, and they produced Champion Salgray's Battle Chief. In his turn, along with many personal achievements in the show ring, Chief sired the unforgettable

Salgray "F" litter, from Champion Marquam Hills Flamingo. The "F" litter grew up to become Champion Salgray's Fashion Plate, Champion Salgray's Fanfare, Champion Salgray's Frolic, Champion Salgray's Flamecrest, Champion Salgray's Flaming Ember, and Champion Salgray's Flying High.

The members of this litter distinguished themselves in many ways. Along with having sensational show careers, Fashion Plate and Flying High accounted for a stunning list of championships, and high honors-winning progeny. Four members of the "F" litter became Best in Show dogs. Champion Salgray Flying Ember, one of the Best in Show littermates, was bred to litter-brother Flying High with Champion Salgray's Auntie Mame and Champion Salgray's Ambush as the results. Auntie Mame, handled by Stan Flowers, won twelve Bests in Show and forty-three Working Groups. Champion Salgray's Ovation, out at the same period, in 1969 alone won twenty-three Bests in Show and forty-one Working Groups. Champion Salgray's Double Talk and

Ch. Salgray's Valentino, by Ch. Salgray's Bojangles ex Salgray's Poppin Fresh, is one of the consistent winners handled by Stan Flowers for Mr. and Mrs. Daniel M. Hamilburg, Plymouth, Massachusetts.

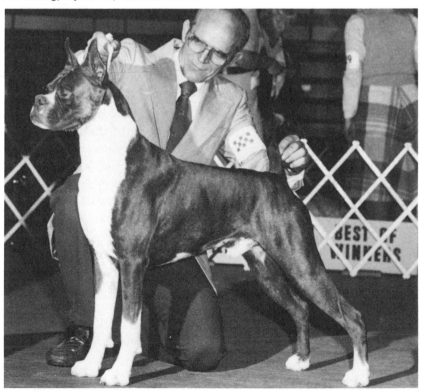

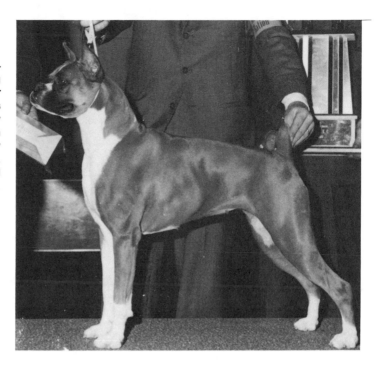

Ch. Salgray's Flaming Ember taking Best in Show under judge Robert Waters at Mad River Valley all the way back in 1962, handled by Stan Flowers for Mr. and Mrs. Daniel Hamilburg.

Champion Salgray's Double Play made their presence felt, as did Champion Salgray's Chances Are, Champion Salgray's Jitterbug, Champion Salgray's V.I.P., and all the other distinguished winners from this kennel.

The honors won by Salgray Boxers over the past thirty or so years add up to a staggering total, and include every category of competition. Breeder of the Year—Stud Dog of the Year—Brood Bitch of the Year—Top Best in Show Dog—Top Working Dog—Top Best of Breed Dog; and the bitch, too, at one time or another in all these categories. You name it, and almost certainly Salgray has won it, not just once but on repeated occasions. These are true *Breeders:* the type who form the background of our fancy, and Salgray takes its place as the continuation of the great producers Mazelaine, Barmere, and Sirrah Crest in carrying on the tradition which built the breed here.

Phyllis and Dan Hamilburg recently sold their big kennel and moved to smaller, more convenient quarters, turning over the responsibility of Salgray's future to their daughter and her husband. Jane Hamilburg has grown up a Boxer person, sharing her parents' love for and interest in the breed, so Salgray should continue to flourish. Phyllis and Dan are every bit as interested as ever in the dogs, and very definitely continuing their participation.

Shilo

Shilo Boxers at Mechanicsville, Virginia are owned by Paul and Shirley O'Donohue who had no sooner become Boxer owners when they decided that they would also like to become exhibitors.

Their purchase of Sam El's Maker's Mark, a Shadrack grandson, did his new owners proud when he gained his first points from the American-bred Class of the New Jersey Boxer Club Specialty, judged by the late Alice Wood. Before he had reached eighteen months of age, Mark was a champion and then, although shown as a Special on a very limited basis, he proceeded to bring home an all-breed Best in Show, a Specialty Best of Breed, plus first in five Working Groups, which was certainly good going! Mark was sold to the O'Donohues by Sam and Eleanor Jordan, owners of the Sam El Kennels.

Mark is now proving himself to be as excellent a sire as show dog. So far he has three champions to his credit, with several others pointed so on the way.

Pictured winning one of his five Working Groups (he is also an all-breed Best in Show and a Specialty winner), Ch. Sam-El's Maker's Mark, a Shadrack grandson, was bred by Sam and Eleanor Jordan and is owned by Paul and Shirley O'Donahue, Mechanicsville, Virginia.

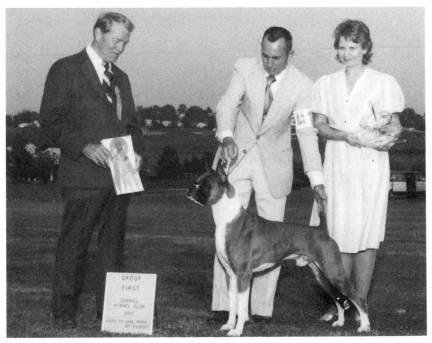

96

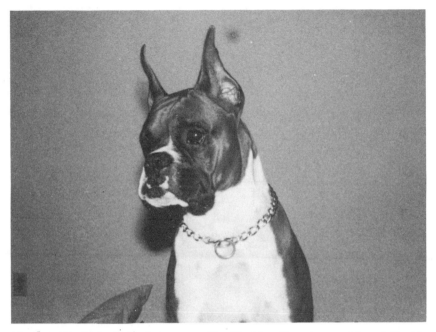

Ch. Sam-El's Maker's Mark has won five Working Groups, an all-breed Best in Show, and a Specialty Show although shown on a very limited basis. Owned by Paul and Shirley O'Donahue, Mechanicsville, Virginia.

Presently the O'Donohues are showing Abbie of Woodcrest, a Mark daughter out of U-All of Woodcrest. She was Winners Bitch at the Indian River Boxer Club Specialty three months after having puppies. One of her daughters, by Champion Aracrest's Talisman, will be the first of their homebred bitches whom the O'Donohues plan on breeding back to Mark, which will truly start the Shilo line on its way.

Treceder

Treceder Boxers were founded by the late Hollyce Stewart in 1946, and operated until her death in 1972. Thereupon her sister, Bobbee Owens, who had also been active in the kennel for several years, joined forces with Mrs. Ann Harr of Houston, Texas, who had been a Boxer breeder since the mid-sixties under the Harmony prefix. The two of them took over as owners of Treceder, thus carrying on one of the earlier important kennels in the breed.

Bobbee Owens passed away in 1981, thus Ann Harr is now the full owner of Treceder.

Since her earliest days in Boxers, Ann Harr has owned Boxers of the Treceder line. Her first champion was purchased from the "old" Treceder back in 1956, Champion Treceder's Shady Lady, and Mrs. Harr was also the breeder of Champion Treceder's Sequel and Treceder's Sequence. Champion Treceder's Sequel sired 23 champions while Champion Treceder's Sequence produced three.

At the time my earlier Boxer book (*The Book of the Boxer*, co-authored with Joan Brearley) went to press, Champion Phil-Dee's Prompt Appointment was chief among the "young hopefuls" at Treceder, a son of Champion Cajon Calling Card, who was a Sequence son. Now the principal mainstay of the kennel is the handsome Champion Treceder's Ho-

Ch. Treceder's Dynamo, by Phil-Dee's Prompt Appointment ex Cava Lane's Shady Mist, was bred and is owned by Ann Harr, Houston, Texas.

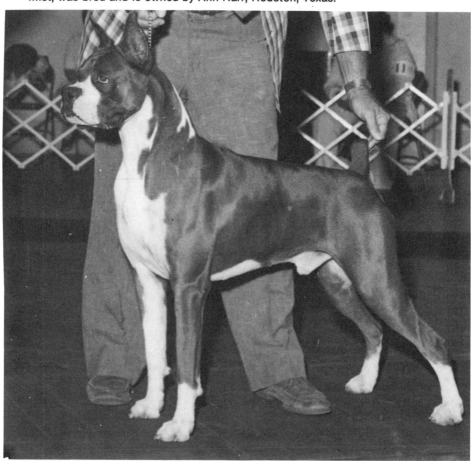

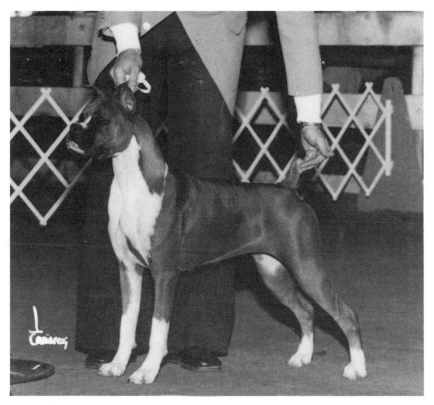

Ch. Treceder's Candy Cane, by Phil-Dee's Prompt Appointment ex Cava Lane's Shady Mist, winning Best of Winners and Best of Opposite Sex for a four-point major at ten months of age. Bred and owned by Treceder Kennels, Houston, Texas.

ly Smoke, a son of Champion Ringmaster's Olimpian ex Treceder's Special Edition, bred by Mary Surasky, whose progeny include the stunning youngster, Champion Treceder's Up In Smoke. Also some very beautiful Prompt Attention progeny are figuring in the show and breeding program, among them the bitch Champion Treceder's Sweet Stuff, another lovely bitch, Champion Treceder's Candy Cane, and a handsome dog, Champion Treceder's Dynamo.

Other recent winner from Treceder lines are Champion Treceder's Heartbreak U.S.A., owned by Ernst and Patricia Dorsch; Champion Treceder's Cover Girl (Linda Leidt); Champion Treceder Liberty Bell (Treceder); Champion Treceder's Avalanche Rodonna (owned by Treceder, Canadian-bred by Donna Cole), Champion Laurel Hills Rudolf (bred by Bruce and Jeanne Korson, purchased by Treceder), and Champion Treceder's Gibraltar (Ginny Crippen).

Vihabra

Vihabra Boxers are owned by Dr. Harry and Virginia Bradley of Los Altos Hills, California. Harry earned his Doctorate at Washington State University and has been a Dean of Students in the Community College System in California since 1967. Virginia, too, is a teacher, "retired" now from the classroom to teach piano at home, play the organ at church, and raise her beautiful Boxer puppies.

The Bradleys purchased their first Boxer, a male, as a pet, in 1968. This dog was so greatly enjoyed that the following year the Bradleys decided to get a companion for him, in this case a lovely red brindle who became their foundation bitch. She was an eighteen-month-old Champion Canzonet's Musical Matinee daughter, Brig's Daisy Mae, and, bred to the original dog, Gee Whizz Von Walt Siete, presented the Bradleys with their first Boxer litter, six dogs and six bitches, all well and husky. That litter really did it! The Bradleys were "hooked" on the pleasure of having Boxer puppies around, and since that time have bred ten litters.

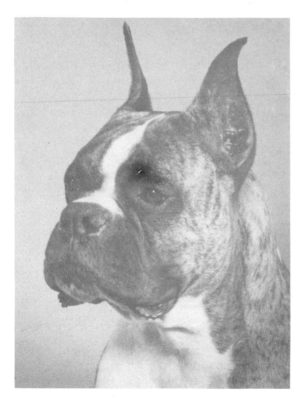

Ch. Merrilane's Vihabra Gold'N Key, by Ch. Merrilane's Happy To Meet You ex Merrilane's Touchdown Benroe, owned by Dr. H.L. and Mrs. V.J. Bradley, Los Altos Hills, California.

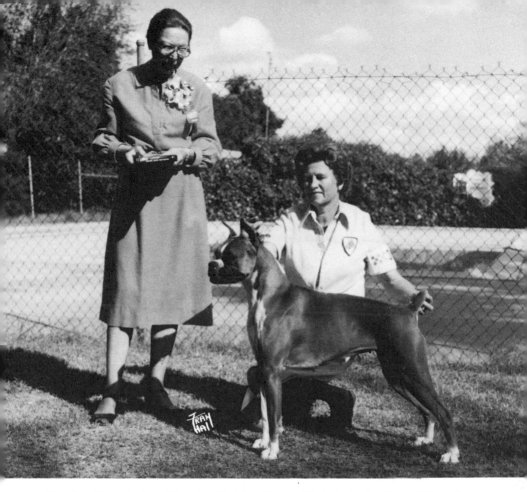

Vagabond's Lady Sunshine, handled by Eleanor Linderholm for Dr. and Mrs. H. Bradley, taking Winners Bitch under judge Phoebe Harris for a three-point major.

For her next breeding, Champion Bold Impulse of Ben Hame was selected for Daisy, and a bitch, Windsong, kept from this litter was eventually bred to Champion Merrilane's Holiday Fashion. This produced Merrilane's Touchdown Monroe, who is now the dam of three American Kennel Club champions and one Philippine champion; Champion Merrilane's Vihahbra Gold'N Key, Champion Vihabra's Star Dust, Champion Vihabra's Mister Gold Dust, and Philippine Champion Vihabra's Arrowhead.

Mrs. Bradley notes that prior to 1978 they did not have a kennel name, using the name of their street, Ben Roe, to identify the dogs. Then as they became more involved, they decided that they must select one, and so Vihabra was coined from VIrginia, HArry and BRAdley.

101

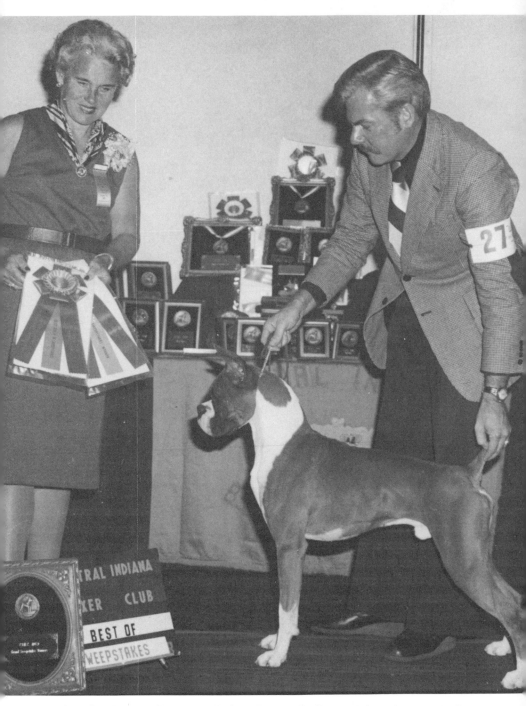

Can. Ch. Iremanor Pinepaths Hudson Bay, Junior Sweepstakes winner at the Central Indiana Boxer Club, October 1979, with owner-handler Jack Ireland and judge Jane Forsyth.

Chapter 4

Boxers in Canada

Thinking back over Canadian Boxers of the past couple of decades, three kennels come to mind whose accomplishments in the early part of this period certainly did their bit to set the stage for the progress enjoyed by this breed.

A lady who came from England, first to the United States where she had been hired to manage a well-known Pekingese kennel in Virginia, then to Canada when the association with the Peke breeder did not work out, was the person to have bred and owned the first Boxer in Canada to win a Best in Show there. The breeder was Miss Jean F. Grant of Blossomlea Kennels, and the Boxer who attained this prestigious honor was Champion Painted Besom of Blossomlea, who represented several generations of Miss Grant's own breeding program.

It was around 1950 when Miss Grant bred one of her bitches to American Champion The Toolmaker, a very lovely dog who was owned by Marjorie and Bill Rankin, prominent Boxer breeders of that period whose Huck Hill Kennels were at Brookfield, Connecticut. A bitch from this litter was kept by Miss Grant, growing up to become Champion Truly Fair of Blossomlea. Bred to Champion Jack's Zebedes, Truly Fair produced Champion Painted Besom, who gained the exciting Best in Show award.

Painted Besom had other contributions to make as well as those in the show ring! She was bred to Champion Bang Away of Sirrah Crest, becoming the dam of Champion Chat Away of Blossomlea, who, bred to Champion Jered's Spellbinder produced Champion Fireside Chat of Blossomlea; Fireside Chat in turn, bred to Champion Salgray's Flying High produced Champion Bobby Pin of Blossomlea, who became the dam of Champion Salgray's Double Talk.

Jean Grant passed away not long before we are writing this book. She was a dedicated and knowledgeable breeder who certainly contributed well to Canadian Boxers!

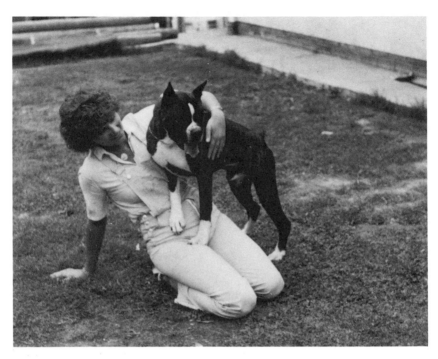

The syndicated Canadian import, Am. and Can. Ch. Tradonalee's Tradewin, shown with syndicate member Lorraine Harris on his release from the quarantine station in South Australia. An extrovert, a dog of great style, excellent type and temperament. He is now making his mark as a new stud force in Australia to complement bitches from the Salgray's Minuteman stock, as well as existing lines.

Then we have Michael Millan, who came to Canada from Yugoslavia in the early 1950's. This gentleman, who had shown Boxers in four countries, bred his bitch, American, Canadian and Bermudian Champion Gaymitz Jet Action, to the Hamilburgs' Champion Salgray's Fashion Plate, and wound up the breeder of that most remarkable and dominant sire, International Champion Millan's Fashion Hint. To bring you a full list of Fashion Hint's progeny and their accomplishments would fill a book in itself. Suffice to say that this dog's progeny and their descendants are to be found in a vast majority of both American and Canadian winning Boxers of the 1970's, and that this will undoubtedly remain the case for many years to come. A truly memorable and very great dog!

Another person from Yugoslavia, Vera Bartel, founded the Memorylane Kennels, also in Ontario (as were both Jean Grant and Michael Millan) and made considerable impact on the breed. Among

104

her outstanding dogs, International Champion Memorylane Fashion Escort, plus at least a dozen other worthy champions. Memorylane dogs are in successful kennels in both Canada and the United States.

Jim and Norah McGriskin, whose activity in Boxers dates back to the late sixties, started the Aracrest Kennels, another familiar and prestigious establishment dedicated to Boxers. The McGriskins got off to what one might call a sensational start in the breed when they bred, in their very first litter, International Champion Aracrest's Jered, American and Canadian Champion Aracrest's Trinkett, American and Canadian Champion Aracrest's Kaylib, and Canadian Champion Aracrest's Brocade. The dam of this litter was Canadian Champion Jocolu's Charming Fashion, who was a Fashion Hint daughter. The sire was Canadian Champion Scher Khoun's Shadrack.

The McGriskins, also, in addition to being top Boxer breeders, are highly successful professional handlers and have had the lead on many a Best in Show Boxer during recent years.

Two of Canada's most dedicated Boxer breeders, fanciers, and exhibitors are the Stanley Whitmores who own the very notable dog, Champion Diamondaire's Dealer's Choice. Bred by Mr. and Mrs. C. King, this son of Champion Haviland's Count Royal ex Verwood's Nina Never Knew, was born September 15th 1978 and has amassed an imposing array of top awards under knowledgeable judges.

Mr. and Mrs. Jack Ireland, who own the Pinepaths Boxers at Fingal, Ontario, are in their fourth generation of homebred winning Boxers who trace their ancestry back to Champions Scher Khoun's Meshak and Shadrack, thus into Champion Millan's Fashion Hint and the Salgray Heritage.

Canadian and American Champion Tri-Manor Pinepaths Hudson Bay unfortunately died in July 1983 at only five and a half years of age, his death caused by commercial feed spray—a heartbreaking loss to his owners. His show career in both Canada and the United States had been highly successful (including Grand Sweepstakes Winner at the Central Indiana Boxer Club Specialty), while as a sire he had already produced sixteen Canadian Champions and two with titles in the United States. Several more by him are pointed, and fortunately he did leave some handsome sons behind to carry on his line.

One of the latter is Canadian Champion Pinepaths Union Jack, who in turn is the sire of a most promising youngster, seven-months-old Pinepaths Palumbo, who went Reserve Winners his first two times in the ring.

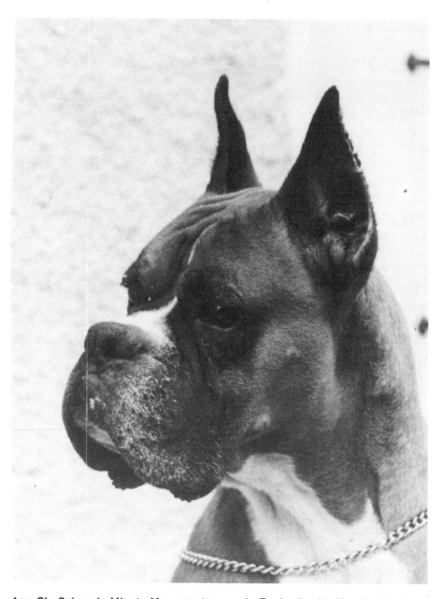

Am. Ch. Salgray's Minute Man spent a year in England, with Mrs. Pat Heath as owner, en route to his new home in Australia, where he belongs to Mr. T. Carter, making his mark as a sire.

Chapter 5

Boxers in Australia

We are very much impressed by the beauty and quality of the Boxers owned and produced in Australia, and are proud at having so representative a group of breeders to tell you about in these pages. A study of the accompanying illustrations will back up the reasons for my admiration of these dogs and the many words of praise for the Boxers from "down under" which have reached my ears from American judges returning home after fulfilling assignments in that country.

Considerable rapport exists between the Australian fancy and ours here in the United States. It is quite usual nowadays for at least several judges each year from here to go there and vice versa. This is good both ways, as it enlarges our true scope of what is taking place worldwide within the breeds of interest to us, and the exchange of ideas and opinions is certainly beneficial to all concerned.

The Australian Standard is based upon the English one. You will note that cropping of ears does not take place in that country, either, and I personally find the expression and heads of the uncropped dogs to be attractive.

Australian breeders are using bloodlines from both England and the United States in their breeding programs, combining them judiciously and advantageously with their own. Achievement of a championship title in Australia is far from easy owing to the many top grade dogs and keen competition found there.

Following is a resume of some of the leading Australian Boxer kennels.

Innsbruck

Innsbruck Boxers are owned by Mrs. Nea E. Evans who resides at Annangrove in New South Wales, Australia. Mrs. Evans has had dogs all her life, but, as she puts it, "during the past 25 years Boxers have BEEN my life." Her kennel is a small one by some standards, making it all the more noteworthy that as of March 1984 she has made up 23 champions.

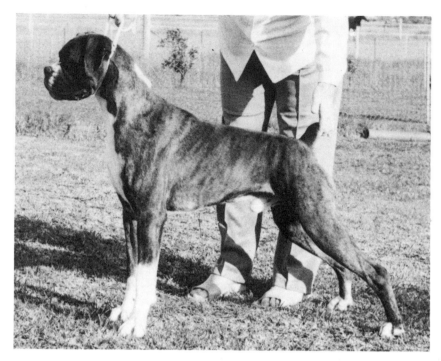

Aust. Ch. Skelder Game Chip, by Eng. Ch. Tyegarth Famous Grouse ex Crisp and Dry of Skeldon, is an import from the United Kingdom, bred by Mrs. M.J. Malcolm and owned by Mrs. Nea Evans, Innsbruck Boxers, Annangrove, New South Wales, Australia.

Over the years, Mrs. Evans has imported seven Boxers from the United Kingdom, from the late Mrs. Jane Thornley of the Cherryburton Boxer Kennels in Yorkshire. During the past seven years her imported dogs have come from Mrs. M.J. Malcolm of the Skelder Boxer Kennels in Dorset, England. The Boxers from both these kennels, together with the homebreds, have won numerous awards up to and including all-breed Bests in Show.

Most notable of the current winners at Innsbruck is Australian Champion Skelder Game Chip, one of the imports, a spectacular brindle dog who within just four weeks, during September and October 1983, achieved the following record: Best in Show at the Boxer Association of Victoria Championship Show, judged by Pat Heath, Seefeld Kennels, United Kingdom, in an entry of 179. Best of Breed at the Royal Agricultural Society Kennel Control Spring Fair, judged by the famous Boxer authority Jane Forsyth, 179 entries. Best in Show at the Western District Boxer Club Championship Show, judges R. Townsend and B. Mason, Australia.

Game Chip's earlier wins had included Reserve Challenge Certificate and Best Junior in Show at the Western District Boxer Club May Championship Show, judge Lily Potts (United Kingdom) and Reserve Dog Challenge Certificate and Best Junior in Show at the Boxer Club of New South Wales June Championship Show, judge Mrs. E. Fraser (Canada).

This record, attained exclusively under breed specialist judges, was climaxed when Game Chip scored in the Major Point Score of the Boxer Club of New South Wales (both dog and bitch) winning of the Dog Division.

Another of Mrs. Evans' Boxers, the stylish, much admired four-year-old bitch, Australian Champion Skelder Weather Wise won the Bitch Division of the Major Point Score of the Boxer Club of New South Wales in 1981 and 1982.

Aust. Ch. Skelder Weather Wise, U.K. import, by Eng. Ch. Gremlin Summer Storm ex Skelder Burnt Amber, born April 1979, was bred by Mrs. M.J. Malcom and is owned by Mrs. M. Evans, Annangrove, New South Wales, Australia.

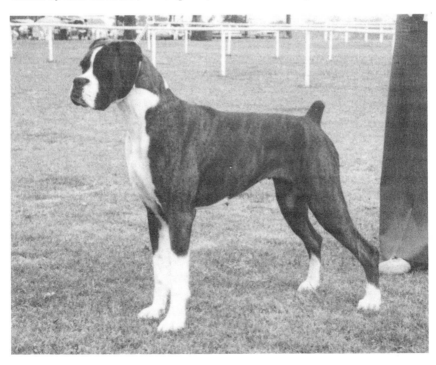

During her show career she was awarded Challenge Certificates by S. Dangerfield (United Kingdom), Fred Young (United States), R. Tongren (United States), and Dr. Wm. Houpt (United States), to add to her Best in Show at the New South Wales Boxer Club Championship Show (October 1982), Best in Group awards, and runner-up to Best in Show all-breeds.

Other famous Boxers at Innsbruck include Australian Champion Double Deal of Skelder, imported, and Australian Champion Innsbruck Dark Eclipse (runner-up to Best in Show, Royal Agricultural Society Spring Fair 1981); also Australian Champion Innsbruck Trevallion, Reserve Challenge Winner at the 1982 and 1983 Sydney Royals.

Intrends

Judy Horton started showing Boxers in 1965 when she purchased a dog who became Australian Champion Jaywick Copperplate and won two Bests in Show along with becoming the sire of three champions. She did not, however, actually start breeding until 1968 and then in partnership with Arakoola Kennels. When one of the partners moved from the state in 1972, Judy registered the kennel prefix, Intrends.

One of the foundation bitches was a daughter of Copperplate, who was linebred Rainey Lane, out of Australian Champion Topline Thomasina, from Panfield and Mazelaine lines. She was Australian Champion Arakoola Autumn Haze, a lovely mahogany brindle with a beautiful head and expression, and she was a top winner in her day. Never a prolific producer, she whelped only six pups in two litters, all by Caesarean birth. Nonetheless she made an important contribution as the grandam of Australian Champion Intrends Be Dazzled.

The second of the brood bitches was a half-sister of Autumn Haze, Australian Champion Arakoola Kiss 'n' Tell also from Thomasina but sired by a son of English Champion Wardrobes Morning Canter, imported from the United Kingdom. She had five puppies, another disappointing producer, but even so, she too left her mark by a gorgeous and successful grandchild, Australian Champion Intrends Superman, who has a Royal Challenge and an all-breed Best in Show to his credit, And there is a puppy out of Superman's sister close to her title in Queensland.

The third foundation bitch was linebred Wardrobes, by a grandson of Morning Canter from a daughter of English Champion Wardrobes Cherryburton Bumblebee (imported from the United Kingdom). She was Australian Champion Atone's Mujuba, a lovely deer red and an

110

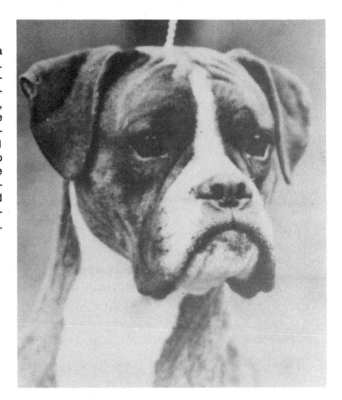

Aust. Ch. Arakoola Autumn Haze, by Aust. Ch. Jaywick Copperplate ex Aust. Ch. Topline Thomasina, whelped May 1970. The top winning bitch in Victoria during late 1971 and 1972, who was to become one of the three foundation bitches at Intrends Kennels. Owned and bred by Judy Horton, Australia.

outstanding winner. She won two Boxer Specialties and a Royal Challenge plus numerous Group wins. Her most successful daughter was from a half-brother to half-sister breeding which produced Intrends Pot O'Gold, the dam of five champions to date. A dog from this mating also gained his obedience title.

From 1972 until 1978, Judy built up her bloodlines by breeding to sons and grandsons of the Wardrobes imports, resulting in some quality bitches who were strongly linebred. While on a visit to England in 1978, she met and fell in love with English Champion Gremlin Summer Storm, so on her return home she mated her bitch, Pot O'Gold, to Summer Storm's son in Australia, Champion Gremlin's Great Gale. This mating produced four bitches, three of which have become champions. One is a multiple Best in Show winner, two are Boxer Specialty Challenge and Royal winners, and the third is the dam of the Victorian Top Boxer of 1983 competition, another Best in Show winner.

In 1980 Judy mated Pot O'Gold to Summer Storm's brother, New Zealand Champion Gremlin Summer Spree; this produced a champion daughter. In 1981 she repeated the Great Gale mating and one

111

champion son was produced. He has gone on to win three Bests in Show and numerous Groups.

Judy Horton spent the following year overseas, which curtailed her breeding program, and necessitated reducing the size of her kennel. Left with only three bitches with whom to continue breeding, she is now in the process of rebuilding where she left off, and now has three young bitches by American and Canadian Champion Tradonalees Trade Win, one out of Pot O'Gold who is continuing on in the tradition of her older sisters and brother by winning Best in Show from the classes at only ten months of age, and two from her half-sister, Australian Champion Intrends Wind Song (Great Gale-Pot O'Gold). Also a young imported bitch by English Champion Kimbra Uncle Sam of Winiwuk from a daughter of Winiwuk Milray's Red Baron of

Aust. Ch. Atones Mujuba, born October 1972, by Aust. Ch. Cudgewa Gaylord ex Wowey Athena, was bred by R. Eaton and is owned by Judy Horton. A great winner and an excellent producer, "Angie" made her presence felt in the ring during 1973 and 1974, winning a Royal Challenge Certificate, two Boxer Specialties, and many Group wins. Photo by Max Neilson.

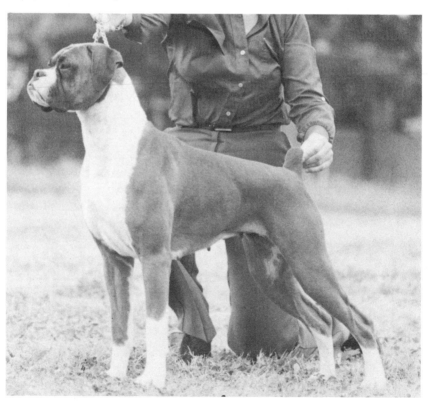

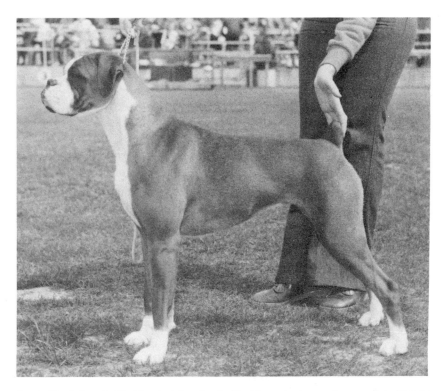

Aust. Ch. Intrends Be Dazzled, by Aust. Ch. Phoenix Jason Argonaut ex Hagge-sled Harlequin, born 1977, won Best Puppy in Show at her first Boxer Specialty, then won four Royal Challenges, two all-breed Bests in Show, and many Group wins. She is the dam of Aust. Ch. Phoenix Shiloh, Best In Show at two Boxer Specialties and a Royal Challenge winner, her latest at almost six years of age and six weeks in whelp. Shown by her breeder, Mrs. Judy Horton, until 1980, then sold to Maxine and Terry Carter and Ron and Jenny Lee in co-ownership.

Valvay who is linebred to Shadrack has been purchased. With the out-cross of her present lines to the Shadrack line, Judy is hoping to get the style that is present in the American Boxer of today together with the quality and substance of her present line.

Judy comments "A big thrill for me last year was viewing the line-up of the champions in the Victorian Top Boxer Competition in which two Boxers bred by her were competing and another two were from Intrends bitches." Only ten dogs are eligible to compete.

She also notes her good fortune as a judge in being able to travel ex-tensively and see the stud dogs available in the country first hand, enabling her to choose the most suitable sire for each of her bitches.

Intrends Kennels are at Ormond, Victoria, Australia.

Pinetop

Pinetop Boxers are owned by K. and L.J. Harris at Welland, South Australia.

This is the home of some very famous and high quality dogs, among them Australian Champion Phoenix Shiloh, whelped November 25th 1980, by Australian Champion Phoenix Peter Paint Pot ex Australian Champion Intrends Bedazzled whose exciting wins include Best in Show under Lois Mathews at the Boxer Club of Tasmania Specialty in 1983; Best in Show under David K. Roche at the Boxer Club of South Australia Specialty 1982; Dog Challenge Certificate winner at the prestigious Melbourne Royal Show in 1982 under specialist judge Kari Jarvinen of Finland, plus numerous Best in Group and in Show awards. He is currently Top Dog in South Australia, 1983-84, undefeated to date among the males.

Australian Champion Pinetop Liberation was born November 9th 1980, by Australian and New Zealand Champion Seefeld Don

Aust. Ch. Pinetop Liberation, by Aust. and N.Z. Ch. Seefeld Don Zachary (U.K. import) ex Pinetop Tantalisa, owned by Pinetop Boxers, Kevin and Lorraine Harris, Welland, South Australia.

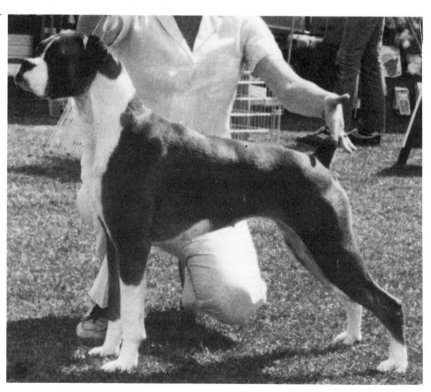

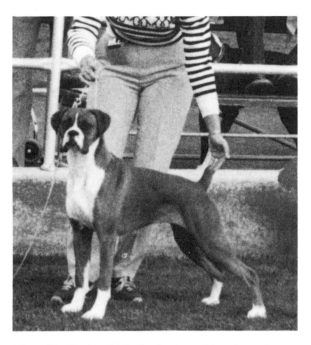

Aust. Ch. Pinetop Timepiece, by Am. Ch. Salgray's Minute Man (American import) ex Pinetop Tantalisa, pictured taking Best in Show at the Boxer Club of Victoria Parade Specialty at ten months old. Owned by Kevin and Lorraine Harris, Welland, South Australia.

Syndicated import Am. and Can. Ch. Tradonalee's Tradewin on his release from quarantine in Australia. Shown with syndicate members (back row, *left to right*) Ron Rudd, Terry Carter, Mick Hart, Rhonda Rudd, Peter Foster, Kevin Harris. (Front row, *left to right*) Lesley Hart, Maxine Carter, Hilda Foster, and Lorraine Harris.

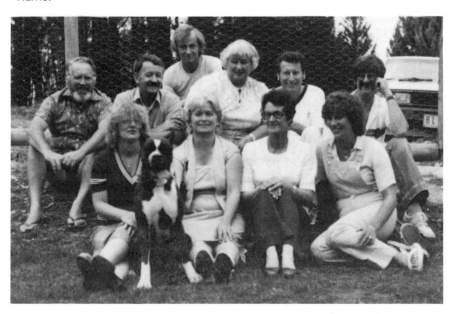

115

Zachary (United Kingdom import) ex Pinetop Tantalisa. He has won many Best in Group, from best Baby Puppy to best Exhibit; Baby Best in Show, Boxer Parade 1981; Opposite Sex in Show, all-breeds, on two occasions; Reserve Bitch winner to her sister, Pinetop Timepiece, under Robert Forsyth at Boxer Club of South Australia 1983 Specialty.

Australian Champion Pinetop Timepiece was whelped July 27th 1982, by American Champion Salgray's Minute Man (United States import) ex Pinetop Tantalisa. Her achievements include many in-Group and in-Show wins, from Minor to Puppy and best Exhibit; Best in Show Boxer Parade (Victoria); Best Opposite Sex and runner up to Best in Show under Robert Forsyth, Boxer Club of South Australia 1983; undefeated bitch winner at the time of the writing of this book; and bitch Challenge Certificate winner at Adelaide Royal 1983. All achieved in a span of fifteen months of limited exhibiting.

Pinetop Dark Omen is an unshown six-month-old bitch puppy for whom hopes for future success are high. She was born August 10th 1983, and is by American and Canadian Champion Tradonalees Tradewin (imported from Canada) ex Australian Champion Pinetop Liberation.

American and Canadian Champion Tradonalee's Tradewin was brought to Australia by a syndicate of Boxer breeders to be used as a stud dog. Those involved include Ron Rudd, Terry Carter, Mick Hart, Rhonda Rudd, Peter Foster, Keven Harris, Lesley Hart, Maxine Carter, Hilda Foster, Lorraine Harris, Kate and Jim Black and Judy Horton. It is believed that he will prove a tremendous asset to the breed there, as his first puppies look extremely exciting.

Rosemullion

The Rosemullion Boxers are owned by Les and Cleone Baker at North Turramurra, New South Wales.

A dog of particular note from there is Australian Champion Rosemullion Regal, which was bred by the Bakers and is now owned by their close friends Athol and Lorraine Smitherengale. Regal is a son of Australian Champion Lalaguli Woowookurung from the Bakers' bitch, Sabari Sari Minta, who is of Wardrobes stock together with Gremlin and Treceder (American) bloodlines.

Most of the breeding at this kennel has been based on those lines and on Cherryburton, but in the early 1980's the Bakers introduced, along with the Guntop Boxers in New South Wales, the American-bred dog Salgray's Minuteman who was imported about three years ago.

116

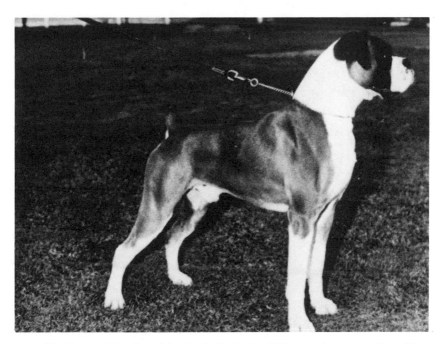

Aust. Ch. Rosemullion Regal, by Aust. Ch. Lalaguli Woowookurung ex Sabari Sari Minta, bred by Les and Cleone Baker, North Turramurra, New South Wales, Australia. Owned by Athol and Lorraine Smitherengale.

Regal started his show career at eight months of age, taking Best of Breed, Champion Puppy in Group, and Minor Puppy Class Entry in Show. Now at age three years he has to his credit six Bests in Show, three Reserves in Show, eleven Bests in Group, Five Reserves in Group, Dog Challenge at Melbourne Royal 1981, Dog Challenge at Toowoomba Royal 1982, and Dog Challenge at Sydney Royal 1982. Regal also was Runner Up Boxer of the Year for 1980 in Queensland, and Top Dog of the Year 1981 in both Queensland and New South Wales Point Score Competition. The Bakers tell us that this is the first time a Boxer has taken this award in both States in the one year.

Sjecoin

Sjecoin Boxers, formerly Anisor Boxers, are owned by Mrs. Rosina Olifent-Brace at Mont Albert, Melbourne, Australia, and is an especially successful establishment with a great many major show awards under International judges to their credit.

The leader of the team is the illustrious Australian Champion Sjecoin Fashion Parade, born in October 1979. She has won nine Bests in

117

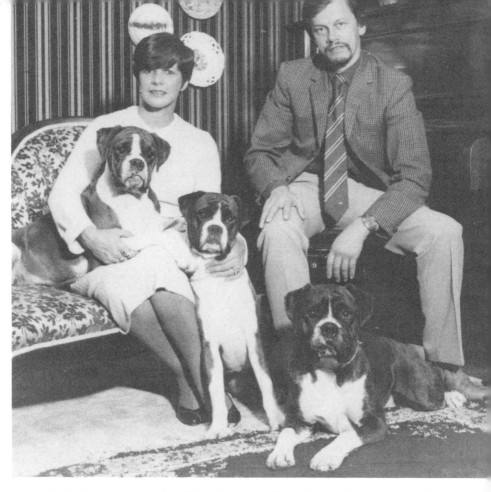

David Brace and Rosina Olifent-Brace of Mont Albert, Victoria, Australia, with three of their famous Australian Boxer Champions Sjecoin Hey Look Me Over, Sjecoin Fashion Parade, and Sjecoin Dash of Fire.

Show, all breeds; twelve times has been Best of Opposite Sex to Best in Show; and has 25 Groups to her credit. She is by Champion Gremlin Great Gale (imported from United Kingdom) ex Champion Sjecoin Super Duper, a daughter of Champion Anisor Super Star.

Top male and stud dog is Australian Champion Sjecoin Dash O'Fire, born January 1980, by Fire Ball of Winuwuk (imported from the United Kingdom), who is a son of Champion Kreyon's Back In Town, from Australian Champion Sjecoin My-T Sweet, a Super Star daughter.

The current show star is Australian Champion Sjecoin Winter Forecast, born June 1982, by Australian and New Zealand Champion Assissi Summer Splurge (Gremlin Summer Spree son) ex Sjecoin P'sonality Plus.

The bloodlines of the modern Sjecoin Kennel are from the foundation laid by crossing Gremlin and Wardrobes lines. The outstanding show and brood bitch from that period was Champion Anisor Super Star, one of the truly great modern winners in Australia and the dam of the marvelous producer Australian Champion Sjecoin My-T Sweet, sired by Rainey-Lane's Grand Slam. She has six champions to her credit, and from her most of the top Sjecoin Boxers have descended.

In recent years, the original Gremlin/Wardrobes bloodlines have been crossed with American influences, specifically Kreyon's Back In Town and Winuwuk Milray's Red Baron of Valvay. These have produced the recent winners, Australian Champions Sjecoin Hey Look Me Over, Raggedy Ann, and Winter-Forecast, who exhibit not only the sound and typey English-European features but the American style and elegance, including arch of neck and animation.

Aust. Ch. Sjecoin Winter Forecast owned by Rosina Olifent-Brace, Mont Albert, Victoria, Australia.

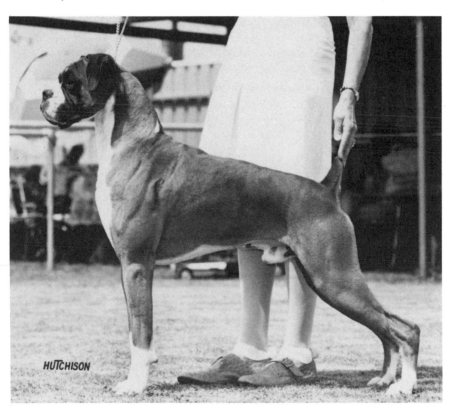

Thasrite

Thasrite Boxers are owned by David A. Strachan at Murrumbateman, New South Wales, Australia.

Top dog here is the English importation, Australian Champion That's Right of Panfield, red and white son of English Champion Steynmere Summer Gold ex English Champion Gold Bangle of Panfield, and he was bred by Major S.W. Somerfield, Panfield Boxers, United Kingdom.

That's Right has enjoyed an outstanding show career in Australia, where he has gone Best Exhibit in Show six times and been Runner-Up to Best Exhibit in Show five times, plus being a Specialty Best in Show dog.

In England, That's Right gained his Junior Warrant and five Reserve Challenge Certificates before going to Australia.

Impeccably linebred to the cream of English stock, this dog is a double grandson of English Champion Seefeld Goldsmith and four times great-grandson of the United Kingdom's top Boxer sire, International Champion Seefeld Picasso. Also a great-grandson of the American-bred bitch, Black Rose of Cherokee Oaks.

That's Right is the sire of twelve champions to date in three countries—England, Australia, and New Zealand. His son, English Champion Steynmere Night Rider, was Top Stud Dog in the United Kingdom for 1983, and his grandson, English Champion Norwatch Blockbuster was Top Dog the same year.

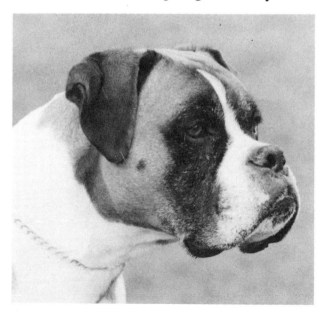

Aust. Ch. That's Right of Panfield, a United Kingdom import, at five and a half years. Owned by Mr. D.A. Strachan, Murrumbateman, N.S.W., Australia.

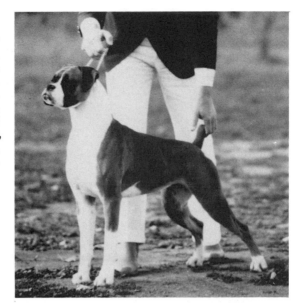

Then there is the stunning bitch Australian Champion Seefeld Sheer Delight, also imported from the United Kingdom, who is a daughter of English Champion Seefeld Shadowfax ex Shebacrest Sunbeam. She was bred by Mrs. Pat Heath, of the Seefeld Boxers, and was brought to Australia primarily as a mate for Champion That's Right of Panfield. Her short show career was brilliant. On her first outing she captured a Best Exhibit in Group, and just prior to retirement for maternal duties three months later, she went Best in Show at a Boxer Specialty.

Sheer Delight has had two litters by That's Right, and is now nursing her third. She is so far the dam of two champions.

The handsome young homebred, Australian Champion Thasrite Sheer Magic, is one of those from That's Right and Sheer Delight. She was a prolific winner from the puppy class, finished her championship at eleven months of age, winning Best Exhibit In Group that same day.

At 21 months of age, Sheer Magic has had a Best in Show and multi-Bests in Group to her credit. Other highlights include Puppy Bitch of the Day at the 1983 Sydney Royal and a maximum point (25) Challenge Certificate at nine months of age against some of the cream of the Australian bitches under American judge Jane Kay at the 1983 Easter Expo. Considering her youth and her early successes, Sheer Magic would seem destined for a truly spectacular show career.

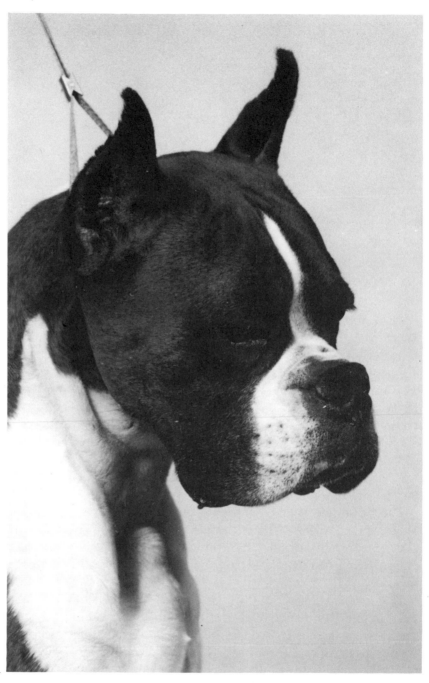

Braz. and Int. Ch. Burke of Cair Paravel, famed sire and Best in Show dog, is owned by Hexastar Boxers, Sao Paulo, Brazil.

Chapter 6

Boxers in Brazil

Sao Paulo, Brazil, is the home of one of the world's foremost Boxer kennels, Hexastar, which is a family affair that began when Agnes Buchwald and her brother Peter Paul Gridali, became interested admirers of the breed, back in the early 1970's. Peter decided to return to the University again and his many occupations as an industrial business man and student kept him so busy that he regretfully gave up his partnership in the kennel. Even so, since he will always be a dog lover, his household is enriched with the presence of a sweet and gentle Whippet.

At this time, Agnes Buchwald's two sons, Jean and Daniel, who since the beginning were active in all facets of the kennel, helping in the breeding, nursing, grooming, and also showing of the dogs, took their uncle's place as partners, and nowadays when someone mentions the Hexastar name, it's just normal to think about the mother and the sons (both of the latter are veterinary medical students).

In ten years of activity as a kennel, and about thirty homebred Brazilian and International champions, all are very proud of the dogs and important victories already scored by Hexastar, and look forward to the future.

The first of the Buchwalds' homebred champions was International Champion Hexastar's Candle Light, a Specialty Show and multi-Group winner, followed by Champion Hexastar's Holly Hock, also a Specialty winner and a dam of Merit as well.

American, Brazilian, Uruguayan and International Champion Hexastar's In Legacy of Ruhlend was bred by the Buchwalds, finishing with a five-point major at a Specialty Show, and a Group winner in Brazil and Uruguay. American and Brazilian Champion Hexastar's Legend of Xanadu was a Best of Breed winner in the United States, and a Group winner in Brazil.

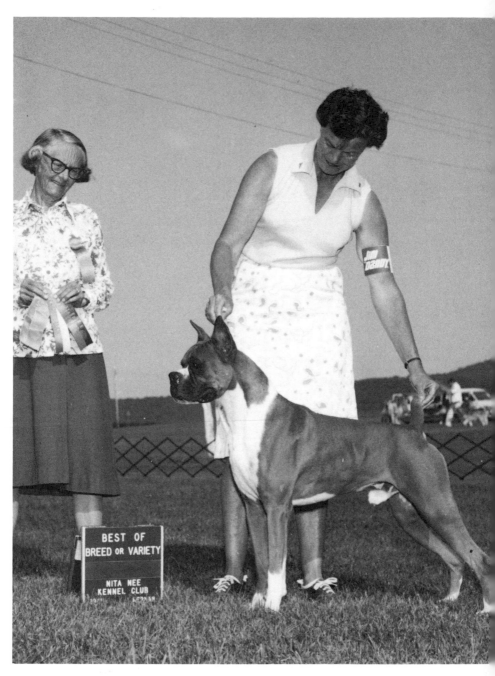

Am. and Braz. Ch. Hexastar's Legend of Xanadu, a Specialty winner and a Group winner, handled here in the United States by Miss Damara Bolte for owner Hexastar Boxers, Mrs. Agnes Buchwald, Brazil.

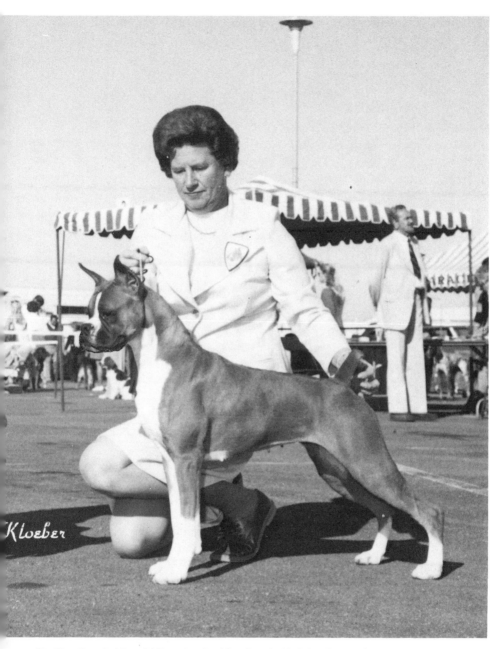

Ch. Merrilane's Kiss Of Fire, by Ch. Merrilane's Holiday Fashion from a daughter of Ch. Eldic's Crusader of Shur Jim (double Landlord breeding), is currently owned by Agnes Buchwald, Hexastar Kennels, Sao Paulo, Brazil. "Kisses" is the dam of Int. Ch. Hexastar's Legend of Xanadu. Eleanor Linderholm Wood handling, and breeder.

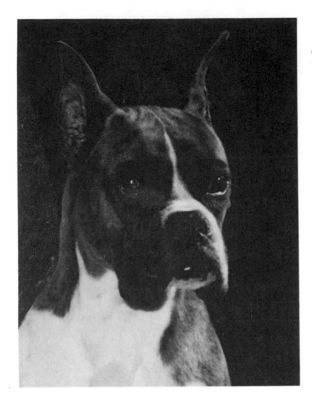

Braz. Ch. Hexastar's Holly Hock, Specialty winner and dam of champions, owned by Hexastar Boxers, Sao Paulo, Brazil.

Then there have been three great bitches brought to Brazil for Hexastar. American, Brazilian and International Champion Merrilane's Kiss of Fire, herself a Best in Show winner, is the dam of Group winners. Champion Ruhlend's Contessa of Abaro, a multi-Best of Breed winner is the dam of three American champions in three litters, and a multi-Group and Best in Show winner, and Champion To-Rini's Allegria's Sequel, a Group winner, is the dam of three Group winners and a multi-Best in Show winner.

The Buchwalds are filled with enthusiasm and future plans. The dogs, as we write, have just been moved to their gorgeous new kennel and now, with the additional room thus provided, it will be possible for Hexastar to expand its breeding program.

Agnes Buchwald is a popular judge both at home and in the United States, making trips to the States pretty much on an annual basis to fulfill her assignments.

126

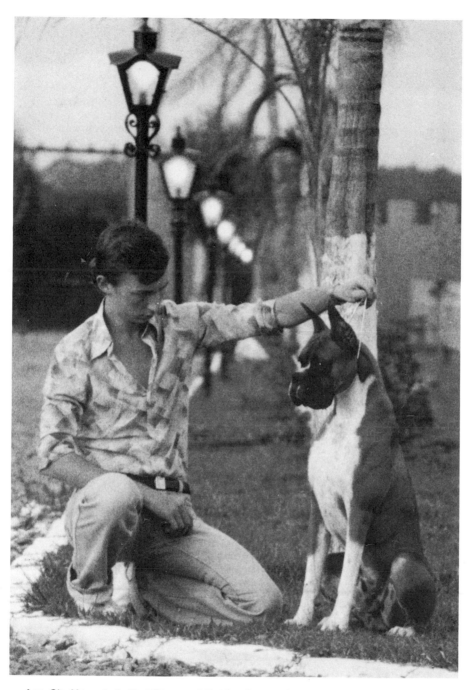

Am. Ch. Hexastar's Ted Stamp of Ruhlend at twelve months of age with Daniel Buchwald, at Hexastar Kennels in Sao Paulo, Brazil.

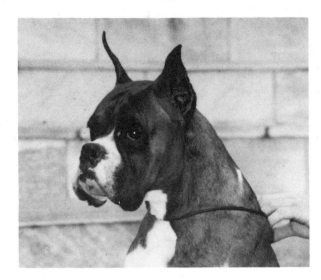

Am. and Braz. Ch. Hexastar's American Graffiti, an all-breed Best in Show winner, owned by Hexastar's Boxers, Mrs. Agnes Buchwald, Sao Paulo, Brazil.

American, Brazilian and International Champion Hexastar's Native Dancer of Ruhlend during 1982 was Number One Brazilian-bred Dog, all breeds, Number One Working Dog, and Number Five all breeds.

Brazilian Champion Hexastar's Royal Mark is a multi-Group winner and the first Brazilian Boxer to be exported to the United States, where his owner is Mr. R. Frohock.

American Champion Hexastar's Ted Stamp of Ruhlend is a multi-Best of Breed winner in the United States. He is from a repeat breeding of that which produced Native Dancer.

American and Brazilian Champion Hexastar's American Graffiti is a Best of Breed winner in the United States and a multi-Best in Show winner, all breeds, in Brazil.

The Buchwalds founded their kennel on some very carefully selected importations. These included Champion Pinebrook's Trade Mark, a Group winner and the sire of more than forty Brazilian champions, including Best in Show and Group winners; also International Champion Burke of Cair Paravel, a Best in Show winner, sire of more than twenty champions in Brazil, the United States and Uruguay, including seven Group winners and two Best in Show winners.

American, Brazilian, International Champion Arriba's Command Performance is a very famous Boxer, the sire of over twenty champions including some in Brazil and the United States; sire of the Number One Boxer in Brazil 1982; sire of Group and Best in Show winners.

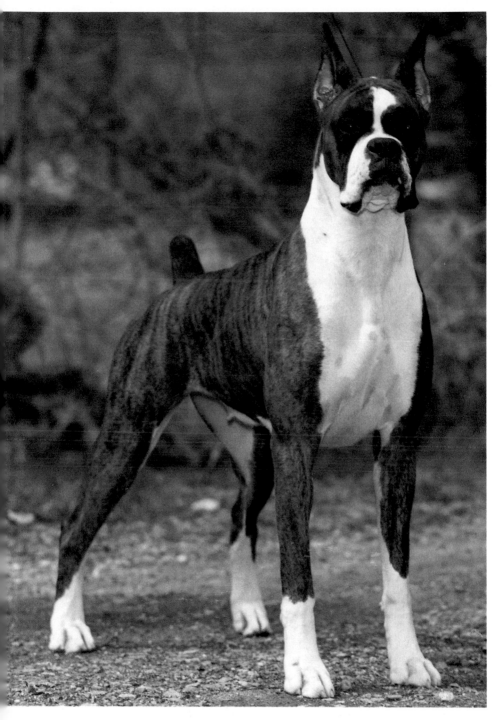

Ch. Turo's Cachet belongs to Leonard Magowitz, New York City, and has an imposing record in hottest eastern competition. Handled by Chic Ceccarini, Westbury, New York.

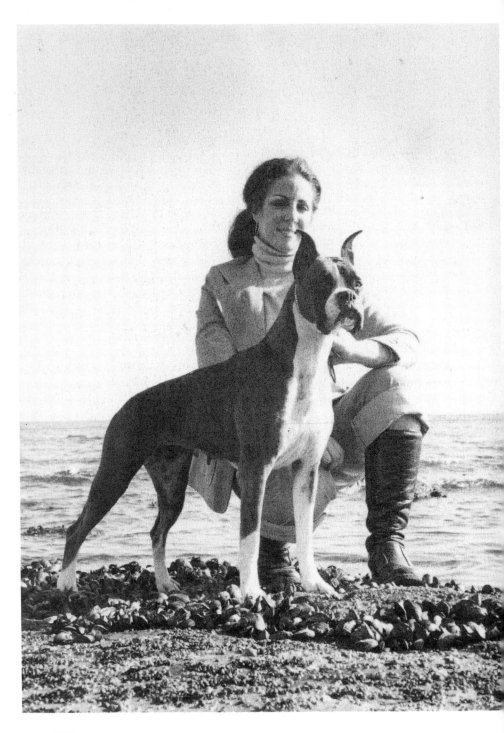

Chapter 7

Standards of the Breed

The *standard of the breed* to which one sees and hears such frequent reference wherever purebred dogs are written of or discussed, is the word picture of what is considered to be the ideal specimen of the breed in question. It outlines, in minute detail, each and every feature of that breed, both in physical characteristics and in temperament, accurately describing the dog from whisker to tail, creating a clear impression of what is to be considered correct or incorrect, the features comprising *breed type,* and the probable temperament and behavior patterns of typical members of that breed.

The standard is the guide for breeders endeavoring to produce quality dogs and for fanciers wishing to learn what is considered beautiful in these dogs; and it is the tool with which judges evaluate and make their decisions in the ring. The dog it describes is the one which we seek, and to which we compare in making our evaluations. It is the result of endless hours spent in dedicated work by knowledgeable members of each breed's parent Specialty Club, resulting from the combined efforts of the club itself, its individual members, and finally the American Kennel Club, by whom official approval must be granted prior to each standard's acceptance, or that of any amendments or changes to it, in the United States. Breed standards are based on intensive study of breed history, earlier standards in the States or in the countries where the dogs originated, or were recognized, prior to introduction to the United States, and the purposes for which the breed was originally created and developed. All such factors have played their part in the drawing up of our present standards.

Opposite: Am. and Can. Ch. Hi-Hat's Cameo of Donessle pictured with Eileen Kaplan, daughter of the owners, is by Ch. Gray Roy's Minstrel Boy ex Can. Ch. Donessle's Miss Fancy (Shadrack daughter). She was the first champion and foundation brood bitch at Hi-Hat Kennels, Jerry and Leni Kaplan, Hamden, Connecticut.

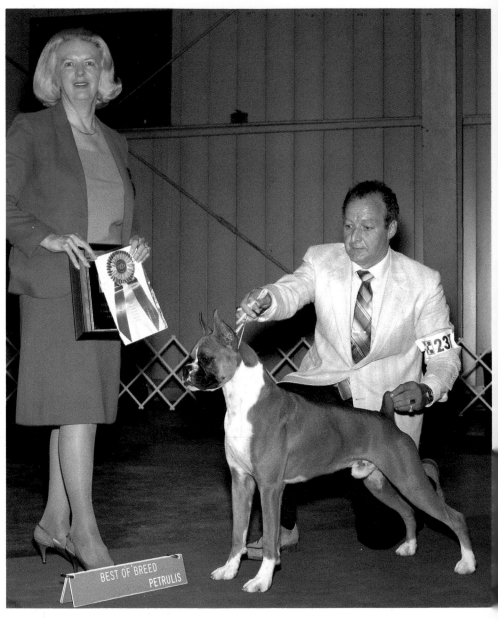

Ch. Hollycrest's Southern Gent winning the breed under judge Mrs. Betty Moore. Owned by Cheryl Colby and Leon De Priest, Hollycrest Boxers, Riverside, Illinois.

Opposite page: Ch. Hi-Hat Nite Star V Cidar Hill owned by Mr. and Mrs. Jerry Kaplan, Hamden, Connecticut. This was the first time Jerry Kaplan had ever handled a dog, and the dog's first show. They took a four-point major that day, which was nice going.

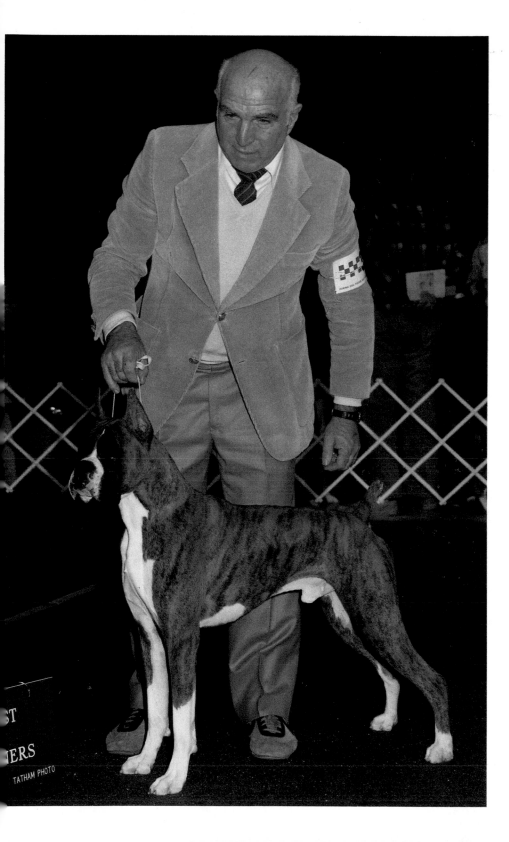

Official American Standard for the Boxer

GENERAL APPEARANCE: The Boxer is a medium-sized, sturdy dog, of square build, with short back, strong limbs, and short, tight-fitting coat. His musculation, well developed, should be clean, hard and appear smooth (not bulging) under taut skin. His movements should denote energy. The gait is firm yet elastic (springy), the stride free and ground-covering, the carriage proud and noble. Developed to serve the multiple purposes of guard, working and escort-dog, he must combine elegance with substance and ample power, not alone for beauty but to ensure the speed, dexterity and jumping ability essential to arduous hike, riding expedition, police or military duty. Only a body whose individual parts are built to withstand the most strenuous efforts, assembled as a complete and harmonious whole, can respond to these combined demands. Therefore, to be at his highest efficiency he must never be plump or heavy and, while equipped for great speed, he must never be racy.

The head imparts to the Boxer a unique individual stamp, peculiar to him alone. It must be in perfect proportion to the body, never small in comparison to the over-all picture. The muzzle is his most distinctive feature, and great value is to be placed on its being of correct form and in absolute proper proportion to the skull.

In judging the Boxer, first consideration should be given to general appearance; next, over-all balance, including the desired proportions of the individual parts of the body to each other, as well as the relation of substance to elegance—to which an attractive color or arresting style may contribute. Special attention is to be devoted to the head, after which the dog's individual components are to be examined for their correct construction and function, and efficiency of gait evaluated.

General Faults: Head not typical, plump, bulldoggy appearance, light bone, lack of balance, bad condition, lack of noble bearing.

HEAD: The beauty of the head depends upon the harmonious proportion of the muzzle to the skull. The muzzle always should appear powerful, never small in its relationship to the skull. The head should be clean, not showing deep wrinkles. Folds will normally appear upon the forehead when the ears are erect, and they are always indicated from the lower edge of the stop running downward on both sides of the muzzle. The dark mask is confined to the muzzle and is in distinct contrast to the color of the head. Any extension of the mask to the skull, other than dark shading around the eyes, creates a somber,

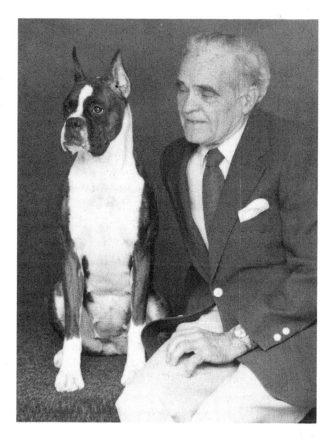

Ch. Turo's Cachet with her friend and handler Chic Ceccarini who piloted her to Number One Boxer in the country while she was being campaigned.

undesirable expression. When white replaces any of the black mask, the path of any upward extension should be between the eyes. The muzzle is powerfully developed in length, width and depth. It is not pointed, narrow, short or shallow. Its shape is influenced first through the formation of both jawbones, second through the placement of the teeth, and third through the texture of the lips.

The Boxer is normally undershot. Therefore, the lower jaw protrudes beyond the upper and curves slightly upward. The upper jaw is broad where attached to the skull and maintains this breadth except for a very slight tapering to the front. The incisor teeth of the lower jaw are in a straight line, the canines preferably up front in the same line to give the jaw the greatest possible width. The line of incisors in the upper jaw is slightly convex toward the front. The upper corner incisors should fit snugly back of the lower canine teeth on each side, reflecting the symmetry essential to the creation of a sound, non-slip bite.

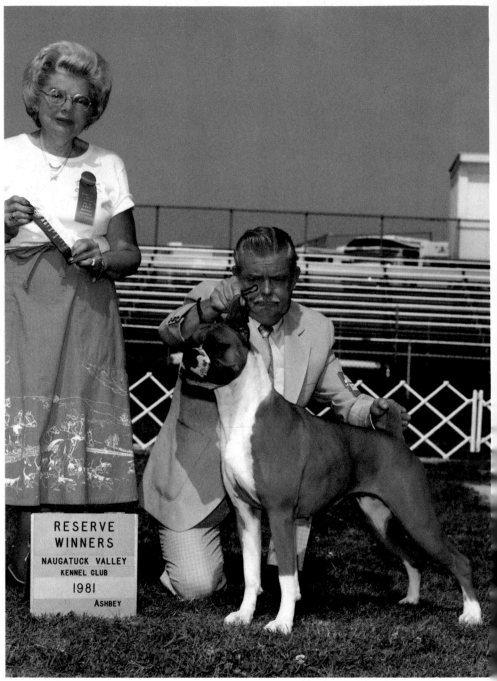

Ch. Flying Apache Uprising, by Ch. Flying Apache Regal Roccoco ex Ch. Brier-court's Independence, winning under judge Anna Katherine Nicholas. Bred by Patricia Adams, owned and handled by Russell K. Anderson.

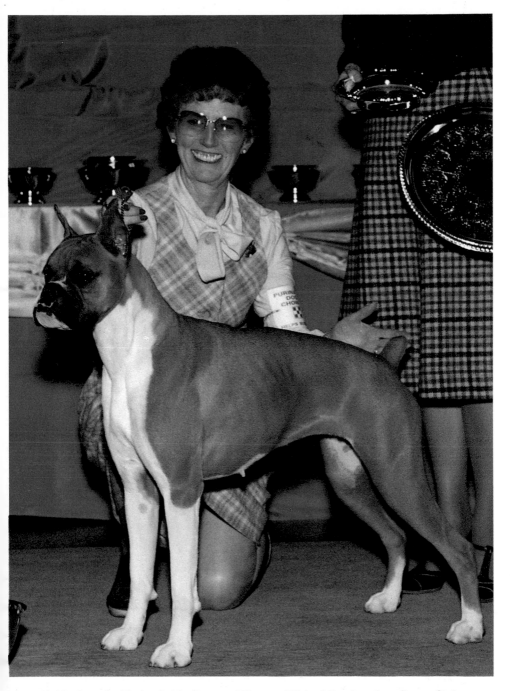

Heldenbrand's Blythe Spirit, Reserve Winners Bitch at the American Boxer Club Regional 1981, daughter of Ch. Holly Lane's Dream Peddler, C.D. ex Holly Lane's Aureate Halo, C.D. Owner-handled by Elvinia Heldenbrand, Manhattan, Kansas.

The lips, which complete the formation of the muzzle, should meet evenly. The upper lip is thick and padded, filling out the frontal space created by the projection of the lower jaw. It rests on the edge of the lower lip and, laterally, is supported by the fangs (canines) of the lower jaw. Therefore these fangs must stand far apart, and be of good length so that the front surface of the muzzle is broad and squarish and, when viewed from the side, forms an obtuse angle with the topline of the muzzle. Over-protrusion of the overlip or underlip is undesirable. The chin should be perceptible when viewed from the sides as well as from the front without being over-repandous (rising above the bite line) as in the Bulldog. The Boxer must not show teeth or tongue when the mouth is closed. Excessive flews are not desirable.

The top of the skull is slightly arched, not rotund, flat, nor noticeably broad and the occiput not too pronounced. The forehead forms a distinct stop with the topline of the muzzle, which must not be forced back into the forehead like that of a Bulldog. It should not slant down (down-faced), nor should it be dished, although the tip of the nose should lie somewhat higher than the root of the muzzle. The forehead shows just a slight furrow between the eyes. The cheeks, though covering powerful masseter muscles compatible with the strong set of teeth, should be relatively flat and not bulge, maintaining the clean lines of the skull. They taper into the muzzle in a slight, graceful curve. The ears are set at the highest points to the sides of the skull, cut rather long without too broad a shell, protruding or deep-set, are encircled by dark hair, and should impart an alert, intelligent expression. Their mood-mirroring quality combined with the mobile skin furrowing of the forehead gives the Boxer head its unique degree of expressiveness. The nose is broad and black, very slightly turned up; the nostrils broad with the nasolabial line running between them down through the upper lip, which, however, must not be split.

Faults: Lack of nobility and expression, somber face, unserviceable bite. Pinscher or Bulldog head, sloping topline of muzzle, muzzle too light for skull, too pointed a bite (snipy). Teeth or tongue showing with mouth closed, driveling, split upper lip. Poor ear carriage, light ("Bird of Prey") eyes.

NECK: Round, of ample length, not too short; strong, muscular and clean throughout, without dewlap; distinctly marked nape with an elegant arch running down to the back. *Fault:* Dewlap.

BODY: In profile, the build is of square proportions in that a horizontal line from the front of the forechest to the rear projection of the upper thigh should equal a vertical line dropped from the top of the withers to the ground.

CHEST AND FOREQUARTERS: The brisket is deep, reaching down to the elbows; the depth of the body at the lowest point of the brisket equals half the height of the dog at the withers. The ribs, extending far to the rear, are well arched but not barrel-shaped. Chest of fair width and forechest well defined, being easily visible from the side. The loins are short and muscular; the lower stomach line, lightly tucked up, blends into a graceful curve to the rear. The shoulders are long and sloping, close-lying and not excessively covered with muscle. The upper arm is long, closely approaching a right angle to the shoulder-blade. The forelegs, viewed from the front, are straight, stand parallel to each other and have strong, firmly joined bones. The elbows should not press too closely to the chest wall or stand off visibly from it. The forearm is straight, long and firmly muscled. The pastern joint is clearly defined but not distended. The pastern is strong and distinct, slightly slanting, but standing almost perpendicular to the ground. The dewclaws may be removed as a safety precaution. Feet should be compact, turning neither in nor out, with tightly arched toes (cat feet) and tough pads. *Faults:* Chest too broad, too shallow or too deep in front; loose or over-muscled shoulders; chest hanging between the shoulders; tied-in or bowed-out elbows; turning feet; hare feet; hollow flanks; hanging stomach.

BACK: The withers should be clearly defined as the highest point of the back; the whole back short, straight and muscular with a firm topline. *Faults:* Roach back, sway back, thin lean back, long narrow loins, weak union with croup.

HINDQUARTERS: Strongly muscled with angulation in balance with that of forequarters. The thighs broad and curved, the breech musculature hard and strongly developed. Croup slightly sloped, flat and broad. Tail attachment high rather than low. Tail clipped, carried upward. Pelvis long and, in females especially, broad. Upper and lower thigh long, leg well angulated with a clearly defined, well-letdown hock joint. In standing position, the leg below the hock joint (metatarsus) should be practically perpendicular to the ground, with a slight rearward slope permissible. Viewed from behind, the hind legs should be straight, with the hock joints leaning neither in nor out. The metatarsus should be short, clean and strong, supported by powerful rear pads. The rear toes just a little longer than the front toes, but similar in all other respects. Dewclaws, if any, may be removed.

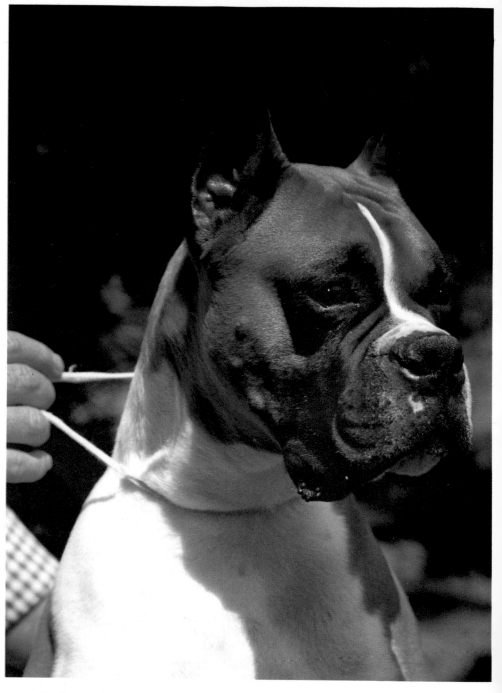

Ch. Sunset Spirit of Five T's owned by Bruce and Jeannie Korsan, Laurel Hill Boxers, Oyster Bay, New York.

Opposite page: Ch. Sunset Spirit of Five T's owned by Bruce and Jeannie Korsan, Laurel Hill Boxers, Oyster Bay, New York.

Ch. Sakura's Cinnamon Spice owned by Donald W. Edwards, M.D., Fullerton, California.

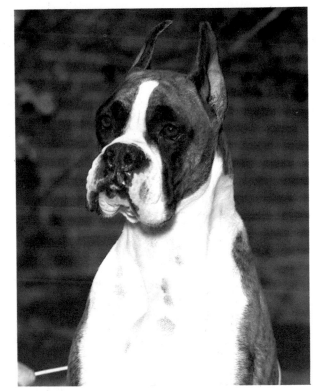

Ch. Spring Willow's Suzy Q, foundation bitch at Evergreen Kennels, the dam of three champions, owned by Jane Nolt Flowers. Handled by Ramon and Dorothy McNulty.

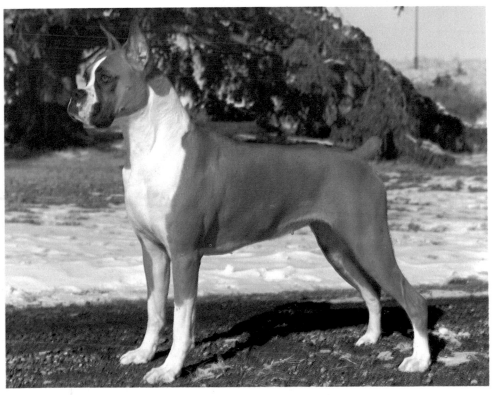

Faults: Too rounded, too narrow, or falling off of croup; low-set tail; higher in back than in front; steep, stiff, or too slightly angulated hindquarters; light thighs; bowed or crooked legs; cowhocks; over-angulated hock joints (sickle hocks); long metatarsus (high hocks); hare feet; hindquarters too far under or too far behind.

GAIT: Viewed from the side, proper front and rear angulation is manifested in a smoothly efficient, level-backed, ground-covering stride with powerful drive emanating from a freely operating rear. Although the front legs do not contribute impelling power, adequate "reach" should be evident to prevent interference, overlap, or "sidewinding" (crabbing). Viewed from the front, the shoulders should remain trim and the elbows not flare out. The legs are parallel until gaiting narrows the track in proportion to increasing speed, then the legs come in under the body but should never cross. The line from the shoulder down through the leg should remain straight, although not necessarily perpendicular to the ground. Viewed from the rear, a Boxer's breech should not roll. The hind feet should "dig in" and track relatively true with the front. Again, as speed increases, the normally broad rear track will become narrower. *Faults:* Stilted or inefficient gait, pounding, paddling or flailing out of front legs, rolling or waddling gait, tottering hock joints, crossing over or interference—front or rear, lack of smoothness.

HEIGHT: Adult males — 22½ to 25 inches; females — 21 to 23½ inches at the withers. Males should not go under the minimum nor females over the maximum.

COAT: Short, shiny, lying smooth and tight to the body.

COLOR: The colors are fawn and brindle. Fawn in various shades from light tan to dark deer red or mahogany, the deeper colors preferred. The brindle variety should have clearly defined black stripes on fawn background. White markings on fawn or brindle dogs are not to be rejected and are often very attractive, but must be limited to one third of the ground color and are not desirable on the back of the torso proper. On the face, white may replace a part or all of the otherwise essential black mask. However, these white markings should be of such distribution as to enhance and not detract from true Boxer expression.

CHARACTER AND TEMPERAMENT: These are of paramount importance in the Boxer. Instinctively a "hearing" guard dog, his bearing is alert, dignified and self-assured, even at rest. In the show ring, his behavior should exhibit constrained animation. With family and friends, his temperament is fundamentally playful, yet patient and stoical with children. Deliberate and wary with strangers, he will exhibit curiosity, but, most importantly, fearless courage and tenacity if threatened. However, he responds promptly to friendly overtures when honestly rendered. His intelligence, loyal affection, and tractability to discipline make him a highly desirable companion. *Faults:* Lack of dignity and alertness, shyness, cowardice, treachery and viciousness (belligerency toward other dogs should not be considered viciousness). DISQUALIFICATION: Boxers with white or black ground color, or entirely white or black, or any color other than fawn or brindle. (White markings, when present, must not exceed one third of the ground color.)

Approved December 12th 1967

Ch. Box M Tropic Storm, by Ch. Merrilane's April Showers ex Box M Happy Hawaiian, winning Best in Show at the Windward Hawaiian Dog Fanciers Association judged by Fernandez Cartwright, Roland Adameck presenting the trophy, Mrs. Wood handling and owned by Lois Matthews of Kailua, Hawaii, and Eleanor Linderholm Wood of California.

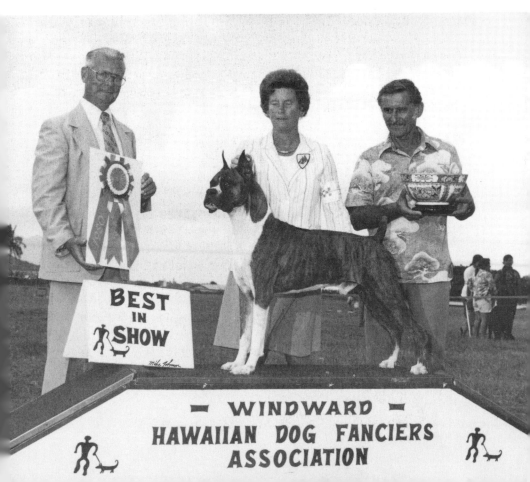

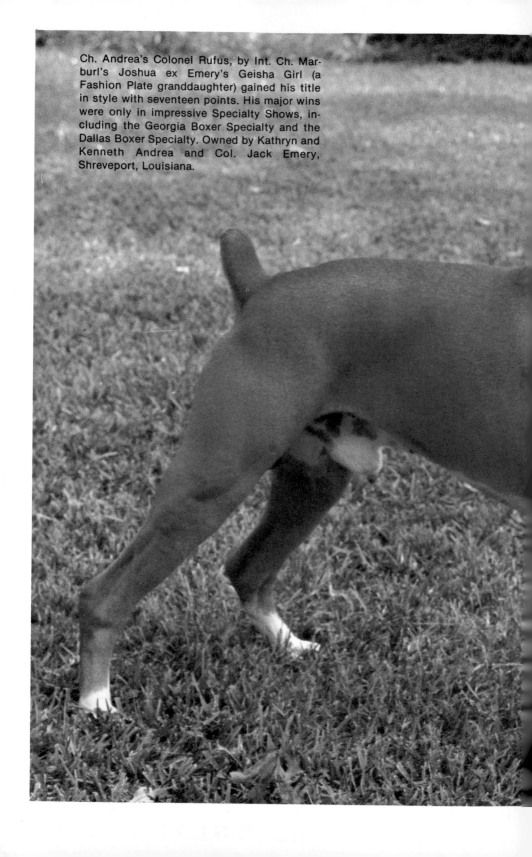

Ch. Andrea's Colonel Rufus, by Int. Ch. Marburl's Joshua ex Emery's Geisha Girl (a Fashion Plate granddaughter) gained his title in style with seventeen points. His major wins were only in impressive Specialty Shows, including the Georgia Boxer Specialty and the Dallas Boxer Specialty. Owned by Kathryn and Kenneth Andrea and Col. Jack Emery, Shreveport, Louisiana.

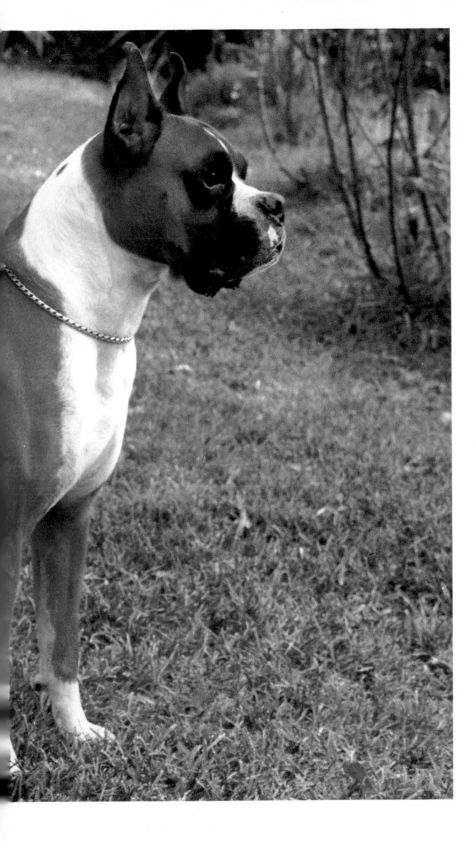

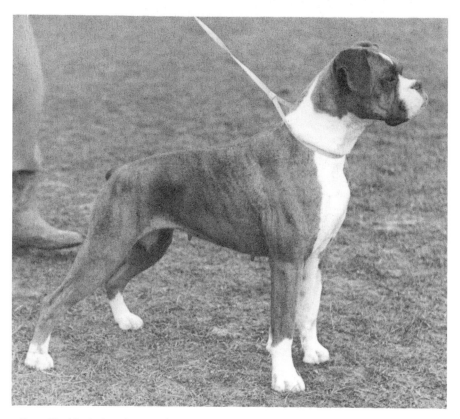

Eng. Ch. Marbelton Pewter Pot, sire Ch. Marbleton Top Mark, owned by Mrs. M. Hambleton, Ormskirk, Lancs, England.

Kennel Club (Great Britain) Standard for the Boxer

CHARACTERISTICS: The character of the Boxer is of the greatest importance and demands the most careful attention. He is renowed from olden times for his great love and faithfulness to his master and household, his alertness and fearless courage as a defender and protector. The Boxer is docile but distrustful of strangers. He is bright and friendly in play but brave and determined when roused. His intelligence and willing tractability, his modesty, and cleanliness make him a highly desirable family dog and cheerful companion. He is the soul of honesty and loyalty. He is never false or treacherous even in his old age.

146

GENERAL APPEARANCE: The Boxer is a medium sized, sturdy, smooth haired dog of short square figure and strong limb. The musculation is clean and powerfully developed, and should stand out plastically from under the skin. Movement of the Boxer should be alive with energy. His gait, although firm, is elastic. The stride free and roomy; carriage proud and noble. As a service and guard dog he must combine a considerable degree of elegance with the substance and power essential to his duties; those of an enduring escort dog whether with horse, bicycle or carriage and as a splendid jumper. Only a body whose individual limbs are built to withstand the most strenuous "mechanical" effort and assembled as a complete and harmonious whole, can respond to such demands. Therefore to be at its highest efficiency, the Boxer must never be plump or heavy. Whilst equipped for great speed, it must not be racy. When judging the Boxer the first thing to be considered is general appearance, the relation of substance to elegance and the desired relationship of the individual parts of the body to each other. Consideration, too, must be given to colour. After these, the individual parts should be examined for their correct construction and their functions. Special attention to be devoted to the head.

HEAD AND SKULL: The head imparts to the Boxer a unique individual stamp peculiar to the breed. It must be in perfect proportion to his body; above all it must never be too light. The muzzle is the most distinctive feature. The greatest value is to be placed on its being of correct form and in absolute proportion to the skull. The beauty of the head depends upon the harmonious proportion between the muzzle and the skull. From whatever direction the head is viewed, whether from the front, from the top or from the side, the muzzle should always appear in correct relationship to the skull. That means that the head should never appear too small or too large. The length of the muzzle to the whole of the head should be as 1 is to 3. The head should not show deep wrinkles. Normally wrinkles will spring up on the top of the skull when the dog is alert. Folds are always indicated from the root of the nose running downwards on both sides of the muzzle. The dark mask is confined to the muzzle. It must be in distinct relief to the colour of the head so that the face will not have a "sombre" expression. The muzzle must be powerfully developed in length, in breadth and in height. It must not be pointed or narrow; short or shallow. Its shape is influenced through the formation of both jaw-bones, the placement of teeth in the jaw-bones, and through the

147

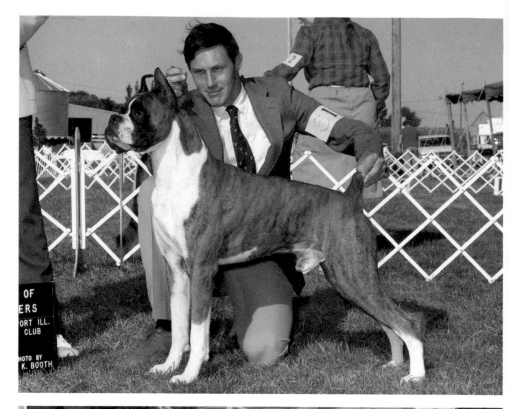

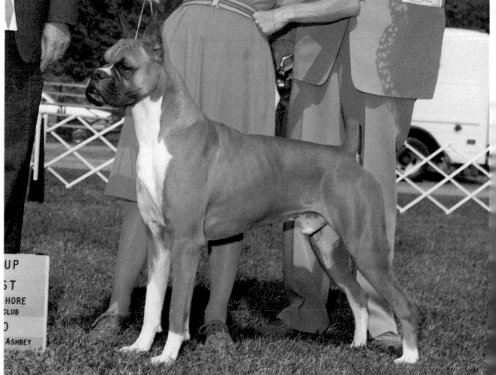

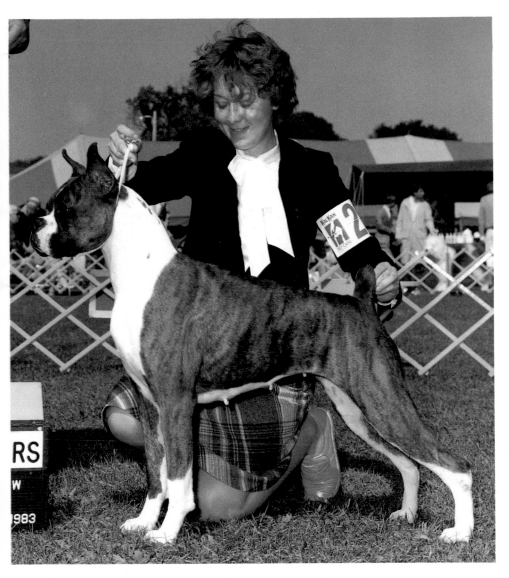

Ch. Jacquet's Dancing Star, by Ch. Jacquet's Zephan ex Susan's Lucy Mid-nightstar, taking Best of Winners for Dr. Hideaki Nakazawa, Tokyo, Japan.

Opposite page: *(Top)* Vihabra's Magnificent Obsession, by Ch. Merrilane's Vihabra Gold'n Key ex Shur Jim's Spitfire, has fifteen points but needs a major to finish as we go to press. Handled by Brian Meyer and co-owned by Maxine and Don Evans, St. Paul, Minnesota, with Virginia Bradley, Vihabra Boxers. *(Bottom)* Ch. Moreleen's Meralota V Imladris, by Ch. Sir Lancelot of Box Run ex Moreleen's ESP, winning the Group at North Shore in 1980. Bred by Moreleen Goneau. Co-owned by Susan J. Campbell and Gerard F. Hughes.

quality of the lips. The top of the skull should be slightly arched. It should not be so short that it is rotund, too flat, or too broad. The occiput should not be too pronounced. The forehead should form a distinct stop with the top line of the muzzle, which should not be forced back into the forehead like that of a Bulldog. Neither should it slope away (downfaced). The tip of the nose should lie somewhat higher than the root of the muzzle. The forehead should show a suggestion of furrow which, however, should never be too deep, especially between the eyes. Corresponding with the powerful set of teeth, the cheeks accordingly should be well developed without protruding from the head with "too bulgy" an appearance. For preference they should taper into the muzzle in a slight, graceful curve. The nose should be broad and black, very slightly turned up. The nostrils should be broad with a naso-labial line between them. The two jaw-bones should not terminate in a normal perpendicular level in the front but the lower jaw should protrude beyond the upper jaw and bend slightly upwards. The Boxer is normally undershot. The upper jaw should be broad where attached to the skull, and maintain this breadth except for a very slight tapering to the front.

EYES: The eyes should be dark brown; not too small or protruding; not deep set. They should disclose an expression of energy and intelligence, but should never appear gloomy, threatening or piercing. The eyes must have a dark rim.

EARS: Some American and Continental Boxers are cropped and are ineligible for competition under Kennel Club Regulations. The Boxer's natural ears are defined as: moderate in size (small rather than large), thin to the touch, set on wide apart at the highest points of the sides of the skull and lying flat and close to the cheek when in repose. When the dog is alert the ears should fall forward with a definite crease.

MOUTH: The canine teeth should be as widely separated as possible. The incisors (6) should all be in one row, with no projection of the middle teeth. In the upper jaw they should be slightly concave. In the lower they should be in a straight line. Both jaws should be very wide in front; bite powerful and sound, the teeth set in the most normal possible arrangement. The lips complete the formation of the muzzle. The upper lip should be thick and padded and fill out the hollow space in front formed by the projection of the lower jaw and be supported by the fangs of the jaw. These fangs must stand as far apart as possible and be of good length so that the front surface of the muzzle becomes broad and almost square; to form an obtuse (rounded) angle with the

150

top line of the muzzle. The lower edge of the upper lip should rest on the edge of the lower lip. The repandous (bent upward) part of the under-jaw with the lower lip (sometimes called the chin) must not rise above the front of the upper lip. On the other hand it should not disappear under it. It must, however, be plainly perceptible when viewed from the front as well as the side, without protruding and bending upward as in the English Bulldog. The teeth of the under-jaw should not be seen when the mouth is closed, neither should the tongue show when the mouth is closed.

NECK: The neck should be not too thick and short but of ample length, yet strong, round, muscular and clean-cut throughout. There should be a distinctly marked nape and an elgant arch down to the back.

FOREQUARTERS: The chest should be deep and reach down to the elbows. The depth of the chest should be half the height of the dog at the withers. The ribs should be well arched but not barrel-shaped. They should extend far to the rear. The loins should be short, close and taut and slightly tucked up. The lower stomach line should blend into an elegant curve to the rear. The shoulders should be long and sloping, close lying but not excessively covered with muscle. The upper arm should be long and form a right-angle to the shoulder-blade. The forelegs when seen from the front should be straight, parallel to each other and have strong, firmly articulated (joined) bones. The elbows should not press too closely to the chest-wall or stand off too far from it. The underarm should be perpendicular, long and firmly muscled. The pastern joint of the foreleg should be clearly defined, but not distended. The pastern should be short, slightly slanting and almost perpendicular to the ground.

BODY: The body viewed in profile should be of square appearance. The length of the body from the front of the chest to the rear of the body should equal the height from the ground to the top of the shoulder, giving the Boxer a short-coupled, square profile. The torso rests on trunk-like straight legs with strong bones. The withers should be clearly defined. The whole back should be short, straight, broad, and very muscular.

HINDQUARTERS: The hindquarters should be strongly muscled. The musculation should be hard and stand out plastically through the skin. The thighs should not be narrow and flat but broad and curved. The breech musculation should also be strongly developed. The croup should be slightly sloped, flat arched and broad, the pelvis should be long and, in females especially, broad. The upper and lower thighs

151

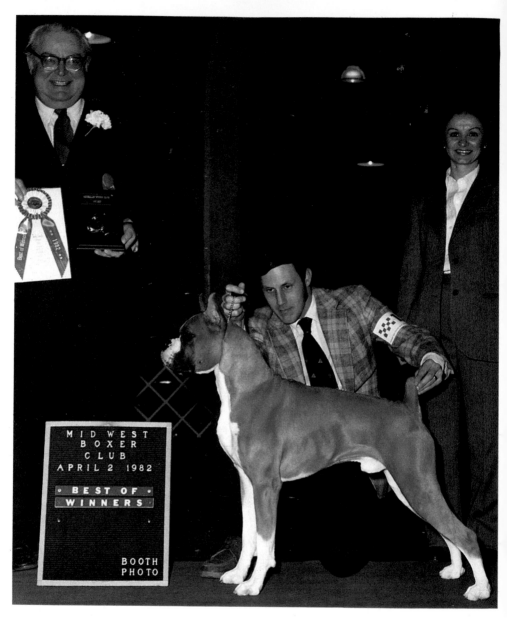

Ch. C.C. Bobber of Bethal, by Ch. Regail Bo-Jack ex Bethal's Pretty Direct, was bred by M. Dunnan and B. Guerra. Owned by Cheryl Colby, Hollycrest Boxers, Riverside, Illinois. Handled here by Brian Meyer to Best of Winners at the Mid-West Boxer Club Specialty in April 1982.

Opposite page: Ch. Treceder's Sweet Stuff, by Phil-Dee's Prompt Appointment ex Ch. Treceder's Candy Cane, completed her championship with all major wins. Bred by Treceder Kennels. Owned by Ginny Crippen.

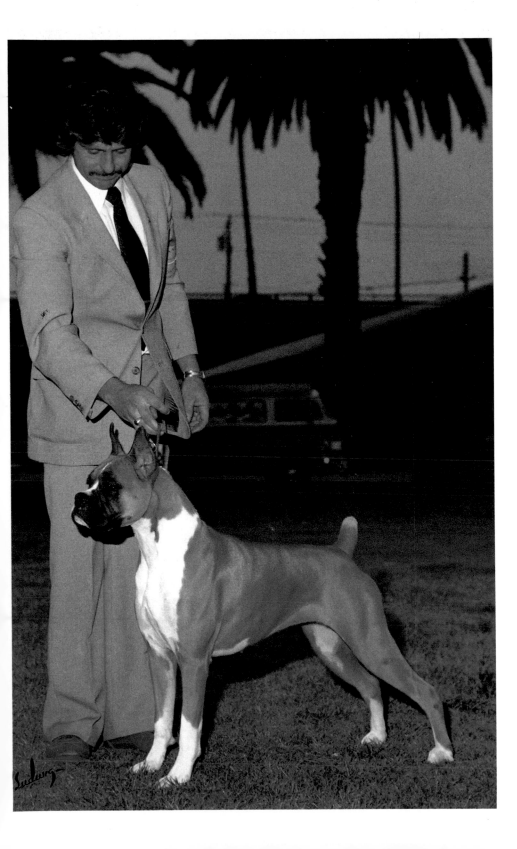

should be long. The hip and knee joints should have as much angle as possible. In a standing position the knee should reach so far forward that it would meet a vertical line drawn from the hip protuberance to the floor. The hock angle should be about 140 degrees; the lower part of the foot at a slight slope of about 95 to 100 degrees from the hock joint to the floor; that is, not completely vertical. Seen from behind, the hind legs should be straight. The hocks should be clean and not distended, supported by powerful rear pads.

FEET: The feet should be small with tightly-arched toes (cat feet) and hard soles. The rear toes should be just a little longer than the front toes, but similar in all other respects.

TAIL: The tail attachment should be high. The tail should be docked and carried upwards and should not be more than 2 inches long.

COAT: The coat should be short and shiny, lying smooth and tight to the body.

Ch. Marbelton Don't Dilly Dally, sire Australian Ch. Marbelton Van Der Veer, owned by Mrs. M. Hambleton, Ormskirk, Lancashire, England.

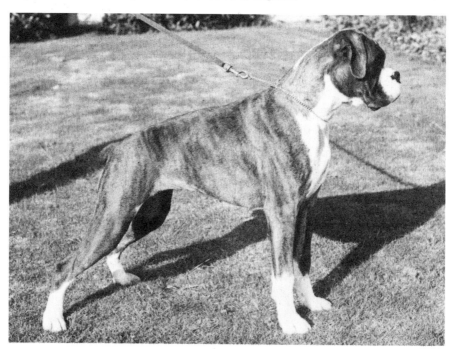

COLOUR: The permissible colours are fawn, brindle and fawn in various shades from light yellow to dark deer red. The brindle variety should have black stripes on a golden-yellow or red-brown background. The stripes should be clearly defined and above all should not be grey or dirty. Stripes that do not cover the whole of the top are not desirable. White markings are not undesirable, in fact, they are often very attractive in appearance. The black mask is essential but when white stretches over the muzzle, naturally that portion of the black mask disappears. It is not possible to get black toe-nails with white feet. It is desirable, however, to have an even distribution of head markings.

WEIGHT AND SIZE: Dogs: 22 to 24 inches at the withers. Bitches: 21 to 23 inches at the withers. Heights above or below these figures not to be encouraged. Dogs around 23 inches should weigh about 66 lbs. and Bitches of about 21 inches should weigh about 62 lbs.

FAULTS: Viciousness; treachery; unreliability; lack of temperament; cowardice. Head: a head that is not typical. A plump, bulldoggy appearance. Light bone. Lack of proportion. Bad physical condition. Lack of nobility and expression. "Sombre" face. Unserviceable bite whether due to disease or to faulty tooth placement. Pinscher or Bulldog head. Showing the teeth or the tongue. A sloping top line of the muzzle. Too pointed or too light a bite (snipy). Eyes: visible conjunctiva (Haw). Light eyes. Ears: flying ears; rose ears; semi-erect or erect ears. Neck: dewlap. Front: too broad and low in front; loose shoulders; chest hanging between the shoulders; hare feet; turned legs and toes. Body: carp (roach) back; sway back; thin, lean back; long narrow, sharp-sunken in loins. Weak union with the croup, hollow flanks; hanging stomach. Hindquarters: a falling off or too arched or narrow croup. A low-set tail; higher in back than in front; steep, stiff or too little angulation of the hindquarters; light thighs; cow-hocks; bow-legs; hind dewclaws; soft hocks, narrow heel, tottering, waddling gait; hare's feet; hindquarters too far under or too far behind. Colour; Boxers with white or black ground colour, or entirely white or black or any other colour than fawn or brindle. (White markings are allowed but must not exceed one-third [⅓] of the ground colour).

NOTE: Male animals should have two apparently normal testicles fully descended into the scrotum.

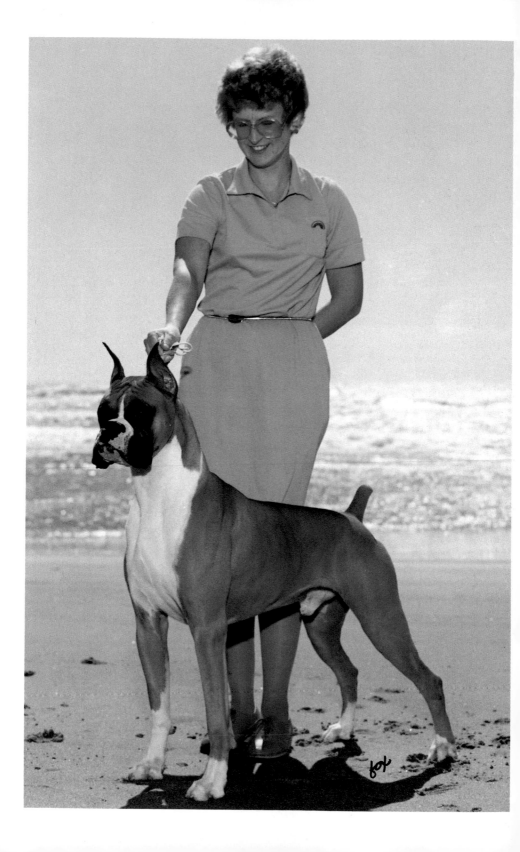

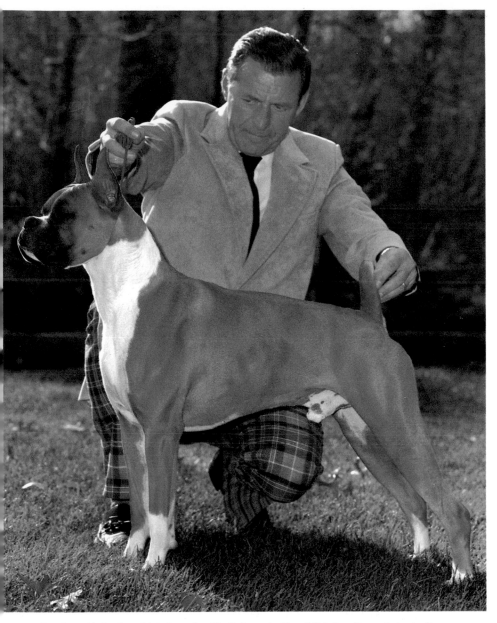

Ch. Cher Kei's Son-Of-A-Gun, by Ch. Salgray's Good Grief ex Baron's Lady Come Lately, owned by Cheryl and Keith Robbins. Photo courtesy of Robert S. Forsyth.

Opposite page: Ch. Merrilane's Salute To April, Reserve Winners at the American Boxer Club Specialty in May 1981, was by Ch. Merrilane's April Holiday ex daughter of Champion Aracrest Jered; current owner, Paul Scott, Kennel Formula, Stabekk, Norway.

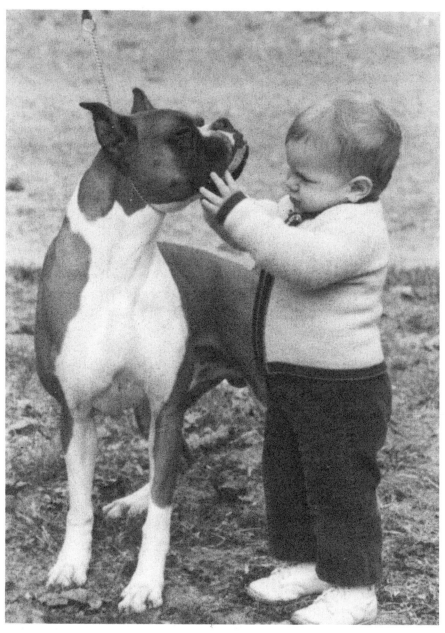

Andrew Korsan, Bruce and Jeannie Korsan's young son, with his good friend "Bosco" (Ch. Sunset Image of Five T's).

Chapter 8

Versatility of the Boxer

The Boxer is a very adaptable and pleasant dog to have around. He is quiet and easy going, while at the same time full of fun and seeming almost to possess a sense of humor; but he does not "bug" you for attention, and is not hyperactive as is the case with some breeds.

It would be impossible to improve upon a Boxer as an all-around family dog. He loves people and becomes deeply devoted to his family, and seems to adapt himself perfectly to your every mood. He is a formidable watch dog, and a reliable one, at the same time being extremely manageable by his family; but his size and dignity can be quite impressive and the sight of him on guard duty so to speak is a fine deterrent to those who are bent on mischief. Also an alert dog, he is quick to sound the alarm should he sense danger.

Boxers are not in the least destructive. They love family life and conduct themselves accordingly. Although they enjoy snoozing on the sofa, you are not at all likely to come home and find parts of it eaten— that just is not how a Boxer behaves.

Boxers are not quarrelsome and seldom start problems with other animals, although the construction of their powerful jaws makes them formidable opponents should some other dog be so imprudent as to start something with them. They associate well with other pets in your own household, very seldom permit themselves to engage in hostilities with neighboring animals. That sort of thing is just beneath their dignity!

Whether you live in the city, suburbs or country, Boxers adapt themselves to share your life. They are an easy dog to keep in town as they are quiet and walking with you on the street behave sedately, while at the same time providing you with excellent protection by their very presence. If one must walk a dog on city streets, especially at night, it is comforting to have one who bears an air of warning not to approach you should any prospective muggers happen along!

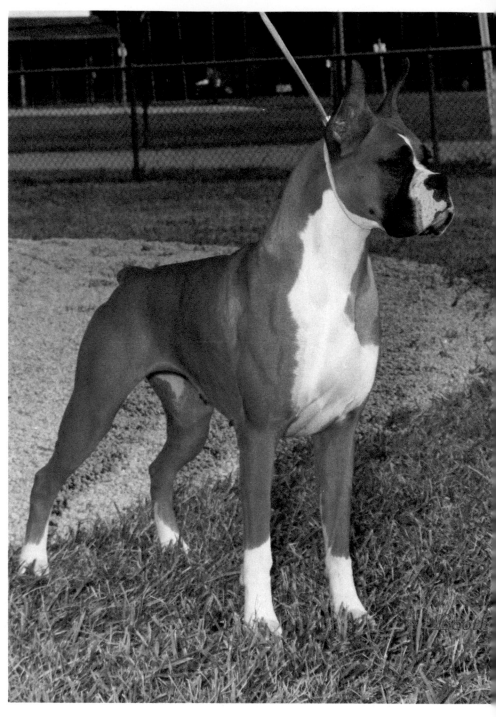

The current big winner owned by Mr. and Mrs. Daniel Hamilburg is Champion Salgray's Showstopper, handled to an impressive Group and Best in Show record by Stanley Flowers.

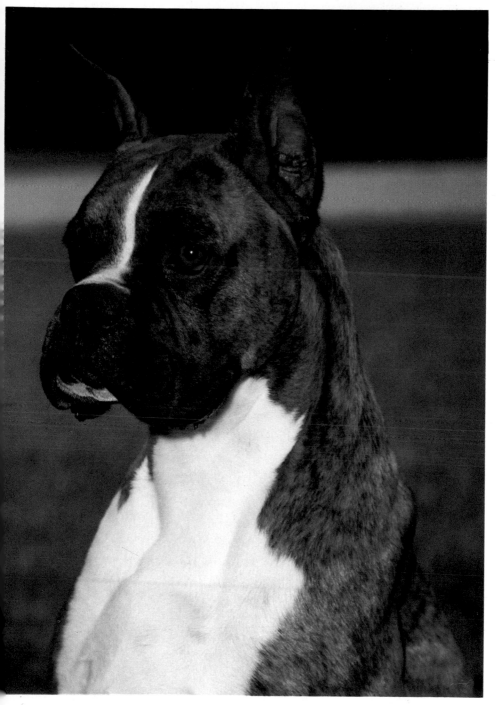

Ch. Laurel Hill's Arabian Knight, by Ch. Merrilane's April Fashion ex Brayshaw's Lady Brat, owned by Bruce and Jeannie Korsan, Laurel Hill Boxers, Oyster Bay, New York.

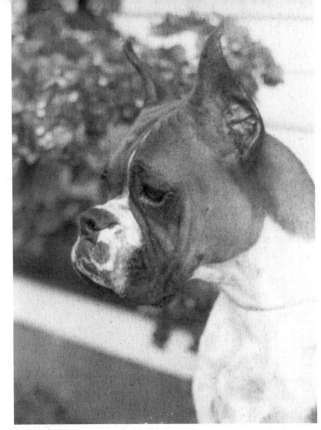

Head study of Ch. Beau Monde Boquet of Box M owned by Richard Beauchamp of Hollywood, California and Lois Matthews of Kailua, Hawaii.

Aust. Ch. That's Right of Panfield, United Kingdom import, by Eng. Ch. Steynmere Summer Gold ex Eng. Ch. Gold Bangle of Panfield is owned by Mr. D.A. Strachan, Thasrite Boxers, Murrumbateman, New South Wales, Australia.

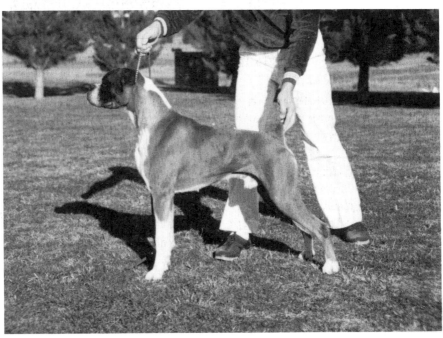

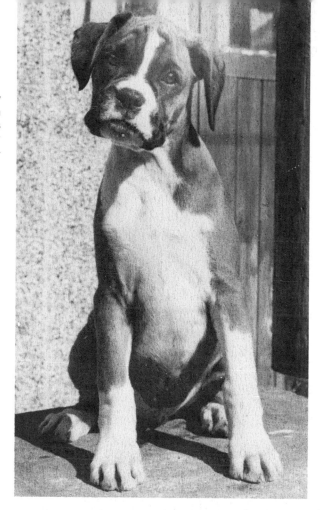

Winuwuk Samson, by Ch. Kinbra Uncle Sam of Winuwuk, was bred and is owned by M. and I. Ward-Davies.

Boxers are great dogs with children, seeming utterly devoted to them. You will note how many youngsters show the breed in Junior Showmanship as an example. But even simply as pets, they are super companions for a youngster, patient and gentle and amazingly keen about sensing danger should any arise, and alerting you to it.

Boxers are very trainable, being intelligent and anxious to please. They do well in obedience for this reason, making working with them fun, and they are a nice breed to show, being docile and easily manageable.

They have been successful in guide dog work and have proven very adaptable in this regard.

As frosting on the cake, there is the pride of ownership in having so handsome a dog as the Boxer. Certainly he is a beautiful animal, with his unique and noble head, his striking coloring, and his well balanced powerful elegance.

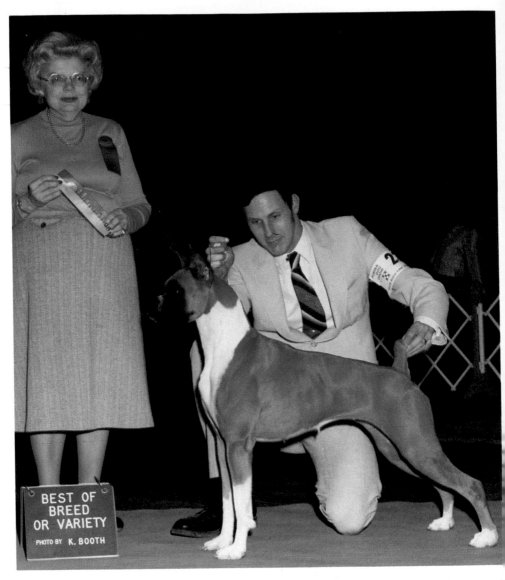

BEST OF
BREED
OR VARIETY

PHOTO BY K. BOOTH

Ch. Holly Lane's Sunflower, here winning Best of Breed under judge Anna Katherine Nicholas, was bred by Mr. and Mrs. John Deckard and is owned by Lorraine C. Meyer, My-R Boxers, Rockford, Illinois and Eileen McClintock, Holly Lane, Topeka, Kansas.

Opposite page: Ch. Mac-A-Nor's Sirocco Suzi Q had a great show record on the West Coast from 1979 through 1982, including Group and Specialty Show wins and 38 Bests of Breed. A daughter of Ch. Notelrac's Sirocco ex Diamond's Gay Mitzi of Mac-A-Nor, she was born in May 1977. Breeders, C.N. Elnora McLean; owners, Robert H. and Shirley L. Hickam; and handler Cheryl Cates.

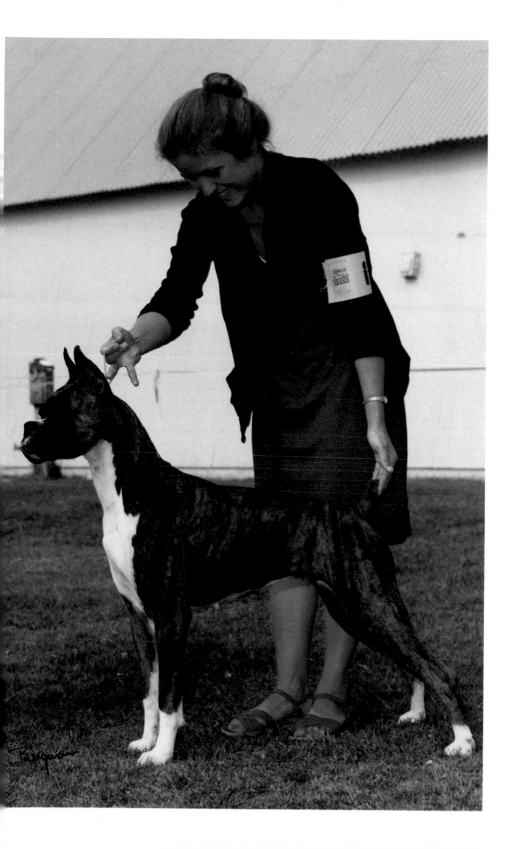

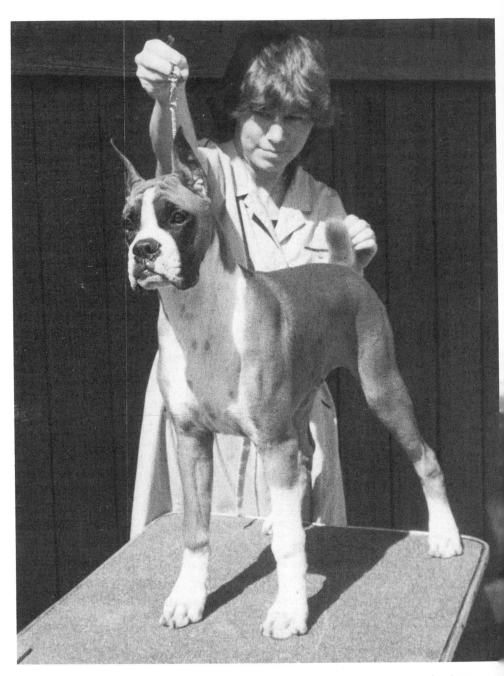

Seawest Yuri-Nuff, by Ch. Box M Irving de Keefo ex Box M Sabra de Keefer, is a most promising four month old puppy owned by Lois Matthews and Donna Keefer, Kailua, Hawaii.

Chapter 9

The Purchase of Your Boxer

Careful consideration should be given to what breed of dog you wish to own prior to your purchase of one. If several breeds are attractive to you, and you are undecided which you prefer, learn all you can about the characteristics of each before making your decision. As you do so, you are thus preparing yourself to make an intelligent choice; and this is very important when buying a dog who will be, with reasonable luck, a member of your household for at least a dozen years or more. Obviously since you are reading this book, you have decided on the breed—so now all that remains is to make a good choice.

It is never wise to just rush out and buy the first cute puppy who catches your eye. Whether you wish a dog to show, one with whom to compete in obedience, or one as a family dog purely for his (or her) companionship, the more time and thought you invest as you plan the purchase, the more likely you are to meet with complete satisfaction. The background and early care behind your pet will reflect in the dog's future health and temperament. Even if you are planning the purchase purely as a pet, with no thoughts of showing or breeding in the dog's or puppy's future, it is essential that if the dog is to enjoy a trouble-free future you assure yourself of a healthy, properly raised puppy or adult from sturdy, well-bred stock.

Throughout the pages of this book you will find the names and locations of many well-known and well-established kennels in various areas. Another source of information is the American Kennel Club (51 Madison Avenue, New York, New York 10010) from whom you can obtain a list of recognized breeders in the vicinity of your home. If you plan to have your dog campaigned by a professional handler, by all means let the handler help you locate and select a good dog. Through their numerous clients, handlers have access to a variety of interesting show prospects; and the usual arrangement is that the handler re-sells

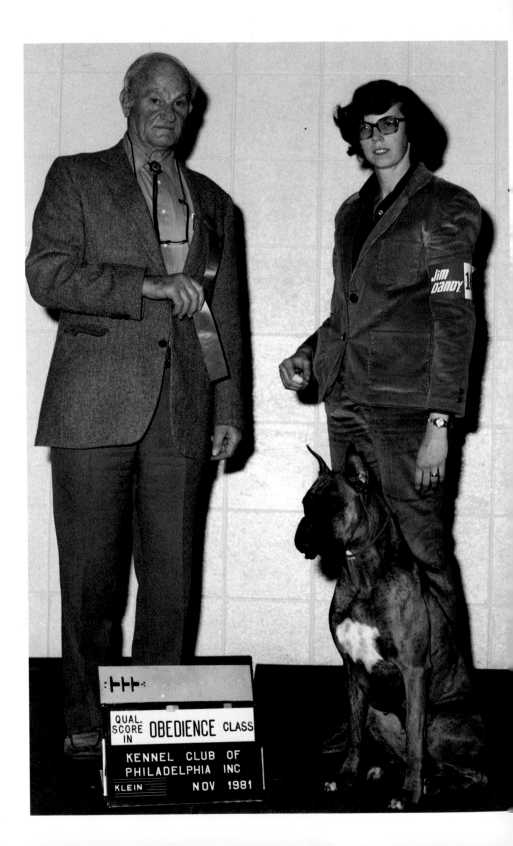

QUAL.
SCORE IN **OBEDIENCE** CLASS

KENNEL CLUB OF
PHILADELPHIA INC

KLEIN NOV 1981

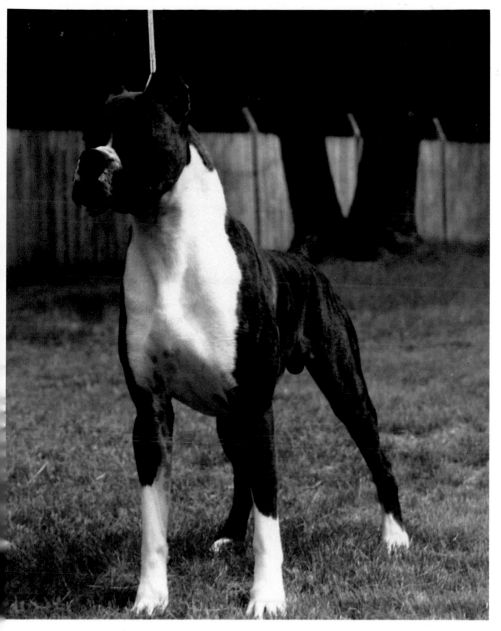

Ch. Salgray's Valentino, important winning Boxer owned by Mr. and Mrs. Daniel Hamilburg, Plymouth, Massachusetts. Handled by Stanley Flowers.

Opposite page: Jacquet's Mischief Maker, C.D., winning the third leg in three shows with score of 197 at the Kennel Club of Philadelphia. Sired by Ch. Jacquet's Zephan, Mischief Maker was trained, owned and shown by Carole Brower, Glen Rock, New Jersey.

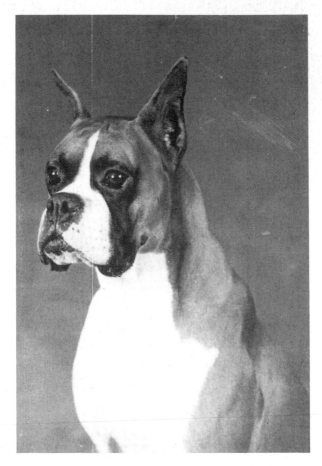

Ch. Jacquet's Bransto, by Ch. Merrilane's April Fashion ex Jacquet Perigal (American Boxer Club Dam of Merit) is owned by Bernie and Georgine Schwerdtfeger and Richard Tomita, Jacquet Boxers, Paramus, New Jersey.

the dog to you for what his cost has been, with the agreement that the dog be campaigned for you by him throughout the dog's career. I most strongly recommend that prospective purchasers follow these suggestions, as you thus will be better able to locate and select a satisfactory puppy or dog.

Your first step in searching for your puppy is to make appointments at kennels specializing in the chosen breed, where you can visit and inspect the dogs, both those available for sale and the kennel's basic breeding stock. You are looking for an active, sturdy puppy with bright eyes and intelligent expression and who is friendly and alert; avoid puppies who are hyperactive, dull, or listless. The coat should be clean and thick, with no sign of parasites. The premises on which he was raised should look (and smell) clean and be tidy, making it ob-

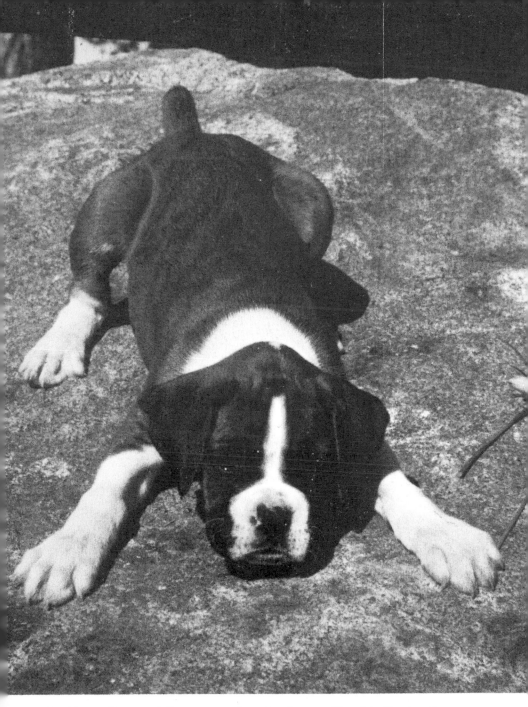

Ch. Magen Monten of Evergreen at 8 weeks. Owners, Al and Jo Monten, Burnsville, Minnesota. Handler, Stan Flowers.

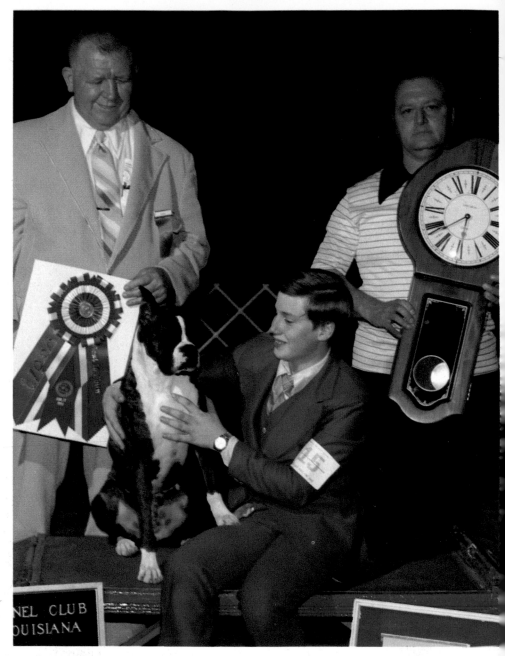

Ch. Turo's Angel Fire of D.J., by Ch. Turo's Dancer ex Turo's Cross Fire, winning **Best in Show** at Alexandria Kennel Club under judge James Vaughters, Sr. Breeder, Turo's Boxers. Owners, Dick and Jenna Dunn, Grangerland, Texas. This splendid dog has won two all-breed Bests in Show and a Best of Breed at Westminster, among numerous other honors.

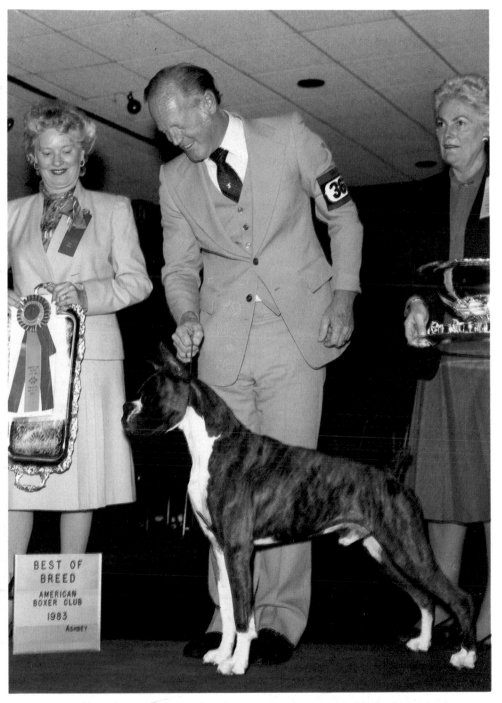

BEST OF
BREED
AMERICAN
BOXER CLUB
1983
ASHBEY

Ch. Richaire's Domino, by Ch. Telstar's Highflyer ex Tiffany of Brookwood, winning Best of Breed at the American Boxer Club Specialty in May 1983 judged by Mrs. Alice Downey. Richard Mysyiwiec handling for Richard and Claire Tolagian, Tucson, Arizona.

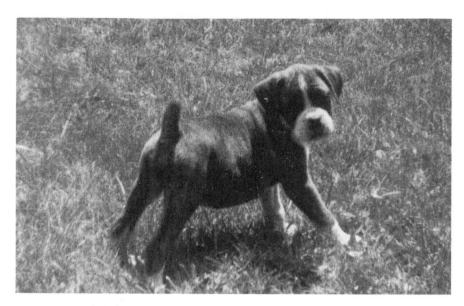

Hi-Hat's Cameo Jewel, by Ch. Hi-Hat Nitewind V Cidar Hill ex Ch. He-Hat's Cameo of Donessle. A promising show puppy owned by Mr. and Mrs. Jerry Kaplan, Hamden, Connecticut.

Ch. Merrilane's April Fashion enjoys his comfort on the road. Co-owned by Eleanor Linderholm Wood and Lois Matthews.

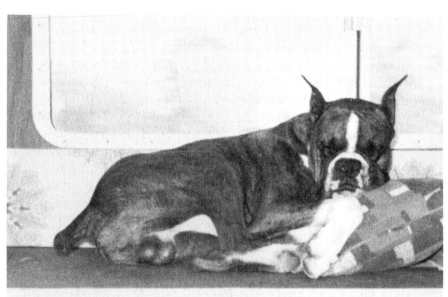

vious that the puppies and their surroundings are in capable hands. Should the kennels featuring the breed you intend owning be sparse in your area or not have what you consider attractive, do not hesitate to contact others at a distance and purchase from them if they seem better able to supply a puppy or dog who will please you *so long as it is a recognized breeding kennel of that breed.* Shipping dogs is a regular practice nowadays, with comparatively few problems when one considers the number of dogs shipped each year. A reputable, well-known breeder wants the customer to be satisfied; thus he will represent the puppy fairly. Should you not be pleased with the puppy upon arrival, a breeder such as I have described will almost certainly permit its return. A conscientious breeder takes real interest and concern in the welfare of the dogs he or she causes to be brought into the world. Such a breeder also is proud of a reputation for integrity. Thus on two counts, for the sake of the dog's future and the breeder's reputation, to such a person a *satisfied* customer takes precedence over a sale at any cost.

If your puppy is to be a pet or "family dog," I feel the earlier the age at which it joins your household the better. Puppies are weaned and ready to start out on their own, under the care of a sensible new owner, at about six weeks old; and if you take a young one, it is often easier to train it to the routine of your household and your requirements of it than is the case with an older dog which, even though still a puppy technically, may have already started habits you will find difficult to change. The younger puppy is usually less costly, too, as it stands to reason the breeder will not have as much expense invested in it. Obviously, a puppy that has been raised to five or six months old represents more in care and cash expenditure on the breeder's part than one sold earlier and therefore should be and generally is priced accordingly.

There is an enormous amount of truth in the statement that "bargain" puppies seldom turn out to be that. A "cheap" puppy, cheaply raised purely for sale and profit, can and often does lead to great heartbreak including problems and veterinarian's bills which can add up to many times the initial cost of a properly reared dog. On the other hand, just because a puppy is expensive does not assure one that is healthy and well reared. I know of numerous cases where unscrupulous dealers have sold for several hundred dollars puppies that were sickly, in poor condition, and such poor specimens that the breed of which they were supposedly members was barely recognizable. So one cannot always judge a puppy by price alone. Common sense must guide a prospective purchaser, plus the selection of a *reliable*, well-

Ch. Marburl's Rahab of Wesan, by Ch. Marburl's Joshua ex Ch. Wesan's Dark Apache Miss (Winners Bitch at the A.B.C. Regional in 1975), was bred by Wesley and Ann Tomhave and is owned by Rufus and Mary Burleson. A champion at eleven months of age, this lovely bitch won her first Best in Show at fourteen months and went on to six All-Breed Bests in Show plus Best of Breed at the American Boxer Club Specialty in 1980.

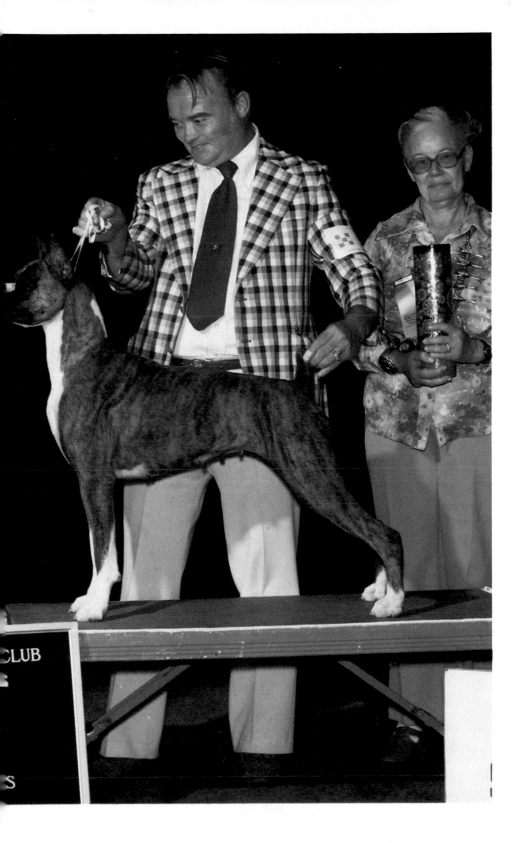

CLUB

S

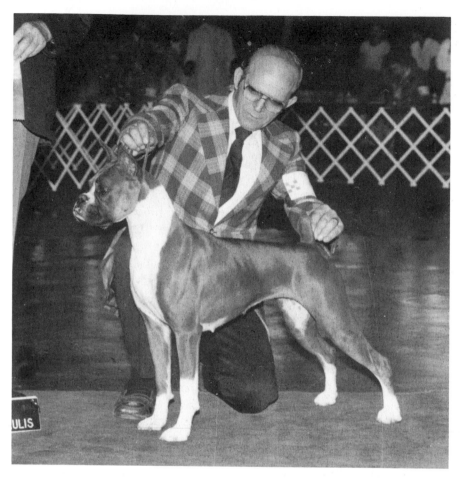

Ch. Evergreen's Cassiopeia winning Best of Breed at Mid-Continent in November 1980. Breeder-owner, Jane Nolt Flowers. Handler, Stan Flowers, Buffalo, Minnesota.

recommended dealer whom you know to have well satisfied customers or, best of all, a specialized breeder. You will probably find the fairest pricing at the kennel of a breeder. Such a person, experienced with the breed in general and with his or her own stock in particular, through extensive association with these dogs has watched enough of them mature to have obviously learned to assess quite accurately each puppy's potential—something impossible where such background is non-existent.

One more word on the subject of pets. Bitches make a fine choice for this purpose as they are usually quieter and more gentle than the males, easier to house train, more affectionate, and less inclined to roam. If you do select a bitch and have no intention of breeding or showing her, by all means have her spayed, for your sake and for hers. The advantages to the owner of a spayed bitch include avoiding the nuisance of "in season" periods which normally occur twice yearly, with the accompanying eager canine swains haunting your premises in an effort to get close to your female, plus the unavoidable messiness and spotting of furniture and rugs at this time, which can be annoying if she is a household companion in the habit of sharing your sofa or bed. As for the spayed bitch, she benefits as she grows older because this simple operation almost entirely eliminates the possibility of breast cancer ever occurring. I personally believe that all bitches should eventually be spayed—even those used for show or breeding when their careers are ended—in order that they may enjoy a happier, healthier old age. Please take note, however, that a bitch who has been spayed (or an altered dog) *cannot be shown at American Kennel Club Dog shows once this operation has been performed.* Be certain that you are *not* interested in showing her before taking this step.

Also in selecting a pet, never underestimate the advantages of an older dog, perhaps a retired show dog or a bitch no longer needed for breeding, who may be available quite reasonably priced by a breeder anxious to place such a dog in a loving home. These dogs are settled and can be a delight to own, as they make wonderful companions, especially in a household of adults where raising a puppy can sometimes be a trial.

Everything we have said about careful selection of your pet puppy and its place of purchase applies, but with many further considerations, when you plan to buy a show dog or foundation stock for a future breeding program. Now is the time for an in-depth study of the breed, starting with every word and every illustration in this book and all others you can find written on the subject. The standard of the breed now has become your guide, and you must learn not only the words but also how to interpret them and how they are applicable in actual dogs before you are ready to make an intelligent selection of a show dog.

If you are thinking in terms of a dog to show, obviously you must have learned about dog shows and must be in the habit of attending them. This is fine, but now your activity in this direction should be increased, with your attending every single dog show within a reasonable distance from your home. Much can be learned about a breed at

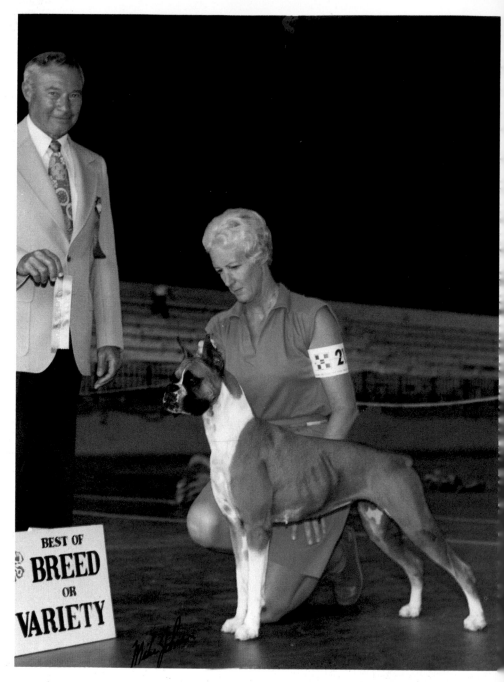

Ch. Beau Monde Boquet of Box M, by Ch. Box M Hawaiian Commander ex Marburl's Upper Class, here is winning the Working Group at Hilo Kennel Club in October 1983. "Boki" won three Working Groups during that year, and an American Boxer Club Award for the bitch winning most Groups. Owned by Richard Beaumont, editor of *Kennel Review,* North Hollywood, California, and Lois Matthews, Kailua, Hawaii.

Future Champion Hi Hill's Rave Review as a puppy. This lovely youngster finished her title at nine months of age in only thirteen months. Owned by Cheryl Colby and Leon De Priest, Hollycrest Boxers, Riverside, Illinois.

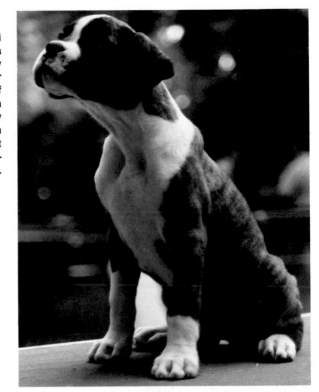

"That's a long step, Mom" would seem to be what Seawest Yuri Nuff of Box M is thinking when at five weeks of age he tries his first *big* step. Owned by Lois Matthews, Kailua, Hawaii. Photo taken by Rich Keefer.

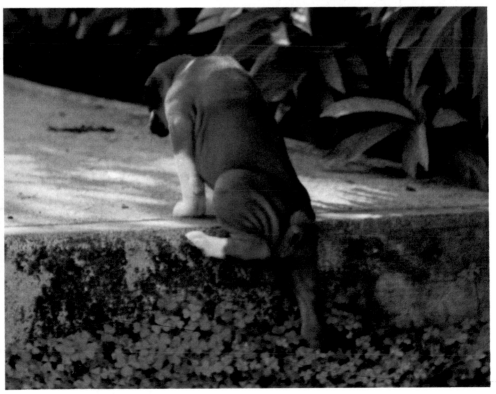

ringside at these events. Talk with the breeders who are exhibiting. Study the dogs they are showing. Watch the judging with concentration, noting each decision made and attempt to follow the reasoning by which the judge has reached it. Note carefully the attributes of the dogs who win and, for your later use, the manner in which each is presented. Close your ears to the ringside know-it-alls, usually novice owners of only a dog or two and very new to the Fancy, who have only derogatory remarks to make about all that is taking place unless they happen to win. This is the type of exhibitor who "comes and goes" through the Fancy and whose interest is usually of very short duration owing to lack of knowledge and dissatisfaction caused by the failure to recognize the need to learn. You, as a fancier who we hope will last and enjoy our sport over many future years, should develop independent thinking at this stage; you should learn to draw your own conclusions about the merits, or lack of them, seen before you in the ring and thus, sharpen your own judgment in preparation for choosing wisely and well.

Note carefully which breeders campaign winning dogs, not just an occasional isolated good one but consistent, homebred winners. It is from one of these people that you should select your own future "star."

If you are located in an area where dog shows take place only occasionally or where there are long travel distances involved, you will need to find another testing ground for your ability to select a worthy show dog. Possibly, there are some representative kennels raising this breed within a reasonable distance. If so, by all means ask permission of the owners to visit the kennels and do so when permission is granted. You may not necessarily buy then and there, as they may not have available what you are seeking that very day, but you will be able to see the type of dog being raised there and to discuss the dogs with the breeder. Every time you do this, you add to your knowledge. Should one of these kennels have dogs which especially appeal to you, perhaps you could reserve a show-prospect puppy from a coming litter. This is frequently done, and it is often worth waiting for a puppy, unless you have seen a dog with which you are truly greatly impressed and which is immediately available.

We have already discussed the purchase of a pet puppy. Obviously this same approach applies in a far greater degree when the purchase involved is a future show dog. The only place at which to purchase a show prospect is from a breeder who raises show-type stock; otherwise, you are almost certainly doomed to disappointment as the puppy

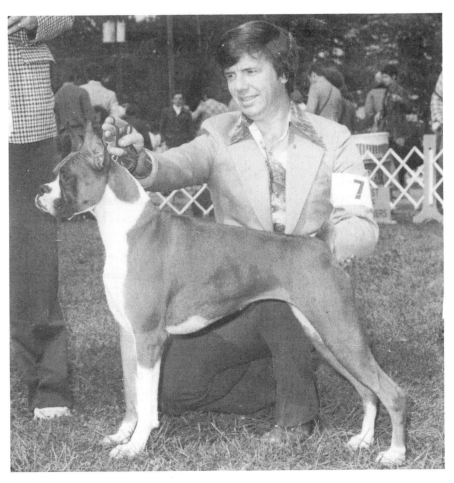

Ch. Woodcrest Alicia finishing her title at Rock Creek-Potomac specialty in October 1975 with Don Simmons handling. Alicia succumbed to an attack of bloat while still nursing her "X" litter. Woodcrest on both sides, she was a Shadrack granddaughter. Owned by Woodcrest Kennels, Carl Wood, La Selva Beach, California.

matures. Show and breeding kennels obviously cannot keep all of their fine young stock. An active breeder-exhibitor is, therefore, happy to place promising youngsters in the hands of people also interested in showing and winning with them, doing so at a fair price according to the quality and prospects of the dog involved. Here again, if no kennel in your immediate area has what you are seeking, do not hesitate to contact top breeders in other areas and to buy at long distance. Ask for pictures, pedigrees, and a complete description. Heed the breeder's advice and recommendations, after truthfully telling exactly what your

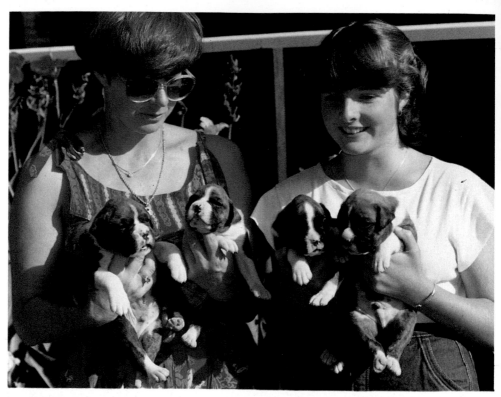

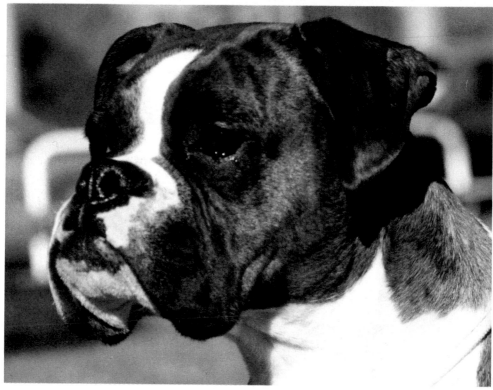

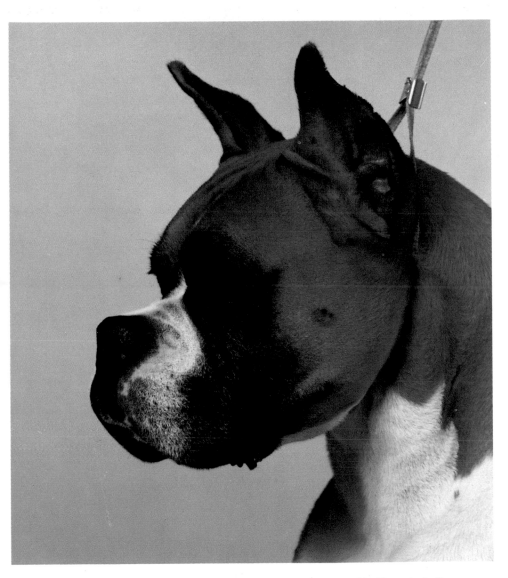

Am., Braz., and Int. Ch. Arriba's Command Performance owned by Hexastar's Kennels and Domingos Aliperti, Jr., Brazil.

Opposite page: *(Top)* Australian Boxer breeder Rosina Olifent-Brace and her daughter, Denise, with a crop of youngsters at three-and-a-half weeks of age, double Am. and N.Z. Ch. My-T Sweet grandchildren. *(Bottom)* Aust. Ch. Intrends Winds' O'Chance, born May 1979, by Aust. Ch. Gremlin Great Gale (U.K. import) ex Intrends Pot O'Gold, never unplaced during her show career at any Royal or Specialty Show, doing most of her top winning under specialist judges. She has won a Royal Challenge and a Victorian Boxer Specialty. Bred by Judy Horton; owned by Mr. and Mrs. D.C. Rawnsley, Cordoba Kennels.

expectations are for the dog you purchase. Do you want something with which to win just a few ribbons now and then? Do you want a dog who can complete his championship? Are you thinking of the real "big time" (*i.e.,* seriously campaigning with Best of Breed, Group wins, and possibly even Best in Show as your eventual goal)? Consider it all carefully in advance; then honestly discuss your plans with the breeder. You will be better satisfied with the results if you do this, as the breeder is then in the best position to help you choose the dog who is most likely to come through for you. A breeder selling a show dog is just as anxious as the buyer for the dog to succeed, and the breeder will represent the dog to you with truth and honesty. Also, this type of breeder does not lose interest the moment the sale has been made but when necessary will be right there ready to assist you with beneficial advice and suggestions based on years of experience.

As you make inquiries of at least several kennels, keep in mind that show-prospect puppies are less expensive than mature show dogs, the latter often costing close to four figures, and sometimes more. The reason for this is that, with a puppy, there is always an element of chance, the possibility of its developing unexpected faults as it matures or failing to develop the excellence and quality that earlier had seemed probable. There definitely is a risk factor in buying a show-prospect puppy. Sometimes all goes well, but occasionally the swan becomes an ugly duckling. Reflect on this as you consider available puppies and young adults. It just might be a good idea to go with a more mature, though more costly, dog if one you like is available.

When you buy a mature show dog, "what you see is what you get"; and it is not likely to change beyond coat and condition which are dependent on your care. Also advantageous for a novice owner is the fact that a mature dog of show quality almost certainly will have received show ring training and probably match show experience, which will make your earliest handling ventures far easier.

Frequently it is possible to purchase a beautiful dog who has completed championship but who, owing to similarity in bloodlines, is not needed for the breeder's future program. Here you have the opportunity of own-ing a champion, usually in the two- to five-year-old range, which you can enjoy campaigning as a "special" (for Best of Breed competition) and which will be a settled, handsome dog for you and your family to enjoy with pride.

If you are planning foundation for a future kennel, concentrate on acquiring one or two really superior bitches. These need not necessarily be top show-quality, but they should represent your breed's finest producing bloodlines from a strain noted for producing quality, generation after generation. A proven matron who is already the dam of show-type puppies is, of course, the ideal selection; but these are usually difficult to obtain, no one being anxious to part with so valuable an asset. You just might strike it lucky, though, in which case you are off to a flying start. If you cannot find such a matron available, select a young bitch of finest background from top producing lines who is herself of decent type, free of obvious faults, and of good quality.

Great attention should be paid to the pedigree of the bitch from whom you intend to breed. If not already known to you, try to see the sire and dam. It is generally agreed that someone starting with a breed should concentrate on a fine collection of top-flight bitches and raise a few litters from these before considering keeping one's own stud dog. The practice of buying a stud and then breeding everything you own or acquire to that dog does not always work out well. It is better to take advantage of the many noted sires who are available to be used at stud, who represent all of the leading strains, and in each case carefully to select the one who in type and pedigree seems most compatible to each of your bitches, at least for your first several litters.

To summarize, if you want a "family dog" as a companion, it is best to buy it young and raise it to the habits of your household. If you are buying a show dog, the more mature it is, the more certain you can be of its future beauty. If you are buying foundation stock for a kennel, then bitches are better, but they must be from the finest *producing* bloodlines.

When you buy a purebred dog that you are told is eligible for registration with the American Kennel Club, you are entitled to receive from the seller an application form which will enable you to register your dog. If the seller cannot give you the application form you should demand and receive an identification of your dog consisting of the name of the breed, the registered names and numbers of the sire and dam, the name of the breeder, and your dog's date of birth. If the litter of which your dog is a part is already recorded with the American Kennel Club, then the litter number is sufficient identification.

Do not be misled by promises of papers at some later date. Demand a registration application form or proper identification as described above. If neither is supplied, do not buy the dog. So warns the American Kennel Club, and this is especially important in the purchase of show or breeding stock.

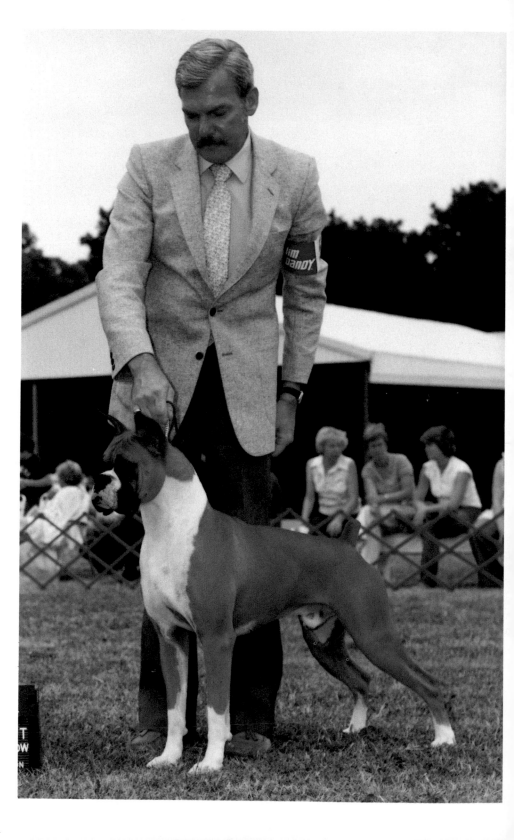

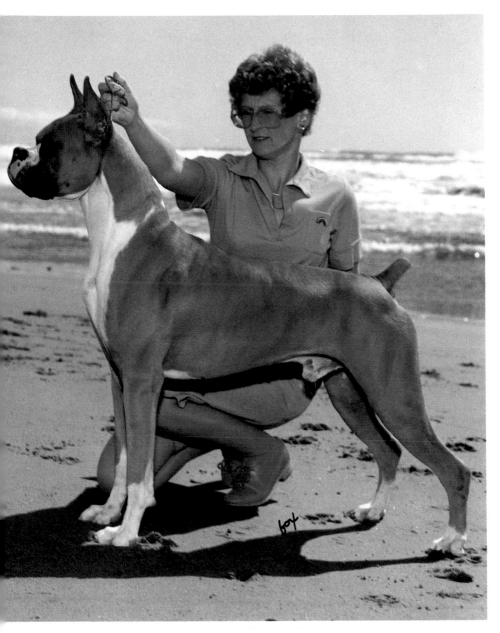

Ch. Merrilane's It Must Be Him, by Ch. Merrilane's April Holiday ex a daughter of Ch. Merrilane's Silver Dollar, is a full brother to Ch. Merrilane's Silver 'n Gold. Current owner, Thomas and Joan Greenwood, Johannesburg, South Africa.

Opposite page: Am. and Can. Ch. Tri-Manor Pinepaths Hudson Bay, by Ch. Pinepaths Gemini ex Pinepaths Fair Cleopatra, the sire of sixteen champions, owned by Mr. and Mrs. Jack Ireland, Fingal, Ontario.

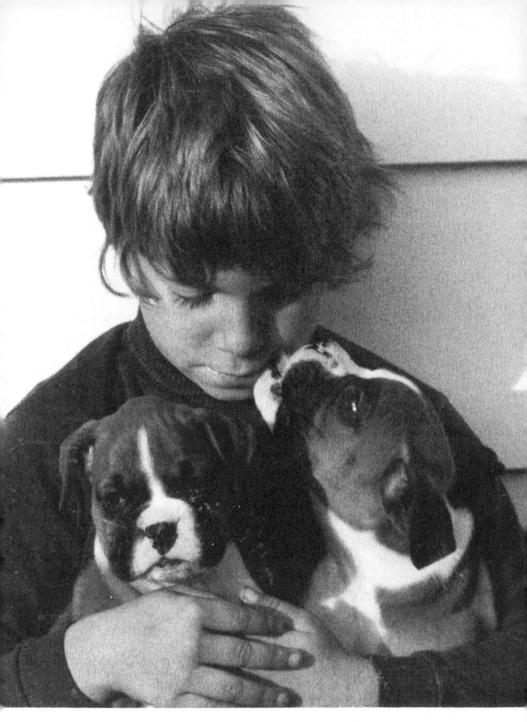

Mathew and friends at Hollycrest Kennels, Riverside, Illinois.

190

Chapter 10

The Care of Your Boxer Puppy

Preparing for Your Puppy's Arrival

The moment you decide to be the new owner of a puppy is not one second too soon to start planning for the puppy's arrival in your home. Both the new family member and you will find the transition period easier if your home is geared in advance for the arrival.

The first things to be prepared are a bed for the puppy and a place where you can pen him up for rest periods. I am a firm believer that every dog should have a crate of its own from the very beginning, so that he will come to know and love it as his special place where he is safe and happy. It is an ideal arrangement, for when you want him to be free, the crate stays open. At other times you can securely latch it and know that the pup is safely out of mischief. If you travel with him, his crate comes along in the car; and, of course, in travelling by plane there is no alternative but to have a carrier for the dog. If you show your dog, you will want him upon occasion to be in a crate a good deal of the day. So from every consideration, a crate is a very sensible and sound investment in your puppy's future safety and happiness and for your own peace of mind.

The crates I recommend are the wooden ones with removable side panels, which are ideal for cold weather (with the panels in place to keep out drafts) and in hot weather (with the panels removed to allow better air circulation). Wire crates are all right in the summer, but they give no protection from cold or drafts. I intensely dislike aluminum crates due to the manner in which aluminum reflects surrounding temperatures. If it is cold, so is the metal of the crate; if it is hot, the crate becomes burning hot. For this reason I consider aluminum crates neither comfortable nor safe.

When you choose the puppy's crate, be certain that it is roomy enough not to become outgrown. The crate should have sufficient

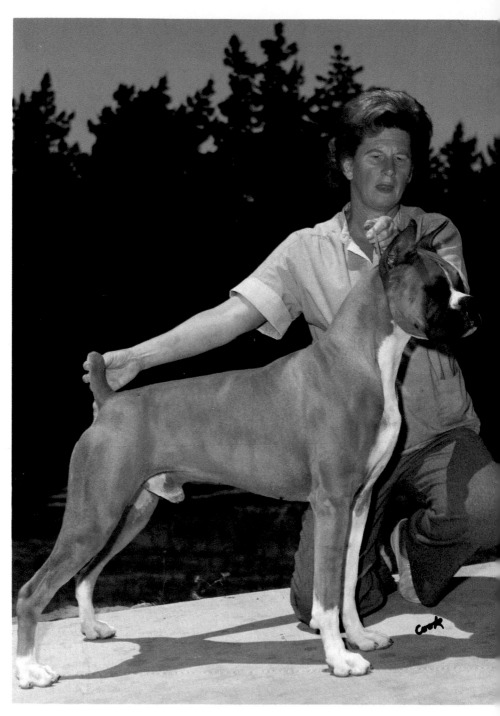

Ch. Merrilane's Silver 'n Gold, a multi-Specialty Best in Show winner, by Ch. Merrilane's April Holiday from a daughter of Ch. Merrilane's Silver Dollar, is the sire of an international champion. Owner, Eleanor Linderholm Wood, La Selva Beach, California.

height so the dog can stand up in it as a mature dog and sufficient area so that he can stretch out full length when relaxed. When the puppy is young, first give him shredded newspaper as a bed; the papers can be replaced with a mat or turkish towels when the dog is older. Carpet remnants are great for the bottom of the crate, as they are inexpensive and in case of accidents can be quite easily replaced. As the dog matures and is past the chewing age, a pillow or blanket in the crate is an appreciated comfort.

Sharing importance with the crate is a safe area in which the puppy can exercise and play. If you are an apartment dweller, a baby's playpen for a toy dog or a young puppy works out well; for a larger breed or older puppy use a portable exercise pen which you can then use later when travelling with your dog or for dog shows. If you have a yard, an area where he can be outside in safety should be fenced in prior to the dog's arrival at your home. This area does not need to be huge, but it does need to be made safe and secure. If you are in a suburban area where there are close neighbors, stockade fencing works out best as then the neighbors are less aware of the dog and the dog cannot see and bark at everything passing by. If you are out in the country where no problems with neighbors are likely to occur, then regular chain-link fencing is fine. For added precaution in both cases, use a row of concrete blocks or railroad ties inside against the entire bottom of the fence; this precludes or at least considerably lessens the chances of your dog digging his way out.

Be advised that if yours is a single dog, it is very unlikely that it will get sufficient exercise just sitting in the fenced area, which is what most of them do when they are there alone. Two or more dogs will play and move themselves around, but from my own experience, one by itself does little more than make a leisurely tour once around the area to check things over and then lies down. You must include a daily walk or two in your plans if your puppy is to be rugged and well. Exercise is extremely important to a puppy's muscular development and to keep a mature dog fit and trim. So make sure that those exercise periods, or walks, a game of ball, and other such activities, are part of your daily program as a dog owner.

If your fenced area has an outside gate, provide a padlock and key and a strong fastening for it, and use them, so that the gate can not be opened by others and the dog taken or turned free. The ultimate convenience in this regard is, of course, a door (unused for other purposes) from the house around which the fenced area can be enclosed,

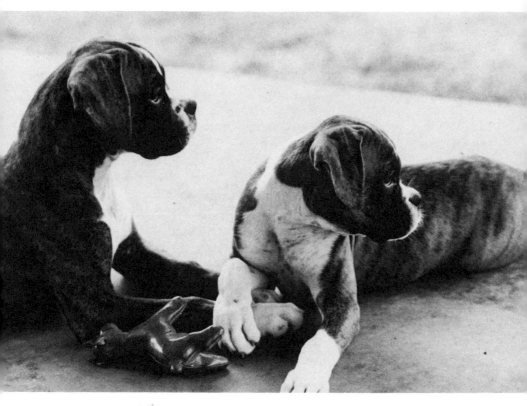

Boxer puppies at play. These owned by Lois Matthews, Box M Kennels, Kailua, Hawaii.

so that all you have to do is open the door and out into his area he goes. This arrangement is safest of all, as then you need not be using a gate, and it is easier in bad weather since then you can send the dog out without taking him and becoming soaked yourself at the same time. This is not always possible to manage, but if your house is arranged so that you could do it this way, I am sure you would never regret it due to the convenience and added safety thus provided. Fencing in the entire yard, with gates to be opened and closed whenever a caller, deliveryman, postman, or some other person comes on your property, really is not safe at all because people not used to gates and their importance are frequently careless about closing and latching gates *securely*. I know of many heartbreaking incidents brought about by someone carelessly only half closing a gate which the owner had thought to be firmly latched and the dog wandering out. For greatest security a fenced *area* definitely takes precedence over a fenced *yard.*

The puppy will need a collar (one that fits now, not one to be grown into) and lead from the moment you bring him home. Both should be an appropriate weight and type for his size. Also needed are a feeding dish and a water dish, both made preferably of unbreakable material. Your pet supply shop should have an interesting assortment of these and other accessories from which you can choose. Then you will need grooming tools of the type the breeder recommends and some toys. One of the best toys is a beef bone, either rib, leg, or knuckle (the latter the type you can purchase to make soup), cut to an appropriate size for your puppy dog. These are absolutely safe and are great exercise for the teething period, helping to get the baby teeth quickly out of the way with no problems. Equally satisfactory is Nylabone® , a nylon bone that does not chip or splinter and that "frizzles" as the puppy chews, providing healthful gum massage. Rawhide chews are safe, too, *IF made in the United States.* There was a problem a few years back owing to the chemicals with which some foreign rawhide toys had been treated, since which time we have carefully avoided giving them to our own dogs. Also avoid plastics and any sort of rubber toys, *particularly* those with squeakers which the puppy may remove and swallow. If you want a ball for the puppy to use when playing with him, select one of very hard construction made for this purpose and do not leave it alone with him because he may chew off and swallow bits of the rubber. Take the ball with you when the game is over. This also applies to some of those "tug of war" type rubber toys which are fun when used with the two of you for that purpose but again should *not* be left behind for the dog to work on with his teeth. Bits of swallowed rubber, squeakers, and other such foreign articles can wreak great havoc in the intestinal tract—do all you can to guard against them.

Too many changes all at once can be difficult for a puppy. For at least the first few days he is with you, keep him on the food and feeding schedule to which he is accustomed. Find out ahead of time from the breeder what he feeds his puppies, how frequently, and at what times of the day. Also find out what, if any, food supplements the breeder has been using and recommends. Then be prepared by getting in a supply of the same food so that you will have it there when you bring the puppy home. Once the puppy is accustomed to his new surroundings, then you can switch the type of food and schedule to fit your convenience, but for the first several days do it as the puppy expects.

Your selection of a veterinarian also should be attended to before the puppy comes home, because you should stop at the vet's office for the puppy to be checked over as soon as you leave the breeder's premises. If the breeder is from your area, ask him for recommendations. Ask your dog-owning friends for their opinions of the local veterinarians, and see what their experiences with those available have been. Choose someone whom several of your friends recommend highly, then contact him about your puppy, perhaps making an appointment to stop in at his office. If the premises are clean, modern, and well equipped, and if you like the veterinarian, make an appointment to bring the puppy in on the day of purchase. Be sure to obtain the puppy's health record from the breeder, including information on such things as shots and worming that the puppy has had.

Joining The Family

Remember that, exciting and happy an occasion as it is for you, the puppy's move from his place of birth to your home can be, for him, a traumatic experience. His mother and littermates will be missed. He quite likely will be awed or frightened by the change of surroundings. The person on whom he depended will be gone. Everything should be planned to make his arrival at your home pleasant—to give him confidence and to help him realize that yours is a pretty nice place to be after all.

Never bring a puppy home on a holiday. There just is too much going on with people and gifts and excitement. If he is in honor of an "occasion," work it out so that his arrival will be a few days earlier or, perhaps even better, a few days later than the "occasion." Then your home will be back to its normal routine and the puppy can enjoy your undivided attention. Try not to bring the puppy home in the evening. Early morning is the ideal time, as then he has the opportunity of getting acquainted and the initial strangeness should wear off before bedtime. You will find it a more peaceful night that way, I am sure. Allow the puppy to investigate as he likes, under your watchful eye. If you already have a pet in the household, keep a careful watch that the relationship between the two gets off to a friendly start or you may quickly find yourself with a lasting problem. Much of the future attitude of each toward the other will depend on what takes place that first day, so keep your mind on what they are doing and let your other activities slide for the moment. Be careful not to let your older pet become jealous by pay-

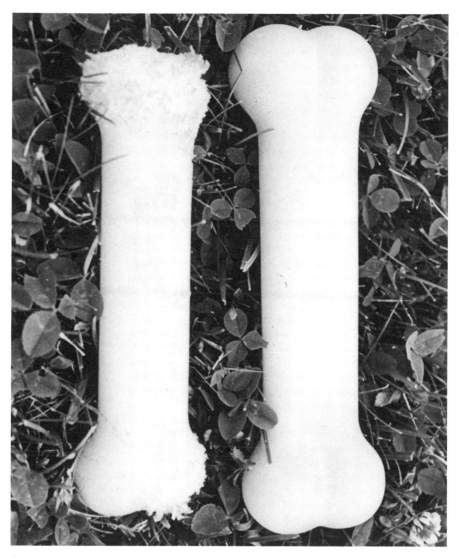

Nylabone can provide your Boxer with hours of safe chewing throughout his life. Start with the petite type for a puppy and offer the regular size when fully grown.

ing more attention to the puppy than to him, as that will start a bad situation immediately.

If you have a child, here again it is important that the relationship start out well. Before the puppy is brought home, you should have a talk with the youngster about puppies, so that it will be clearly understood that puppies are fragile and can easily be injured;

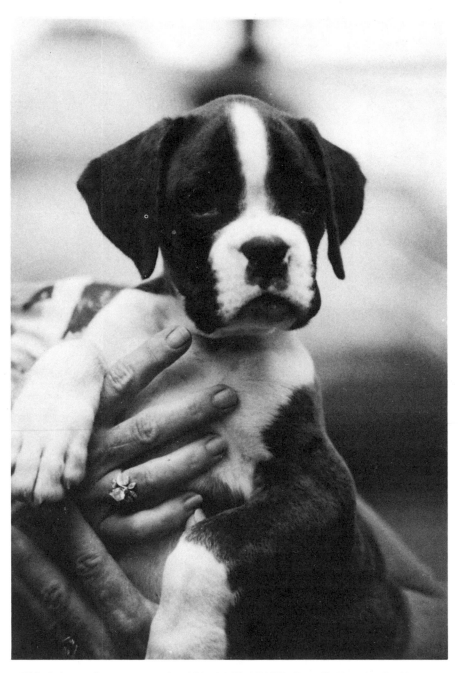

This is how a Boxer puppy should look! Ch. Hi Hill's Rave Review, by Ch. Heldenbrand's K's Kid by Peddler ex Hi-Hill's Summer Shadows, bred by Donna Titus and owned by Cheryl Colby and Leon De Priest. A champion at nine months of age.

therefore, they should not be teased, hurt, mauled, or overly rough-housed. A puppy is not an inanimate toy; it is a living thing with a right to be loved and handled respectfully, treatment which will reflect in the dog's attitude toward your child as both mature together. Never permit your children's playmates to mishandle the puppy, as I have seen happen, tormenting the puppy until it turns on the children in self-defense. Children often do not realize how rough is too rough. You, as a responsible adult, are obligated to assure that your puppy's relationship with children is a pleasant one.

Do not start out by spoiling your puppy. A puppy is usually pretty smart and can be quite demanding. What you had considered to be "just for tonight" may be accepted by the puppy as "for keeps." Be firm with him, strike a routine, and stick to it. The puppy will learn more quickly this way, and everyone will be happier at the result. A radio playing softly or a dim night light are often comforting to a puppy as it gets accustomed to new surroundings and should be provided in preference to bringing the puppy to bed with you—unless, of course, you intend him to share the bed as a permanent arrangement

Socializing and Training Your New Puppy

Socialization and training of your puppy should start the very day of his arrival in your home. Never address him without calling him by name. A short, simple name is the easiest to teach as it catches the dog's attention quickly, so avoid elaborate call names. Always address the dog by the same name, not a whole series of pet names; the latter will only confuse the puppy.

Using his name clearly, call the puppy over to you when you see him awake and wandering about. When he comes, make a big fuss over him for being such a good dog. He thus will quickly associate the sound of his name with coming to you and a pleasant happening.

Several hours after the puppy's arrival is not too soon to start accustoming him to the feel of a light collar. He may hardly notice it; or he may struggle, roll over, and try to rub it off his neck with his paws. Divert his attention when this occurs by offering a tasty snack or a toy (starting a game with him) or by petting him. Before long he will have accepted the strange feeling around his neck and no longer appear aware of it. Next comes the lead. Attach it and then immediately take the puppy outside or otherwise try to divert his attention with things

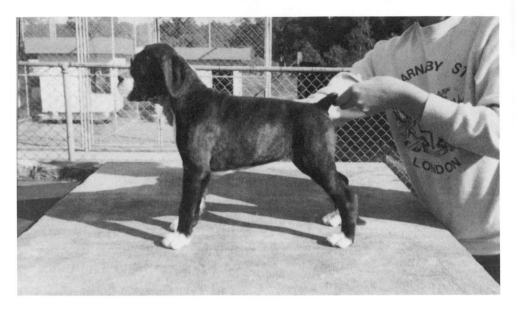

Innsbruck Boxer puppy, eight weeks old, by Innsbruck Sweet Talk, is typical of those being raised at this noted Australian kennel. Mrs. Nea Evans.

Australian Boxer babies, by Aust. Ch. Intrends Great Gatsby ex Intrends Bewitched, were born March 1983. The middle pup is Intrends Bewitched, owned by Sanshur Kennels in Queensland. Bred by Judy Horton, Ormond, Victoria.

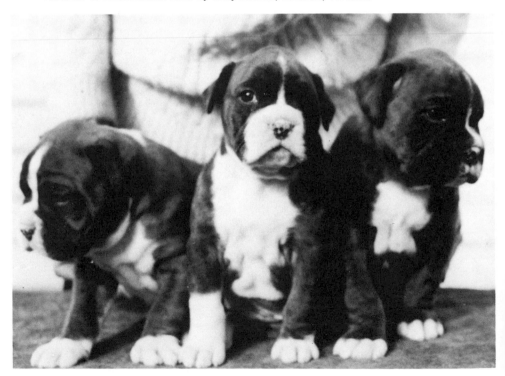

to see and sniff. He may struggle against the lead at first, biting at it and trying to free himself. Do not pull him with it at this point; just hold the end loosely and try to follow him if he starts off in any direction. Normally his attention will soon turn to investigating his surroundings if he is outside or you have taken him into an unfamiliar room in your house; curiosity will take over and he will become interested in sniffing around the surroundings. Just follow him with the lead slackly held until he seems to have completely forgotten about it; then try with gentle urging to get him to follow you. Don't be rough or jerk at him; just tug gently on the lead in short quick motions (steady pulling can become a battle of wills), repeating his name or trying to get him to follow your hand which is holding a bite of food or an interesting toy. If you have an older lead-trained dog, then it should be a cinch to get the puppy to follow along after *him*. In any event, the average puppy learns quite quickly and will soon be trotting along nicely on the lead. Once that point has been reached, the next step is to teach him to follow on your left side, or heel. Of course this will not likely be accomplished all in one day but should be done with short training periods over the course of several days until you are satisfied with the result.

During the course of house training your puppy, you will need to take him out frequently and at regular intervals: first thing in the morning directly from the crate, immediately after meals, after the puppy has been napping, or when you notice that the puppy is looking for a spot. Choose more or less the same place to take the puppy each time so that a pattern will be established. If he does not go immediately, do not return him to the house as he will probably relieve himself the moment he is inside. Stay out with him until he has finished; then be lavish with your praise for his good behavior. If you catch the puppy having an accident indoors, grab him firmly and rush him outside, sharply saying "No!" as you pick him up. If you do not see the accident occur, there is little point in doing anything except cleaning it up, as once it has happened and been forgotten, the puppy will most likely not even realize why you are scolding him.

With a small or moderate size breed, especially if you live in a big city or are away many hours at a time, having a dog that is trained to go on paper has some very definite advantages. To do this, one proceeds pretty much the same way as taking the puppy outdoors, except now you place the puppy on the newspaper at the proper time. The paper should always be kept in the same spot. An easy way to paper train a puppy if you have a playpen for it or an exercise pen is to line the area with newspapers; then gradually, every day or so, remove a section of newspaper until you are down to just one or two. The puppy acquires the habit of using the paper; and as the prepared area grows smaller, in the majority of cases the dog will continue to use whatever paper is still available. My own experience, with dogs of small or moderate size is that this works out well. It is pleasant, if the dog is alone for an excessive length of time, to be able to feel that if he needs it the paper is there and will be used.

The puppy should form the habit of spending a certain amount of time in his crate, even when you are home. Sometimes the puppy will do this voluntarily, but if not it should be taught to do so, which is accomplished by leading the puppy over by his collar, gently pushing him inside, and saying firmly "Down" or "Stay." Whatever expression you use to give a command, stick to the very same one each time for each act. Repetition is the big thing in training—and so is association with what the dog is expected to do. When you mean "Sit" always say exactly that. "Stay" should mean *only* that the dog should remain where he receives the command. "Down" means something else again. Do not confuse the dog by shuffling the commands, as this will create training problems for you.

As soon as he has had his immunization shots, take your puppy with you whenever and wherever possible. There is nothing that will build a self-confident, stable dog like socialization, and it is extremely important that you plan and give the time and energy necessary for this whether your dog is to be a show dog or a pleasant, well-adjusted family member. Take your puppy in the car so that he will learn to enjoy riding and not become carsick as dogs may do if they are infrequent travelers. Take him anywhere you are going where you are certain he will be welcome: visiting friends and relatives (if they do not have housepets who may resent the visit), busy shopping centers (keeping him always on lead), or just walking around the streets of your town. If someone admires him (as always seems to happen when we are out with puppies), encourage the stranger to pet and talk with him. Socialization of this type brings out the best in your puppy and helps him to grow up with a friendly outlook, liking the world and its inhabitants. The worst thing that can be done to a puppy's personality is to overly shelter him. By keeping him always at home away from things and people unfamiliar to him you may be creating a personality problem for the mature dog that will be a cross for you to bear later on.

202

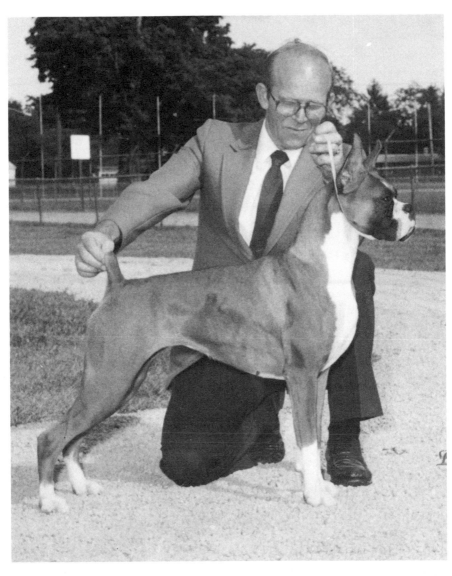

Ch. Salgray's Showstopper, winner of two Bests in Show to date, is a daughter of Ch. Salgray's Market Wise ex Salgray's Special Edition. Owners, Mr. and Mrs. Daniel Hamilburg, Plymouth, Massachusetts. Handler, Stan Flowers, Buffalo, Minnesota.

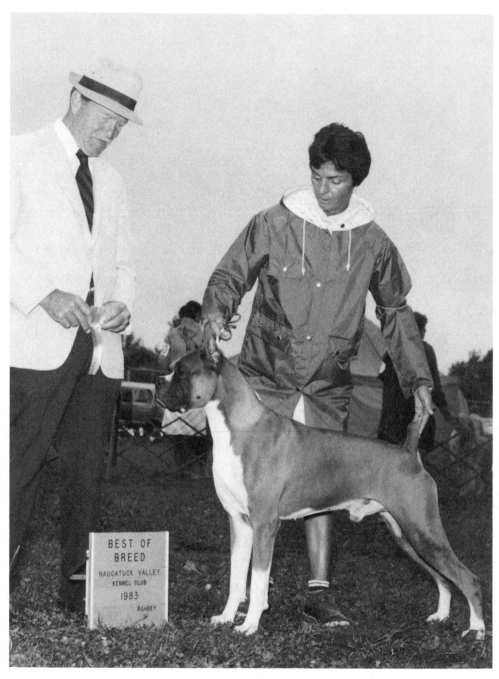

Ch. Sunset Spirit of Five T's owned by Mr. and Mrs. Bruce Korsan, Laurel Hill Boxers, Oyster Bay, New York. Handled by Terry Lazzaro.

Feeding Your Dog

Time was when providing nourishing food for our dogs involved a far more complicated procedure than people now feel is necessary. The old school of thought was that the daily ration must consist of fresh beef, vegetables, cereal, egg yolks, and cottage cheese as basics with such additions as brewer's yeast and vitamin tablets on a daily basis.

During recent years, however, many minds have changed regarding this procedure. We still give eggs, cottage cheese, and supplements to the diet, but the basic method of feeding dogs has changed; and the change has been, in the opinion of many authorities, definitely for the better. The school of thought now is that you are doing your dogs a favor when you feed them some of the fine commercially prepared dog foods in preference to your own home-cooked concoctions.

The reason behind this new outlook is easily understandable. The dog food industry has grown to be a major one, participated in by some of the best known and most respected names in the American way of life. These trusted firms, it is agreed, turn out excellent products, so people are feeding their dog food preparations with confidence and the dogs are thriving, living longer, happier, and healthier lives than ever before. What more could we want?

There are at least half a dozen absolutely top-grade dry foods to be mixed with broth or water and served to your dog according to directions. There are all sorts of canned meats, and there are several kinds of "convenience foods," those in a packet which you open and dump out into the dog's dish. It is just that simple. The "convenience" foods are neat and easy to use when you are away from home, but generally speaking we prefer a dry food mixed with hot water or soup and meat. We also feel that the canned meat, with its added fortifiers, is more beneficial to the dogs than the fresh meat. However, the two can be alternated or, if you prefer and your dog does well on it, by all means use fresh ground beef. A dog enjoys changes in the meat part of his diet, which is easy with the canned food since all sorts of beef are available (chunk, ground, stewed, and so on), plus lamb, chicken, and even such concoctions as liver and egg, just plain liver flavor, and a blend of five meats.

There also is prepared food geared to every age bracket of your dog's life, from puppyhood on through old age, with special additions or modifications to make it particularly nourishing and beneficial. Our grandparents, and even our parents, never had it so good where the canine dinner is concerned, because these commercially prepared foods are tasty and geared to meeting the dog's gastronomic approval.

Additionally, contents and nutrients are clearly listed on the labels, as are careful instructions for feeding just the right amount for the size, weight, and age of each dog.

With these foods we do not feel the addition of extra vitamins is necessary, but if you do there are several kinds of those, too, that serve as taste treats as well as being beneficial. Your pet supplier has a full array of them.

Of course there is no reason not to cook up something for your dog if you would feel happier doing so. But it seems to us unnecessary when such truly satisfactory rations are available with so much less trouble and expense.

How often you feed your dog is a matter of how it works out best for you. Many owners prefer to do it once a day. I personally think that two meals, each of smaller quantity, are better for the digestion and more satisfying to the dog, particularly if yours is a household member who stands around and watches preparations for the family meals. Do

Lunch time for the six-week olds at Mrs. Nea Evans's famous Boxer kennel in Australia. These youngsters, by Aust. Ch. Cherryburton Playboy ex Aust. Ch. Innsbruck Sunbonnet, were imported from the United Kingdom.

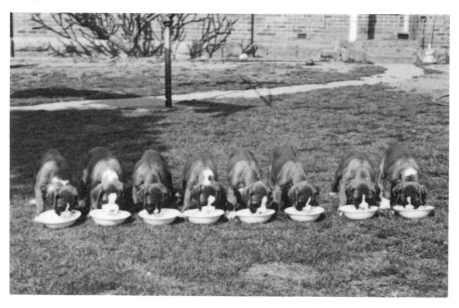

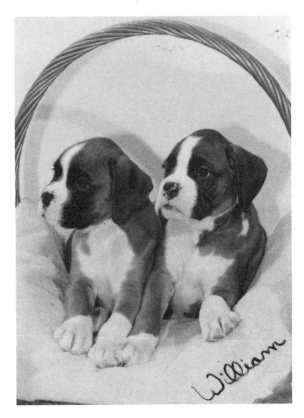

Flirt and Torch, daughters of Ch. Heldenbrand's Kansas Twister ex Holly-crest's Double Trouble. Heldenbrand Boxers, Manhattan, Kansas.

not overfeed. That is the shortest route to all sorts of problems. Follow directions and note carefully how your dog is looking. If your dog is overweight, cut back the quantity of food a bit. If the dog looks thin, then increase the amount. Each dog is an individual and the food intake should be adjusted to his requirements to keep him feeling and looking trim and in top condition.

From the time puppies are fully weaned until they are about twelve weeks old, they should be fed four times daily. From three months to six months of age, three meals should suffice. At six months of age the puppies can be fed two meals, and the twice daily feedings can be continued until the puppies are close to one year old, at which time feeding can be changed to once daily if desired.

If you do feed just once a day, do so by early afternoon at the latest and give the dog a snack, or biscuit or two, at bedtime.

Remember that plenty of fresh water should always be available to your puppy or dog for drinking. This is of utmost importance to his health.

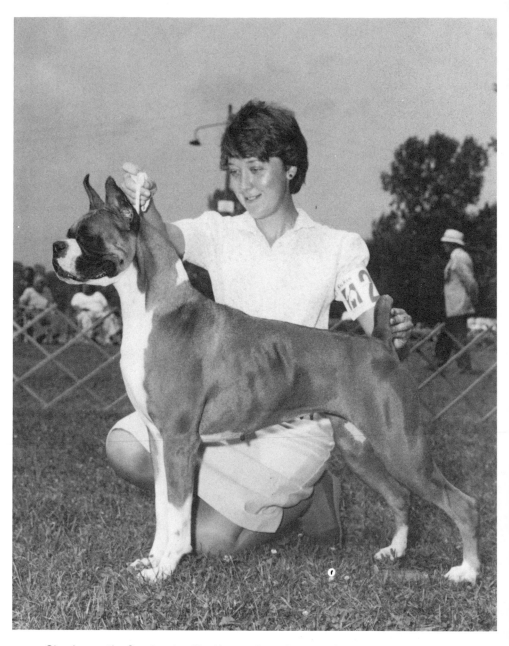

Ch. Jacquet's Garnier, by Ch. Happy Ours Fortune de Jacquet ex Jacquet's Brandywine, was bred by Richard Tomita and James Lally and is owned by Sandy Powell and Richard Tomita. This champion was rated Number Five Boxer during 1983 and the Winner Puppy Winning Most Blue Ribbons Award, A.B.C. that same year.

208

Chapter 11

The Making of a Show Dog

If you have decided to become a show dog exhibitor, you have accepted a very real and very exciting challenge. The groundwork has been accomplished with the selection of your future show prospect. If you have purchased a puppy, we assume that you have gone through all the proper preliminaries concerning good care, which should be the same if the puppy is a pet or future show dog with a few added precautions for the latter.

General Considerations

Remember the importance of keeping your future winner in trim, top condition. Since you want him neither too fat nor too thin, his appetite for his proper diet should be guarded, and children and guests should not be permitted to constantly be feeding him "goodies." The best treat of all is a small wad of raw ground beef or a packaged dog treat. To be avoided are ice cream, cake, cookies, potato chips, and other fattening items which will cause the dog to put on weight and may additionally spoil his appetite for the proper, nourishing, well-balanced diet so essential to good health and condition.

The importance of temperament and showmanship cannot possibly be overestimated. They have put many a mediocre dog across while lack of them can ruin the career of an otherwise outstanding specimen. From the day your dog joins your family, socialize him. Keep him accustomed to being with people and to being handled by people. Encourage your friends and relatives to "go over" him as the judges will in the ring so this will not seem a strange and upsetting experience. Practice showing his "bite" (the manner in which his teeth meet) quickly and deftly. It is quite simple to slip the lips apart with your fingers, and the puppy should be willing to accept this from you or the judge without struggle. This is also true of further mouth examination when necessary. Where the standard demands examination of the roof of the mouth and the tongue, accustom the dog to having his jaws opened wide in order for the judge to make this required examination. When missing teeth must be noted, again, teach the dog to permit his jaws to be opened wide and his side lips separated as judges will need to check them one or both of these ways.

Some judges prefer that the exhibitors display the dog's bite and other mouth features themselves. These are the considerate ones, who do not wish to chance the spreading of possible infection from dog to dog with their hands on each one's mouth—a courtesy particularly appreciated in these days of virus epidemics. But the old-fashioned judges still persist in doing it themselves, so the dog should be ready for either possibility.

Take your future show dog with you in the car, thus accustoming him to riding so that he will not become carsick on the day of a dog show. He should associate pleasure and attention with going in the car, or van or motor home. Take him where it is crowded: downtown, to the shops, everywhere you go that dogs are permitted. Make the expeditions fun for him by frequent petting and words of praise; do not just ignore him as you go about your errands.

Do not overly shelter your future show dog. Instinctively you may want to keep him at home where he is safe from germs or danger. This can be foolish on two counts. The first reason is that a puppy kept away from other dogs builds up no natural immunity against all the things with which he will come in contact at dog shows, so it is wiser actually to keep him well up to date on all protective shots and then let him become accustomed to being among dogs and dog owners. Also, a dog who never is among strange people, in strange places, or among strange dogs, may grow up with a shyness or timidity of spirit that will cause you real problems as his show career draws near.

Keep your show prospect's coat in immaculate condition with frequent grooming and daily brushing. When bathing is necessary, use a mild baby shampoo or whatever the breeder of your puppy may suggest. Several of the brand-name products do an excellent job. Be sure to rinse thoroughly so as not to risk skin irritation by traces of soap left behind and protect against soap entering the eyes by a drop of castor oil in each before you lather up. Use warm water (be sure it is not uncomfortably hot or chillingly cold) and a good spray. A hair dryer is a real convenience for the heavily coated breeds and can be used for

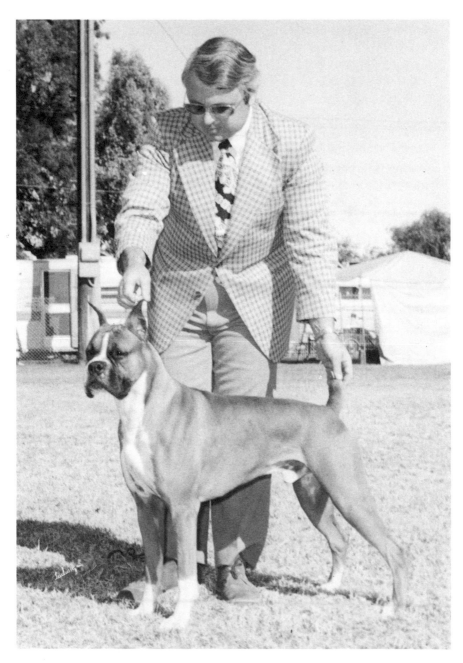

Ch. Braemerwood Bishop Jaggers, by Ch. Peablo's Black Bishop ex Braemerwood's Comin Thru, at the time of becoming a champion was owned by Ruth F. and Wm. J. Leek, Gig Harbor, Washington. After finishing this Boxer was sold to William Cook.

thorough drying after first blotting off the excess moisture with a turkish towel. A wad of cotton in each ear will prevent water entering the ear cavity.

Toenails also should be watched and trimmed every few weeks. It is important not to permit nails to grow excessively long, as they will ruin the appearance of both the feet and pasterns.

Assuming that you will be handling the dog yourself, or even if he will be professionally handled, a few moments each day of dog show routine is important. Practice setting him up as you have seen the exhibitors do at the shows you've attended, and teach him to hold this

Aust. Ch. Seefeld Sheer Delight, imported from the United Kingdom, is by Eng. Ch. Seefeld Shadowfax ex Shebacrest Sunbeam. Bred by Mrs. Pat Heath, Seefeld Kennels, England and owned by Dave Strachan, Thasrite Boxers, Australia.

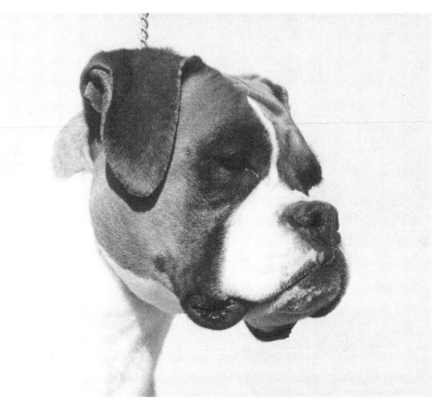

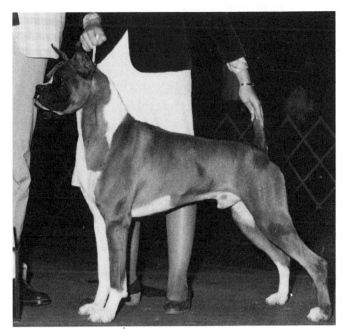

position once you have him stacked to your satisfaction. If he is a small breed that judges examine on a table, accustom him to this. Make the learning period pleasant by being firm but lavish in your praise when he responds correctly. Teach him to gait at your side at a moderate rate on a loose lead. When you have mastered the basic essentials at home, then hunt out and join a training class for future work. Training classes are sponsored by show-giving clubs in many areas, and their popularity is steadily increasing. If you have no other way of locating one, perhaps your veterinarian would know of one through some of his other clients; but if you are sufficiently aware of the dog show world to want a show dog, you will probably be personally acquainted with other people who will share information of this type with you.

Accustom your show dog to being in a crate (which you should be doing with a pet dog as well). He should relax in his crate at the shows "between times" for his own well being and safety.

A show dog's teeth must be kept clean and free of tartar. Hard dog-biscuits can help toward this, but if tartar accumulates, see that it is removed promptly by your veterinarian. Bones are not suitable for show dogs as they tend to damage and wear down the tooth enamel.

Match Shows

Your show dog's initial experience in the ring should be in match show competition for several reasons. First, this type of event is intended as a learning experience for both the dog and the exhibitor. You will not feel embarrassed or out of place no matter how poorly your puppy may behave or how inept your attempts at handling may be, as you will find others there with the same type of problems. The important thing is that you get the puppy out and into a show ring where the two of you can practice together and learn the ropes.

Ch. Laurel Hill's Rudolf, by Ch. Sunset Spirit of Five T's ex Laurel Hill's Jingle Bells, pictured going Winners Dog, Best of Winners, and Best of Opposite Sex (over two Best in Show dogs) at the Sir Francis Drake Kennel Club in 1983. Co-owned by the breeders, Bruce and Jeannie Korsan, and by Ann Herr of Treceder Boxers.

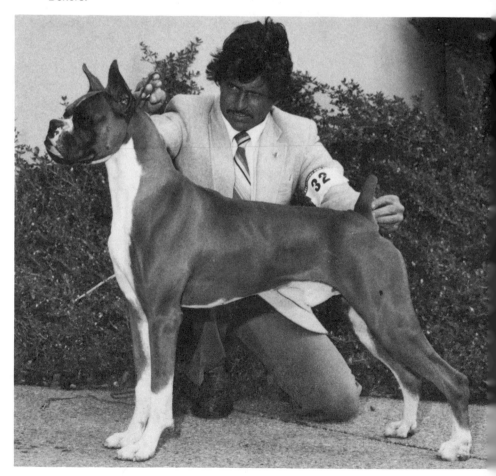

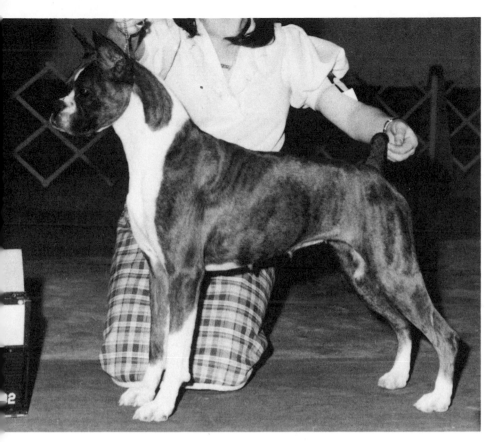

Ch. Laurel Hill's Call Me Brat taking Winners Bitch at North Country in 1982 for Jeannie and Bruce Korsan, Oyster Bay, N.Y.

Only on rare occasions is it necessary to make match show entries in advance, and even those with a pre-entry policy will usually accept entries at the door as well. Thus you need not plan several weeks ahead, as is the case with point shows, but can go when the mood strikes you. Also there is a vast difference in the cost, as match show entries only cost a few dollars while entry fees for the point shows may be over ten dollars, an amount none of us needs to waste until we have some idea of how the puppy will behave or how much more pre-show training is needed.

Match shows very frequently are judged by professional handlers who, in addition to making the awards, are happy to help new exhibitors with comments and advice on their puppies and their presentation of them. Avail yourself of all these opportunities before heading out to the sophisticated world of the point shows.

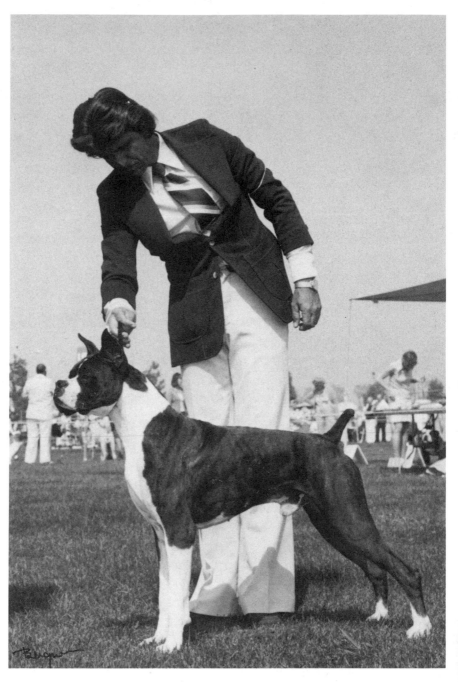

Ch. Treceder's Holy Smoke, by Ch. Ringmaster's Olimpian ex Treceder's Special Edition, owned by Treceder Kennels, bred by Mary Surasky.

216

Ch. Jondem's Jason, by Ch. Treceder Selection ex Summerdale Showboat (imported from England), figures strongly in the background of most of the present day Box M Kennels stock of Lois Matthews, Kailua, Hawaii. Headstudy by Patience Birley.

This lovely bitch is the consistent winner Ch. My Cyn's Winter Wheat taking one of her Working Group firsts for Mr. and Mrs. Judson L. Streicher, Scarsdale, New York, under judge Henry Stoecker and Jane Forsyth handling.

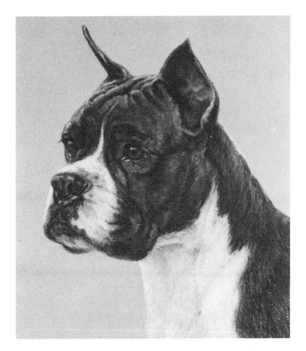

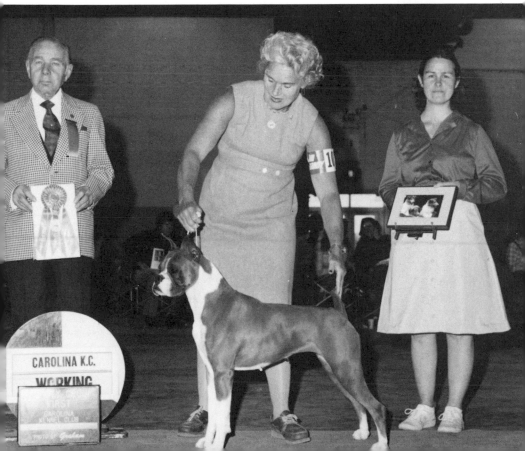

Point Shows

As previously mentioned, entries for American Kennel Club point shows must be made in advance. This must be done on an official entry blank of the show-giving club. The entry must then be filed either personally or by mail with the show superintendent or the show secretary (if the event is being run by the club members alone and a superintendent has not been hired, this information will appear on the premium list) in time to reach its destination prior to the published closing date or filling of the quota. These entries must be made carefully, must be signed by the owner of the dog or the owner's agent (your professional handler), and must be accompanied by the entry fee; otherwise they will not be accepted. Remember that it is not when the entry leaves your hands that counts but the date of arrival at its destination. If you are relying on the mails, which are not always dependable, get the entry off well before the deadline to avoid disappointment.

A dog must be entered at a dog show in the name of the actual owner at the time of the entry closing date of that specific show. If a registered dog has been acquired by a new owner, it must be entered in the name of the new owner in any show for which entries close after the date of acquirement, regardless of whether the new owner has or has not actually received the registration certificate indicating that the dog is recorded in his name. State on the entry form whether or not transfer application has been mailed to the American Kennel Club, and it goes without saying that the latter should be attended to promptly when you purchase a registered dog.

In filling out your entry blank, type, print, or write clearly, paying particular attention to the spelling of names, correct registration numbers, and so on.

The Puppy Class is for dogs or bitches who are six months of age and under twelve months, were whelped in the United States, and are not champions. The age of a dog shall be calculated up to and inclusive of the first day of a show. For example, the first day a dog whelped on January 1st is eligible to compete in a Puppy Class at a show is July 1st of the same year; and he may continue to compete in Puppy Classes up to and including a show on December 31st of the same year, but he is *not* eligible to compete in a Puppy Class at a show held on or after January 1st of the following year.

Can. Ch. Pinepaths
Union Jack, son of Am.
and Can. Ch. Tremenor
Pinepaths Hudson Bay,
Union Jack 13 months
old in this photo. Owned
by Jack and Cathryn
Ireland, Fingal, Ontario,
Canada.

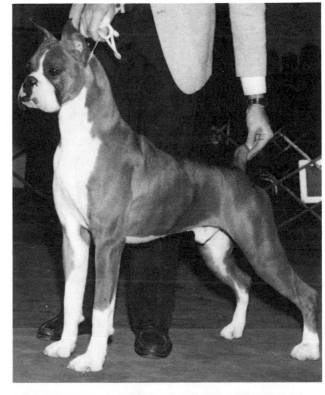

Ch. Box M Royal
Hawaiian, by Ch. My-R's
Imperial ex Ch. Box M
Sparkle, a Makiki
daughter was Best of
Breed at the Boxer Club
of Hawaii Specialty in
1974. Lois Matthews,
owner, Box M Kennels,
Kailua, Hawaii.

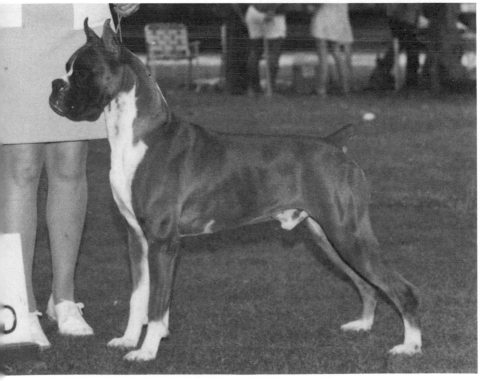

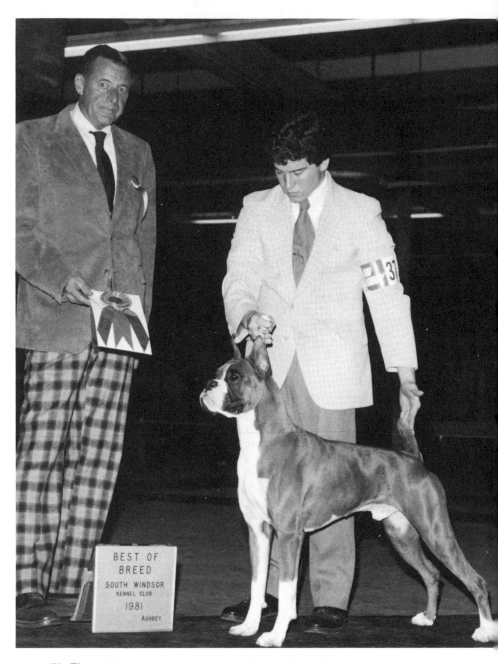

Ch. Thorn Hill's Country Squire by Ch. Yuri Nuff of Z Best ex Talisman's Southern Belle, was Best of Breed at South Windsor K.C. in 1981. Handled by George Russell. Owners, Marian and Norman Scribner.

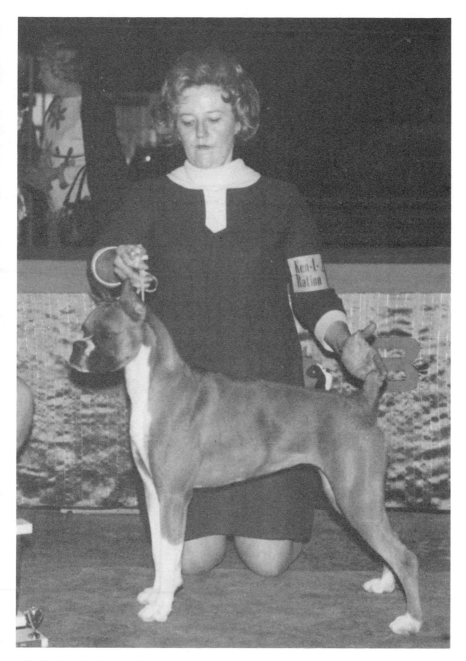

Ch. Ruhland's Swiss Miss on her first ring appearance, nine months old, in March 1969 at the Heart of America Boxer Club. Handled by Carol Howell to Best of Winners for a five-point major and Best Puppy for owners Ruth and Bill Leek, Gig Harbor, Washington.

The Puppy Class is the first one in which you should enter your puppy. In it a certain allowance will be made for the fact that they *are* puppies, thus an immature dog or one displaying less than perfect showmanship will be less severely penalized than, for instance, would be the case in Open. It is also quite likely that others in the class will be suffering from these problems, too. When you enter a puppy, be sure to check the classification with care, as some shows divide their Puppy Class into a 6-9 months old section and a 9-12 months old section.

The Novice Class is for dogs six months of age and over, whelped in the United States or Canada, who *prior to the official closing date for entries* have *not* won three first prizes in the Novice Class, any first prize at all in the Bred-by-Exhibitor, American-bred, or Open Classes, or one or more points toward championship. The provisions for this class are confusing to many people, which is probably the reason exhibitors do not enter in it more frequently. A dog may win any number of first prizes in the Puppy Class and still retain his eligibility for Novice. He may place second, third or fourth not only in Novice on an unlimited number of occasions but also in Bred-by-Exhibitor, American-bred and Open and still remain eligible for Novice. But he may no longer be shown in Novice when he has won three blue ribbons in that class, when he has won even one blue ribbon in either Bred-by-Exhibitor, American-bred, or Open, or when he has won a single championship point.

In determining whether or not a dog is eligible for the Novice Class, keep in mind the fact that previous wins are calculated according to the official published date for closing of entries, not by the date on which you may actually have made the entry. So if in the interim, between the time you made the entry and the official closing date, your dog makes a win causing him to become ineligible for Novice, change your class *immediately* to another for which he will be eligible, preferably such as either Bred-by-Exhibitor or American-bred. To do this, you must contact the show's superintendent or secretary, at first by telephone to save time and at the same time confirm it in writing. The Novice Class always seems to have the fewest entries of any class, and therefore it is a splendid "practice ground" for you and your young dog while you are getting the "feel" of being in the ring.

Bred-by-Exhibitor Class is for dogs whelped in the United States or, if individually registered in the American Kennel Club Stud Book, for dogs whelped in Canada who are six months of age or older, are not champions, and are owned wholly or in part by the person or by the spouse of the person who was the breeder or one of the breeders of

Ch. Wheatland's Bluestone Buffie, a daughter of Ch. Heldenbrand's Kansas Twister, going Grand Sweepstakes Winner.

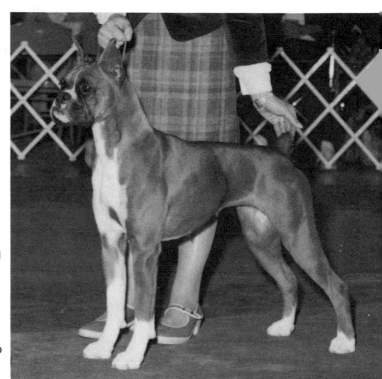

Ch. Baroque's Dorable Dulcimer owned by Robert and Kathryn Billings, Newington, Connecticut, finished June 1980 at Del Otse Nango and was the American Boxer Club First Prize Futurity winner in May 1980.

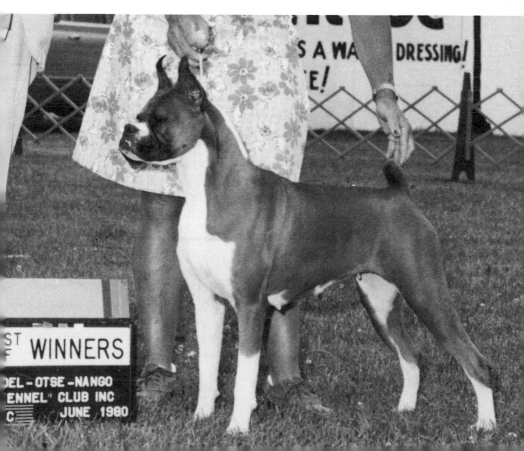

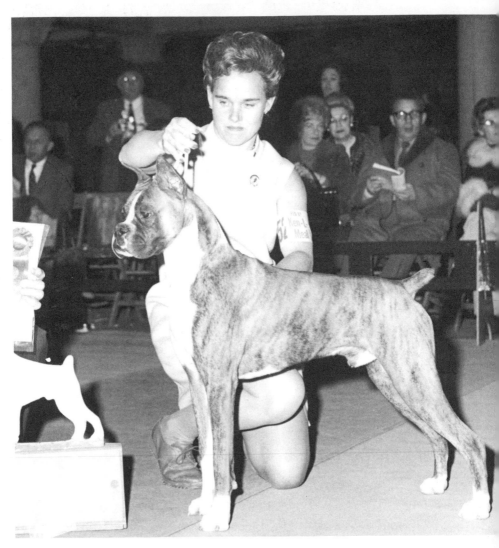

Ch. Salgray's Double Talk owned by Mr. and Mrs. Daniel Hamilburg, Jane Forsyth handling.

Opposite page: Ch. Evening Star of Heritage pictured taking Winners Bitch at the Boomer Boxer Club at the age of seven months. Born March 22nd 1975, by Ch. Quisto's Cornerstone ex Holly Lane's Captivating Wind, was the first of three litter sisters to finish, doing so at eight months and fifteen days with three majors. Her other two sisters also did a lot of puppy class winning. Bred and owned by Jane G. Moog, East Aurora, New York. Handled by Charles E. Steele.

224

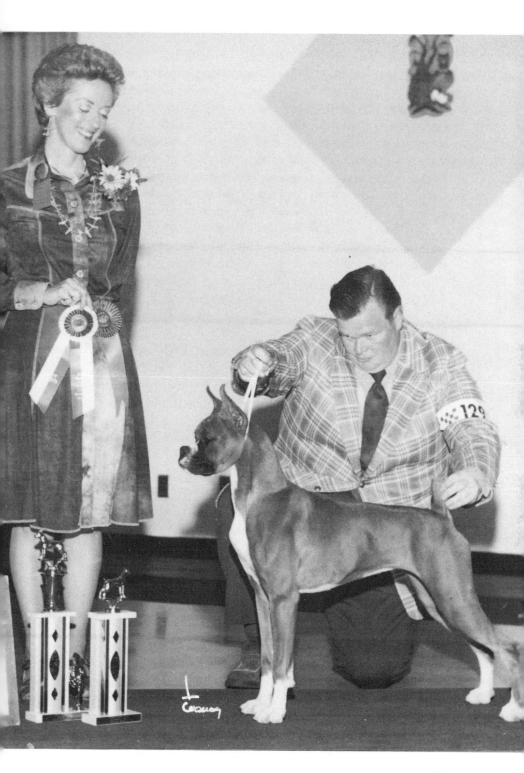

record. Dogs entered in this class must be handled in the class by an owner or by a member of the immediate family of the owner. Members of an immediate family for this purpose are husband, wife, father, mother, son, daughter, brother or sister. This is the class which is really the "breeders' showcase," and the one which breeders should enter with particular pride to show off their achievements.

The American-bred Class is for all dogs excepting champions, six months of age or older, who were whelped in the United States by reason of a mating which took place in the United States.

The Open Class is for any dog six months of age or older (this is the only restriction for this class). Dogs with championship points compete in it, dogs who are already champions are eligible to do so, dogs who are imported can be entered, and, of course, American-bred dogs compete in it. This class is, for some strange reason, the favorite of exhibitors who are "out to win." They rush to enter their pointed dogs in it, under the false impression that by doing so they assure themselves of greater attention from the judges. This really is not so, and in my opinion to enter in one of the less competitive classes, with a better chance of winning it and thus earning a second opportunity of gaining the judge's approval by returning to the ring in the Winners Class, can often be a more effective strategy.

One does not enter for the Winners Class. One earns the right to compete in it by winning first prize in Puppy, Novice, Bred-by-Exhibitor, American-bred, or Open. No dog who has been defeated on the same day in one of these classes is eligible to compete for Winners, and every dog who has been a blue-ribbon winner in one of them and not defeated in another, should he have been entered in more than one class, (as occasionally happens) *must* do so. Following the selection of the Winners Dog or the Winners Bitch, the dog or bitch receiving that award leaves the ring. Then the dog or bitch who placed second in that class, unless previously beaten by another dog or bitch in another class at the same show, re-enters the ring to compete against the remaining first-prize winners for Reserve. The latter award indicates that the dog or bitch selected for it is standing "in reserve" should the one who received Winners be disqualified or declared ineligible through any technicality when the awards are checked at the American Kennel Club. In that case, the one who placed Reserve is moved up to Winners, at the same time receiving the appropriate championship points.

Winners Dog and Winners Bitch are the awards which carry points toward championship with them. The points are based on the number

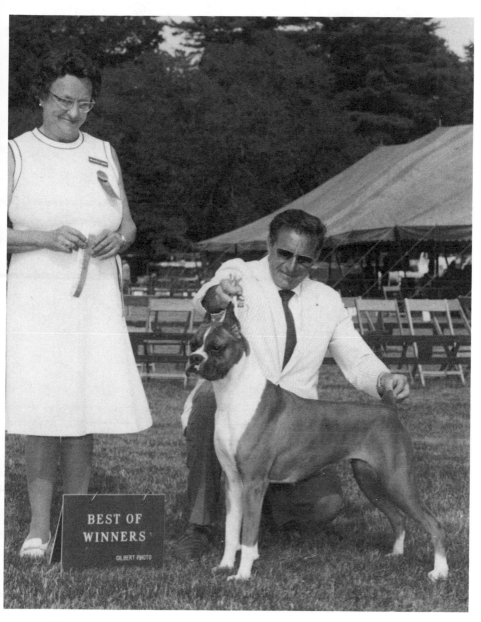

Ch. O'Laiwe's Silk'n'Stuff finished this day with her second major. Owners, Kathy and Bob Billings, handler, Bob Forsyth.

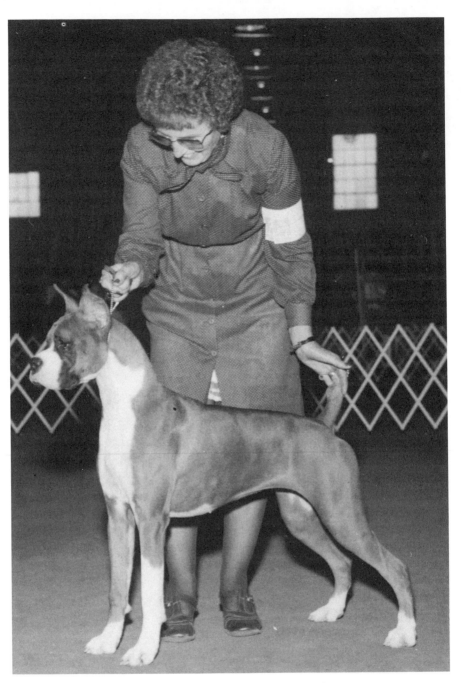

Heldenbrand's Peddler's Dream, daughter of Ch. Holly Lane's Dream Peddler, C.D., ex Holly Lane's Aureate, C.D., winning Grand Sweepstakes at the Wichita Kansas Boxer Club Specialty. Elvinia Heldenbrand, owner-handler, Manhattan, Kansas.

of dogs or bitches actually in competition, and the points are scaled one through five, the latter being the greatest number available to any one dog or bitch at any one show. Three-, four-, or five-point wins are considered majors. In order to become a champion, a dog or bitch must have won two majors under two different judges, plus at least one point from a third judge, and the additional points necessary to bring the total to fifteen. When your dog has gained fifteen points as described above, a championship certificate will be issued to you, and your dog's name will be published in the champions of record list in the *Pure-Bred Dogs/American Kennel Gazette,* the official publication of the American Kennel Club.

The scale of championship points for each breed is worked out by the American Kennel Club and reviewed annually, at which time the number required in competition may be either changed (raised or lowered) or remain the same. The scale of championship points for all breeds is published annually in the May issue of the *Gazette,* and the current ratings for each breed within that area are published in every show catalog.

When a dog or bitch is adjudged Best of Winners, its championship points are, for that show, compiled on the basis of which sex had the greater number of points. If there are two points in dogs and four in bitches and the dog goes Best of Winners, then *both* the dog and the bitch are awarded an equal number of points, in this case four. Should the Winners Dog or the Winners Bitch go on to win Best of Breed or Best of Variety, additional points are accorded for the additional dogs and bitches defeated by so doing, provided, of course, that there were entries specifically for Best of Breed Competition or Specials, as these specific entries are generally called.

If your dog or bitch takes Best of Opposite Sex after going Winners, points are credited according to the number of the same sex defeated in both the regular classes and Specials competition. If Best of Winners is also won, then whatever additional points for each of these awards are available will be credited. Many a one-or two-point win has grown into a major in this manner.

Moving further along, should your dog win its Variety Group from the classes (in other words, if it has taken either Winners Dog or Winners Bitch), you then receive points based on the greatest number of points awarded to any member of any breed included within that Group during that show's competition. Should the day's winning also include Best in Show, the same rule of thumb applies, and your dog or bitch receives the highest number of points awarded to any other dog of any breed at that event.

Best of Breed competition consists of the Winners Dog and the Winners Bitch, who automatically compete on the strength of those awards, in addition to whatever dogs and bitches have been entered specifically for this class for which champions of record are eligible. Since July 1980, dogs who, according to their owner's records, have completed the requirements for a championship after the closing of entries for the show, but whose championships are unconfirmed, may be transferred from one of the regular classes to the Best of Breed competition, provided this transfer is made by the show superintendent or show secretary *prior to the start of any judging at the show.*

This has proved an extremely popular new rule, as under it a dog can finish on Saturday and then be transferred and compete as a Special on Sunday. It must be emphasized that the change *must* be made *prior* to the start of *any* part of the day's judging, not for just your individual breed.

In the United States, Best of Breed winners are entitled to compete in the Variety Group which includes them. This is not mandatory, it is a privilege which exhibitors value. (In Canada, Best of Breed winners *must* compete in the Variety Group, or they lose any points already won.) The dogs winning *first* in each of the seven Variety Groups *must* compete for Best in Show. Missing the opportunity of taking your dog in for competition in its Group is foolish as it is there where the general public is most likely to notice your breed and become interested in learning about it.

Non-regular classes are sometimes included at the all-breed shows, and they are almost invariably included at Specialty Shows. These include Stud Dog Class and Brood Bitch Class, which are judged on the basis of the quality of the two offspring accompanying the sire or dam. The quality of the latter two is beside the point and should not be considered by the judge; it is the youngsters who count, and the quality of *both* are to be averaged to decide which sire or dam is the best and most consistent producer. Then there is the Brace Class (which, at all-breed shows, moves up to Best Brace in each Variety Group and then Best Brace in Show), which is judged on the similarity and evenness of appearance of the two members of the brace. In other words, the two dogs should look like identical twins in size, color, and conformation and should move together almost as a single dog, one person handling with precision and ease. The same applies to the Team Class competi-

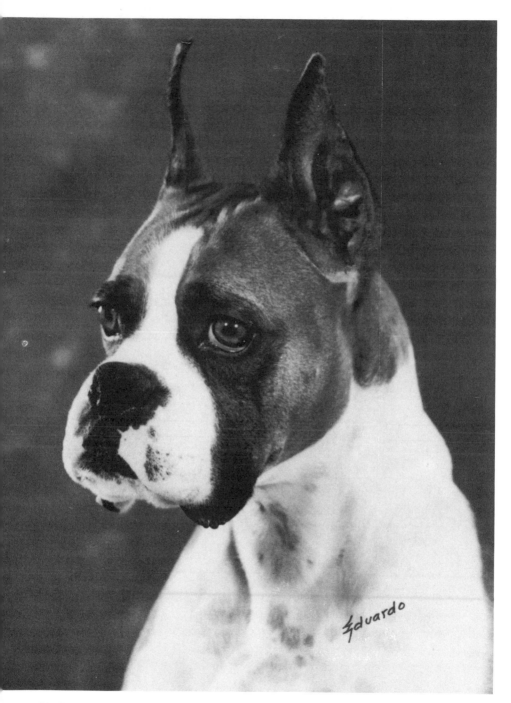

Ch. Evergreen's Delight owned by Jane Nolt Flowers, Buffalo, Minnesota.

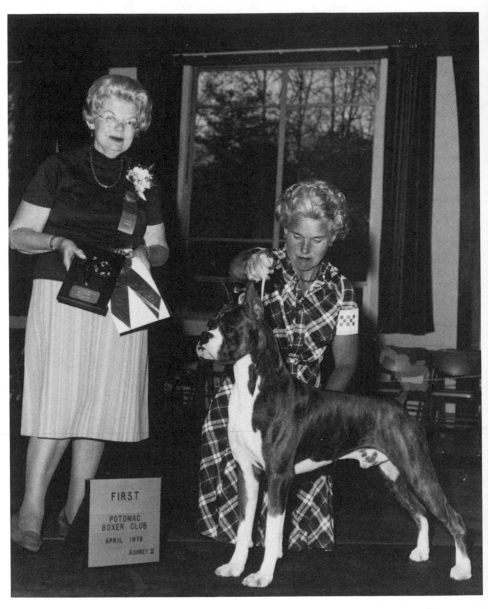

Ch. Cava Lanes Sgt. Pepper, owned by Dr. F. Gusmano, at the Potomac Boxer Club Specialty in 1979, under judge Anna Katherine Nicholas. Jane Forsyth handling.

tion, except that four dogs are involved and, if necessary, two handlers.

The Veterans Class is for the older dogs, the minimum age of whom is seven years. This class is judged on the quality of the dogs, as the winner competes in Best of Breed competition and has, on a respectable number of occasions, been known to take that top award. So the point is *not* to pick out the oldest dog, as some judges seem to believe, but the best specimen of the breed, exactly as in the regular classes.

Then there are Sweepstakes and Futurity Stakes sponsored by many Specialty clubs, sometimes as part of their regular Specialty Shows and sometimes as separate events on an entirely different occasion. The difference between the two stakes is that Sweepstakes entries usually include dogs from six to eighteen months age with entries made at the same time as the others for the show, while for a Futurity the entries are bitches nominated when bred and the individual puppies entered at or shortly following their birth.

If you already show your dog, if you plan on being an exhibitor in the future, or if you simply enjoy attending dog shows, there is a book, written by me, which you will find to be an invaluable source of detailed information about all aspects of show dog competition. This book is *Successful Dog Show Exhibiting* (T.F.H. Publications, Inc.) and is available wherever the one you are reading was purchased.

Junior Showmanship Competition

If there is a youngster in your family between the ages of ten and sixteen, I can suggest no better or more rewarding hobby than becoming an active participant in Junior Showmanship. This is a marvelous activity for young people. It teaches responsibility, good sportsmanship, the fun of competition where one's own skills are the deciding factor of success, proper care of a pet, and how to socialize with other young folks. Any youngster may experience the thrill of emerging from the ring a winner and the satisfaction of a good job well done.

Entry in Junior Showmanship Classes is open to any boy or girl who is at least ten years old and under seventeen years old on the day of the show. The Novice Junior Showmanship Class is open to youngsters who have not already won, at the time the entries close, three firsts in this class. Youngsters who have won three firsts in Novice may compete in the Open Junior Showmanship Class. Any junior handler who wins his third first-place award in Novice may participate in the Open Class at the same show, provided that the Open Class has at least one other junior handler entered and competing in it that day. The Novice

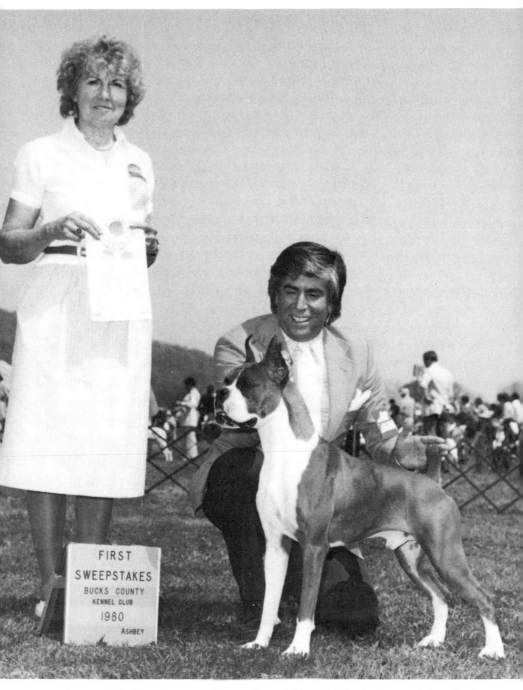

Laurel Hill's Pipe Dream, a "Bosco" son, taking first in the Sweepstakes, Bucks County K.C. in 1980, handled by co-breeder-owner Bruce Korsan, Laurel Hill Boxers, Oyster Bay, N.Y.

234

and Open Classes may be divided into Junior and Senior Classes. Youngsters between the ages of ten and twelve, inclusively, are eligible for the Junior division; and youngsters between thirteen and seventeen, inclusively, are eligible for the Senior division.

Any of the foregoing classes may be separated into individual classes for boys and for girls. If such a division is made, it must be so indicated on the premium list. The premium list also indicates the prize for Best Junior Handler, if such a prize is being offered at the show. Any youngster who wins a first in any of the regular classes may enter the competition for this prize, provided the youngster has been undefeated in any other Junior Showmanship Class at that show.

Junior Showmanship Classes, unlike regular conformation classes in which the quality of the dog is judged, are judged solely on the skill and ability of the junior handling the dog. Which dog is best is not the point—it is which youngster does the best job with the dog that is under consideration. Eligibility requirements for the dog being shown in Junior Showmanship, and other detailed information, can be found in *Regulations for Junior Showmanship,* available from the American Kennel Club.

A junior who has a dog that he or she can enter in both Junior Showmanship and conformation classes has twice the opportunity for success and twice the opportunity to get into the ring and work with the dog, a combination which can lead to not only awards for expert handling but also, if the dog is of sufficient quality, for making a conformation champion.

Pre-Show Preparations for Your Dog and You

Preparation of the items you will need as a dog show exhibitor should not be left until the last moment. They should be planned and arranged for at least several days in advance of the show in order for you to remain calm and relaxed as the countdown starts.

The importance of the crate has already been mentioned, and we hope it is already part of your equipment. Of equal importance is the grooming table, which very likely you have also already acquired for use at home. You should take it along with you to the shows, as your dog will need last minute touches before entering the ring. Should you have not yet made this purchase, folding tables with rubber tops are made specifically for this purpose and can be purchased at most dog shows, where concession booths with marvelous assortments of "doggy" necessities are to be found, or at your pet supplier. You will also need a sturdy tack box (also available at the dog show concessions) in which to carry your grooming tools and equipment. The latter should include brushes, comb, scissors, nail clippers, whatever you use for last minute clean-up jobs, cotton swabs, first-aid equipment, and anything you are in the habit of using on the dog, including a leash or two of the type you prefer, some well-cooked and dried-out liver or any of the small packaged "dog treats" for use as bait in the ring, an atomizer in case you wish to dampen your dog's coat when you are preparing him for the ring, and so on. A large turkish towel to spread under the dog on the grooming table is also useful.

Take a large thermos or cooler of ice, the biggest one you can accommodate in your vehicle, for use by "man and beast." Take a jug of water (there are lightweight, inexpensive ones available at all sporting goods shops) and a water dish. If you plan to feed the dog at the show, or if you and the dog will be away from home more than one day, bring food for him from home so that he will have the type to which he is accustomed.

You may or may not have an exercise pen. Personally I think one a *must*, even if you only have one dog. While the shows do provide areas for the exercise of the dogs, these are among the most likely places to have your dog come in contact with any illnesses which may be going around, and I feel that having a pen of your own for your dog's use is excellent protection. Such a pen can be used in other ways, too, such as a place other than the crate in which to put the dog to relax (that is roomier than the crate) and a place in which the dog can exercise at motels and rest areas. These, too, are available at the show concession stands and come in a variety of heights and sizes. A set of "pooper scoopers" should also be part of your equipment, along with a package of plastic bags for cleaning up after your dog.

Bring along folding chairs for the members of your party, unless all of you are fond of standing, as these are almost never provided anymore by the clubs. Have your name stamped on the chairs so that there will be no doubt as to whom the chairs belong. Bring whatever you and your family enjoy for drinks or snacks in a picnic basket or cooler, as show food, in general, is expensive and usually not great. You should always have a pair of boots, a raincoat, and a rain hat with you (they should remain permanently in your vehicle if you plan to attend shows regularly), as well as a sweater, a warm coat, and a change of shoes. A smock or big cover-up apron will assure that you remain tidy as you prepare the dog for the ring. Your overnight case should include a small sewing kit for emergency repairs, bandaids, headache

236

Pinetop Dark Omen, by Am. and Can. Ch. Tradonalees Tradewin (Canadian import) ex Aust. Ch. Pinetop Liberation at six months of age. Owned by Kevin and Lorraine Harris, Pinetop Boxers, Welland, South Australia.

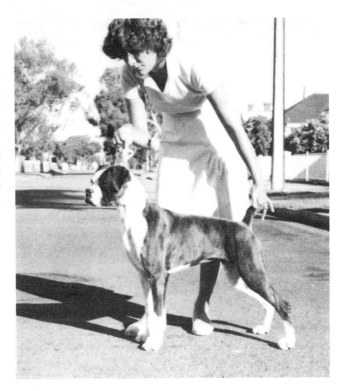

Aust. Ch. Intrends Wind Song began her show career winning Best Puppy in Show at the 1979 Victoria Boxer Specialty under Tom Perret, taking Challenge Certificate Bitch the next year at this same Specialty. She also has won Challenge Bitch at the South Australian Boxer Specialty in 1982 and has two Bests in Show, all-breeds, to her credit. Bred by Judy Horton and owned by Mr. and Mrs. J. Dickinson.

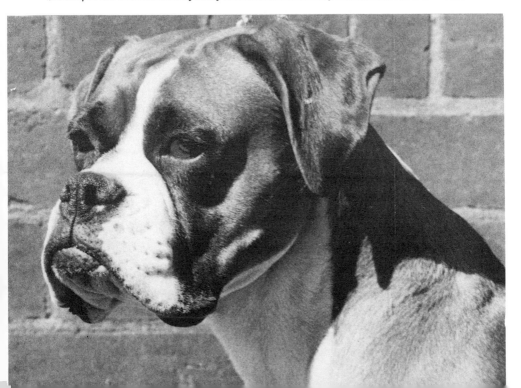

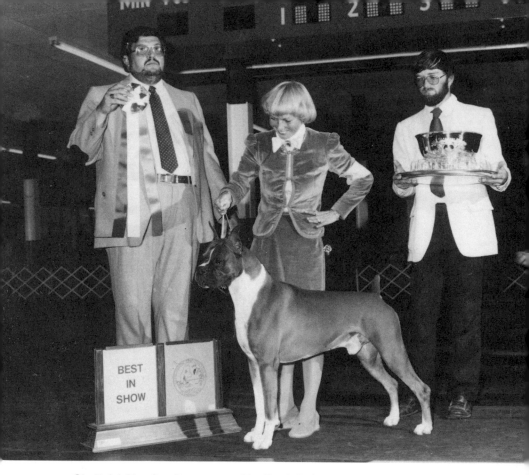

Ch. Kojak Von San Remo, owned by Frank O. Scelfo and Liane Dimitroff winning Best in Show at Vacationland Dog Club, October 8th 1983. Judge, Dr. Esporite. Handler, Carmen Skinner.

and indigestion remedies, and any personal products or medications you normally use.

In your car you should always carry maps of the area where you are headed and an assortment of motel directories. Generally speaking, we have found Holiday Inns to be the nicest about taking dogs. Ramadas and Howard Johnsons generally do so cheerfully (with a few exceptions). Best Western generally frowns on pets (not always, but often enough to make it necessary to find out which do). Some of the smaller chains welcome pets. The majority of privately owned motels do not.

Have everything prepared the night before the show to expedite your departure. Be sure that the dog's identification and your judging program and other show information are in your purse or briefcase. If you are taking sandwiches, have them ready. Anything that goes into

238

the car the night before the show will be one thing less to remember in the morning. Decide upon what you will wear and have it out and ready. If there is any question in your mind about what to wear, try on the possibilities before the day of the show; don't risk feeling you may want to change when you see yourself dressed a few moments prior to departure time!

In planning your outfit, make it something simple that will not detract from your dog. Remember that a dark dog silhouettes attractively against a light background and vice-versa. Sport clothes always seem to look best at dog shows, preferably conservative in type and not overly "loud" as you do not want to detract from your dog, who should be the focus of interest at this point. What you wear on your feet is important. Many types of flooring can be hazardously slippery, as can wet grass. Make it a habit to wear rubber soles and low or flat heels in the ring for your own safety, especially if you are showing a dog that likes to move out smartly.

Your final step in pre-show preparation is to leave yourself plenty of time to reach the show that morning. Traffic can get amazingly heavy as one nears the immediate area of the show, finding a parking place can be difficult, and other delays may occur. You'll be in better humor to enjoy the day if your trip to the show is not fraught with panic over fear of not arriving in time!

Enjoying the Dog Show

From the moment of your arrival at the show until after your dog has been judged, keep foremost in your mind the fact that he is your reason for being there and that he should therefore be the center of your attention. Arrive early enough to have time for those last-minute touches that can make such a great difference when he enters the ring. Be sure that he has ample time to exercise and that he attends to personal matters. A dog arriving in the ring and immediately using it as an exercise pen hardly makes a favorable impression on the judge.

When you reach ringside, ask the steward for your arm-card and anchor it firmly into place on your arm. Make sure that you are where you should be when your class is called. The fact that you have picked up your arm-card does not guarantee, as some seem to think, that the judge will wait for you. The judge has a full schedule which he wishes to complete on time. Even though you may be nervous, assume an air of calm self-confidence. Remember that this is a hobby to be enjoyed, so approach it in that state of mind. The dog will do better, too.

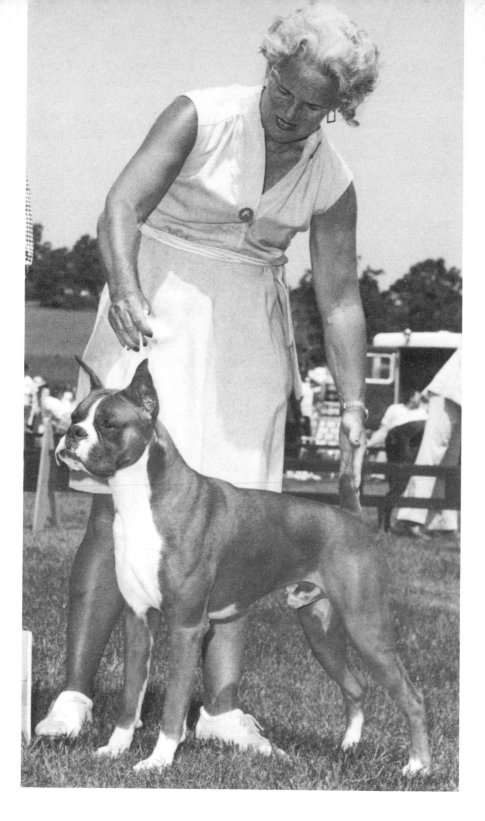

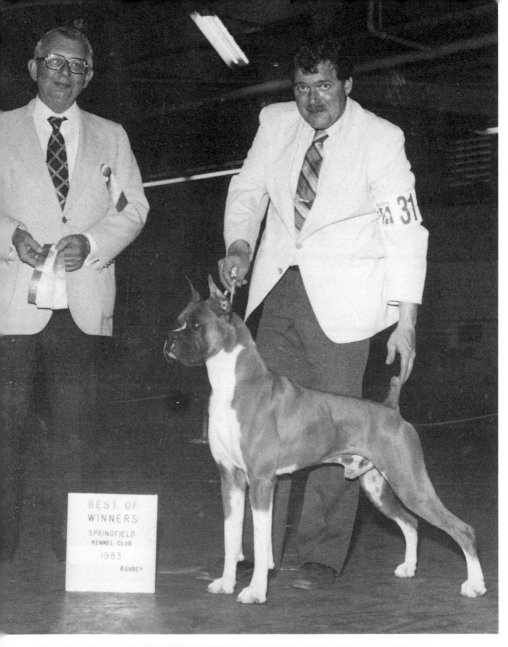

Am. Ch. Hexastar's Ted Stamp of Ruhlend, by Ch. Arriba's Command Performance ex Ch. Ruhlend's Contessa of Abaro, finishing his title the weekend following the American Boxer Club Specialty. A multi-Best of Breed winner, "Teddy" is handled by Douglas R. Holloway, Jr., for Dick Frohock and Hexastar Kennels.

Opposite page: Doris and Thomas McMillen own this handsome Boxer, Ch. Lu-N's Diamond Jim of Hawknest. Jane Forsyth handling,

Always show your dog with an air of pride. If you make mistakes in presenting him, don't worry about it. Next time you will do better. Do not permit the presence of more experienced exhibitors to intimidate you. After all, they, too, once were newcomers.

The judging routine usually starts when the judge asks that the dogs be gaited in a circle around the ring. During this period the judge is watching each dog as it moves, noting style, topline, reach and drive, head and tail carriage, and general balance. Keep your mind and your eye on your dog, moving him at his most becoming gait and keeping your place in line without coming too close to the exhibitor ahead of you. Always keep your dog on the inside of the circle, between yourself and the judge, so that the judge's view of the dog is unobstructed.

Calmly pose the dog when requested to set up for examination whether on the ground or on a table. If you are at the head of the line and many dogs are in the class, go all the way to the end of the ring before starting to stack the dog, leaving sufficient space for those behind you to line theirs up as well as requested by the judge. If you are not at the head of the line but between other exhibitors, leave sufficient space ahead of your dog for the judge to examine him. The dogs should be spaced so that the judge is able to move among them to see them from all angles. In practicing to "set up" or "stack" your dog for the judge's examination, bear in mind the importance of doing so quickly and with dexterity. The judge has a schedule to meet and only a few moments in which to evaluate each dog. You will immeasurably help yours to make a favorable impression if you are able to "get it all together" in a minimum amount of time. Practice at home before a mirror can be a great help toward bringing this about, facing the dog so that you see him from the same side that the judge will and working to make him look right in the shortest length of time.

Listen carefully as the judge describes the manner in which the dog is to be gaited, whether it is straight down and straight back; down the ring, across, and back; or in a triangle. The latter has become the most popular pattern with the majority of judges. "In a triangle" means the dog should move down the outer side of the ring to the first corner, across that end of the ring to the second corner, and then back to the judge from the second corner, using the center of the ring in a diagonal line. Please learn to do this pattern without breaking at each corner to twirl the dog around you, a senseless maneuver we sometimes have noted. Judges like to see the dog in an uninterrupted triangle, as they are thus able to get a better idea of the dog's gait.

It is impossible to overemphasize that the gait at which you move your dog is tremendously important, and considerable study and thought should be given to the matter. At home, have someone move the dog for you at different speeds so that you can tell which shows him off to best advantage. The most becoming action almost invariably is seen at a moderate gait, head up and topline holding. Do not gallop your dog around the ring or hurry him into a speed atypical of his breed. Nothing being rushed appears at its best; give your dog a chance to move along at his (and the breed's) natural gait. For a dog's action to be judged accurately, that dog should move with strength and power but not excessive speed, holding a straight line as he goes to and from the judge.

As you bring the dog back to the judge, stop him a few feet away and be sure that he is standing in a becoming position. Bait him to show the judge an alert expression, using whatever tasty morsel he has been trained to expect for this purpose or, if that works better for you, use a small squeak-toy in your hand. A reminder, please, to those using liver or treats. Take them with you when you leave the ring. Do not just drop them on the ground where they will be found by another dog.

When the awards have been made, accept yours graciously, no matter how you actually may feel about it. What's done is done, and arguing with a judge or stomping out of the ring is useless and a reflection on your sportsmanship. Be courteous, congratulate the winner if your dog was defeated, and try not to show your disappointment. By the same token, please be a gracious winner; this, surprisingly, sometimes seems to be still more difficult.

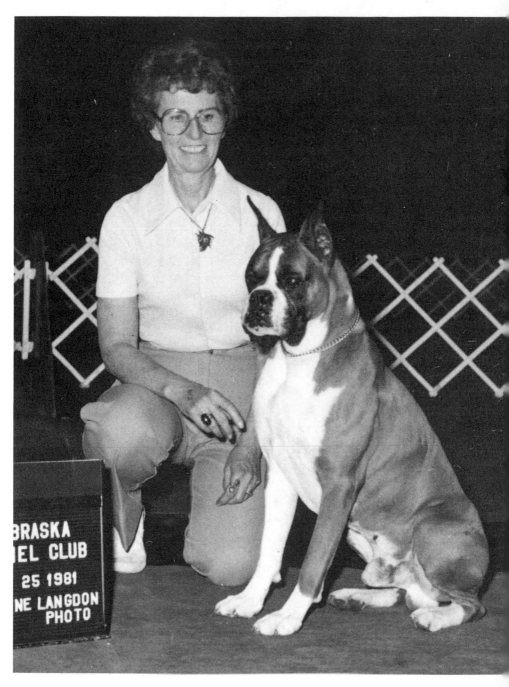

Ch. Holly Lane's Dream Peddler, C.D. earning his C.D. degree under judge Joan
Johnson. Trained and handled by owner Elvinia Heidenbrand, Manhattan, Kansas.

244

Chapter 12

Your Boxer and Obedience

For its own protection and safety, every dog should be taught, at the very least, to recognize and obey the commands "Come," "Heel," "Down," "Sit," and "Stay." Doing so at some time might save the dog's life and in less extreme circumstances will certainly make him a better behaved, more pleasant member of society. If you are patient and enjoy working with your dog, study some of the excellent books available on the subject of obedience and then teach your canine friend these basic manners. If you need the stimulus of working with a group, find out where obedience training classes are held (usually your veterinarian, your dog's breeder, or a dog-owning friend can tell you) and you and your dog can join up. Alternatively, you could let someone else do the training by sending the dog to class, but this is not very rewarding because you lose the opportunity of working with your dog and the pleasure of the rapport thus established.

If you are going to do it yourself, there are some basic rules which you should follow. You must remain calm and confident in attitude. Never lose your temper and frighten or punish your dog unjustly. Be quick and lavish with praise each time a command is correctly followed. Make it fun for the dog and he will be eager to please you by responding correctly. Repetition is the keynote, but it should not be continued without recess to the point of tedium. Limit the training sessions to ten- or fifteen-minute periods at a time.

Formal obedience training can be followed, and very frequently is, by entering the dog in obedience competition to work toward an obedience degree, or several of them, depending on the dog's aptitude and your own enjoyment. Obedience trials are held in conjunction with the majority of all-breed conformation dog shows, with Specialty shows, and frequently as separate Specialty events. If you are working alone with your dog, a list of trial dates might be obtained from your

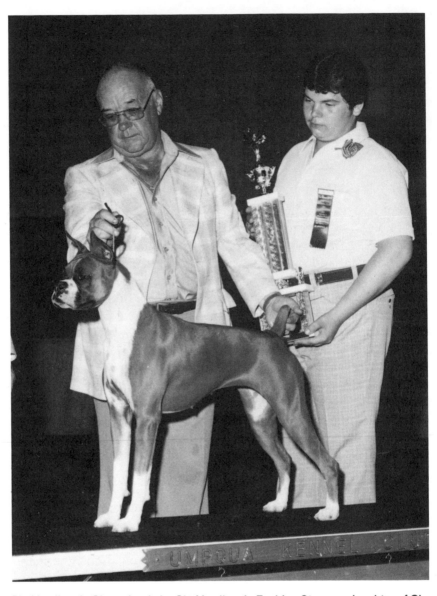

Ch. Merrilane's Closer Look, by Ch. Merrilane's Fashion Star ex a daughter of Ch. Benjamin of Five T's, a Specialty Best in Show and multi-Group winner. Owned by Gordon J. and Edith Turner, Sacramento, California.

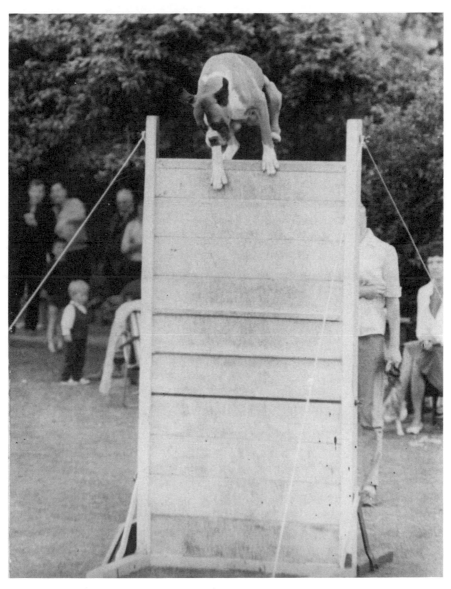

Eng. Ch. Seefeld Holbein, C.D.(Ex) scaling six feet in competition. Mrs. Pat Heath, owner, Seefeld Boxer Kennels, Axbridge, Somerset, England.

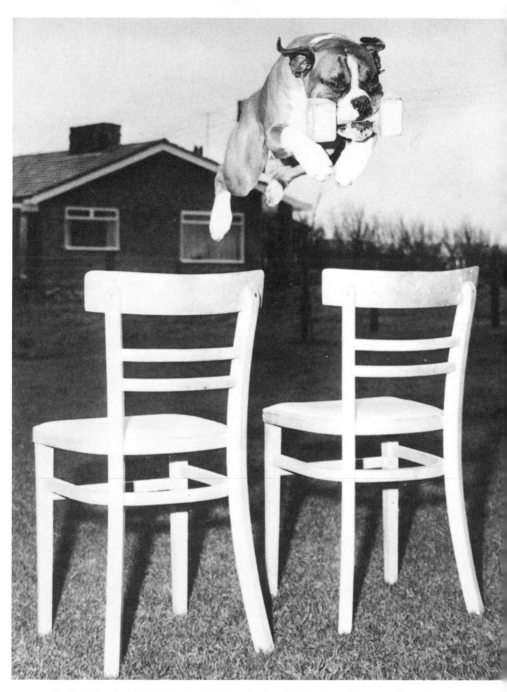

English Ch. Seefeld Holbein, C.D.(Ex), by Seefeld Radden Rembrandt ex Mixonne Mitzi Moonbeam, the sire of the great Int. Ch. Seefeld Picasso, is the only show champion Boxer in the U.K. to qualify at Working Trials, a first prize obedience winner, and the sire of champions. Breeder, Mrs. Harris. Owner, Mrs. Pat Heath, Seefeld Boxers, England.

dog's veterinarian, your dog breeder, or a dog-owning friend; the A.K.C. *Gazette* lists shows and trials to be scheduled in the coming months; and if you are a member of a training class, you will find the information readily available.

The goals for which one works in the formal A.K.C. Member or Licensed Trials are the following titles: Companion Dog (C.D.), Companion Dog Excellent (C.D.X.), and Utility Dog (U.D.). These degrees are earned by receiving three "legs," or qualifying scores, at each level of competition. The degrees must be earned in order, with one completed prior to starting work on the next. For example, a dog must have earned C.D. prior to starting work on C.D.X.; then C.D.X. must be completed before U.D. work begins. The ultimate title attainable in obedience work is Obedience Trial Champion (O.T.Ch.).

When you see the letters "C.D." following a dog's name, you will know that this dog has satisfactorily completed the following exercises: heel on leash, heel free, stand for examination, recall, long sit and long stay. "C.D.X." means that tests have been passed on all of those just mentioned plus heel free, drop on recall, retrieve over high jump, broad jump, long sit, and long down. "U.D." indicates that the dog has additionally passed tests in scent discrimination (leather article), scent discrimination (metal article), signal exercises, directed retrieve, directed jumping, and group stand for examination. The letters "O.T.Ch." are the abbreviation for the only obedience title which precedes rather than follows a dog's name. To gain an obedience trial championship, a dog who already holds a Utility Dog degree must win a total of one hundred points and must win three firsts, under three different judges, in Utility and Open B Classes.

There is also a Tracking Dog title (T.D.) which can be earned at tracking trials. In order to pass the tracking tests the dog must follow the trail of a stranger along a path on which the trail was laid between thirty minutes and two hours previously. Along this track there must be more than two right-angle turns, at least two of which are well out in the open where no fences or other boundaries exist for the guidance of the dog or the handler. The dog wears a harness and is connected to the handler by a lead twenty to forty feet in length. Inconspicuously dropped at the end of the track is an article to be retrieved, usually a glove or wallet, which the dog is expected to locate and the handler to pick up. The letters "T.D.X." are the abbreviation for Tracking Dog Excellent, a more difficult version of the Tracking Dog test with a longer track and more turns to be worked through.

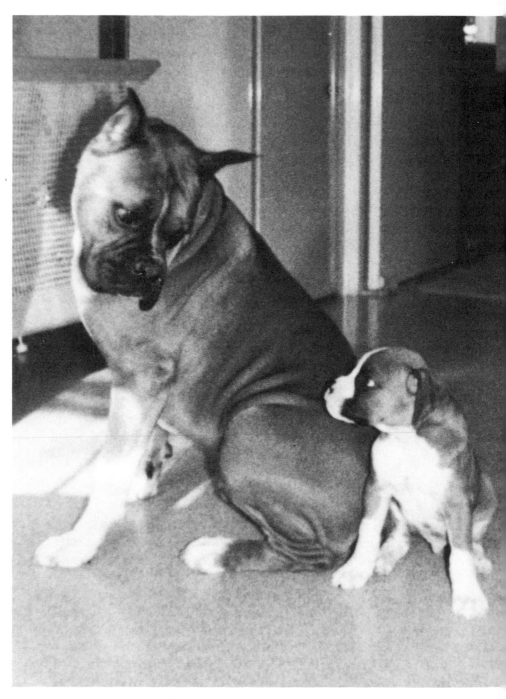

Firppo and Giacco at Cheryl Colby's Hollycrest Kennels, Riverside, Illinois.

250

Chapter 13

Breeding Your Boxer

The Boxer Brood Bitch

We have in an earlier chapter discussed selection of a bitch you plan to use for breeding. In making this important purchase, you will be choosing a bitch who you hope will become the foundation of your kennel. Thus she must be of the finest producing bloodlines, excellent in temperament, of good type, and free of major faults or unsoundness. If you are offered a "bargain" brood bitch, be wary, as for this purchase you should not settle for less than the best and the price will be in accordance with the quality.

Conscientious breeders feel quite strongly that the only possible reason for producing puppies is the ambition to improve and uphold quality and temperament within the breed—definitely *not* because one hopes to make a quick cash profit on a mediocre litter, which never seems to work out that way in the long run and which accomplishes little beyond perhaps adding to the nation's heartbreaking number of unwanted canines. The only reason ever for breeding a litter is, with conscientious people, a desire to improve the quality of dogs in their own kennel or, as pet owners, because they wish to add to the number of dogs they themselves own with a puppy or two from their present favorites. In either case breeding should not take place unless one has definitely prospective owners for as many puppies as the litter may contain, lest you find yourself with several fast-growing young dogs and no homes in which to place them.

Bitches should not be mated earlier than their second season, by which time they should be from fifteen to eighteen months old. Many breeders prefer to wait and first finish the championships of their show bitches before breeding them, as pregnancy can be a disaster to a show coat and getting the bitch back in shape again takes time. When you have decided what will be the proper time, start watching at least several months ahead for what you feel would be the perfect mate to best complement your bitch's quality and bloodlines. Subscribe to the magazines which feature your breed exclusively and to some which cover all breeds in order to familiarize yourself with outstanding stud dogs in areas other than your own for there is no necessity nowadays to limit your choice to a nearby dog unless you truly like him and feel that he is the most suitable. It is quite usual to ship a bitch to a stud dog a distance away, and this generally works out with no ill effects. The important thing is that you need a stud dog strong in those features where your bitch is weak or lacking and of bloodlines compatible to hers. Compare the background of both your bitch and the stud dog under consideration, paying particular attention to the quality of the puppies from bitches with backgrounds similar to your bitch's. If the puppies have been of the type and quality you admire, then this dog would seem a sensible choice for yours, too.

Stud fees may be a few hundred dollars, sometimes even more under special situations for a particularly successful sire. It is money well spent, however. Do *not* ever breed to a dog because he is less expensive than the others unless you honestly believe that he can sire the kind of puppies who will be a credit to your kennel and your breed.

Contacting the owners of the stud dogs you find interesting will bring you pedigrees and pictures which you can then study in relation to your bitch's pedigree and conformation. Discuss your plans with other breeders who are knowledgeable (including the one who bred your own bitch). You may not always receive an entirely unbiased opinion (particularly if the person giving it also has an available stud dog), but one learns by discussion so listen to what they say, consider their opinions, and then you may be better qualified to form your own opinion.

As soon as you have made a choice, phone the owner of the stud dog you wish to use to find out if this will be agreeable. You will be asked about the bitch's health, soundness, temperament, and freedom from serious faults. A copy of her pedigree may be requested, as might a picture of her. A discussion of her background over the telephone may be sufficient to assure the stud's owner that she is suitable for the stud dog and of type, breeding, and quality herself to produce puppies of the quality for which the dog is noted. The owner of a top-quality stud is often extremely selective in the bitches permitted to be bred to his dog,

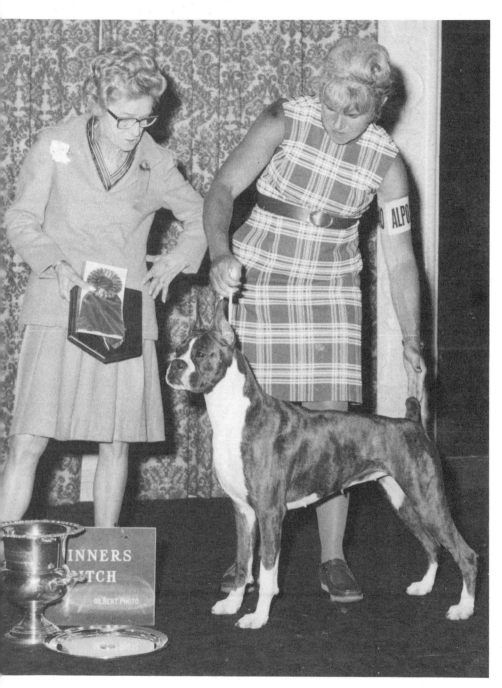

Ch. Weber's Hustling Black Garter, owned by Jim and Lu Jackson, was Winners Bitch and Best of Winners at the 1974 A.B.C. Specialty. Jane Forsyth handling.

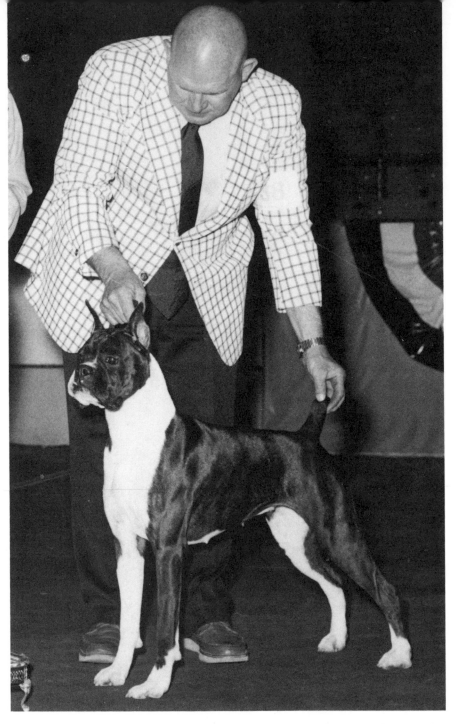

Ch. Treceder's Up In Smoke, by Ch. Treceder's Holy Smoke ex Treceder's Luscious, winning second major at Houston Boxer Club Specialty in March 1981. Bred and owned by Treceder Kennels, Houston, Texas.

in an effort to keep the standard of his puppies high. The owner of a stud dog may require that the bitch be tested for brucellosis, which should be attended to not more than a month previous to the breeding.

Check out which airport will be most convenient for the person meeting and returning the bitch if she is to be shipped and also what airlines use that airport. You will find that the airlines are also apt to have special requirements concerning acceptance of animals for shipping. These include weather limitations and types of crates which are acceptable. The weather limits have to do with extreme heat and extreme cold at the point of destination, as some airlines will not fly dogs into temperatures above or below certain levels, fearing for their safety. The crate problem is a simple one, since if your own crate is not suitable, most of the airlines have specially designed crates available for purchase at a fair and moderate price. It is a good plan to purchase one of these if you intend to be shipping dogs with any sort of frequency. They are made of fiberglass and are the safest type to use for shipping.

Normally you must notify the airline several days in advance to make a reservation, as they are able to accommodate only a certain number of dogs on each flight. Plan on shipping the bitch on about her eighth or ninth day of season, but be careful to avoid shipping her on a weekend, when schedules often vary and freight offices are apt to be closed. Whenever you can, ship your bitch on a direct flight. Changing planes always carries a certain amount of risk of a dog being overlooked or wrongly routed at the middle stop, so avoid this danger if at all possible. The bitch must be accompanied by a health certificate which you must obtain from your veterinarian before taking her to the airport. Usually it will be necessary to have the bitch at the airport about two hours prior to flight time. Before finalizing arrangements, find out from the stud's owner at what time of day it will be most convenient to have the bitch picked up promptly upon arrival.

It is simpler if you can plan to bring the bitch to the stud dog. Some people feel that the trauma of the flight may cause the bitch to not conceive; and, of course, undeniably there is a slight risk in shipping which can be avoided if you are able to drive the bitch to her destination. Be sure to leave yourself sufficient time to assure your arrival at the right time for her for breeding (normally the tenth to fourteenth day following the first signs of color); and remember that if you want the bitch bred twice, you should allow a day to elapse between the two matings. Do not expect the stud's owner to house you while you are there. Locate a nearby motel that takes dogs and make that your headquarters.

Just prior to the time your bitch is due in season, you should take her to visit your veterinarian. She should be checked for worms and should receive all the booster shots for which she is due plus one for parvo virus, unless she has had the latter shot fairly recently. The brucellosis test can also be done then, and the health certificate can be obtained for shipping if she is to travel by air. Should the bitch be at all overweight, now is the time to get the surplus off. She should be in good condition, neither underweight nor overweight, at the time of breeding.

The moment you notice the swelling of the vulva, for which you should be checking daily as the time for her season approaches, and the appearance of color, immediately contact the stud's owner and settle on the day for shipping or make the appointment for your arrival with the bitch for breeding. If you are shipping the bitch, the stud fee check should be mailed immediately, leaving ample time for it to have been received when the bitch arrives and the mating takes place. Be sure to call the airline making her reservation at that time, too.

Do not feed the bitch within a few hours before shipping her. Be certain that she has had a drink of water and been well exercised before closing her in the crate. Several layers of newspapers, topped with some shredded newspaper, make a good bed and can be discarded when she arrives at her destination; these can be replaced with fresh newspapers for her return home. Remember that the bitch should be brought to the airport about two hours before flight time as sometimes the airlines refuse to accept late arrivals.

If you are taking your bitch by car, be certain that you will arrive at a reasonable time of day. Do not appear late in the evening. If your arrival in town is not until late, get a good night's sleep at your motel and contact the stud's owner first thing in the morning. If possible, leave children and relatives at home, as they will only be in the way and perhaps unwelcome by the stud's owner. Most stud dog owners prefer not to have any unnecessary people on hand during the actual mating.

After the breeding has taken place, if you wish to sit and visit for awhile and the stud's owner has the time, return the bitch to her crate in your car (first ascertaining, of course, that the temperature is comfortable for her and that there is proper ventilation. She should not be permitted to urinate for at least one hour following the breeding. This is the time when you get the business part of the transaction attended to. Pay the stud fee, upon which you should receive your breeding certificate and, if you do not already have it, a copy of the stud dog's

256

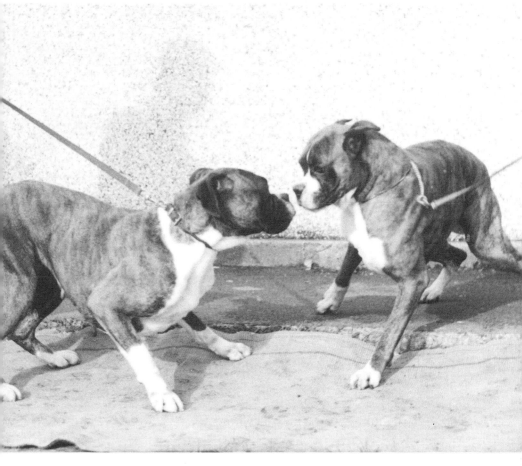

A bitch in season welcomes the attention of a prospective mate. The sense of smell plays a big role in the premating behavior of dogs.

pedigree. The owner of the stud dog does not sign or furnish a litter registration application until the puppies have been born.

Upon your return home, you can settle down and plan in happy anticipation a wonderful litter of puppies. A word of caution! Remember that although she has been bred, your bitch is still an interesting target for all male dogs, so guard her carefully for the next week or until you are absolutely certain that her season has entirely ended. This would be no time to have any unfortunate incident with another dog.

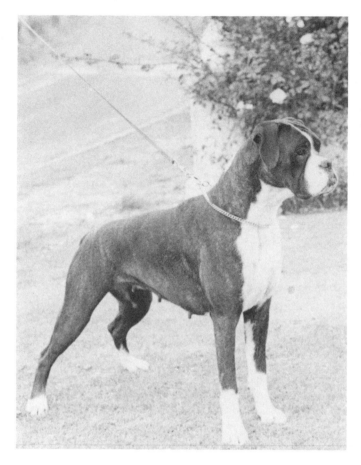

Eng. Ch. Marbelton
Tyzack Misty Blue.
Sire Marbelton Hasty
Harry. Owned by
Mrs. M. Hambleton,
Ormskirk, Lanca-
shire, England.

The Boxer Stud Dog

Choosing the best stud dog to complement your bitch is often very difficult. The two principal factors to be considered should be the stud's conformation and his pedigree. Conformation is fairly obvious; you want a dog that is typical of the breed in the words of the standard of perfection. Understanding pedigrees is a bit more subtle since the pedigree lists the ancestry of the dog and involves individuals and bloodlines with which you may not be entirely familiar.

To a novice in the breed, then, the correct interpretation of a pedigree may at first be difficult to grasp. Study the pictures and text of this book and you will find many names of important bloodlines and members of the breed. Also make an effort to discuss the various dogs behind the proposed stud with some of the more experienced breeders, starting with the breeder of your own bitch. Frequently these folks will be personally familiar with many of the dogs in question, can offer opinions of them, and may have access to additional pictures which you would benefit by seeing.

It is very important that the stud's pedigree should be harmonious with that of the bitch you plan on breeding to him. Do not rush out and breed to the latest winner with no thought of whether or not he can produce true quality. By no means are all great show dogs great producers. It is the producing record of the dog in question and the dogs and bitches from which he has come which should be the basis on which you make your choice.

Breeding dogs is never a money-making operation. By the time you pay a stud fee, care for the bitch during pregnancy, whelp the litter, and rear the puppies through their early shots, worming, and so on, you will be fortunate to break even financially once the puppies have been sold. Your chances of doing this are greater if you are breeding for a show-quality litter which will bring you higher prices as the pups are sold as show prospects. Therefore, your wisest investment is to use the best dog available for your bitch regardless of the cost; then you should wind up with more valuable puppies. Remember that it is equally costly to raise mediocre puppies as top ones, and your chances of financial return are better on the latter. To breed to the most excellent, most suitable stud dog you can find is the only sensible thing to do, and it is poor economy to quibble over the amount you are paying in stud fee.

It will be your decision which course you decide to follow when you breed your bitch, as there are three options: linebreeding, inbreeding, and outcrossing. Each of these methods has its supporters and its detractors! Linebreeding is breeding a bitch to a dog belonging originally to the same canine family, being descended from the same ancestors, such as half-brother to half-sister, grandsire to granddaughters, niece to uncle (and vice-versa) or cousin to cousin. Inbreeding is breeding father to daughter, mother to son, or full brother to sister. Outcross breeding is breeding a dog and a bitch with no or only a few mutual ancestors.

Linebreeding is probably the safest course, and the one most likely to bring results, for the novice breeder. The more sophisticated inbreeding should be left to the experienced, long-time breeders who thoroughly know and understand the risks and the possibilities involved with a particular line. It is usually done in an effort to intensify some ideal feature in that strain. Outcrossing is the reverse of inbreeding, an effort to introduce improvement in a specific feature needing correction, such as a shorter back, better movement, more correct head or coat, and so on.

It is the serious breeder's ambition to develop a strain or bloodline of their own, one strong in qualities for which their dogs will become distinguished. However, it must be realized that this will involve time, patience, and at least several generations before the achievement can be claimed. The safest way to embark on this plan, as we have mentioned, is by the selection and breeding of one or two bitches, the best you can buy and from top-producing kennels. In the beginning you do *not* really have to own a stud dog. In the long run it is less expensive and sounder judgment to pay a stud fee when you are ready to breed a bitch than to purchase a stud dog and feed him all year; a stud dog does not win any popularity contests with owners of bitches to be bred until he becomes a champion, has been successfully Specialed for awhile, and has been at least moderately advertised, all of which adds up to a quite healthy expenditure.

The wisest course for the inexperienced breeder just starting out in dogs is as I have outlined above. Keep the best bitch puppy from the first several litters. After that you may wish to consider keeping your own stud dog if there has been a particularly handsome male in one of your litters that you feel has great potential or if you know where there is one available that you are interested in, with the feeling that he would work in nicely with the breeding program on which you have embarked. By this time, with several litters already born, your eye should have developed to a point enabling you to make a wise choice, either from one of your own litters or from among dogs you have seen that appear suitable.

The greatest care should be taken in the selection of your own stud dog. He must be of true type and highest quality as he may be responsible for siring many puppies each year, and he should come from a line of excellent dogs on both sides of his pedigree which themselves are, and which are descended from, successful producers. This dog should have no glaring faults in conformation; he should be of such quality that he can hold his own in keenest competition within his breed. He should be in good health, be virile and be a keen stud dog, a proven sire able to transmit his correct qualities to his puppies. Need I say that such a dog will be enormously expensive unless you have the

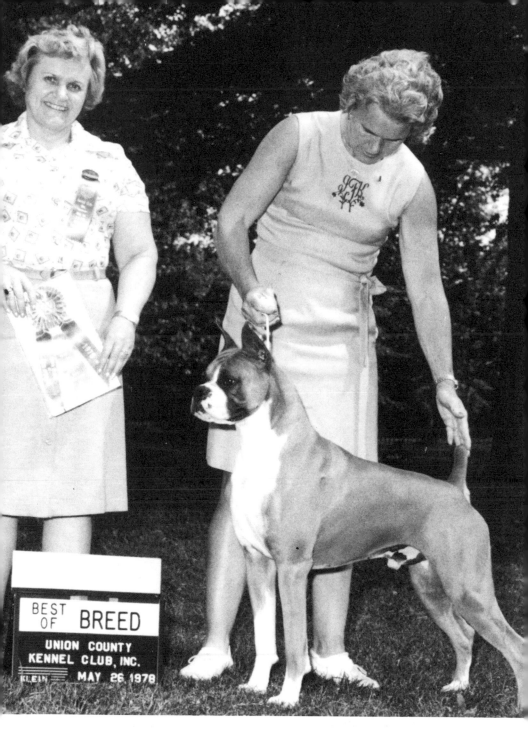

The famous Best in Show and Group winning Boxer, Ch. Merrilane's April Fashion, in May 1978 with his handler, Jane Forsyth. Owned by Coleman Cook, Grove City, Ohio. This dog is the Top Living Boxer Sire at the present time.

good fortune to produce him in one of your own litters? To buy and use a lesser stud dog, however, is downgrading your breeding program unnecessarily since there are so many dogs fitting the description of a fine stud whose services can be used on payment of a stud fee.

You should *never* breed to an unsound dog or one with any serious standard or disqualifying faults. Not all champions by any means pass along their best features; and by the same token, occasionally you will find a great one who can pass along his best features but never gained his championship title due to some unusual circumstances. The information you need about a stud dog is what type of puppies he has produced and with what bloodlines and whether or not he possesses the bloodlines and attributes considered characteristic of the best in your breed.

If you go out to buy a stud dog, obviously he will not be a puppy but rather a fully mature and proven male with as many of the best attributes as possible. True, he will be an expensive investment, but if you choose and make his selection with care and forethought, he may well prove to be one of the best investments you have ever made.

Of course, the most exciting of all is when a young male you have decided to keep from one of your litters due to his tremendous show potential turns out to be a stud dog such as we have described. In this case he should be managed with care, for he is a valuable property that can contribute inestimably to his breed as a whole and to your own kennel specifically.

Do not permit your stud dog to be used until he is about a year old, and even then he should be bred to a mature, proven matron accustomed to breeding who will make his first experience pleasant and easy. A young dog can be put off forever by a maiden bitch who fights and resists his advances. Never allow this to happen. Always start a stud dog out with a bitch who is mature, has been bred previously, and is of even temperament. The first breeding should be performed in quiet surroundings with only you and one other person to hold the bitch. Do not make it a circus, as the experience will determine the dog's outlook about future stud work. If he does not enjoy the first experience or associates it with any unpleasantness, you may well have a problem in the future.

Your young stud must permit help with the breeding, as later there will be bitches who will not be cooperative. If right from the beginning you are there helping him and praising him whether or not your assistance is actually needed, he will expect and accept this as a matter of course when a difficult bitch comes along.

262

Things to have handy before introducing your dog and the bitch are K-Y jelly (the only lubricant which should be used) and a length of gauze with which to muzzle the bitch should it be necessary to keep her from biting you or the dog. Some bitches put up a fight; others are calm. It is best to be prepared.

At the time of the breeding the stud fee comes due, and it is expected that it will be paid promptly. Normally a return service is offered in case the bitch misses or fails to produce one live puppy. Conditions of the service are what the stud dog's owner makes them, and there are no standard rules covering this. The stud fee is paid for the act, not the result. If the bitch fails to conceive, it is customary for the owner to offer a free return service; but this is a courtesy and not to be considered a right, particularly in the case of a proven stud who is siring consistently and whose fault the failure obviously is *not*. Stud dog owners are always anxious to see their clients get good value and to have in the ring winning young stock by their dog; therefore, very few refuse to mate the second time. It is wise, however, for both parties to have the terms of the transaction clearly understood at the time of the breeding.

If the return service has been provided and the bitch has missed a second time, that is considered to be the end of the matter and the owner would be expected to pay a further fee if it is felt that the bitch should be given a third chance with the stud dog. The management of a stud dog and his visiting bitches is quite a task, and a stud fee has usually been well earned when one service has been achieved, let alone by repeated visits from the same bitch.

The accepted litter is one live puppy. It is wise to have printed a breeding certificate which the owner of the stud dog and the owner of the bitch both sign. This should list in detail the conditions of the breeding as well as the dates of the mating.

Upon occasion, arrangements other than a stud fee in cash are made for a breeding, such as the owner of the stud taking a pick-of-the-litter puppy in lieu of money. This should be clearly specified on the breeding certificate along with the terms of the age at which the stud's owner will select the puppy, whether it is to be a specific sex, or whether it is to be the pick of the entire litter.

The price of a stud fee varies according to circumstances. Usually, to prove a young stud dog, his owner will allow the first breeding to be quite inexpensive. Then, once a bitch has become pregnant by him, he becomes a "proven stud" and the fee rises accordingly for bitches that follow. The sire of championship-quality puppies will bring a stud fee

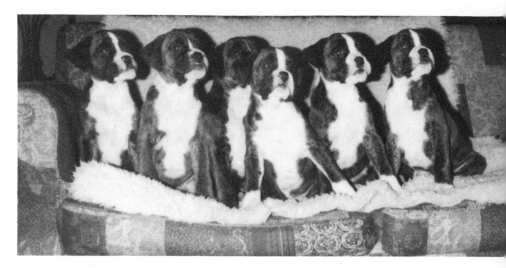

A homebred litter by Skelder Slap and Tickle ex Crisp and Dry of Skelder whose sire is Eng. Ch. Skelder Scorching. The center puppy, Skelder Slapstick, is winning well. Owned by Mrs. Joy Malcolm, Brandford Forum, Dorset, England.

Vihabra's "M" litter, by Ch. Merrilane's Vihabra Gold'n Key ex Shur Jim's Spitfire, owned by Dr. Harry and Virginia Bradley, co-bred by Virginia Bradley and Beverly Chretian-Wik, Los Altos Hills, California.

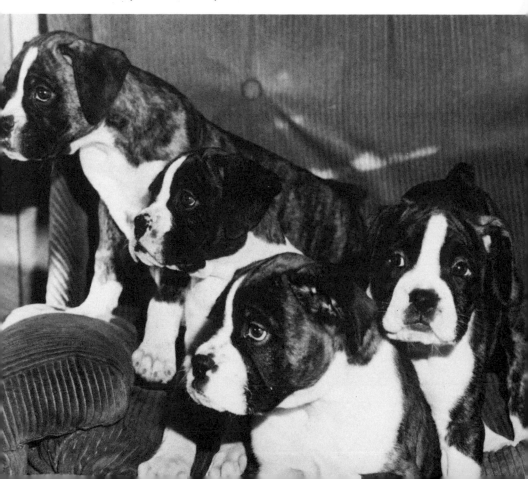

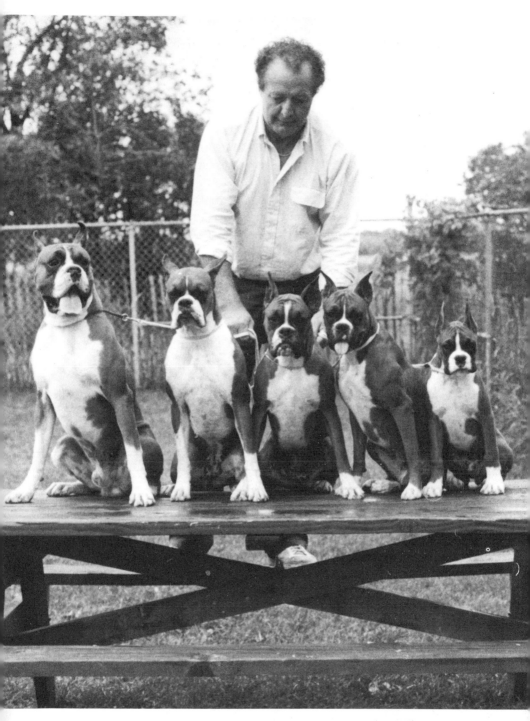

Friends at Hollycrest. Boxers owned by Cheryl J. Colby, Riverside, Illinois.

of at least the purchase price of one show puppy as the accepted "rule-of-thumb." Until at least one champion by your stud dog has finished, the fee will remain equal to the price of one pet puppy. When his list of champions starts to grow, so does the amount of the stud fee. For a top-producing sire of champions, the stud fee will rise accordingly.

Almost invariably it is the bitch who comes to the stud dog for the breeding. Immediately upon having selected the stud dog you wish to use, discuss the possibility with the owner of that dog. It is the stud dog owner's prerogative to refuse to breed any bitch deemed unsuitable for his dog. Stud fee and method of payment should be stated at this time, and a decision reached on whether it is to be a full cash transaction at the time of the mating or a pick-of-the-litter puppy, usually at eight weeks of age.

If the owner of the stud dog must travel to an airport to meet the bitch and ship her for the flight home, an additional charge will be made for time, tolls, and gasoline based on the stud owner's proximity to the airport. The stud fee includes board for the day on the bitch's arrival through two days for breeding, with a day in between. If it is necessary that the bitch remain longer, it is very likely that additional board will be charged at the normal per-day rate for the breed.

Be sure to advise the stud's owner as soon as you know that your bitch is in season so that the stud dog will be available. This is especially important because if he is a dog being shown, he and his owner may be unavailable owing to the dog's absence from home.

As the owner of a stud dog being offered to the public, it is essential that you have proper facilities for the care of visiting bitches. Nothing can be worse than a bitch being insecurely housed and slipping out to become lost or bred by the wrong dog. If you are taking people's valued bitches into your kennel or home, it is imperative that you provide them with comfortable, secure housing and good care while they are your responsibility.

There is no dog more valuable than the proven sire of champions, Group winners and Best in Show dogs. Once you have such an animal, guard his reputation well and do *not* permit him to be bred to just any bitch that comes along. It takes two to make the puppies; even the most dominant stud can not do it all himself, so never permit him to breed a bitch you consider unworthy. Remember that when the puppies arrive, it will be your stud dog who will be blamed for any lack of quality, while the bitch's shortcomings will be quickly and conveniently overlooked.

266

Going into the actual management of the mating is a bit superfluous here. If you have had previous experience in breeding a dog and bitch you will know how the mating is done. If you do not have such experience, you should not attempt to follow directions given in a book but should have a veterinarian, breeder friend, or handler there to help you the first few times. You do not just turn the dog and bitch loose together and await developments, as too many things can go wrong and you may altogether miss getting the bitch bred. Someone should hold the dog and the bitch (one person each) until the "tie" is made and these two people should stay with them during the entire act.

If you get a complete tie, probably only the one mating is absolutely necessary. However, especially with a maiden bitch or one that has come a long distance for this breeding, we prefer following up with a second breeding, leaving one day in between the two matings. In this way there will be little or no chance of the bitch missing.

Once the tie has been completed and the dogs release, be certain that the male's penis goes completely back within its sheath. He should be allowed a drink of water and a short walk, and then he should be put into his crate or somewhere alone where he can settle down. Do not allow him to be with other dogs for a while as they will notice the odor of the bitch on him, and particularly with other males present, he may become involved in a fight.

Pregnancy, Whelping, and the Litter

Once the bitch has been bred and is back at home, remember to keep an ever watchful eye that no other male gets to her until at least the twenty-second day of her season has passed. Until then, it will still be possible for an unwanted breeding to take place, which at this point would be catastrophic. Remember that she actually can have two separate litters by two different dogs, so take care.

In other ways, she should be treated normally. Controlled exercise is good, and necessary for the bitch throughout her pregnancy, tapering it off to just several short walks daily, preferably on lead, as she reaches about her seventh week. As her time grows close, be careful about her jumping or playing too roughly.

The theory that a bitch should be overstuffed with food when pregnant is a poor one. A fat bitch is never an easy whelper, so the overfeeding you consider good for her may well turn out to be the exact opposite. During the first few weeks of pregnancy, your bitch should be fed her normal diet. At four to five weeks along, calcium should be added to her food. At seven weeks her food may be increased if she seems to crave more than she is getting, and a meal of canned milk (mixed with an equal amount of water) should be introduced. If she is fed just once a day, add another meal rather than overload her with too much at one time. If twice a day is her schedule, then a bit more food can be added to each feeding.

A week before the pups are due, your bitch should be introduced to her whelping box so that she will be accustomed to it and feel at home there when the puppies arrive. She should be encouraged to sleep there but permitted to come and go as she wishes. The box should be roomy enough for her to lie down and stretch out but not too large lest the pups have more room than is needed in which to roam and possibly get chilled by going too far away from their mother. Be sure that the box has a "pig rail"; this will prevent the puppies from being crushed against the sides. The room in which the box is placed, either in your home or in the kennel, should be kept at about 70 degrees Fahrenheit. In winter it may be necessary to have an infrared lamp over the whelping box, in which case be careful not to place it too low or close to the puppies.

Newspapers will become a very important commodity, so start collecting them well in advance to have a big pile handy to the whelping

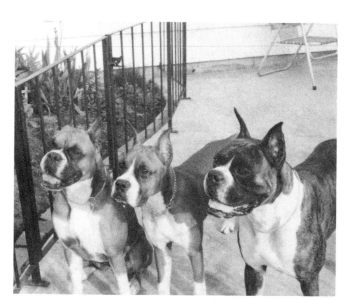

Left to right: Ruhlend's Swiss Miss, Ch. Breamerwood Jitters, and Ch. Peablo's Black Bishop, all owned by Ruth F. Leek, Gig Harbor, Washington.

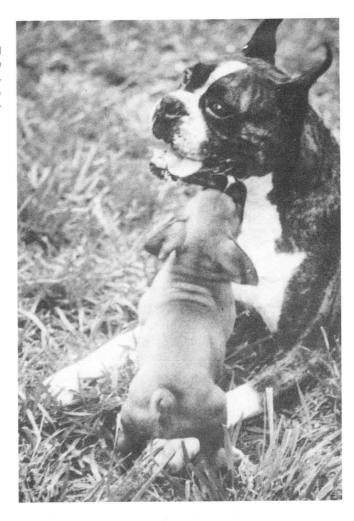

Heldenbrand's Proud Ruler, U.D. with one of the puppies. Heldenbrand Boxers, Manhattan, Kansas.

box. With a litter of puppies, one never seems to have papers enough, so the higher pile to start with, the better off you will be. Other necessities for whelping time are clean, soft turkish towels, scissors, and a bottle of alcohol.

You will know that her time is very near when your bitch becomes restless, wandering in and out of her box and of the room. She may refuse food, and at that point her temperature will start to drop. She will dig at and tear up the newspapers in her box, shiver, and generally look uncomfortable. Only you should be with your bitch at this time. She does not need spectators; and several people, even though they may be family members whom she knows, hanging over her may upset her to the point where she may harm the puppies. You should remain nearby, quietly watching, not fussing or hovering; speak calmly and frequently to her to instill confidence. Eventually she will settle down in her box and begin panting; contractions will follow. Soon thereafter a puppy will start to emerge, sliding out with the contractions. The mother immediately should open the sac, sever the cord with her teeth, and then clean up the puppy. She will also eat the placenta, which you should permit. Once the puppy is cleaned, it should be placed next to the bitch unless she is showing signs of having the next one immediately. Almost at once the puppy will start looking for a nipple on which to nurse, and you should ascertain that it is able to latch on successfully.

If the puppy is a breech (*i.e.*, born feet first), you must watch carefully for it to be completely delivered as quickly as possible and the sac removed quickly so that the puppy does not drown. Sometimes even a normally positioned birth will seem extremely slow in coming. Should this occur, you might take a clean towel and, as the bitch contracts, pull the puppy out, doing so gently and with utmost care. If, once the puppy is delivered, it shows little signs of life, take a rough turkish towel and massage the puppy's chest by rubbing quite briskly back and forth. Continue this for about fifteen minutes, and be sure that the mouth is free from liquid. It may be necessary to try mouth-to-mouth breathing, which is done by pressing the puppy's jaws open and, using a finger, depressing the tongue which may be stuck to the roof of the mouth. Then place your mouth against the puppy's and blow hard down the puppy's throat. Bubbles may pop out of its nose, but keep on blowing. Rub the puppy's chest with the towel again and try artificial respiration, pressing the sides of the chest together slowly and rhythmically—in and out, in and out. Keep trying one method or the other for at least twenty minutes before giving up. You may be rewarded with a live puppy who otherwise would not have made it.

If you are successful in bringing the puppy around, do not immediately put it back with the mother as it should be kept extra warm. Put it in a cardboard box on an electric heating pad or, if it is the time of year when your heat is running, near a radiator or near the fireplace or stove. As soon as the rest of the litter has been born it then can join the others.

An hour or more may elapse between puppies, which is fine so long as the bitch seems comfortable and is neither straining nor contracting. She should not be permitted to remain unassisted for more than an hour if she does continue to contract. This is when you should get her to your veterinarian, whom you should already have alerted to the possibility of a problem existing. He should examine her and perhaps give her a shot of pituitrin. In some cases the veterinarian may find that a Caesarean section is necessary due to a puppy being lodged in a manner making normal delivery impossible. Sometimes this is caused by an abnormally large puppy, or it may just be that the puppy is simply turned in the wrong position. If the bitch does require a Caesarean section, the puppies already born must be kept warm in their cardboard box with a heating pad under the box.

Once the section is done, get the bitch and the puppies home. Do not attempt to put the puppies in with the bitch until she has regained consciousness as she may unknowingly hurt them. But do get them back to her as soon as possible for them to start nursing.

Should the mother lack milk at this time, the puppies must be fed by hand, kept very warm, and held onto the mother's teats several times a day in order to stimulate and encourage the secretion of milk, which should start shortly.

Assuming that there has been no problem and that the bitch has whelped naturally, you should insist that she go out to exercise, staying just long enough to make herself comfortable. She can be offered a bowl of milk and a biscuit, but then she should settle down with her family. Freshen the whelping box for her with fresh newspapers while she is taking this respite so that she and the puppies will have a clean bed.

Unless some problem arises, there is little you must do about the puppies until they become three to four weeks old. Keep the box clean and supplied with fresh newspapers the first few days, but then turkish towels should be tacked down to the bottom of the box so that the puppies will have traction as they move about.

If the bitch has difficulties with her milk supply, or if you should be so unfortunate as to lose her, then you must be prepared to either hand-feed or tube-feed the puppies if they are to survive. We personally prefer tube-feeding as it is so much faster and easier. If the bitch is available, it is best that she continues to clean and care for the puppies in the normal manner excepting for the food supplements you will provide. If it is impossible for her to do this, then after every feeding you must gently rub each puppy's abdomen with wet cotton to make it urinate, and the rectum should be gently rubbed to open the bowels.

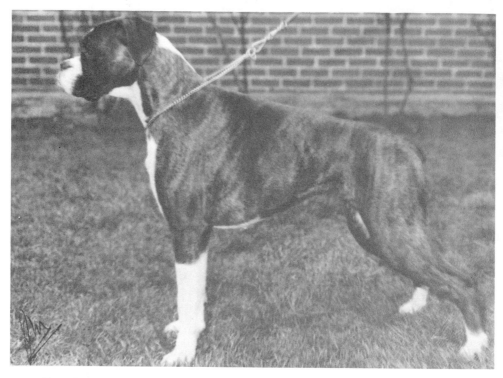

Eng. Ch. Marbelton Tyzack Super Trouper, winner of the Bitch Challenge Certificate at Crufts in 1974, was sired by Eng. Ch. Marbelton Desperate Dan. Owned by Mrs. M. Hambleton, Ormskirk, Lancashire, England.

Newborn puppies must be fed every three to four hours around the clock. The puppies must be kept warm during this time. Have your veterinarian teach you how to tube-feed. You will find that it is really quite simple.

After a normal whelping, the bitch will require additional food to enable her to produce sufficient milk. In addition to being fed twice daily, she should be given some canned milk several times each day.

When the puppies are two weeks old, their nails should be clipped, as they are needle sharp at this age and can hurt or damage the mother's teats and stomach as the pups hold on to nurse.

Between three and four weeks of age, the puppies should begin to be weaned. Scraped beef (prepared by scraping it off slices of beef with a spoon so that none of the gristle is included) may be offered in very small quantities a couple of times daily for the first few days. Then by the third day you can mix puppy chow with warm water as directed on the package, offering it four times daily. By now the mother should be kept away from the puppies and out of the box for several hours at a time so that when they have reached five weeks of age she is left in with them only overnight. By the time the puppies are six weeks old, they should be entirely weaned and receiving only occasional visits from their mother.

Most veterinarians recommend a temporary DHL (distemper, hepatitis, leptospirosis) shot when the puppies are six weeks of age. This remains effective for about two weeks. Then at eight weeks of age, the puppies should receive the series of permanent shots for DHL protection. It is also a good idea to discuss with your vet the advisability of having your puppies inoculated against the dreaded parvovirus at the same time. Each time the pups go to the vet for shots, you should bring stool samples so that they can be examined for worms. Worms go through various stages of development and may be present in a stool sample even though the sample does not test positive in every checkup. So do not neglect to keep careful watch on this.

The puppies should be fed four times daily until they are three months old. Then you can cut back to three feedings daily. By the time the puppies are six months of age, two meals daily are sufficient. Some people feed their dogs twice daily throughout their lifetime; others go to one meal daily when the puppy becomes one year of age.

The ideal age for puppies to go to their new homes is between eight and twelve weeks, although some puppies successfully adjust to a new home when they are six weeks old. Be sure that they go to their new owners accompanied by a description of the diet you've been feeding them and a schedule of the shots they have already received and those they still need. These should be included with the registration application and a copy of the pedigree.

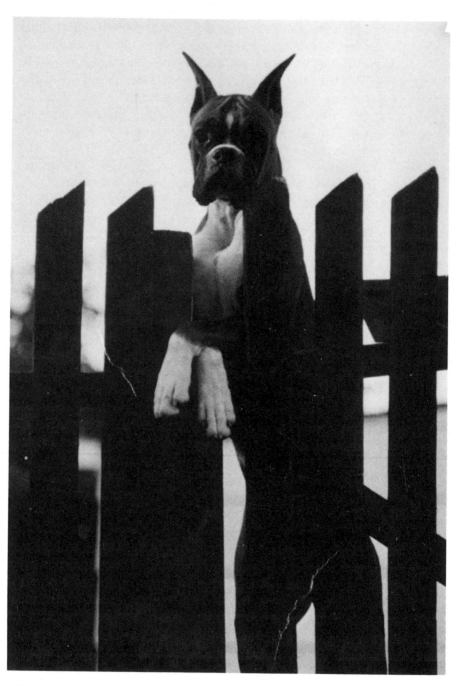

Wagner's Oriana waiting for the family. Mr. and Mrs. Richard Wagner, owners. Photo courtesy of Jane Forsyth.

Chapter 14

Traveling with Your Boxer

When you travel with your dog, to shows or on vacation or wherever, remember that everyone does not share our enthusiasm or love for dogs and that those who do not, strange creatures though they seem to us, have their rights, too. These rights, on which we should not encroach, include not being disturbed, annoyed, or made uncomfortable by the presence and behavior of other people's pets. Your dog should be kept on lead in public places and should recognize and promptly obey the commands "Down," "Come," "Sit," and "Stay."

Take along his crate if you are going any distance with your dog. And keep him in it when riding in the car. A crated dog has a far better chance of escaping injury than one riding loose in the car should an accident occur or an emergency arise. If you do permit your dog to ride loose, never allow him to hang out a window, ears blowing in the breeze. An injury to his eyes could occur in this manner. He could also become overly excited by something he sees and jump out, or he could lose his balance and fall out.

Never, ever under any circumstances, should a dog be permitted to ride loose in the back of a pick-up truck. I have noted, with horror, that some people do transport dogs in this manner, and I think it cruel and shocking. How easily such a dog can be thrown out of the truck by sudden jolts or an impact! And I am sure that many dogs have jumped out at the sight of something exciting along the way. Some unthinking individuals tie the dog, probably not realizing that were he to jump under those circumstances, his neck would be broken, he could be dragged alongside the vehicle, or he could be hit by another vehicle. If you are for any reason taking your dog in an open back truck, please have sufficient regard for that dog to at least provide a crate for him, and then remember that, in or out of a crate, a dog riding under the

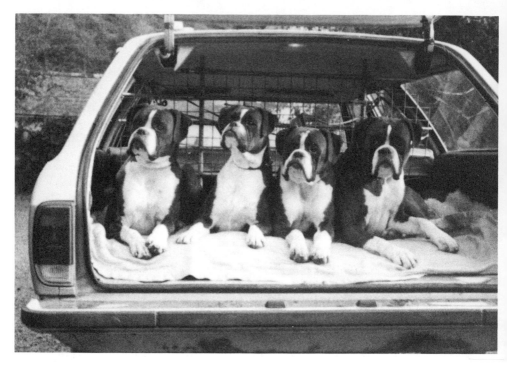

Left to right: Eng. Ch. Skelder Scorching, Eng. Ch. Skelder Burnt Offering, Eng. Ch. Skelder Sky High, and Eng. Ch. Snare Stone Sky Rocket of Skelder are all owned by Mrs. Joy Malcolm, Blandford Forum, Dorset, England.

direct rays of the sun in hot weather can suffer and have his life endangered by the heat.

If you are staying at a hotel or motel with your dog, exercise him somewhere other than in the flower beds and parking lot of the property. People walking to and from their cars really are not thrilled at "stepping in something" left by your dog. Should an accident occur, pick it up with a tissue or a paper towel and deposit it in a proper receptacle; do not just walk off leaving it to remain there. Usually there are grassy areas on the sides of and behind motels where dogs can be exercised. Use them rather than the more conspicuous, usually carefully tended, front areas or those close to the rooms. If you are becoming a dog show enthusiast, you will eventually need an exercise pen to take with you to the show. Exercise pens are ideal to use when staying at motels, too, as they permit you to limit the dog's roaming space and to pick up after him more easily.

276

Never leave your dog unattended in the room of a motel unless you are absolutely, positively certain that he will stay there quietly and not damage or destroy anything. You do not want a long list of complaints from irate guests, caused by the annoying barking or whining of a lonesome dog in strange surroundings or an overzealous watch dog barking furiously each time a footstep passes the door or he hears a sound from an adjoining room. And you certainly do not want to return to torn curtains or bedspreads, soiled rugs, or other embarrassing evidence of the fact that your dog is not really house-reliable after all.

If yours is a dog accustomed to traveling with you and you are positive that his behavior will be acceptable when left alone, that is fine. But if the slightest uncertainty exists, the wise course is to leave him in the car while you go to dinner or elsewhere; then bring him into the room when you are ready to retire for the night.

When you travel with a dog, it is often simpler to take along from home the food and water he will need rather than buying food and looking for water while you travel. In this way he will have the rations to which he is accustomed and which you know agree with him, and there will be no fear of problems due to different drinking water. Feeding on the road is quite easy now, at least for short trips, with all the splendid dry prepared foods and high-quality canned meats available. A variety of lightweight, refillable water containers can be bought at many types of stores.

If you are going to another country, you will need a health certificate from your veterinarian for each dog you are taking with you, certifying that each has had rabies shots within the required time preceding your visit.

Be careful always to leave sufficient openings to ventilate your car when the dog will be alone in it. Remember that during the summer, the rays of the sun can make an inferno of a closed car within only a few minutes, so leave enough window space open to provide air circulation. Again, if your dog is in a crate, this can be done quite safely. The fact that you have left the car in a shady spot is not always a guarantee that you will find conditions the same when you return. Don't forget that the position of the sun changes in a matter of minutes, and the car you left nicely shaded half an hour ago can be getting full sunlight far more quickly than you may realize. So, if you leave a dog in the car, make sure there is sufficient ventilation and check back frequently to ascertain that all is well.

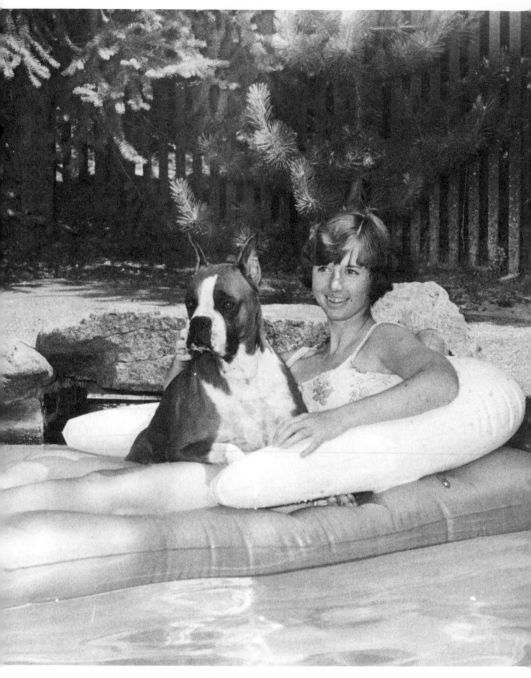

Ch. Jondem's Makiki taking his ease in retirement with Lucille Pomeroy in Puyall-up, Washington. His swim companion is Carol Baumgartner.

278

Chapter 15

Responsibilities of Breeders and Owners

The first responsibility of any person breeding dogs is to do so with care, forethought, and deliberation. It is inexcusable to breed more litters than you need to carry on your show program or to perpetuate your bloodlines. A responsible breeder should not cause a litter to be born without definite plans for the safe and happy disposition of the puppies.

A responsible dog breeder makes absolutely certain, so far as is humanly possible, that the home to which one of his puppies will go is a good home, one that offers proper care and an enthusiastic owner. I have tremendous admiration for those people who insist on visiting (although doing so is not always feasible) the prospective owners of their puppies, to see if they have suitable facilities for keeping a dog, that they understand the responsibility involved, and that all members of the household are in accord regarding the desirability of owning one. All breeders should carefully check out the credentials of prospective purchasers to be sure that the puppy is being placed in responsible hands.

I am certain that no breeder ever wants a puppy or grown dog he has raised to wind up in an animal shelter, in an experimental laboratory, or as a victim of a speeding car. While complete control of such a situation may be impossible, it is at least our responsibility to make every effort to turn over dogs to responsible people. When selling a puppy, it is a good idea to do so with the understanding that should it become necessary to place the dog in other hands, the purchaser will first contact you, the breeder. You may want to help in some way, possibly by buying or taking back the dog or placing it elsewhere. It is not fair just to sell our puppies and then never again give a thought to their welfare. Family problems arise, people may be forced to move where dogs are prohibited, or people just plain grow bored with a dog and its care. Thus the dog becomes a victim. You, as the dog's breeder, should concern yourself with the welfare of each of your dogs and see to it that the dog remains in good hands.

The final obligation every dog owner shares, be there just one dog or an entire kennel involved, is that of making detailed, explicit plans for the future of our dearly loved animals in the event of the owner's death. Far too many of us are apt to procrastinate and leave this very important matter unattended to, feeling that everything will work out or that "someone will see to them." The latter is not too likely, at least

Ch. Turo's Monogram of Sarazak taking Winners Dog, then on to Best of Breed from the classes to finish under judge John Connolly. Owned by Sandra Roberts and Elizabeth Esacove, Turo Boxers, Houston, Texas.

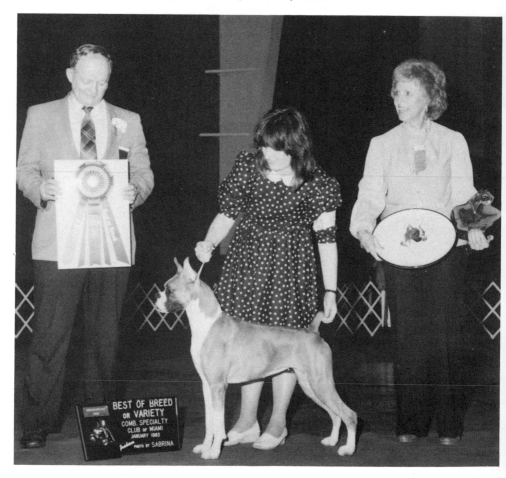

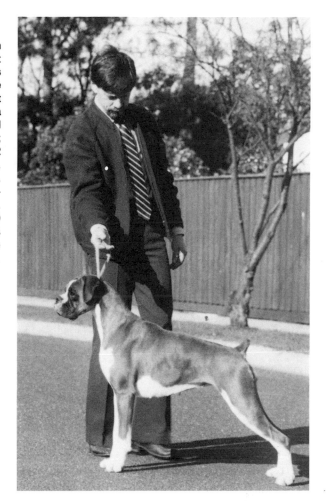

Aust. Ch. Sjecoin Hey Look Me Over at 2 years of age. This winner of Challenge Certificate and Best of Breed 1981 Melba Royal (judge Edd Bivin, U.S.A.); Reserve C.C. 1982 Melba Royal; C.C. Winter Classic; C.C. Boxer Club of Tasmania; C.C. Expo. and Winner of 600 C.C. points was handled by the owner, David Brace.

not to the benefit of the dogs, unless you have done some advance planning which will assure their future well-being.

Life is filled with the unexpected, and even the youngest, healthiest, most robust of us may be the victim of a fatal accident or sudden illness. The fate of our dogs, so entirely in our hands, should never be left to chance. If you have not already done so, please get together with your lawyer and set up a clause in your will specifying what you want done with each of your dogs, to whom they will be entrusted (after first making absolutely certain that the person selected is willing and able to assume the responsibility), and telling the locations of all registration papers, pedigrees, and kennel records. Just think of the possibilities which might happen otherwise! If there is another family member who shares your love of the dogs, that is good and you have less to worry about. But if your heirs are not dog-oriented, they will hardly know how to proceed or how to cope with the dogs themselves, and they may wind up disposing of or caring for your dogs in a manner that would break your heart were you around to know about it.

In our family, we have specific instructions in each of our wills for each of our dogs. A friend, also a dog person who regards her own dogs with the same concern and esteem as we do ours, has agreed to take over their care until they can be placed accordingly and will make certain that all will work out as we have planned. We have this person's name and phone number prominently displayed in our van and car and in our wallets. Our lawyer is aware of this fact. It is all spelled out in our wills. The friend has a signed check of ours to be used in case of an emergency or accident when we are traveling with the dogs; this check will be used to cover her expense to come and take over the care of our dogs should anything happen to make it impossible for us to do so. This, we feel, is the least any dog owner should do in preparation for the time our dogs suddenly find themselves without us. There have been so many sad cases of dogs unprovided for by their loving owners, left to heirs who couldn't care less and who disposed of them in any way at all to get rid of them, or left to heirs who kept and neglected them under the misguided idea that they were providing them "a fine home with lots of freedom." All of us *must* prevent any of these misfortunes befalling our own dogs who have meant so much to us!

Index